SJ
ALLE · ZEIT · WACH · 1842

Helmut Thomä Horst Kächele

Psychoanalytic Practice

2 Clinical Studies

With the Collaboration of
Stephan Ahrens Andreas Bilger Manfred Cierpka
Walter Goudsmit Roderich Hohage Michael Hölzer
Juan Pablo Jiménez Lotte Köhler Martin Löw-Beer
Robert Marten Joachim Scharfenberg Rainer Schors
Wolfgang Steffens Imre Szecsödy Brigitte Thomä
Angelika Wenzel

Translated by M. Wilson

Springer-Verlag
Berlin Heidelberg New York
London Paris Tokyo
Hong Kong Barcelona
Budapest

Professor emeritus Dr. Helmut Thomä
Wilhelm-Leuchner-Str. 11, 7900 Ulm
Federal Republic of Germany

Professor Dr. Horst Kächele
Abteilung Psychotherapie der Universität Ulm
Am Hochsträss 8, 7900 Ulm
Federal Republic of Germany

Translator:

Dr. Michael Wilson
Max-Wolf-Straße 16, 6900 Heidelberg
Federal Republic of Germany

Title of the original German edition:
Lehrbuch der psychoanalytischen Therapie, Band 2 Praxis
© Springer-Verlag Berlin Heidelberg 1988
ISBN-13:978-3-642-71880-9 /0-387-16196-1

ISBN-13:978-3-642-71880-9 e-ISBN-13:978-3-642-71878-6
DOI: 10.1007/978-3-642-71878-6

Library of Congress Cataloging-in-Publication Data (Revised for v. 2).
Thomä, Helmut. Psychoanalytic practice. Translation of: Lehrbuch der psychoanalytischen Therapie. Includes bibliographical references and indexes. Contents: 1. Principles - 2. Clinical studies. 1. Psychoanalysis. I. Kächele, Horst, 1944 - II. Title. [DNLM: 1. Psychoanalytic Therapy. WM 460.6 / T452L]
RC504.T4613 1986 616.89'17 86-28042
ISBN-13:978-3-642-71880-9

Softcover reprint of the hardcover 1st edition 1992

Media conversion: Appl, Wemding, Germany
26/3130-543210 - Printed on acid-free paper

Preface

We are pleased to present the second volume of our study on *Psychoanalytic Practice*, which we entitle *Clinical Studies*. Together, the two volumes fulfill the functions usually expected of a textbook on theory and technique. In fact, some reviewers have asked why such a title was not chosen. One of the reasons for our narrower choice was that our primary concern is focused on those aspects of psychoanalytic theory that are relevant to treatment.

The first volume, entitled *Principles*, has evoked much interest within and outside the professional community, creating high expectations toward its clinical counterpart. After all, psychoanalytic principles must demonstrate their value and efficacy in treatment, i.e., in achieving changes in symptoms and their underlying structures. This is apparent in the clinical studies contained in this book, and in the process of compiling them the senior author has had the opportunity to take stock of his long professional career.

We have willingly let others closely examine how we work, and one consequence of this has been a growing exchange with other psychoanalysts and with scientists from other disciplines and from numerous countries. This cooperation has enriched the contents of this volume. Although not mentioned specifically in the text, both our collaborators from Ulm and our colleagues from other locations have provided drafts of passages and left it to our discretion to use them as we saw fit. Although it would theoretically have been possible to attribute authorship to those who drafted specific sections, our coworkers have agreed to references to their names being omitted in the text as part of our efforts to prepare a uniform and coherent volume.

Our special thanks for their unusual willingness to place their specific knowledge at our disposal for inclusion in this book go to the following psychoanalysts who are not members of our Ulm group: Stephan Ahrens (Hamburg) enriched our knowledge on the state of discussion about alexthymia; Walter Goudsmit (Groningen) reported on his years of experience in treating delinquents; Lotte Köhler (Munich) examined our view of countertransference from the perspective of self psychology; Imre Szecsödy (Stockholm) described and applied his model of supervision. Our conviction that interdisciplinary cooperation has a positive effect on clinical work is demonstrated by several passages of text contributed by scientists from other disciplines. Martin Löw-Beer's (Frankfurt) philosophical comments have extended our understanding of the "good hour" (see Sect. 10.2); Joachim Scharfenberg (Kiel) provided annotations from a theological perspective to a dialogue in which the analyst was confronted with religious problems (see Sect. 10.3.2); and Angelika Wenzel's (Karlsruhe) linguistic interpretations demonstrate how our clinical understanding can profit from the application of other methods to psychoanalytic texts (see Sect. 7.5.2). We are more than merely personally grateful for such contributions because they emphasize how fruitful interdisciplinary cooperation can be.

Of particular value have been the critical comments that numerous colleagues have provided to the drafts of various chapters or sections of the manuscript. Although we are very aware of our sole responsibility for the text we present here, we would like to extend our gratitude to Jürgen Aschoff, Helmut Baitsch, Hermann Beland, Claus Bischoff, Werner Bohleber, Helga Breuninger, Marianne Buchheim, Peter Buchheim, Johannes Cremerius, Joachim Danckwardt, Ulrich Ehebald, Franz Rudolf Faber, Heinz Henseler, Reimer Karstens, Otto F. Kernberg, Joachim P. Kerz, Gisela Klann-Delius, Lisbeth Klöß-Rotmann, Rolf Klüwer, Marianne Leuzinger-Bohleber, Wolfgang Lipp, Adolf-Ernst Meyer, Emma Moersch, Michael Rotmann, Ulrich Rüger, Walter Schmitthenner, Erich Schneider, Almuth Sellschopp, and Ilka von Zeppelin.

We are grateful to the members of the staff of the Department of Psychotherapy in Ulm, whose constant support enabled us to complete the manuscript in a relatively brief period of time. We are also grateful to the staff at Springer-Verlag, who ensured that the preparation of the book proceeded smoothly.

We are especially indebted to our translators, in the case of this English edition to Michael Wilson, who mastered this formidable task authoritatively but sensitively. Our discussions with him (and the translators into other languages) exposed a number of ambiguities and obscurities in the original German text, which we believe have been resolved in this English edition.

We are, finally, most indebted to our patients. It is in the nature of things that advances in psychoanalytic technique are linked to an interpersonal process. The examples that can be found in this book document the significance that we attribute to the critical collaboration of our patients. We hope that this book's descriptions of our clinical experience in psychoanalysis will benefit future patients and be a helpful stimulus to their therapists.

Ulm, May 1991 Helmut Thomä, Horst Kächele

Contents

Introduction

Becoming a psychoanalyst is a unique learning process of getting acquainted with Freud's work and the development of psychoanalytic theories and techniques. Especially for German psychoanalysts, it is fraught with unusual difficulties. This issue must be considered in the context of how each generation attains its own professional identity. Unfortunately, each subsequent generation of psychoanalysts achieves independence much too late. The reasons for this delay can be found both in the overwhelming stature of Freud and in the idiosyncrasies of psychoanalytic training (Thomä, 1991).

In the first volume of our study we have presented our theoretical positions, taking our guiding idea from Balint's two- and three-person psychology, which focuses on what the analyst contributes to the therapeutic process. For reasons rooted in our biographies and because of the general and the specifically German problems we discuss in Vol. 1, our scientific efforts in pursuing our goals have proceeded slowly and hesitatingly. This is especially true for the senior author, who had to travel a long path before reaching his present understanding of psychoanalysis, expressed in these two books. It was Merton Gill who gave him the final stimulus to undertake a critical survey of the theory and practice of psychoanalysis and to contemplate its future.

We can legitimately claim to have set a good example in at least one regard, namely by having made psychoanalytic dialogues - and thus how we really work - accessible to psychoanalysts and other scientists. One consequence of anchoring case reports in audio recordings and transcriptions of sessions is that the therapist exposes himself to the criticism of his colleagues in a unique manner.

The physician's obligation to secure confidentiality requires that we be extraordinarily cautious. In attempting to resolve the problems related to making dialogues accessible to assessment by others, we have left no stone unturned in extending the example Freud suggested for protecting a patient's anonymity, altering everything that might enable a patient to be identified. Such coding, however, cannot go so far as to make it impossible for the patient to recognize himself, should some coincidence lead him to read this book. Yet we also consider it possible that a former patient described here might have some difficulty in recognizing himself. A peculiar type of estrangement results, first, from the alterations we have made in external features and, second, from the one-sided description - restricted to specific problems - of a patient which those around him are very often not aware of. This estrangement is very welcome to us in connection with the issue of confidentiality.

We refer, furthermore, to biographical data - which we "code" in the sense that we replace them with analogous phenomena - only insofar as they are relevant for comprehending events in therapy. One widespread mistake is to believe that in analysis the entire individual becomes visible. In fact, the weak spots, the problems, and the suffering are at the center of the analytic encounter. The other, conflict-free sides of the individual's life are neglected because they do not constitute the primary object of therapy. Although this omission creates a distorted image of the analysand's personality, this one-sided and frequently negative image that a patient presents is welcome from the perspective of facilitating anonymity.

We have spent much thought on the nature of the codes we should employ. No one method is entirely satisfactory. To use a code name based on some prominent feature would attribute particular importance to one aspect. On the other hand, we did not want to use numbers for identifying patients. As pseudonyms we have consequently decided to use (arbitrarily chosen) Christian names together with an X for women and a Y for men, borrowed from the terminology for the chromosomes responsible for determining female and male gender. The anatomical difference between the sexes constitutes the inherent and biological foundation of the life histories of men and of women, regardless of the significance of psychosocial factors for sex role and sense of identitiy. This code thus reflects the tension between the uniqueness of each individual's life and the biological basis of the two sexes. Dimorphism is, after all, the basis for each individual's gender role even if the plasticity of human psychosexuality goes as far as the desire to change the sexual role in the case of transsexualism. We hope that our readers will accept our coding system, the purpose of which is to facilitate the use of the index of patients.

This volume could never have been written without the permission of our patients for us to record therapeutic dialogues and to evaluate and publish them in a form in which their identity is protected. The consent of many patients is linked to their hope that the thorough discussion of problems of analytic technique will benefit other patients. Several patients have provided commentaries to the sections of text related to themselves; we are especially grateful to them.

This willingness to cooperate constitutes a rewarding change in the social and cultural climate, to which psychoanalysis has also contributed. Although Freud may have had good reason to assume that the patients he treated "would not have spoken if it had occurred to them that their admissions might possibly be put to scientific uses" (Freud 1905 e, p. 8), over the past decades many patients have shown us that this is no longer true. It is beyond doubt that psychoanalysis is going through a phase of demystification. It is no coincidence that at the same time that patients are reporting about their analyses autobiographically, the general public is eagerly devouring everything that earlier analysands have to report about Freud's therapies. The literature on the latter is growing and demonstrates that Freud was not a Freudian. Intellectual and social conditions have changed so much in the past decades that analysands - whether patients or prospective analysts - are reporting about their therapies in one form or another. The "other side" is thus finally getting their hearing. We psychoanalysts would be taking the easy way out if we were to dismiss such autobiographic fragments, the quality of writing in which varies considerably, as being the result of negative transference that was not worked through or of exhibitionism and narcissism.

Most reservations against the use of tape recordings and the evaluation of transcripts do not stem from patients but rather from analysts. The fact that research into psychoanalysis must pay special attention to what the therapist has contributed to the course and outcome has gained widespread acceptance. The stress that results from the clinical and scientific discussion does not affect the anonymous patient but rather the analyst, whose name cannot be kept a secret in professional circles.

Such personally motivated reservations, however, cannot alter the fact that the changes mentioned above make it easier for the present generation of psychoanalysts to fulfill obligations toward both the individual patient and research. According to Freud, all patients should profit from the benefits of enlightenment and scientifically grounded generalizations:

> Thus it becomes the physician's duty to publish what he believes he knows of the causes and structure of hysteria, and it becomes a disgraceful piece of cowardice on his part to neglect doing so, as long as he can avoid causing direct personal injury to the single patient concerned. (Freud 1905 e, p. 8)

In this context, personal injury refers to damage that could result from flaws in the coding of confidential material.

Medical confidentiality and coding have often made it impossible for us to provide precise details about a case history. Readers will nonetheless be able to recognize that the majority of our patients suffered from severe chronic symptoms and that we have chosen these cases from a wide spectrum. Somatic symptoms are frequently a concomitant manifestation of psychic suffering. Numerous examples stem from the psychoanalysis of patients with psychosomatic illnesses; we believe we have convincingly demonstrated that psychic factors were a relevant etiological factor.

The critical reappraisal of his psychoanalytic thinking has led to changes in the *practice* of the senior author over the past decades. We include here case histories and reports from over a period of more than thirty years. In many cases we were able to examine the effectiveness of psychoanalyses in long-term follow-up studies.

In one of his aphorisms, Wittgenstein (1984, p. 149) emphasized the significance of examples. It reads about as follows: Rules are not adequate to determine practice; examples are also necessary. Our rules leave backdoors open, and practice has to speak for itself.

Psychoanalytic practice has numerous faces, and we have attempted to portray them by referring to typical examples. Detailed studies from close up illustrate the respective focus of the dialogue, while a bird's eye view is necessary to gain an overview of therapies of long duration. A theoretical framework is necessary to provide orientation, enabling one to see phenomena, hear words, read texts, and comprehend the connections between human experiencing and thinking. On a larger scale, we have presented our theoretical models in the companion volume on *Principles*. On a smaller scale, we provide the reader theoretical information in the passages entitled "Consideration" and "Commentary" that are interspersed in the dialogues in this book. These passages reflect different degrees of distance to the verbal exchanges and facilitate the comprehension of the focus of the respective dialogue. Important in this regard is that the considerations are from the perspective of the treating analyst, and are thus set in the same type of print as the dialogues themselves, while the commentaries are from our own and a more distant point of view. As many of the cases presented here were treated by the authors, the considerations and commentaries might in fact have originated in the same person, although at different times and distances to the actual moment of the therapeutic situation. This is especially true for the senior author and his role as commentator of his own clinical work, which has extended over a long period of time.

Located at another level of abstraction are references to etiologic psychoanalytic theories in general and in particular. They have been included in this volume to facilitate the classification of examples. These supplementary theoretical comments, together with the wide diagnostic spectrum from which we have chosen typical cases, are the reason for the considerable size of this volume.

As a guide for the reader we would like to add that, with the exception of Chaps. 1, 9, and 10, the topics of the chapters in both volumes are the same. The volumes on theory and practice have been so organized that we provide a systematic exposition of theory in the same chapter and section in Vol. 1 as we discuss therapy and technical aspects in this volume. This parallel structure facilitates switching from one volume to another to take both practical and theoretical aspects into consideration. For instance, a case history of a chronic anorexic illustrating the therapeutic management of identity resistance is given in Sect. 4.6, and a theoretical discussion of identity resistance is the topic of Sect. 4.6 in Vol. 1.

The decision to publish a two-volume text and to follow the same organization in this book on clinical practice is, however, linked with the disadvantage that the discussion of phenomena that belong together in the psychoanalytic situation is torn apart. Transference and resistance, for example, often alternate rapidly and are interrelated. Yet it is necessary to identify an object, i. e., call it by its name, in order to discuss it. We provide a theoretical and conceptual clarification of issues in the first volume; here we describe examples of this or that form of transference or of resistance. The detailed subdivision of each chapter supplies a general frame of reference, and the index contains a large number of entries, facilitating the location of connections between different phenomena described in the text.

We have selected typical examples from the analyses of 37 patients, 20 men and 17 women. Following this introduction is a list of the code names that we have assigned to these patients. The topics and section numbers printed in italics refer to passages in which we provide information to general questions concerning the course of a patient's illness and treatment. The therapeutic processes of 14 patients are documented in this book. For the other cases the courses are implicit and the reader can reconstruct some of them; the presentation of these cases serves primarily to explicate important analytic concepts.

We provide information as to frequency of sessions, the length of treatment, and the setting if this has special significance or if topics related to the initiation and termination of therapy are being discussed.

In the dialogues and comments made from the perspective of the analyst providing treatment, *I* is used for the analyst. Of course, in reality this "I" does not always refer to one and the same analyst. Otherwise we refer to analysts or therapists in general.

We employ the terms "analysis," "psychoanalysis," and "therapy" as synonyms. Many of our patients do not distinguish between therapy and analysis, and some even retain their naivety in this regard. In Vol. 1 we have entered into the discussion of the differences in the wide spectrum defined by the assumptions and rules of psychoanalytic theory. Here the point is to reconstruct the lines actually followed in psychoanalytic therapies, an allusion to Freud's publication entitled "Lines of Advance in Psycho-analytic Therapy" (1919 a).

In this book we retain the use of the generic masculine in general discussions, although we obviously direct our comments to patients and psychoanalysts of both sexes. We speak to the former as individual persons who are suffering, and to the latter as those who, on the basis of their professional competence, contribute substantially to the improvement and cure of patients.

Index of Patients' Code Names

In the Introduction we discuss the general principles of coding confidential material. The following is a list of the issues discussed for each patient. The references to sections containing a summary or information about the genesis of the illness are printed in italics. Reading the respective sections in succession can provide insights into the course of treatment.

Amalie X

Beatrice X

Clara X

Dorothea X

1 Case Histories and Treatment Reports

Introduction

The crisis of psychoanalytic theory, which was the central topic of Chap. 1 of the companion volume on the principles of psychoanalytic practice, has inevitably had some effects on psychoanalytic technique. In the last decade it has also become apparent that the perspectives of psychoanalytic therapy rooted in interpersonal theories have caused many concepts relevant to psychoanalytic practice to be reevaluated. It is now essential to distinguish between, on the one hand, the theory of the genesis or the explanation of psychic and psychosomatic illnesses and, on the other, the theory of therapeutic change and how it is brought about. Of course, all assumptions about structural changes depend on the observation of variations and alterations of symptoms.

This chapter's title, "Case Histories and Treatment Reports," reflects the discord in Freud's work between the theory of genesis and that of change. Our reconsideration leads us in the first section of this chapter to reject the notion that he gave adequate scientific consideration to both poles of this discord in his case histories. It is necessary to reformulate his famous assertion about the existence of an inseparable bond between curing and research. A promising new source for regrounding psychoanalytic therapy is for us to take the fact seriously that the theory of repeated traumatization has significance for the structuring of the therapeutic situation.

If we attempt to apply scientific criteria to the preparation of case histories and treatment reports, it is necessary for us to experiment with different schemes for reporting our work. For about three decades we, together with many other analysts, have striven toward the goal of reproducing the psychoanalytic dialogue as precisely as possible. In Sects. 1.2 and 1.3 we refer to important stages in the development of reporting, which we elaborate on in later chapters by providing appropriate examples. We have now reached a new stage. The use of audio recordings enables us to make the verbal exchanges between patient and analyst accessible to third parties in a reliable form. Because of the significance of this technical aid for advanced training and research, in Sect. 1.4 we make the reader familiar with a controversy that has been dragging on for a long time and that the examples we give in Sect. 7.8 should help resolve.

1.1 Back to Freud and the Path to the Future

Freud's case histories frequently fulfill the function of an introduction to his work. Jones emphasizes that the Dora case – the first of Freud's exemplary case histories following his *Studies on Hysteria* –

> for years served as a model for students of psycho-analysis, and although our knowledge has greatly progressed since then, it makes today as interesting reading as ever. It was the first of Freud's post-neurological writings I had come across, at the time of its publication, and I well remember the deep impression the intuition and the close attention to detail displayed in it made on me. Here was a man who not only listened closely to every word his patient spoke, but regarded each such utterance as every whit as definite and as in need of correlation as the phenomena of the physical world. (Jones 1954, p. 288)

This makes it all the more remarkable that it was precisely on this case that Erikson (1962) demonstrated substantial weaknesses in Freud's understanding of etiology and therapy (see Vol.1, Sect. 8.6). The paper he presented to the American Psychoanalytic Association marked the increasing criticism both of Freud's explanations of etiology in his *case histories* and of his technique as described in his *treatment reports*. In view of the growing flood of publications containing such criticism, Arlow (1982, p. 14) has expressed his concern about their ties to objects belonging to the past. He recommended that we should simply say goodbye to these "childhood friends" who served us so well, put them to rest, and get back to work.

That and how Anna O., little Hans, Dora, President Schreber, the Rat Man, and the Wolf Man became our childhood friends is definitely very important, as is knowing the conditions under which each friendship developed. Training institutes mediate these friendships, in this way familiarizing the candidates with Freud's work as a therapist, scientist, and author.

While writing this textbook we have returned to our own childhood friends and have studied several of Freud's large case histories in detail. Even though new elements can be discovered by rereading them, we have hermeneutic reservations about supporting Lacan's (1975, p. 39) call for a "return to Freud." With Laplanche (1989, p. 16), we "prefer to speak of *going back over* Freud, as it is impossible to return to Freud without working on him, without making him the object of work." In our reconsideration we do not meet these old friends in the same form as during our initial encounter with and enthusiasm for Katharina or little Hans. We have always viewed Freud's case histories in a somewhat different light and, unfortunately, have frequently shown too little concern for how Freud himself understood his texts. We were not, after all, introduced to the love for psychoanalysis through Freud alone, but also by spiritual parents who solicited support for their own views. In whom could we then place our trust and confidence in going back to Freud in order to ensure that ideas can be revitalized and point to the future that Arlow and Brenner (1988) and Michels (1988) envisage in their suggestions for reforming psychoanalytic training.

In view of the immensity of our task in determining which items belong to the past, it is impossible to rely on a single individual, not even someone of the stature of Rapaport, who ventured (in 1960) to estimate the probable longevity of important psychoanalytic concepts. Which mediator should we turn to in attempting to master this hermeneutic task? Hermes' name did not provide the etymological source for the concept of hermeneutics, but as messenger and translator between the gods and the mortals he was also a participant in the doings and dealings of the world who always acted according to his own interests. The same is true of those interpreters who try to do justice to Freud's work without losing sight of their own interests. Practicing psychoanalysts are not the only ones who live from Freud's legacy; this is also true of the many authors for whom Freud's legacy is a playground for their criticism.

Can the analyst's acquisition of his own approach be considered a special form of translation? Uncertainty has spread since Brandt (1977) applied the play on the Italian words "traduttore-traditore" to the *Standard Edition* and thus made Strachey the translator into the traitor, and since Bettelheim's (1982) provocative book appeared. Following the criticism of Strachey's translation by Bettelheim (1982), Brandt (1961, 1972, 1977), Brull (1975), Ornston (1982, 1985a, b), Mahoney (1987), Junker (1987), and Pines (1985), nothing could illuminate the difficult situation of Anglo-American psychoanalysts who have relied on the *Standard Edition* better than the ironic title of Wilson's (1987) article, "Did Strachey Invent Freud?" The answer is obvious (see Thomä and Cheshire 1991).

The unjustified and very exaggerated criticism of Strachey's admirable achievement has in the last few years led the discussion onto a side track and distracted attention from the real reasons for the crisis of psychoanalysis. It is consequently more than naive to want to resolve this crisis allegedly caused by the *Standard Edition* with the aid of a new translation. Beyond demonstrating that Strachey made mistakes and distorted passages, which have been correctly pointed out by many authors, the criticism of the *Standard Edition* concerns the hermeneutic question of whether Strachey's translation distorted the work itself. To demonstrate mistakes in translation that distort meaning is a relatively simple matter. Yet we confront difficulties of a more principle nature - and not limited to Freud's works - because hermeneutics, i. e., the theory of the interpretation of texts, does not provide us with rules we can use as a mountain climber would a safety line while climbing a difficult mountain trail. We follow Schleiermacher (1977, p. 94) in assuming that it is possible after all for a reader to equate himself with an author both objectively and subjectively. Equating oneself with the author is one of the preconditions for being able to interpret a text and ultimately to understand the object better than the author himself (see Hirsch 1976, pp.37 ff.). According to Schleiermacher this task can be expressed as follows: "To understand the statement at first as well and later better than the author." Every reading enriches our basic store of knowledge and puts us in a better position to have a better understanding; thus Schleiermacher continues, "It is only with insignificant things that we are satisfied with what we immediately understand" (p.95).

When we read Freud's treatment reports we naturally take our own experience as a basis for comparison, and in time we become more confident that we understand the subject better than the founder of psychoanalysis did. The growth of knowledge on our subject - in our context, the analytic technique - is fed by several sources. One factor is that the critical discussion of Freud's treatment reports has created a distance to them, so that we today view these childhood friends differently than when we had our initial experiences with them. Another factor helping us to make our own experience is the fact that creative psychoanalysts have discovered other and new aspects of the subject that have brought about changes in therapy and theory.

With a view to the many psychoanalysts and other Freud interpreters to whom we ourselves owe a debt of gratitude from our studies of Freud, we request that the reader identify with our interpretation on a trial basis. In this two-volume textbook we believe we have brought our long grappling for the foundations of psychoanalytic theory and its effectiveness as therapy to a preliminary conclusion in that we are able to ground a firm point of view. There is a lot at stake in our attempt to grasp the current crisis of psychoanalysis on the basis of Freud's works and their reception in the psychoanalytic movement and in intellectual history as a whole. We hesitated for a long time to compress our ideas into a limited number of sentences because we are aware that this is a problem with far-reaching implications. It was Freud's grand idea to link, in an *inseparable bond*, the interpretative method he discovered for treating patients with causal explanations, i.e., with the study of the genesis of psychic and psychosomatic illnesses. Yet if proof of the causal relationship requires that the data be independent of suggestion by the therapist, then therapy destroys the science. If the analyst, on the other hand, believes that it is possible to refrain from making any suggestion whatsoever, in order to obtain uncontaminated data by means of pure interpretations, then he ruins the therapy without coming closer to a theoretical explanation if *independence* from the researcher is required. It is obvious that the analyst offering interpretations influences the patient even if he apparently only directs his interpretations to the unconscious and without any further-reaching aims, which is a self-deception as it is impossible. Instead of eliminating manipulations it opens the door to hidden manipulations.

Freud's inseparable bond thus contains a dilemma that has gone largely unrecognized because it suggested that following the rules served therapy and research equally. For decades the magic of this concept exerted a settling influence and appeared to solve the therapeutic and scientific problems of psychoanalysis with a single stroke. Only recently has it become obvious how many methodological problems have to be solved to realize Freud's credo. It implies that therapeutic efficacy, i.e., symptomatic and structural change, as well as the truth of explanatory hypotheses are the two sides of the same coin: the gold of the pure psychoanalytic method without *direct* suggestion. Of course, the scientific and therapeutic problems are the inevitable and necessary indirect influence exerted by the analyst on the patient.

By contrasting the *case history* and the *treatment report* it is possible to demonstrate that the scientific reconstruction of the genesis of psychic and psychosomatic illnesses in the case history follows criteria that differ from those for treatment; the function of these criteria is to ground the theory of therapy and specify the conditions for cure. In Sect. 10.5 of Vol. 1, we have described the individual consequences of loosening the inseparable bond and freeing the analyst from the excessive demands it places on him. To quote the concluding sentence from the first volume, "Freud's theory of technique requires that the analyst distinguish between the following components: *curing, gaining* new hypotheses, *testing* hypotheses, the *truth* of explanations, and the *utility* of knowledge" (p. 371).

With regard to therapeutic theory and its testing, we completely agree with Lorenzer's opinion that

> The goal of psychoanalytic understanding is to *achieve alterations in terms of the patient's suffering*; psychoanalytic theory conceptualizes this suffering and the reactions to it. Psychoanalysis is thus a theory of the therapeutic attitude toward suffering. (1986, p. 17, emphasis added)

One aspect of Lorenzer's definition is that it is very important to possess suitable methods for assessing change. Such investigations are part of therapeutic theory, but this theory raises questions that differ from those raised by the theory describing the etiology of psychic and psychosomatic illnesses.

Our study of the sources has convinced us that Freud grappled with this still unresolved dilemma for his entire life. Much can still be discovered in his works, and each renewed study of them enriched us. Yet the guides that Freud himself provided for satisfying the inseparable bond condition appear to us to be completely inadequate to meet the criteria for research designed to test hypotheses. For decades psychoanalysis was practiced under the cover of Freud's authority, in a manner that led to the stagnation of the therapeutic and scientific potential offered by the psychoanalytic method. It was more than unfortunate that explanatory theories were tied to metapsychology. Many pseudoscientific constructions have resulted from this union and have impeded the study of causal relationships and the attempt to solve the problems associated with the explanatory theory of psychoanalysis. Causal research cannot consist in employing metapsychological terminology to describe clinical phenomena. Grünbaum's interpretation that the study of the causal relationships surrounding the genesis of psychic and psychosomatic illnesses is not tied to metapsychological concepts is convincing. Fara and Cundo (1983, pp.54–55) have shown in an ingenious study that different approaches are combined in all of Freud's works although the mixture of metapsychological models and art of interpretation is always different.

In the first volume we demonstrated that Freud's materialistic monism, which determined his metapsychology, was probably the cause of the subsequent mistakes and confusion. Habermas' claim, however, that Freud fell victim to a "scientistic selfmisunderstanding" not only inaccurately judges the significance of causal research in psychoanalysis, as a result of an unfortunate linkage of such research with metapsychology, but also burdens therapy with a handicap that, as we have demonstrated in detail elsewhere (Thomä et al. 1976), was made even more severe by Lorenzer. Both of these influential authors have filled old wine into new bottles that have impressive labels simply because they were renamed. As *metahermeneutics* or *depth hermeneutics* it has been possible not only for the old metapsychological points of view to survive but also to influence practice indiscriminantly for the first time in the history of psychoanalysis, because they were put in direct relationship with the interpretive process. Neither Habermas nor Lorenzer seems to have recognized that large portions of metapsychology derive from the fact that Freud "psychologized" the "neurophysiological hypotheses" of his time, to use Bartel's (1976) words.

Yet of course not all "self-misunderstandings" are the same. It is possible to distinguish between different kinds of ignorance on the part of authors. Freud was not in a position to have a clear understanding of many of the implications of the therapeutic and scientific applications of his method. In this sense his work has suffered the same fate as that of all discoverers and authors of importance in intellectual history, namely that later researchers have understood some things better than the founder, discoverer, or author himself. As far as we have been able to refer to the relevant literature, we have not found any convincing arguments to justify the thesis of a scientistic self-misunderstanding. Habermas himself has to concede that an analyst bases his interpretations on *explanatory theories.* Freud's error was not his credo in causality but that he based it on the psychophysiology of "psychic energy."

It is an especially urgent task that social science perspectives be taken into consideration in psychoanalytic research, as we point out in our "Introduction" to Chap.2. This could provide psychoanalysis a scientific foundation that leads beyond the polarization between interpretative skill and explanation. We consider ourselves, at any rate, to belong to the group of hermeneuticists whose prime precept is that their interpretations be validated. We speak of an autonomous hermeneutic technology in order to emphasize that the psychoanalytic art of making interpretations is endebted to validations that are of necessity also concerned with the question of causal relationships. Hirsch (1967, 1976), whose understanding of hermeneutics is characterized by sober pragmatism, argues along the same lines. It is surprising that his studies have hardly received any attention in the Anglo-American psychoanalytic literature from authors following a hermeneutic approach. Rubovits-Seitz (1986) was recently the first to emphasize that Hirsch's view of hermeneutics places high demands on the grounding of interpretations.

In summary, it is possible to say that our disentanglement of the inseparable bond is not only useful for research but enables psychoanalytic practice to be innovative. One side effect of the social psychological understanding of the psychoanalytic situation has been the discovery of new aspects of transference and countertransference. Clarifying such distinctions is thus not only essential for research designed to test hypotheses, which is of increasing importance in our time, but also well suited to prepare the ground for new discoveries and new hypotheses. Freud's inseparable bond assertion belonged to a phase in which ingenious analysts were able to make discoveries about psychic relationships in almost every treatment. Today it is far more difficult to discover something truly new and to formulate it in a way meeting the demands raised by research concerned with the *verification of hypotheses.*

A cooperative effort is necessary to move Freud's paradigm into a phase of normal science. Although we definitely cannot expect philosophers to solve our empirical problems, we no longer have any doubt that even the study of extended psychoanalytic dialogues by philosophers would prove more productive than their epistemological criticism of Freud's works. Regardless of the significance of self-reflection in therapy, it would hardly have been possible after the study of several transcripts of tape recorded sessions for Habermas to make psychoanalysis into a purely reflective science. Ricoeur, for his part, could have discovered that psychoanalysts also observe. Finally, Grünbaum would feel confirmed that psychoanalysts search for relationships that may be of causal relevance and might have even discovered that psychoanalysts are today more cautious in claiming to have found the past and unconsciously still active causes of symptoms than Freud was. On the other hand, it is impossible to uphold Grünbaum's view that the influence exerted by the anaylst contaminates the data in a way that cannot be disentangled. The dialogues presented in this volume, for example, make it possible to recognize different degrees of suggestion. It is true, however, that the demands raised by Meehl (1983) - that the large spectrum of means ranging from persuasion to manipulation be registered - have not yet been met. The suggestive elements of the psychoanalytic technique of interpretation are themselves becoming the object of joint reflection, whose goal is to eliminate dependencies. It is surprising that Grünbaum (1985) himself did not point to such useful applications of his epistemological study of the placebo concept. He demonstrated that the discrimination of the *characteristic* and *spurious factors* with regard to the medication for a *syndrome under investigation* depends on the particular theory of therapy. Without wanting to reopen the discussion of nonspecific and specific or general and specific factors that is included in the first volume (Chap.8), we do want to mention that Strupp (1973, p. 35) and Thomä (1981, p. 35) have shown that the valence of the therapeutic influence exercised in a particular situation depends on that situation itself. A reliable and valid clinical classification of characteristic and spurious factors is thus difficult but not impossible. Finally, we believe that the study of the dialogues presented in this volume can also lead the epistemological discussion out of its ivory tower.

Freud (1933a, p. 151) referred to the treatment of patients as the *home-ground* of psychoanalysis. This is the source of the interpretative method of therapy that, in contrast to hermeneutics in theology and the humanities (Szondi 1975), systematically examines the unconscious psychic life of patients who come to analysts hoping for an *end* to their suffering. This therapeutic goal distinguishes psychoanalytic hermeneutics significantly from other hermeneutic disciplines. Works of art cannot in general be damaged by an interpretation, and a dead artist can only metaphorically turn around in his grave if he does not agree with an interpretation. Psychoanalytic interpretations interfere in human destinies. Patients seek help for their symptoms, and whether an improvement or cure is achieved is fundamental to them. Texts are not affected by differing exegeses and interpretations, and cannot make critical comments of their own.

The analyst thus must not only justify his therapeutic actions in the individual case, but also has the responsibility of continuously examining the accuracy of his theoretical ideas about the unconscious and about human experience and behavior. In contrast to hermeneutics in theology and the humanities the founder of psychoanalysis linked the art of making therapeutic interpretations to explanatory theories. Freud assumed that his theory of psychogenesis had causal *relevance* and raised the demand that the analyst differentiate between the *necessary* and the *sufficient* conditions regarding the genesis and course of psychic and psychosomatic illnesses. Later reconstructions have shown them to be postdictions. For this reason Freud's concept of *restrospective attribution* (*Nachträglichkeit*) assumes a significance that has been largely underestimated, as we show in Sects. 3.3 and 6.3.

The analytic dialogue is doubtlessly concerned with words. These words mean something, and this something is nothing exclusively sensory or linguistic. The words "connection," "relation," "relationship," "synthesis" etc. appear in Freud's works for the term "explain," in accordance with the scientific usage of the time.

Freud (1901a, p. 643) spoke, for example, with regard to the conditions under which the manifest dream is constituted, of its "regular relations" with the latent dream thoughts. In principle he was concerned with clarifying causal relationships; in individual cases he was mistaken regarding the question of empirical proof and on the whole underestimated the problems posed by research concerned with verifying hypotheses.

Clinical psychoanalysis is subject to research about its course and results. Freud's explanatory theories were based on his therapy, and they in turn have had a lasting influence on the interpretive method. Therefore interpretations are wrong if they are derived from a component of the theory that has been refuted. For example, in view of the results of recent research on mother-child interaction and of epidemiology, many assumptions of the general and specific theories of neurosis are questionable (Lichtenberg 1983). It is especially essential for therapeutic theory to be revised.

In revising the technique we can proceed from several of Freud's assumptions that have been ignored. It is especially with this thought in mind that we have given this section the heading "Back to Freud and the Path to the Future." According to Freud (1937c, p.250), "the business of analysis is to secure the best possible psychological conditions for the functions of the ego; with that it has discharged its task." If we relate this statement to the treatment situation and not only to the patient's ultimate ability to master the difficulties of everyday life without developing symptoms, then it is possible to formulate the following general thesis: Favorable conditions for the resolution of conflicts in the treatment situation are those that make it possible for the patient to transform the passive suffering from the original pathogenic traumas into independent action. This is a generalization of Freud's trauma theory; at its center is *helplessness*, at least since Freud's article "Inhibitions, Symptoms, and Anxiety" (1926d; see Vol.1, Sect. 8.7). We agree with Freud (1926d, p. 167) that "the ego, which experienced the trauma passively, now repeats it actively in a weakened version, in the hope of being able itself to direct its course. It is certain that children behave in this fashion towards every distressing impression they receive, by reproducing it in their play. In thus changing from passivity to activity they attempt to master their experiences psychically." This thesis can be generalized even further: "Through this means of going from passivity to activity [man] seeks to master psychically his life's impressions" (G. Klein 1976, pp.259 ff.). Klein has shown convincingly that the neurotic and psychotic repetition compulsion described by Freud takes place for psychological reasons, both affective and cognitive. This exacerbates the patient's feeling of passive helplessness, which continuously makes it more difficult for him to overcome past conditions of anxiety. Such unconscious expectations have the function of filtering perception in the sense of a negative self-fulfilling prophecy, so that that patient either does not have positive experiences or brackets out pleasant experiences and empties them of meaning. Sacrifices, punishments, and hurt feelings in the distant past - in short, all traumatic experiences - are not only conserved in this way, but enlarge cumulatively in everyday life and even in therapy if the course is unfavorable. We believe that we do justice to viewing psychogenesis as an ongoing process by expanding the theory of cumulative traumatization inaugurated by Khan (1963) to apply to the entire life cycle.

The life histories of many people are structured, for unconscious reasons, in ways that lead predispositions to be confirmed and new traumatic experiences to occur continuously. For example, "jealous and persecutory paranoics . . .project outwards on to others what they do not wish to recognize in themselves . . ..but they do not project it into the blue, so to speak, where there is nothing of the sort already . . ..they, too, take up minute indications with which these other, unknown, people present them and use them in their delusions of reference" (Freud 1922b, p.226). In one of his late works Freud emphasized the fundamental significance of such processes:

> The adult's ego, with its increased strength, continues to defend itself against dangers which no longer exist in reality; indeed, it finds itself compelled to seek out those situations in reality which can serve as an approximate substitute for the original danger, so as to be able to justify, in relation to them, its maintaining its habitual modes of reaction. Thus we can easily understand how the defensive mechanisms, by bringing about an ever more extensive alienation from the external world and a permanent weakening of the ego, pave the way for, and encourage, the outbreak of neurosis. (1937c, p. 238)

In such a process symptoms can be given new contents. This age-old discovery of Freuds (1895d, p. 133) is theoretically grounded in particular in Hartmann's concept of change in function, but its relevance to technique has not been systematically worked out. For this reason we put special emphasis, in Sect. 4.4 of Vol.1, on how symptoms can maintain themselves in a vicious circle that becomes increasingly strong on its own. Every day it is possible for situations of helplessness and hopelessness to develop whose contents are very different from the original traumas. A sure sign of this process is an increasing sensitivity to feeling offended, which enhances the patient's receptiveness to all kinds of stimuli. Finally, events that seem banal when viewed superficially can have drastic consequences for oversensitive people - and the feeling of being offended is a heavy burden on all interpersonal relations.

As a result of such repetitions, which we understand on the basis of the extension of the theory of trauma, it is also possible for a patient to feel offended in therapy. Such events, which must be taken very seriously, occur despite the analyst's efforts to create a friendly atmosphere. An unfavorable effect can even result if the analyst believes that it is possible to produce a kind of psychoanalytic incubator, i. e., constant conditions enabling undisturbed psychic growth to take place. The patient can also feel offended as a result of the setting and of the misunderstandings that inevitably occur, and the traumatic effects are stronger the less it is called by name, and recognized and interpreted as such (see Vol.1, Chap.7 and Sect. 8.4).

For a long time analysts did not recognize the severity of the trauma that can occur as a consequence of transferences that are associated with a repetition of old oedipal or preoedipal frustrations and that, moreover, can also affect the adult patient in new way. The traumatic consequences of transference were probably not discovered until late because the frustration theory of therapy seemed to justify it. In an unpublished speech held at the Budapest congress in 1987, Thomä emphasized the fact that traumatic events can be an unintended side effect of transference. At that time the profound discoveries that Ferenczi (1988) had recorded in his diary in 1932 were largely unknown. He described how professional attitudes and psychoanalytic rules can have new traumatic consequences of their own and revive traumas that analysis is supposed to help the patient overcome.

The consquences we draw from the rediscovery that traumatization is a constituent element of the analytic situation differ from Ferenczi's. We believe that our readiness to let the patient take part in the process of interpretation and, if necessary, in countertransference helps to overcome new and old traumas. Balint's two and more person psychology extended Freud's definition of helplessness to characterize the traumatic situation and drew attention to the unintentional and antitherapeutic microtraumas in the psychoanalytic situation. It could be of fundamental importance that this basic problem of technique led to the polarization into schools - on the one hand, the mirroring analyst who apparently cannot be injured or offended and, on the other hand, the loving analyst who, as a person, attempts to compensate for deficiencies.

A new era was initiated when Weiss and Sampson (1986) refuted the frustration theory on the basis of an experimental design, in favor of the mastery theory of therapy. The analyst must display great determination in considering every possibility at his disposal for countering the patient's repeated feelings of being offended during the analysis of transference, including its unfavorable effects on the patient's self-esteem and self-confidence. First steps in this direction are Klauber's emphasis on spontaneity as an antidote to traumatization in transference and Cremerius' (1981b) detailed description of the therapeutic significance of naturalness in the analyses Freud conducted.

Some aspects of Kohut's self-psychological technique indicate how strongly the frustration theory has established itself, to the detriment of the therapeutic effectiveness of psychoanalysis and in promoting a pseudoscientific idolatry. Kohut believed it is only possible for the analyst, as part of his adherence to analytic abstinence or neutrality, to provide narcissistic gratification and not true confirmation. This retention of a misunderstood concept of neutrality by Kohut removes the emotional basis from the confirmation and encouragement that are therapeutically so important, thus not strengthening the patient's realistic self-esteem but creating an as-if situation. According to Kohut's selfobject theory, confirmation does not even come from a significant other, but represents a kind of narcissistic self-confirmation - a reflection of the patient's own self.

The fear that acknowledgment might lead to oedipal seduction and incestuous wish fulfillment will continue to diminish in the new era of psychoanalytic therapy. Genuine acceptance substantially limits the occurrence of traumas from transference and considerably improves the therapeutic effectiveness of psychoanalysis. A constant theme running through all the chapters of this book is the question of how the analyst creates the conditions in his office that are most conducive to therapeutic change. The issue is to further the growth of the patient in ways so that he can cope and master old and new situations of helplessness and anxiety. The concept of working through conflicts must be subordinated to the comprehensive theory of mastering. Previously neglected therapeutic potential can be derived from the psychoanalytic theory of anxiety, which we recapitulate in Sect. 9.1, if the mechanisms of defense are understood from the perspective of coping in the here and now.

1.2 Case Histories

In the case histories that he published, Freud pursued the goal of demonstrating the connection between illness and life history. The conclusion he reached was that the genesis of psychic and psychosomatic illnesses should be understood as a *complemental series.* There must be a convergence of many factors for neurotic disturbances to develop and become chronic. An individual's capacity to cope with stress in a critical phase of life depends on his disposition, which he acquires as a result of formative influences and conflicts in childhood and in adolescence, which he in turn acquires on the basis of an innate reaction readiness. Oedipal conflicts have far-reaching implications for everyone's life history because, first, it is in them that the basic structuring of *psychosexual differentiation* takes place and, second, the acceptance of the specific psychosocially defined sex role - which is subjectively experienced as a feeling of identity that refers and is tied to one's sex - is elementary. Whether and how these conflicts subside or whether they form an unconscious structure that can be diagnosed on the basis of typical forms of behavior and experiencing depends in turn on many sociocultural and familial constellations.

The phenomenon referred to as the overdetermination of symptoms and the fact that pathological processes are maintained by subsequent unfavorable events have remarkable consequences for therapy. Overdetermination makes it possible for the therapeutic effects of the analyst's interventions to spread via the network of these very conditions. These therapeutic consequences extending beyond the immediate focus are the result of the role of overdetermination in the etiology of neuroses, or in Freud's words, "their genesis is as a rule overdetermined, [and] several factors must come together to produce this result" (1895d, p.263). Overdetermination does not refer to a multiple determination in the sense that each condition or each individual cause in itself would cause an event, a parapraxis, a slip of the tongue, or a symptom. On the contrary, it is the *convergence* of several motives in speech disturbances that Wilhelm Wundt described and that Freud incorporated in the concept of overdetermination (1901b, p. 60). The assumption of overdetermination makes it necessary, with regard to the genesis of psychic and psychosomatic illnesses, to establish a hierarchy of factors and to distinguish the conditions into those which are *necessary* and those which are *sufficient.* Accordingly, we have to start from the possibility that the causal factors can be combined in various ways, e.g., necessary, sufficient, sometimes necessary, sometimes sufficient, together necessary, together sufficient, etc. The discussion that Eagle (1973a,b) and Rubinstein (1973) initiated following the publication of Sherwood's book *The Logic of Explanation in Psychoanalysis* (1969) shows that Freud, who translated several works by J.S. Mill into German, advocated a philosophically well-grounded theory of causality (Thomä and Cheshire 1991; Cheshire and Thomä 1991). The following passage from one of Freud's early publications refers to several important concepts within a causal theory:

(a) *Precondition*, (b) *Specific Cause*, (c) *Concurrent Causes*, and, as a term which is not equivalent to the foregoing ones, (d) *Precipitating or Releasing Cause.*

In order to meet every possibility, let us assume that the aetiological factors we are concerned with are capable of a quantitative change - that is of increase or decrease.

If we accept the idea of an aetiological equation of several terms which must be satisfied if the effect is to take place, then we may characterize as the *precipitating* or releasing cause the one which makes its appearance last in the equation, so that it immediately precedes the emergence of the effect. It is this chronological factor alone which constitutes the essential nature of a precipitating cause. Any of the other causes, too, can in a particular case play the role of precipitating cause; and [the factor playing] this role can change within the same aetiological combination.

The factors which may be described as *preconditions* are those in whose absence the effect would never come about, but which are incapable of producing the effect by themselves alone, no matter in what amount they may be present. For the specific cause is still lacking.

The *specific cause* is the one which is never missing in any case in which the effect takes place, and which moreover suffices, if present in the required quantity or intensity, to achieve the effect, provided only that the preconditions are also fulfilled.

As *concurrent causes* we may regard such factors as are not necessarily present every time, nor able, whatever their amount, to produce the effect by themselves alone, but which operate alongside of the preconditions and the specific cause in satisfying the aetiological equation.

The distinctive character of the concurrent, or auxiliary, causes seems clear; but how do we distinguish between a precondition and a specifc cause, since both are indispensable and yet neither suffices alone to act as a cause?

The following considerations seem to allow us to arrive at a decision. Among the '*necessary causes*' we find several which reappear in the aetiological equations concerned in many other effects and thus exhibit no special relationship to any one particular effect. One of these causes, however, stands out in contrast to the rest from the fact that it is found in no other aetiological equation, or in very few; and this one has a right to be called the *specific* cause of the effect concerned. Furthermore, preconditions and specific causes are especially distinct from each other in those cases in which the preconditions have the characteristic of being long-standing states that are little susceptible to alteration, while the specific cause is a factor which has recently come into play. (1895f, pp.135-136)

These four factors have to converge to create a complete "aetiological equation." The complexity of causes poses a difficult task because different sufficient or necessary causes can be linked or replace each other. An exception is the specific cause, which by itself is sufficient if there is a certain predisposition. The context of the Freud quotation shows that the model for this cause and effect relationship is the *specific* pathogen that is responsible for an infectious disease and that can be deduced by pathologists from very particular transformations of tissue that are also referred to as specific.

In psychic and psychosomatic illnesses the disposition that develops in the course of an individual's life history takes on a special significance as the necessary condition, in contrast to the external "stimulus" which is the precipitating factor. These two factors, i. e., the necessary conditions, therefore play a correspondingly large role in Freud's model of scientific explanation. We will return to these problems when we discuss the specificity hypothesis in psychosomatic medicine (Sect. 9.7), yet in the context of Freud's case histories it should be noted that his explanatory model has proven itself to be exceptionally productive, even though the *validity* of many individual causal assumptions must be doubted today. The logic of the causal schema has not been refuted, rather the relationships discovered in individual cases have turned out to be wrong or have had to be relativized. We must keep this distinction in mind. Freud linked his model of *complemental series* to the causal theories of Hume and Mill (Eimer 1987). The interrelatedness of the factors makes it possible for the effects of therapeutic interventions to be reproduced via the above-mentioned network, the "nodal points" (Freud 1895d).

Freud's *causal* model of the etiology of psychic illnesses is complemented by a corresponding understanding of therapy. In order for an individual to find solutions to the problems later posed by life and to be able to discover connections between very different human activities, it may be necessary to descend "into the deepest and most primitive strata of mental development" (Freud 1918b, p. 10; see Vol.1, Sect. 10.2).

Freud's case histories are reconstructions that proceed from an individual's present situation and attempt to find the roots and typical conditions of symptoms in the individual's past. With regard to the symptoms of psychic and psychosomatic illnesses, time does appear to stand still - the past is present. The phobic is just as afraid of a completely harmless object today as he was 10 or 20 years ago, and compulsive thoughts and actions are repeated ritually in the same way for years.

Neurotic symptoms are so embedded in the patient's life history that knowledge of it is essential for comprehending the specific pathogenesis. "Case histories of this kind are intended to be judged like psychiatric ones; they have, however, one advantage over the latter, namely an intimate connection between the story of the patient's sufferings and the symptoms of his illness" (Freud 1895d, p. 161).

Of special significance is the case history of the Wolf Man, which Freud published under the title *From the History of an Infantile Neurosis* (1918b). A very substantial secondary literature has appeared on this patient alone, which in 1984 had amounted to about 150 articles (Mahony 1984). Despite many reservations about the demonstration or validation of psychoanalytic explanations, Perrez (1972) concludes that the description of the Wolf Man is beyond doubt a grand attempt to explain the puzzles that this case presented in the form of a narrative. The designation "narrative," introduced by Farrell (1961), acknowledges an aspect of the case histories that filled Freud with a certain sense of uneasiness - namely, "that the case histories I write should read like *short stories*" (Freud 1895d, p. 160). He sought recognition as a scientist and was concerned that his description of the fates of human beings might "lack the serious stamp of science" (Freud 1895d, p. 160). The Goethe Prize honored Freud the author, whose style has attracted students of literature from Muschg (1930) to Mahony (1987; see Schönau 1968).

The special tension contained in Freud's case histories results, in our opinion, from the fact that all the descriptions in them have the goal of making the background of the patients' thoughts and actions plausible in order to be able to present explanatory outlines of their history.

> Of special importance is the fact that the analysis of one of Freud's case presentations clearly shows that Freud was not only concerned with *describing* the history of a neurosis. He was concerned most of all with *explaining* it, and apparently in the form of a *genetic historical explanation.* The genetic historical form of explanation not only attempts to describe a chain of events, but also to show *why* one state leads to the next. For this reason it makes use of certain laws of probability, and in the case of Freud's narratives this is not always made explicit. (Perrez 1972, p. 98)

However unclear the etiology may be in an individual case and however insufficiently statistical probabilities and laws may be validated, the general result still holds that schemata of experiencing and behavior anchored in the unconscious develop over a very long period of time. Thus there is not only the danger that repeated adverse experiences can lead to the formation and maintenance of stereotypes, but also always a good chance that positive experiences can alter motivational schemata. Freud's conversation with Katharina may have opened new perspectives for this young girl, who consulted him in passing in an alpine lodging. Noteworthy is that this conversation provides an especially precise view into how Freud conducted diagnostic-therapeutic interviews (Argelander 1978).

The uniqueness of each life history links the psychoanalytic method to the rationale of the "single case study" (Edelson 1985). *Scientific* aims, of course, go beyond single case studies and are directed at postulating generalizations; Freud therefore emphasized in his report on the Wolf Man that generalizations can only be gained with regard to certain assumptions about pathogenesis by presenting numerous cases that have been thoroughly and deeply analyzed (Freud 1918b).

Since the primary purpose of Freud's case histories was to reconstruct the psychogenesis, i.e., to demonstrate that symptoms have repressed unconscious causes, the description of therapeutic technique took second place. Freud did not discuss *technical* rules systematically in his treatment reports. He only mentioned in a rather fragmentary way what he felt, thought, interpreted, or otherwise did in a particular session.

Freud distinguished between *case histories,* which he occasionally referred to as the histories of illnesses, and *treatment histories.* We have adopted this distinction, except that we prefer the designation *treatment reports* because of the significance of the different forms of documentation. Freud pointed out the difficulties confronting suitable reporting in an early publication:

> The difficulties are very considerable when the physician has to conduct six or eight psychotherapeutic treatments of the sort in a day, and cannot make notes during the actual session with the patient for fear of shaking the patient's confidence and of disturbing his own view of the material under observation. Indeed, I have not yet succeeded in solving the problem of how to record for publication the history of a treatment of long duration. (Freud 1905e, pp.9-10)

He was referring in this instance to Dora, whose case history and treatment he described in the *Fragment of an Analysis of a Case of Hysteria.* His task of reporting this case was eased by two circumstances, namely the brevity of the treatment and the fact that "the material which elucidated the case was grouped around two dreams (one related in the middle of the treatment and one at the end). The wording of these dreams was recorded immediately after the session, and they thus afforded a secure point of attachment for the chain of interpretations and recollections which proceeded from them" (Freud 1905e, p. 10).

Freud did not write the case history itself, the core of the publication, until after the cure; he did it from memory but claimed it had a high degree of precision. According to his own words, he accepted incompleteness with regard to the *treatment history* as a given:

> I have as a rule not reproduced the process of interpretation to which the patient's associations and communications had to be subjected, but only the results of that process. Apart from the dreams, therefore, the technique of the analytic work has been revealed in only a very few places. My object in this case history was to demonstrate the intimate structure of a neurotic disorder and the determination of its symptoms; and it would have led to nothing but hopeless confusion if I had tried to complete the other task at the same time. Before the technical rules, most of which have been arrived at empirically, could be properly laid down, it would be necessary to collect material from the *histories* of a large number of *treatments.* (Freud 1905e, pp.12-13, emphasis added)

Freud did not assign any special weight to the abbreviated form of this description because transference "did not come up for discussion during the short treatment," which only lasted three months (1905e, p. 13). A similar predominance of the case history at the expense of the treatment history can be found in all of the case reports Freud published.

Freud's reason for putting the genesis of neurotic symptoms at the center of his published case histories was his view that clarifying the genesis and achieving more insight are the factors that create the best preconditions for therapeutic interventions. A representative quotation reads: "We want something that is sought for in all scientific work - to understand the phenomena, to establish a correlation between them and, in the latter end, if it is possible, to enlarge our power over them" (Freud 1916/17, p. 100).

Not Freud's case histories, but his five technical works are, according to Greenson (1967, p. 17), the source from which an analyst can learn to create the best conditions for therapeutic change. Considering Freud's unique position in psychoanalysis, the fact that he did not provide a synoptic description of his technique comprising both theory *and* practice has had lasting consequences. His case histories acquired exemplary character for the psychoanalytic theories describing the conditions of genesis, and were referred to in this way by, for example, Sherwood (1969), Gardiner (1971), Niederland (1959), Perrez (1972), Schalmey (1977), and Mahony (1984, 1986). Freud was more concerned with specifying rules of research to clarify the genesis rather than with making these rules the object of study to determine whether they provide the patient the necessary and sufficient *conditions for change* (see Vol.1, Sects. 7.1 and 10.5).

At the beginning of therapy the *neurosis* becomes the *transference neurosis* regardless of how deep its roots reach back into and are anchored in the patient's life history (see Vol.1, Sect. 2.4). Even if the domain referred to by this concept has not been sufficiently defined, as is assumed by prominent analysts in the controversial discussion edited by London and Rosenblatt (1987), we cannot overlook the fact that the analyst makes a substantial contribution to determining the nature of the transference. In this sense, school-specific transference neuroses even develop, contradicting to Freud's idea that simple observance of the rules of treatment lead transference neuroses to develop uniformly. This extension of the theory of transference and countertransference follows from the recognition of the analyst's influence. These developments were eased by the fact that it has become possible in recent years to acquire some insight into Freud's own practice, deepening our understanding of the case histories he reconstructed and also extending our knowledge of how he applied technical rules.

In Vol.1 we referred to the fact that the increasing amount of literature about Freud's practice has facilitated the critical reapraisal of the history of the psychoanalytic technique (Cremerius 1981b; Beigler 1975; Kanzer and Glenn 1980). When necessary, Freud gave patients board, lent them money, or even gave it to them. Yet it would, of course, be naive to want to find solutions to today's problems by identifying with Freud's natural and humane attitude in the consulting room as he apparently disregarded the consequences of transference.

It is characteristic of Freud's case histories that they, on the one hand, report the concrete analysis of an individual case while, on the other hand, containing far-reaching hypotheses that attempt to present the entire wealth of clinical observations in condensed form and to put them in a causal connection.

According to Jones (1954), Charcot's nosographic method exerted a lasting influence on Freud's goals with regard to the reconstruction of the genesis and course of psychogenic illnesses. Freud did not study the technical rules primarily to determine whether they provide the best conditions for therapeutic change. He instead wanted his technical recommendations to secure the scientific foundation for the psychoanalytic method: "We have a right, or rather a duty, to carry on our research without consideration of any immediate beneficial effect. In the end - we cannot tell where or when - every litte fragment of knowledge will be transformed into power, and into therapeutic power as well" (Freud 1916/17, p. 255). The rules Freud set down were supposed to guarantee the objectivity of the results and to limit the analyst's influence on the data as much as possible. The documentation of the phenomena observed in interviews was oriented around the statements made by patients that were incorporated into the case histories because of their assumed causal relevance. The material is structured by the method, according to Freud's fundamental thesis:

> What characterizes psycho-analysis as a science is not the material which it handles but the technique with which it works. It can be applied to the history of civilization, to the science of religion and to mythology, no less than to the theory of the neuroses, without doing violence to its essential nature. What it aims at and achieves is nothing other than the uncovering of what is unconscious in mental life. (Freud 1916/17, p. 389)

Of course it makes an immense difference whether the psychoanalytic method is applied to cultural history or is practiced as a form of therapy, because the patient comes to the analyst expecting a lessening or cure of his suffering. By providing therapy the analyst assumes a responsibility that does not arise in the interpretation of mythology or in other applications of the psychoanalytic method. Most importantly, however, the patient is a critical witness of the analyst's actions.

1.3 Treatment Reports

Attention was so focused on the dialogue between patient and analyst in the metamorphosis from the case history to the treatment report that the preparation of protocols according to *selective* criteria has become the object of intense interest. Freud's literarily stimulating description of the Rat Man, of which Mahoney (1986) recently presented a linguistic interpretation, owes its wealth of details to the daily notes that Freud was accustomed to making from memory. The protocols about the Rat Man were first published in 1955, in Vol.10 of the *Standard Edition.*

When Zetzel, while preparing an article, turned to the *Standard Edition* instead of to the *Collected Papers*, she found Freud's protocols, which until then had gone largely unnoticed. They are instructive particularly with regard to his therapeutic technique, yet also provide important additional information about the genesis of the symptoms. Freud's notes contain over 40 references to a highly ambivalent mother-son relationship, which were not given adequate consideration in the case history published in 1909 (Zetzel 1966). Freud (1909, p. 255 himself noted, "After I had told him my terms, he said he must consult his mother." This important reaction by the patient is not mentioned in the case history. Since these protocols have become known, the case history of the Rat Man has been reinterpreted by Shengold (1971) and Holland (1975), in addition to the others named above.

Like all psychoanalysts, Freud prepared his protocols according to some criteria, i. e., selectively; they guided what he selected from his notes. Freud used the individual cases to describe examples of typical connections and processes in psychic life.

The notes Freud made about the Rat Man have aroused attention because the founder of psychoanalysis did not observe - neither then nor later on - the technical recommendatons that were later incorporated into the system of psychoanalytic rules. Yet as we outlined above and explained in Vol.1, the solution to technical problems cannot be found in a return to Freud's unorthodox style of treatment.

We see a sign of radical change in the fact that analysts are devoting more attention to the dyadic nature of the analytic situation while preparing protocols of treatment, both for shorter and longer periods. Influential psychoanalysts from all the different schools have contributed to this change toward the adoption of an interpersonal point of view in presenting case material.

The criteria that must be applied in order to write a convincing case history, i. e., a reconstruction of the conditions of genesis, are different from those for the description in a treatment report. Treatment reports focus on determining whether change has occurred and which conditions led to the change. Freud could be satisfied with making relatively rough distinctions that left a lot to subsequent research. From today's point of view, however, Freud's case histories are not suited to serve either as a model for a reconstruction of the etiology or as a paradigm for protocols of psychoanalytic treatment. The task of creating the most favorable conditions for change and of investigating the therapeutic process is a very challenging one. Similarly, etiological research that is designed to provide evidence to test hypotheses demands too much of the individual analyst. Following Grünbaum's (1984) criticism, Edelson (1986) drafted an ideal model according to which a case history and a treatment report would have to be written today in order to make it possible for hypotheses to be tested.

Insights can be gained into Freud's technique by reading any of his case histories. The emphasis in each of them is on reconstructing the genesis of the particular neurosis. Freud also gave some examples of therapeutic interventions, sometimes even word for word. We recommend that anyone reading one of Freud's case histories consult a representative book from the secondary literature for critical guidance.

The post-Freudian development of the preparation of case histories and treatment reports has in fact been characterized by an increase in the number of large-scale case reports (Kächele 1981). In the last few years there has been an unmistakable and growing tendency for more and more analysts to make their clinical work accessible to readers. Given adequate preparation, this can put the critical discussion within the profession on a sound footing. However, in the psychoanalytic literature the "vignette" is still the primary form of presentation. A vignette is characterized by unity, subtlety, and refinement (see discussion in Thomä and

Hohage 1981) and serves to illustrate typical psychodynamic connections. In it the implications for the analyst's therapeutic actions are secondary in comparison with this focus of interest. Greenson (1973, p. 15) has also criticized older textbooks, including those by Sharpe (1930), Fenichel (1941), Glover (1955), and Menninger and Holzman (1977), for hardly describing how the analyst actually works and what he feels, thinks, and does.

Thus we are justified in joining Spillius (1983) in complaining-as she did in her critical survey of new developments in the Kleinian therapeutic technique - about the lack of availability of representative treatment reports prepared by leading analysts. Everywhere case reports are primarily supplied by candidates in training, who submit them for admission into the psychoanalytic societies; because of their compromising character, these reports are of dubious value, as Spillius rightly emphasized. This state of affairs is confirmed by the exceptions, and we do not want to miss the opportunity of favorably mentioning a few examples of them.

Shortly before her death M. Klein completed a comprehensive treatment report of the 4-month analysis of a 10-year-old boy (from 1941), whom she named Richard; it was published in 1961.

> In presenting the following case-history, I have several aims in view. I wish first of all to illustrate my technique in greater detail than I have done formerly. The extensive notes I made enable the reader to observe how interpretations find confirmation in the material following them. The day-to-day movement in the analysis, and the continuity running through it, thus become perceptible. (Klein 1961, p. x)

There is hardly another treatment report in which the analyst's theoretical assumptions as clearly determine his actions as in this report, which reproduces all 93 sessions in detail. In addition to the reviews by Geleerd (1963) and Segal and Meltzer (1963), there is also a thorough study by Meltzer (1978) that contains a detailed reappraisal of the course of the case.

Another treatment report, a large one by Winnicott (1972) entitled "Fragment of an Analysis," was also published posthumously, in a volume edited by Giovacchini (1972). The interactive nature of the exchange of thoughts between this patient and Winnicott irritated the French analyst A. Anzieu (1977, p. 28) because, according to her argument, the large number of Winnicott's interpretations made it impossible to perceive what the patient had said. Analysts in Lacan's sphere of influence are often extremely reticent, one of the items that Lang (1986) criticized. Lacan himself has not provided detailed clinical descriptions, and there are no empirical studies either, especially linguistic ones, although it would seem natural for such studies to be conducted considering his particular theses. Only a few indications of Lacan's treatment can be drawn from the published version (1982) of Lacan's diagnostic interview of a psychotic patient that was recorded. He merely explored the patient's symptoms by using the traditional psychiatric technique of clarifying the psychopathology by questions.

In strong contrast to this is Dewald's (1972) description of a psychoanalytic process. He bases his account, just as Wurmser (1987) later did, on protocols of sessions recorded in shorthand, which provided Lipton (1982) an excellent basis for his criticism of Dewald's technique (see Vol.1, Chap.9).

An ideal example is also provided by a discussion that Pulver (1987) edited under the title "How Theory Shapes Technique: Perspectives on a Clinical Study." The basis of the discussion is a collection of an analyst's (Silverman) notes. The analyst prepared a protocol containing his thoughts and feelings in addition to the interpretations he made and the patient's reactions in three sessions. This clinical material was examined by ten analysts who are prominent representatives of the various psychoanalytic schools. Shane (1987) and Pulver (1987) summarized the results of the discussion, in which each of the analysts naturally started from his own personal point of view. Silverman, the treating analyst, is known as an adherent of structural theory.

After an evaluation of the material by Brenner (structural theory), Burland (Mahler's school), Goldberg (self psychology), and Mason (Kleinian perspective), Shane concluded in resignation:

> First, we cannot help observing that each panelist found in the patient important diagnostic features best explained by his particular frame of reference... .In summary, I would say that the diversity of opinions regarding the diagnosis and dynamics of Silverman's patient would suggest that one's theoretical stance takes precedence over other considerations. The presentations amply demonstrate that each theory can sound highly convincing, which makes absolute judgment almost impossible and personal choice inevitable. (Shane 1987, pp.199, 205)

Schwaber (1987, p. 262) also showed convincingly that the models employed by the participants in this discussion even frequently have a distorting effect on the gathering of data. For this reason she argues that theoretical models should be used in a more appropriate manner.

> Modern science teaches us that the observer's participation is an essential and fascinating element of the data. I make no argument for an atheoretical orientation, even if that were possible. I argue, rather, for our recognition that no matter what theory we espouse, we run the risk of using it to foreclose rather than to continue inquiry, to provide an answer rather than to raise a new question... .Our models are not simply interchangeable, matters of personal preference. We must seek that model which best explains the data and best expands our perceptual field. (Schwaber 1987, pp.274, 275)

These critical insights into an on-going treatment illuminate the numerous problems that the participation of third parties, whether they be specialists, scientists from other disciplines, or lay people, can make apparent. It was therefore logical for Pulver (1987) to be particularly concerned with the question of how a protocol should be prepared.

Pulver enthusiastically welcomed the frankness of the reporting analyst. It is remarkable, in fact, that analysts still deserve our special praise when they attempt to precisely record in a protocol - prepared during or after the session - what the patient said and what they themslelves felt, thought, or said, fully aware that this protocol will form the basis for a discussion with colleagues from other psychoanalytic schools and approaches. There are several reasons for the increasing willingness of analysts to let colleagues look over their shoulder. Without a doubt, psychoanalysis itself is going through a phase of demystification and shattering of illusions; although psychoanalysis has played a major role in the enlightenment, for a long time it did not subject itself to the same critical self-criticism. Institutionalized psychoanalysis is in danger of transforming itself into an ideology. Freud became a mythical figure. It is consequently no coincidence that a large public eagerly absorbs everything that Freud's analysands report about his work. Thus the rhetorical question expressed in the title of an article by Momogliano – "Was Freud a Freudian?" – can be answered clearly: "He was not" (Momogliano 1987).

The fear of publicity has declined sufficiently in recent decades to encourage many analysands, whether patients or prospective analysts, to report in one form or another about their treatments (Anzieu 1986; Guntrip 1975). In addition to the well-known stories and diaries by Anais Nin, Marie Cardinale, Hannah Green, Erica Jong, Dörte von Drigalski, and Tilmann Moser, there are also joint publications containing the individual reports of both participants, for example that by Yalom and Elkin (1974). They take the old motto – *audiatur et altera pars* – seriously that it is important to hear both sides. The psychoanalytic community makes it too easy for itself if it reduces such autobiographic fragments of varying quality prose to someone's hurt feelings, to negative transference that has not been analyzed, or to excessive exhibitionism and narcissism.

Systematically planned empirical research on therapy is one of the factors contributing, to an increasing degree, to these changes in climate in psychoanalysis that, in turn, have initiated this demystification in psychoanalysis (see for example Masling 1983, 1986; Dahl et al. 1988). This then leads to further changes, which are very valuable precisely because the arguments employed in the clinical literature have been relatively naive. For example, Pulver stated, in the article referred to above, that each of the very experienced and distinguished analysts are equally successful despite holding divergent views about a case. In fact, however, the sessions presented by Silverman took a rather unfavorable course, so the fact that the protocols were not examined for curative factors might be traced back to a case of special consideration among colleagues. Of course, it is still unclear how many of the general and specific factors that are taken to be curative on the basis of the results of research on therapy must converge qualitatively and quantitatively in an individual case in order to achieve a significant improvement or cure (Kächele 1988). Thus it is entirely possible that the effectiveness of psychodynamic therapies is more the result of similarities with regard to a few fundamental principles than of the differences separating them with regard to the meaning of interpretations. Joseph (1979) listed some of these basic assumptions, including unconscious processes, resistance, transference, free associations, the genetic derivation of problems, the therapeutic efforts to understand and to interpret, and the assumption that there are conflicts. Pulver went even further when he said that the differences of opinion between the participants in the discussion are more apparent than real.

> The therapists may be saying essentially the same thing to the patient, but in different words. The patients, once they get used to the therapist's words, in fact *do feel understood.* For instance, this patient might feel that her ineffable feeling of defectiveness was understood by a Kleinian who spoke of her envy at not having a penis, a self-psychologist who spoke of her sense of fragmentation, and a structural theorist who spoke of her sense of castration. (Pulver 1987, p. 298)

Thus Pulver assumed that this patient could have had insights that could have been expressed in different sets of terminology, yet that the latter would simply represent metaphoric variations of the same processes. Joseph (1984) argued in a similar vein by referring to unconscious linkages; for example, an interview covering anxiety and loss touches both on unconscious preoedipal separation anxiety and on castration anxiety. Every individual does in fact recall many experiences in response to the word "loss" that may be interrelated but that belong to separate subgroups. Which narrative develops in a treatment is therefore not arbitrary or insignificant (Spence 1982, 1983; Eagle 1984). Although it is definitely important for both participants, patient and analyst, to reach some agreements, the purpose is not to find or invent an arbitrary "language game" that metaphorically links everything together. The patient wants to be cured of his defects, after all. He would like to master his specific conflicts and their roots, not just to recognize them. Furthermore, independent persons are able to determine whether the alterations in symptoms are really there.

The phenomena that occur in analytic treatment can, as Eagle has convincingly demonstrated, make a special contribution

> to a theory of therapy, that is, an understanding of the relationship between certain kinds of operations and interventions and the occurrence or failure of occurrence of certain kinds of specific changes. It seems to me ironic that psychoanalytic writers attempt to employ clinical data for just about every purpose but the one for which they are most appropriate - an evaluation and understanding of therapeutic change. (Eagle 1988, p. 163)

From today's perspective, the summary of a course of treatment is, if for no other reason than because of its incompleteness, of problematic value for the task of scientific validation. Yet the nature of the subject itself dictates that completeness cannot be achieved. It is possible, however, to fulfill one important demand today, namely that detailed documentation be provided at the level of observation, from which generalizations are made. The model that Mitscherlich introduced for systematic case histories was an early attempt in this direction, even if very few case histories of this kind were actually written (Thomä 1954, 1957, 1961, 1978; de Boor 1965). Important was the demand that the abstraction and conceptualization that were the basis for classification be grounded. The Hampstead Index attempted to achieve something similar, namely to make it possible to clarify the major psychoanalytic concepts by means of a systematic documentation (Sandler 1962; Bolland and Sandler 1965). The Mitscherlich model was of great didactic value because it facilitated reflection during the phase in which specific hypotheses are made in psychosomatic medicine; its systematization also eased comparison. Its design pointed the direction for subsequent developments. Mitscherlich emphasized the significance of the doctor-patient relationship for diagnosis and therapy by also adopting the interview scheme of the Tavistock Clinic for purposes of documentation. The changes in symptoms that result from the analyst's interventions became the center of interest in descriptions of the course of a psychoanalytic treatment.

Going beyond the technical aspects of interpretation and the question of what should be interpreted in what way at what time, Bernfeld (1941) was innovative in concerning himself with the topic of the scientific validity and the truth of interpretations. This problem was further discussed in the 1950s by Glover (1952), Kubie (1952), and Schmidl (1955).

The studies of interpretations conducted at the Psychosomatic Clinic of the University of Heidelberg and in cooperation with the staff of the Sigmund Freud

Institute in Frankfurt - both institutions headed for longer periods by A. Mitscherlich - in the mid-1960s pursued the ambitious goal of validating the theory that was the basis of the individual analyst's therapeutic actions. Important impulses for this attempt came from the manner in which Balint structured his seminars on treatment technique, which assigned just as much significance to the thoughts of the analyst before he made a given interpretation as to the patient's reaction.

In order to do justice to the numerous thoughts that are part of the analyst's evenly suspended attention, Balint recommended that items which were merely thought should also be included in the notes about the session. The inclusion in the analyst's protocol of what the analyst considered - in addition to his actual interventions - and of information about the emotional and rational context in which interpretations originated was an important intermediate step. It became evident from this form of keeping records that it is of great importance to let the patient take part in the thoughts that are the basis of the analyst's interventions or interpretations. This is in fact a result of experience that was first discovered long ago and that Freud (1940a, p. 178) had already referred to. He emphasized that the patient must be made an accomplice, i. e., must have some knowledge of the analyst's constructions, specifically about how the analyst arrives at his interpretations and what the reasons for them are. According to the reports available to us today, Freud did in fact acquaint his patients with his thoughts in detail, i. e., with the context of his interpretations. According to him, it is not unusual for the case to be divided into two distinctly separate phases:

> In the first, the physician procures from the patient the necessary information, makes him familiar with the premises and postulates of psycho-analysis, and unfolds to him the reconstruction of the genesis of his disorder as deduced from the material brought up in the analysis. In the second phase the patient himself gets hold of the material put before him; he works on it, recollects what he can of the apparently repressed memories, and tries to repeat the rest as if he were in some way living it over again. In this way he can confirm, supplement, and correct the inferences made by the physician. It is only during this work that he experiences, through overcoming resistances, the inner change aimed at, and acquires for himself the convictions that make him independent of the physician's authority. (Freud 1920a, p. 152)

The danger of intellectualization that is associated with this can be avoided. Explaining the rational context of interpretations generally elicits a strong affective echo from the patient and provides additional information, giving the patient the opportunity to critically consider the analyst's perspective. The patient achieves a greater freedom to understand the analyst's views and what appeared to be his mysterious role. An exact examination of what is termed the patient's identification with the analyst's functions also depends on whether the exchange processes are documented in a detailed manner (see Sect. 2.4).

Thomä and Houben (1967) attempted - by examining interpretations--to identify the important aspects of an analyst's technique and its theoretical foundation, and - by studying patient's reactions - to estimate its therapeutic effectiveness. While conducting these studies we slowly became aware of the problems concerning the *effectiveness* of interpretations and the *truth* of theories.

In order to systematically study interpretations, we followed a recommendation made by Isaacs (1939) and designed a report scheme. It required the psychoanalyst preparing the protocol to locate interpretations between observation and theory and to describe the patient's reactions. Periods of treatment were distinguished according to the following points:

1. Associations, forms of behavior, and the patient's dreams that led the analyst to focus on a specific topic in one period for working through (*psychodynamic hypotheses*)
2. The analyst's thoughts, based on the theory of neuroses and his technique, that preceded individual interpretations
3. The goal of the interpretation
4. The formulation of the interpretation
5. The patient's immediate reaction
6. All the rest of the analyst's interpretations and the patient's reactions (associations, forms of behavior, dreams, changes in mood and affective state, etc.) that appear to be relevant for the topic to be worked through
7. Was the goal achieved?
8. Reference to material that does not agree with the hypotheses

While working on this project it became clear that the question of validation can only be answered within the complex sphere of research into the course and outcome of psychoanalysis, which was far beyond our possibilities at the time. The reporting scheme is, however, still a suitable means for providing important information for clinical discussion, as Pulver (1987) demonstrated 25 years later. It is enormously productive for the analyst to prepare protocols of his feelings, thoughts, and interventions in a way that enables a third party to develop an alternative perspective or that facilitates this task (for an example, see Chap.8). The clarifications we have summarized in Vol.1 (Chap.10), are necessary to promote clinical research and to be able to reach a better scientific grounding for psychoanalytic practice.

Our special interest in the effects that interpretations have led us, in preparing those protocols, to pay insufficient attention to the role of the emotional aspects of the relationship. The loss of the emotional context forming the background of analysis makes interpretations and reactions appear far more intellectual than they in reality are. Insight and experience, interpretation and relationship, and the verbal and nonverbal aspects of the dialogue interact (Thomä 1983; see also Vol.1, Sect. 8.6). While making or reconstructing interpretations, analysts also move into the depths of countertransference, which is easier to talk about than to write about.

These two examples of attempts to write treatment reports were concerned with obtaining data regarding what the analyst felt, thought, and did in the presence of his patient that is as accurate as possible. Glover (1955) also assigned special value to the analyst preparing a protocol of what he told the patient. This is important because many of the so-called narratives are, as Spence (1986) criticized, typical narratives constructed by psychoanalysts according to hidden psychodynamic perspectives and without it being possible to recognize the analysts' own contributions.

The tape recording of analyses has finally put the development outlined here on a firm footing, both for research into the course and outcome of treatment and for further training (Thomä and Rosenkötter 1970; Kächele et al. 1973). Almost 30 years after the introduction of the Mitscherlich model the *systematic single case study* has proven itself to be very fruitful. The methodology of such studies has been the focus of discussion for some time (Bromley 1986; Edelson 1988; Petermann 1982). Such case studies provide a means to satisfy the demands placed today on research testing psychoanalytic hypotheses (Weiss and Sampson 1986; Neudert et al. 1987).

1.4 Approximating the Dialogue: Tape Recordings and Transcriptions

The idea of employing technical aids should be given very careful consideration. Although tape recordings document the verbal dialogue, this technological "third ear" does not register the thoughts and feelings that go unspoken or that fill unspoken space with meaning and affects. It would be superfluous to make special reference to this fact if this deficiency were not given such weight in the literature. It is possible, after all, to "hear" more of the tone that makes the music when reading transcripts or, particularly, listening to the original recordings than by reading publications based on protocols. An analyst's attention can be distracted if he takes a protocol during a session, and the analyst is more selective if he reports key words after the session, as Freud recommended. In selecting the phenomena to be described, the analyst follows his own subjective theoretical perspective, and who appreciates discovering that his own expectations and assumptions have been refuted! It is not only the patients who draw pleasure and hope from confirmation. Research testing hypotheses is a burden on all psychotherapists because it of necessity questions preferred convictions (Bowlby 1982). For this reason we like to share this task with cooperating scientists not participating directly in the therapy.

After becoming chairman of the department of psychotherapy and director of the psychoanalytic institute in Ulm in 1967, the senior author initiated the tape recording of psychoanalytic therapies. In the following years these recordings, together with those of therapies conducted by some of his associates, became the core of the transcripts of psychoanalytic therapies stored in the "Ulm Textbank," that in the meantime has been made available to a large number of scientists from around the world (Mergenthaler 1985).

It took years before we learned to sufficiently appreciate the enormously profitable effects of listening to dialogues and reading verbatim transcripts of our own clinical work for us to overcome all of our earlier reservations. The struggle to introduce corresponding technical aids into the analytic interview was begun by E. Zinn in 1933 (Shakow and Rapaport 1964, p.138). Although it is not over yet, the opportunities offered by the tape recording of analyses for psychoanalytic training and practice were first mentioned in positive terms by McLaughlin at the International Psychoanalytic Congress held in Helsinki in 1982.

In contrast to the followers of C. Rogers, psychoanalysis did not take advantage of these numerous possibilities for a long time. At the core of many misgivings was the concern that the presence of a tape recorder could have consequences similar to those of a third party, namely that the patient "would become silent as soon as he observed a single witness to whom he felt indifferent" (Freud 1916/17, p. 18). Yet it has long been known that patients, with few exceptions, readily give their approval to having the interview recorded, discussed in professional circles, and evaluated scientifically. It is not unusual for patients to - correctly - expect to profit therapeutically from having their analyst concern himself especially intensively with their case. Of course, the patient's initial approval and his motivations are just one aspect; another and decisive question concerns the effects of the tape recording on the psychoanalytic process. In order to make a comparative study of one and the same patient it would have to be possible to treat him twice, once with and once without a recording. Yet it is possible to refer to the large number of psychoanalytic treatments that have been recorded and in which no systematic negative effect has become known. We do not employ the so-called playback technique, but according to Robbins (1988) severely disturbed patients achieve a therapeutically effective "self objectification" (Stern 1970) by listening to their recorded interviews and being able to work through the experiences they thus acquire.

Once recording has been agreed upon, we consider it to be part of the permanent framework on the basis of which everything that happens is interpreted. Of course, the patient can also retract his approval. In Sect. 7.5 we give examples of such cases; they show that it is not only possible but also very productive for these events to be made the object of precise analytic study. At any rate, according to our own experience and the relevant literature the course of the psychoanalytic process is in general such that the recording ultimately becomes a matter of routine that only occasionally has an unconscious significance, just as lying on the couch does. Superego functions can, for example, only be attributed to the tape recording and projected onto the secretary (as a transference figure) as long as such expectations of punishment are virulent. Similarly, in the course of analysis the omnipotent fantasies a patient is ashamed of and whose publication he fears - neurotic fears that they might be identified despite being used anonymously - lose their disturbing force.

After working through, many things become simple and human that initially appeared to be characterized by a unique personal dynamism. Nonetheless, no text of a psychoanalytic dialogue is superficial even though many readers express surprise at how little the text alone says. Occasionally doubts are therefore raised whether the availability of verbatim protocols offers anything new. Yet at least the analyst in question is frequently surprised when he realizes, from hearing his own voice or reading the transcript, how far his interpretations are from what they should be according to the textbooks, i. e., clear and distinct.

It is remarkable how many problems an analyst has to cope with when he gives a colleague the data from his clinical work, in this case a transcribed dialogue, for evaluation. Colleagues confirm more or less bluntly what one's self evaluation actually cannot overlook, namely that there can be a significant discrepancy between one's professional ideal and reality. The tape recorder is without a doubt a neutral receiver that cannot miss something or be selective! Kubie, to whose supervision using tape recordings the senior author owes a debt of gratitude, described in the following quotation painful experiences that every psychoanalyst has to get over when he is directly confronted with his statements in an analytic situation:

When for the first time a student psychiatrist or an experienced analyst hears himself participate in an interview or a psychotherapeutic session, it is always a surprising and illuminating experience. He hears himself outshouting or outwhispering the patient, always louder or always softer. Or he hears himself playing seesaw with his patient - loud when the patient is soft, and soft when the patient is loud. Or with surprise and dismay he hears in his own voice the edge of unintended scorn or sarcasm, or impatience or hostility, or else overtender solicitude and seductive warmth. Or he hears for the first time his own unnoted ticlike noises punctuating and interrupting the patient's stream. From such data as this he and the group as a whole learn a great deal about themselves and about the process of interchange with patients and what this process evokes in them in the form of automatic and therefore indescribable patterns of vocal interplay.

They learn also to watch for and to respect the subtle tricks of forgetting and false recall to which the human mind is prone. At one seminar a young psychiatrist reported that in a previous interview at one point his patient had asked that the recording machine be turned off while he divulged some material which was particularly painful to him. The group discussed the possible reasons for this, basing our discussion on our knowledge of the patient from previous seminars. Then to check the accuracy of our speculative reconstruction, the psychiatrist was asked to play to the group about five minutes of the recorded interview which had preceded the interruption, and then about five or ten minutes which followed when the recording had been resumed. To the amazement of the young psychiatrist and of the group as a whole, as we listened to the recording we discovered that it had been the psychiatrist and not the patient who had suggested that the recording should be interrupted. Of his role in this, the young psychiatrist had not the slightest memory. Furthermore, as we heard the patient's halting speech, his change of pace and volume, the altered pitch and placing of his voice, it became clear to the whole group that the young psychiatrist's intuitive move had been sound: that he had correctly evaluated the patient's mounting tension and had perceived the need for this gesture of special consideration and privacy. The result was that the patient's rapport was more firmly established than before, to such an extent that the psychiatrist could now recall that it had been the patient who had suggested that the recording be resumed after a relatively brief interruption, and who then, with the machine turned on, had continued to discuss frankly and without embarrassment the material about which he had been so touchy before. The illuminating implications of this episode for the data itself and for the transference and countertransference furnished the group with material for reflection and discussion throughout the remaining course of the seminars. These could not have been studied without the recording machine. (Kubie 1958, pp.233-234)

It is difficult to ignore the meaning of this story. It opens a context of discovery that illuminates the always latent danger of reductionism inherent in a condensed and selected report.

Transcripts often seem paltry in comparison to the recollections that the analyst has of the session and that are immediately revitalized when he reads the text. It is the rich emotional and cognitive context that adds vitality to the sentences expressed by the patient and the analyst. This context and the multifaceted background, which are revitalized when the treating analyst reads a transcript, can only be assumed by the reader who did not participate in the interview; it may be possible for the latter to fill in the gaps with the aid of his imagination and his own experience. In the traditional presentation of case material, which in general contains much less original data, this enrichment is provided by the author's narrative comments. Even the use of generalizations, i. e., of the abstract concepts that are regularly employed in clinical narratives, probably contributes to making the reader feel at home. The concepts that are used are filled - automatically, as it were - with the views that the reader associates with them. If a report refers to trauma or orality, we all attribute it a meaning on the basis of our own understanding of these and other concepts that is in itself suited to lead us into an approving or skeptical dialogue with the author.

Uncommented transcripts, in particular, are sometimes rather strange material. It took us some time to get accustomed to them. Yet if you become absorbed in these dialogues and practice on your own texts and those of other analysts, you become able to recognize a wealth of detail. For example, the context clarifies how a patient understood a question and whether he took it as encouragement or criticism. Thus the verbatim transcript at least makes it possible to understand how the tone makes the music. An even preciser method for studying the emotional background is for the analyst to summarize his countertransference during specific sequences or immediately after the session or for him to be questioned afterwards.

This also makes it possible for third parties to examine the theoretical assumptions behind an interpretation. The assumptions they make about the background motives and the goals contained in an interpretation are more reliable if entire sequences can be considered in a transcript. The "thinking-out-loud" approach, which Meyer (1981, 1988) used to examine the thought processes involved in the conclusions drawn by three analysts, leads even further. Finally, listening to the tape recording makes it possible to establish very close contact with the original situation.

Missing in manuscripts of analyses recorded in their entirety are both the silence pauses, which can be very eloquent "comments" for each participant, and descriptions of the mood, which can be remembered during an oral presentation at a seminar on treatment. We would like to raise the question of why it seems to be easier for musicians to hear the music while reading a score than for analysts to make the transcript of a session come alive.

Sandler and Sandler (1984, p. 396) refer to the "major task for future researchers to discover why it is that the transcribed material of other analysts' sessions so often makes one feel that they are very bad analysts indeed." They qualify this by adding that "this reaction is far too frequent to reflect reality" and ask, "can so many analysts really be so bad?" This conclusion is a challenge for us to enlarge the size of the sample available for examination. Apparently only the bad analysts have so far been ready to put the naked facts - the unerring transcripts - on the table. With the examples contained in this volume we considerably enlarge the previous sample size and naturally hope that we do not fall victim to the same verdict. Yet even more bad examples can serve a useful function and encourage renown analysts to finally demonstrate how it should be done by making ideal models of transcripts of dialogues available for discussion. Everyone in the process of learning looks for role models. The great masters of our time should not miss the chance to set a good example. Of course, the naked facts of the verbal exchange are not the last word. By coding intonations and other nonverbal communications it is possible to represent affects better in transcripts than in traditional publications. It requires some practice, however, to be able to follow texts of psychoanalytic dialogues containing such coded information.

Video recordings are essential to examine some issues, for example, to study how affects are expressed in mimicry and intonation (Fonagy 1983), gestures, and the overall expressiveness of posture and movement, i. e., body language (Krause and Lütolf 1988). Of course, they do not lead anywhere if the issues have not been clearly conceptualized or if there is no clearly defined method for evaluating the data. This is the reason that the films of a complete psychoanalytic treatment that have been made (Bergmann 1966) have disappeared into the vaults of the National Institute of Mental Health and have probably been destroyed in the meantime. There are less complicated and costly means to register the nonverbal communication expressed by posture and movement for clinical purposes than to make video recordings of the patient while he is lying on the couch and restricted in movement. In several articles Deutsch (1949, 1952) has pointed to the significance of posture and movement, and McLaughlin (1987) has described how he uses simple marks in the protocol to record the patient's movements on the couch.

On the basis of our experience, we realize that transcribed psychoanalytic dialogues become more meaningful the more the reader can put himself into the situation and add vitality to it by identifying with the participants and reenacting, as it were, the dialogue. There is still a difference, however, between in vivo and in vitro. When the treating analyst reads his own interpretations, his memories add important dimensions. It simply makes a difference whether you read a drama by Shakespeare, sit in the audience and view a stage performance, or help to enact it as an actor or director. Since we will frequently confront the reader with excerpts from transcripts, we request him to make the mental attempt to dramatize the text. We believe that most dialogues can stimulate the reader to make multifaceted and imaginative identifications and, consequently, numerous interpretations. Yet this does not eliminate the difference between the producer and the recipient of a text.

So-called naked facts or raw data have always been couched in personal theories, on the basis of which the observer illuminates the individual fact and assigns it a meaning. This on-going process of attribution makes the talk about registering simple facts appear just as dubious as the related teaching of mere sensations, which William James termed the classic example of the psychologist's fallacy. Yet there are hard facts, as we inevitably discover when we believe we are able to disregard laws of nature. The pain we sense after a fall, which is in accordance with the law of falling bodies (i. e., gravity) but not with the magical belief in being invulnerable, may serve as an example that can be recognized as easily being in agreement with Freud's reality principle. In this example it is very obvious that belief was attributed a power that foundered on the reality principle. The analyst's recognition of both the metaphoric and the literal meaning and of the tension between them makes it possible for him to grasp the deeper levels of the transcribed texts. Of course, the wise Biblical saying "Seek, and ye shall find" also applies here. As an aid we supplement the dialogue with commentaries and further considerations.

The detailed study of verbatim protocols opens new approaches in training at all levels (Thomä and Rosenkötter 1970). On the basis of such protocols supervisions can be very productively organized, especially with regard to technical procedure and developing alternative modes of understanding. For this reason we dedicate an entire section to this topic (Sect. 10.1).

The issue is not to make the tape recording of treatments a routine measure. We are of the opinion that tape recording is linked to certain learning experiences that are difficult to acquire in other ways. The most important one, for us, is that the treating analyst can acquire a realistic picture of his concrete therapeutic procedure; this is only possible to a limited degree in retrospective protocols, for psychological reasons associated with our memory. This limitation has a systematic character since regular omissions creep into such protocols, as we know since the instructive studies by Covner (1942) and Rogers (1942). In the form of supervision common today, the supervisor attempts to discover the candidate's blind spots although these are customarily well hidden as a result of unconscious motives. The frequently observed procedure of participants at seminars of reading the prepared report against the grain, i. e., of searching for alternative interpretations, speaks for the widespread nature of this attitude.

Once the analyst has exposed himself to the confrontation with the tape recorder and has overcome his many inevitable hurt feelings, which regularly occur when he compares his ideals with the reality of his actions, then he can dedicate his entire and undivided attention to the patient in the session. He is not distracted by thoughts of whether and what he should note after the session or of which key words he should note during the session. The analyst's subjective experience is relieved of the responsibility of having to fulfill a scientific function in addition to the therapeutic one. One independent task is, however, reserved for the analyst's free retrospective consideration of the psychoanalytic session, called the inner monologue by Heimann (1969); it obviously cannot be recorded at all. The manner in which analysts look back at their own experiences and ideas constitutes a field of its own in which free reports have an indispensible function; we have studied this question for many years together with A.E. Meyer (Meyer 1981, 1988; Kächele 1985).

In retrospect we can say that the introduction of tape recordings into psychoanalytic treatment was linked with the beginning of a critical reappraisal of therapeutic processes from a perspective directly adjacent to the phenomena themselves. This simple technical tool was and is still today an object of controversy among psychoanalysts; those analysts, however, who are active in research agree that such recordings have become an important instrument in research (e.g., Gill et al. 1968; Gill and Hoffman 1982; Luborsky and Spence 1978). Criticism of research methodology from within the ranks of psychoanalysis began in the 1950s and was initially not taken very seriously (Kubie 1952). Glover (1952) complained, for example, about the lack of sufficient control on the collection of data. Shakow (1960) referred to the view, derived from Freud's assertion of an inseparable bond, that every analyst is per se a researcher as a "naive misunderstanding of the research process." This inseparable bond has in fact only been made possible by the introduction of tape recordings and to the extent that the treating analyst, i. e., his personal theories and their application in therapy, can now be made an object of scientific study. The substantial participation of independent third parties is an essential aspect of such studies to test analysts' hypotheses. Thus Stoller questioned the claim that the psychoanalytic method is scientific as long as one essential element is missing that can be found in other disciplines acknowledged to be sciences:

> To the extent that our data are accessible to no one else, our conclusions are not subject to confirmation. This does not mean that analysts cannot make discoveries, for scientific method is only one way to do that. But it does mean that the process of confirmation in analysis is ramshackle... ..I worry that we cannot be taken seriously if we do not reveal ourselves more clearly. (Stoller 1979, p. xvi)

We think that Stoller's skepticism is unfounded today because the tape recording of sessions provides reliable data about verbal exchange. Insofar we agree with Colby and Stoller (1988, p. 42) that the transcript "is not a record of what happened" but "only of what was recorded." The verbal data can easily be supplemented by additional studies about, for instance, the analyst's countertransference (see our studies referred to above).

Since psychoanalysis quite rightly insists that the clinical situation is its home ground for acquiring clinical data to test theories, it is necessary to arrive at an improved method of observation that does not exclude the analyst as a participant observer but provides him the tools for verifying his "observations." Gill et al. (1968) recommended separating the functions of the clinician and the researcher and introducing additional procedures for systematic observation.

Freud's (1912e, p. 113) own impressive ability to record examples "from memory in the evening after work is over" did not protect him from being selective and forgetful and does not supply sufficient justification for any psychoanalyst to make notes for scientific purposes from memory only. We need to employ some form of externally recording data as a means to support our memories, regardless of how good our unconscious memory is. Gill et al. (1968) have pointed out that the ability to remember is developed to very different degrees. It is probably impossible to "calibrate" our ability to remember in a way which would comply with the standardization of a mechanical recording method. Psychoanalytic training, and especially the training analysis, promotes the apperception and selection characteristic of a specific school more than it does a balanced and critical attitude.

Following the lead of cognitive psychology, models have recently been put forward that demonstrate the complexity of an analyst's patient-specific memory configurations; Peterfreund (1983) has called them working models (see also Moser et al. 1981; Teller and Dahl 1986; Pfeifer and Leuzinger-Bohleber 1986; Meyer 1988). The approaches described in this book suggest that we expect to encounter great variability in the personality-dependent processes of image formation, storage, and retrieval (Jacob 1981).

The method of listening that Freud recommended can facilitate the perception of unconscious processes. There have also been experimental studies that emphasize the heuristic value of nondirected listening (Spence and Lugo 1972). The point of this discussion cannot be to restructure the exclusively subjective protocol, but to acknowledge that it has a limited scope in matters related to research. A clinician working on a specific problem will have to find additional opportunities for observation in order to be able to make any systematic statements. This is exactly the purpose of introducing tape recording into treatment. This technical aid influences - as do many other factors - both the patient and the analyst; the same is true of the presentation of cases by candidates in training and of the consequences that the analyst's life history has on the patient.

We believe that the introduction of research into the psychoanalytic situation is of immediate benefit to the patient because it enables the analyst to draw many stimuli from the scientific issues that are raised. Thus we can return to items we mentioned above to better prepare the reader to study transcripts. We are all used to facts being presented in the light of theories. A transcript creates, in contrast, the impression of being one-dimensional: the analyst's interpretations and the patient's answers do not automatically reflect the latent structures of perception and thinking. Although typical interpretations disclose which school the analyst belongs to, we cannot simply throw his statements into one pot with his theoretical position. In traditional case reports phenomena are united in a psychodynamic structure that satisfies several needs at once. One does not ask, with regard to a good report, whether the items the patient contributed were left in their original form or whether they only fit into the whole after interpretive work was done. To demand that the cognitive process and the consistency of a structure be scrutinized and that the structure be divided into its parts leads us back into the analyst's office, which obviously can only be poorly reflected in a transcript. Yet this is a means to obtain a reasonable approximation of what analysts do in order to satisfy the demands of the day, namely that the clinical practice of psychoanalysis be studied. Insofar the tape recording provides an "independent observer" (Meissner 1989, p. 207). Such an observer is a prerequisite for examining Sandler's thesis that psychoanalysis is what psychoanalysts do.

Before we conclude this chapter we still have to mention several simple facts. It is rather arduous to read a transcript of a session of treatment that has not been edited. We believe that the resulting loss of linguistic accuracy is made up for by the didactic benefit. Texts have to be in a certain linguistic form in order to entice clinically oriented readers to participate in the processes that are described.

In written form it is only possible to approximate complex relational processes. Our previous line of argument indicates which form of protocols we will primarily rely on. We will also refer to notes and protocols made by analysts. In accordance with our basic idea we will, as a rule, dispense with extensive biographical introductions to the episodes of treatment. We want to demonstrate that it is possible to comment on the fundamental principles of therapeutic activity without providing a detailed introduction describing the patient's biography. Both theoretical considerations and therapeutic experience document that, at least in the sphere of symptoms, structures of meaning that play a causal role remain constant through time. Clichees are sustained that are the basis for repetition compulsion. It is not always necessary to resort to detailed descriptions of preceding biographical events in order to be able to understand processes in the here and now.

2 Transference and Relationship

Introduction

The headings of the sections in this chapter do not correspond exactly to those in the second chapter of Vol.1, which is a systematic historical treatise on the all-encompassing themes of transference and relationship. As important as it is to illustrate concepts by referring to precise examples, it is just as important not to lose sight of the fact that concepts do not lead lives of their own but rather place emphasis on significant connections in chains of events. It therefore seems logical to consider several examples of transference from the perspective of resistance (see Chap.4).

In this introduction we will restrict ourselves to a few words about major issues. The initial task in analysis is to create a "helping alliance" (Luborsky 1984); once this has been achieved, the psychoanalytic process is characterized by the interplay between transference and the working alliance (Sect. 2.1). The analyst's contribution toward creating favorable conditions for change is a special object of our interest. It seems obvious that we should choose examples from the initial phase of therapy as it is in this phase that the patient attempts to come to terms with the strange and unsettling situation. The patient's hopes that analysis will help him become better able to cope with the problems in his life are nourished by the experiences he has in the analytic situation.

The interplay of working alliance and transference is described in more detail in Sect. 2.2, and the patient's identification with the psychoanalyst and his functions is illustrated by a detailed example in Sect. 2.4.

The feature specific to the psychoanalytic theory of transference is the revival of past experiences in transference (Sect. 2.3). To live up to its name, the point of this theory must be to find out which earlier, internalized relationship is revived and transferred to the analyst. We therefore speak of father, mother, and sibling transference and mean the actualization of the conflicts and/or unsatisfied wishes and needs that are associated with the prototypical images of these persons and that have become a "cliché" in the sense that Freud used the term.

It would be possible to achieve a slightly different focus by correlating the particular contents of the transference to typical forms of anxiety; the context of the momentary genesis of the latter would of course have to be taken into consideration. In order to be able to comprehend a patient's anxieties both in and outside of transference it is necessary to be familiar with the psychoanalytic theory of anxiety, which we outline in Sect. 9.1.

Examples of the connection between present and past in therapeutic technique are distributed throughout the entire book since movement back and forth along the temporal axis forms the basis of all transference interpretations. For a theoretical introduction we recommend reading Sect. 8.4 in Vol.1, and believe that our examples can help steer the ongoing controversy about transference interpretations that refer to the present and those that refer to the past into more productive directions. The question of how *retrospective* ("then and there") transference interpretations and transference interpretations referring to its *actual* genesis ("here and now") can be combined or supplement one another in order to be therapeutically effective in an individual case is obviously an empirical matter. We introduce this distinction in order to have descriptive adjectives at our disposal, yet it also emphasizes the link between present and past, which led via the observation of repetition to the psychoanalytic theory of transference. The two adjectives "retrospective" and "actual" are not usually employed in the psychoanalytic literature, and it is therefore appropriate that we justify introducting them. Transference interpretations directed to the here and now have required that the analyst provide a circumstantial description indicating that he is hinting at a connection to himself or to the psychoanalytic situation or that he is starting from the manifest level. Actual genesis does not specify the depth to which present experiences are anchored in the past. One consequence of this is that interpretations of the actual development cannot simply be patterned after the stereotype that probably goes back to Groddeck (1977) and is associated with the sentence, "You now mean me" (see Ferenczi 1926, p. 109). We discuss this topic in detail in the introduction to Chap.4.

What we refer to as retrospective transference interpretations are familiar to the reader unter the designation "genetic interpretations." What justification is there for the new term if we adhere to Occam's old dictum, *Entia non sunt multiplicanda praeter necessitatem*? Although we hesitate to further increase the number of psychoanalytic concepts, it is nonetheless useful to introduce the term "*retrospective* transference interpretation"; it is only slightly burdened theoretically, whereas genetic transference interpretations imply the reconstruction of the psychogenesis and claim to be able to explain present behavior and experience with reference to their causes. To look back to predecessors is far less ambitious than to trace certain transferences back to causes in childhood. Retrospective transference interpretations take the principle of retrodictive attribution (*Nachträglichkeit*) seriously (see Sect. 3.3; Thomä and Cheshire 1991).

Hardly any topic stirs feelings to the degree that the debate over the different transference interpretations does. Although this controversy also has to do with therapeutic effectiveness, the bitter polemics seem, as far as they are not motivated by professional politics, to result from differences regarding the psychoanalytic method (Fisher 1987). Gill's (1984) social conception of transference has, if we disregard a few exaggerations that he himself has conceded, the following implications. We must proceed from the fact that influencing is an element of every human interaction. Transference interpretations are, accordingly, two-sided; they act within the sphere of (mutual) influence and take it to a *new* level.

In order to enable the analyst to interpret transference - regardless of the specific contents and forms and regardless of which type of interpretation is preferred - within the helping alliance, it is essential that he not transgress certain limits placed on interaction. This salamonic view taken by Gill (1984) is approved by all sides because the psychoanalytic method obviously requires a framework. We refer the reader to our discussion of the function of rules in Chap.7 of Vol.1.

The reader has the opportunity to retrace, and in a certain sense even to reexamine, our protocols and transcripts of treatment from the perspective of transference interpretation. He will surely find numerous weaknesses that the analyst is responsible for or that we have overlooked. In today's psycho boom there are more than enough repulsive examples of such transgressions that make therapeutically effective interpretations of transference impossible and that should be considered as malpractice. We do not want to contribute anything to them.

Yet where are the differences - which usually escape notice - in the controversy over actual genetic and retrospective transference interpretations, and which Sandler and Sandler (1984), as helpers in a time of emergency, believed they could resolve by introducing the new concept "present unconscious"? According to this concept, transference interpretations emphasizing actual genesis would be directed toward the present unconscious, and the familiar, traditional division into different layers of the unconscious would be extended by a conceptual innovation. Disregarding a few rather terminological finesses, the actual differences between the preconscious and the present unconscious are minor. Gill's passionate argument in favor of transference interpretations of actual genesis is in fact primarily directed at the patient's preconscious perceptions, and he recommends proceeding from their plausibility:

> It is not merely that both patient and analyst contribute to the *relationship* but that both contribute to the *transference*. Furthermore, the social conception of transference is based on a relativistic view of interpersonal reality in contrast to the usual absolutistic one. Transference is not only always contributed to by both participants, but each participant also has a valid, albeit different, perspective on it. Hoffman and I have argued for the rejection of the usual psychoanalytic view that one can dichotomize interpersonal experience in general, and experience in the analytic situation in particular, into veridical and distorted. We see interpersonal experience, instead, as always having a degree of plausibility. (Gill 1984, p. 499)

This rigorous social conception of transference, also pleaded by Stolorow and Lachmann (1984/85), demands that the analyst reflect on his theories of reality and relativize them with regard to the patient. The emphasis put on plausibility is directed against the *dichotomy* of real or realistic experience on the one hand and distorted experience (as the traditional definition of transference) on the other. As a consequence the alleged distortion, i.e., the deviation from a realistic perception of reality, cannot be precisely defined either. Such distortions of perception therefore cover a wide spectrum. The consequences of this point of view for our understanding of transference interpretations are very far-reaching. It is up to the *two participants* to deal with the "cues: the perceptual edge of the transference" (Smith 1990). The task is easy if a patient himself classifies a perception, experience, or manner of behavior as fairly abnormal and the analyst agrees, so that each can start the study with his own tasks, in order to achieve the goal of change desired by the patient. Therapeutically the point is obviously not to conduct an abstract discussion about where the borders of normality are, and also not to continuously discuss differences of opinion in order to overcome them. We simply want to emphasize that it is up to the two participants, the patient and the analyst, to clarify where reality might be distorted in the psychoanalytic situation. Furthermore, the patient and the analyst do not live alone in a world of their own but in a multilayered sociocultural reality in which some average values apply although they lack normative force for the individual's private life. The patient's and analyst's intersubjective determination of a continuum is thus interconnected with the opinions they share with their respective environments.

Associated with the social point of view is the recognition that the analyst exerts a very strong personal influence on the patient, a fact which was also emphasized by Freud when he, while discussing the technique of suggestion, referred to the word's literal meaning. Yet Freud also undertook the vain attempt to use the set of psychoanalytic rules to obtain uncontaminated data. His understanding of the resolution of transference was to attempt to undermine the suggestive force of powerful figures in childhood and their revival in analysis. This orientation toward the *past* has contributed to our neglecting the large influence the analyst has on the present and the actual genesis of all psychic manifestations, including symptoms. The solution of the clinical and scientific problems of psychoanalysis requires first of all that we proceed from the fact that the analyst's influence poses an inevitable contamination of the observed phenomena. This means that it is necessary for all psychoanalytic data to be examined with regard to the analyst's contribution (Meissner 1989; Colby and Stoller 1989).

2.1 Therapeutic Alliance and Transference Neurosis

2.1.1 Promoting the Helping Alliance

In the introductory phase the analyst can make a substantial contribution toward helping the patient quickly come to terms with the unfamiliar situation. Creating hopes at the very beginning and being helpful in developing unused abilities are not the same as promoting dependence and illusions by means of crude suggestion. The growth of the therapeutic alliance and the development of transference can strengthen each other. If the "helping alliance" (Luborsky 1984) is fostered, both the "working alliance" (Greenson 1967) and transference thrive. It is then possible at an early stage to show the patient the neurotic conditions of his behavior and experiencing and, above all, the capacity for change that remains despite all limitations.

In the initial interviews Erna X told me that she suffered from numerous neurotic symptoms and, since childhood, from neurodermatitis. I was recommended to her by friends of hers. She had informed herself about her illness by reading books. Judging from the external and internal conditions it was possible to proceed directly from the interviews to therapy. I formulated the basic rule in accordance with the recommendation made in Vol.1: "Please try to say everything that is on your mind or that you think and feel; it makes the therapy easier."

Erna X began by describing a conflict that had existed for a long time and that she had already mentioned in the initial interviews, namely her indecisive attitude toward a fourth pregnancy. On the one hand, she very much wanted another child, on the other there were numerous objections. In the period since the initial interview she had had a routine examination, and she had seen the wrinkles on her gynecologist's forehead as she had mentioned her desire to have a fourth child. She mentioned her mixed feelings. In response to his question of how she would decide emotionally, she had said her emotions said definitely yes, but her intellect said no.

A: I have the impression that you're torn back and forth. You want to leave it up to chance in order to avoid having to make a decision.

Commentary. This statement implies the tendency of not leaving the decision to chance.

P: At the present I'm entirely prepared for a fourth child. When I go window shopping, it makes me happy to think about being able to buy things for a new baby. But with four children I would have to stop working. Physically I wouldn't be able to take it any more.

Erna X described something similar regarding an allergy test. It had taken her entire courage to interrupt the examination after she had had to wait for hours and hours. She complained about the doctors' lack of willingness to provide information. The examination was supposed to have been repeated three more times, but she couldn't sacrifice a whole afternoon each time. The patient was pleased by her courage: "Courage turned into anger. Being angry, I was able to be courageous."

The patient spoke about her punctuality and about her bad conscience at leaving her children alone. A central theme was that the patient got into situations in which she was in a hurry and that with increasing stress her skin symptoms were joined by situative increases in her blood pressure.

I created an analogy to the session: she was feeling increasingly stressed because of the appointment. The patient emphasized the difference: she expected something from therapy, but nothing from the test.

Erna X talked about her extreme anxiety about blushing: "I often turn dark red, down to the roots of my hair." I made the more precise statement that she apparently suffered from shame anxiety. The patient confirmed that she knew it. She said she was ashamed of everything that had to do with sexuality: "I turn red as soon as I think of my anxiety."

The patient's anxiety about her insecurity triggered her symptoms and led in a typical way to its secondary reinforcement. I made the interpretation that all the feelings were lacking that had originally motivated her blushing and anxiety, and said that it was therefore important to determine which themes underlay her shame anxiety.

Erna X then said that the subject of sexuality had not been talked about at home; sex had never been explained to her. She was uncertain whether she was supposed to laugh or not when a joke was told. She described a shameful situation in which she had been sitting in front of the apprentices at work and turned dark red. She had got mad at herself, exclaiming "Am I stupid!" Her anxiety about blushing was especially strong at work. I returned to the fact that she would be at home more if she had a fourth child and that there would be less of a burden on her.

During her pregnancies she had felt well. Even her skin had been very good after the first one, and she had only taken a little cortisone. She compared her youth to today's 15- to 16-year-old girls who are carefree, and said "Were we dumb!" I described her condition with regard to her other problems: always having to run around with a bad conscience was creating increasing restrictions. The patient noted that for years she had prayed that her parents would not find out anything about her tricks. What other people thought played a decisive role at home. At the moment her mother's biggest worry was that somebody could find out that she was going to a analyst.

It seemed natural to interpret her own worries as an internalization of her mother's values and to make an indirect attempt to support her independence. The question was raised of how far the patient kept her own views to herself in order to please her mother. In contrast to her mother she had a positive attitude toward therapy, which she said had already helped: "I like to lie down. On the way here I thought, 'Am I happy when I can relax.'" She said she was not able to organize her time any better. I asked her about her work schedule, and she described how she put pressure on herself by believing that she always had to do more and more. We talked about her difficulty to adjust and to change a plan, i. e., the compulsiveness of her planning. Her reaction was: "Then everything will fall to pieces and my skin problem will come back right away."

We then considered the real possibilities of her finding household help. Erna X had already looked around. She had a bad conscience toward her children. Now she had to get through a few more weeks, and she wondered whether her neighbor might not be able to help her out. The question of paying the neighbor came up, and in this context we spoke about her family's finances. She had numerous differences of opinion with her husband, and his criticism made her feel very insecure.

It became apparent that she took criticism very seriously. In the course of her marriage Erna X had become even more insecure and self-critical. The fact that her husband considered this entire situation *her* problem annoyed her, and she was happy that she could talk about it here. It was obvious that Erna X was looking for support against her husband's arguments.

I broke a longer period of silence by asking if she was irritated by the silence? Was she waiting for something to happen? She said that she was being considerate and just waiting before continuing although her thoughts had already gone further.

I now made it clear that I would say something on my own if I thought I could contribute something in a given moment. I encouraged the patient to freely say everything that came to her. I then raised the question of whether she had the impression in other aspects of life that she talked too much and did not let the others get a word in. In private conversations, she said, she was rather restrained, an allusion to the distinction between "in here" and "out there," i. e., between the analytic situation and life in general.

Whenever she was waiting for her husband she would think about everything that had happened during the day. Yet if he called to say that he would be late, then everything was over, and when he came on time, he usually did not want to talk. Sometimes she said something anyway, but did not get through to him. It was very unusual for a conversation to be satisfactory if one did develop. She would sometimes call a girl friend to pour out her heart. She was surprised that she so successfully managed to speak freely in the analysis.

The difference between in here and out there was discussed further. I noted that in life we sometimes get answers or that sometimes questions are raised, whereas in analysis I would sometimes not pick up a theme. We considered whether the patient might be disappointed if I did not and remained silent instead.

We went on to discuss the sense in which the fundamental rule provided support. Following it, some aspects of our dialogue would seem unusual and might therefore make her feel insecure, because they are not customary. I emphasized that it was not my intention to make her feel insecure but that this could be an unintentional side effect. This made it clearer to Erna X that she could continue if a pause occurred.

She got caught up on the word "insecurity" and remarked that she continued our talks by herself after the hour was over. For example, after the last session she continued thinking about the subject of adjustment. Because of her insecurity and although she knew better, she would call her husband when she had difficulty making a decision.

P: I shy away from making decisions on my own about very banal matters. It's another aspect of my exaggerated adjustment to my mother.

A: Is this part of the idea that the good Lord knows everything anyway?

P: Yes, I was always possessed by the thought that my mother would hear about it after all, that she would find out sooner or later, and naturally that is how it often turned out. In fact, it often turned out that she was right.

Her husband criticized her because she always turned to her mother. Yet he was frequently not available, and this was *her* criticism of *him*. Erna X emphasized her tendency to follow her mother, with very few exceptions.

Her son Jacob learned bad expressions at kindergarten, and her mother was horrified when she heard them. Erna X said that she would have been spanked if she had done something similar. She defended her children against her mother's moralistic manner. The patient was able, via her identification with her children, to express her right to independence.

Commentary. This early sesson was chosen for prescriptive reasons, because we believe that it displays an exemplary mixture of the different elements constituting the structure of a helping alliance.

2.1.2 Support and Interpretation

In the following example we want to show that interpretations per se can have a supportive effect. The supportive aspect of the psychoanalytic technique is especially strong when interpretations are given in a manner that wakens the patient's hopes of being able to master his difficulties. The establishment of a helping alliance by means of an analysis of transference takes place in the context of interpretations. Particularly in the initial phase, the goal is to create a basis of trust. Although it is necessary to distinguish between the various therapeutic elements and their distribution or mixture in different types of technique (e.g., psychoanalysis, expressive or supportive psychotherapy; Wallerstein 1986), we emphasize here the supportive aspects of psychoanalytic interpretations in their own right.

Daniel Y had suffered for years from numerous neurotic anxieties and hypochondriac fears. He was particularly tormented by his fear of becoming insane. For several reasons it was very difficult for him to decide to undergo therapy. He had also obtained information about behavior therapy. Yet since he not only suffered from his symptoms, but also felt cut off from his life history and was unable to remember hardly anything prior to puberty, he believed that he required psychoanalytic help. Daniel Y's suffering from his anxiety attacks and from the feeling of being separated from his personal roots was so severe that he put aside all his reservations against psychoanalysis.

He was very surprised at the course the treatment had taken. He had neither encountered a silent psychoanalyst nor suffered a worsening of his symptoms, something he had feared the most. He had heard and even observed among his own friends that negative fluctuations initially occur in psychoanalyses and that it was only after having passed through many transitional phases and after resolving conflicts that an improvement might occasionally occur. That I did not leave it to Daniel Y to hold monologues, but made comments that offered him support was in positive contrast to his expectations. In doing this I followed the therapeutic principle of creating the best possible conditions for *mastering* earlier traumas that had been passively incurred. This therapeutic approach made it easier for the patient to verbalize for the first time his dispairing helplessness with regard to overpowering impressions made on him in the present and past and to do something about it. Both the patient and I myself were touched by the intensity of his affects, particularly his crying. My unswerving calmness helped him keep his feeling of shame about his childhood experiences, which were in such complete contrast to his successful carreer, in limits.

Overall a good balance between regressive immersion into affective experience and reflective dialogue had developed in therapy.

Daniel Y's panic attacks, which occurred especially in small rooms, had turned his frequent and routine business trips into a torture, regardless of whether they were by car, train, or airplane. He was surprised that he felt considerably better after only a few weeks and had already been able to manage several long trips by car without any anxiety. I saw one reason for this improvement in the fact that the patient had acquired some confidence and consequently hope. In this sense the improvement could be considered a transference cure in the wider sense of the word. Another reason was that the patient had already been frequently able to experience that, although his helplessness and powerlessness recurred, he was by no means passive and helpless toward all the strain he experienced, and that he in fact was able to actively confront his old, conserved traumas and whatever triggered them in the present. Thus the improvement could also be attributed to the analysis of conflicts.

There had been no reason for me to make the patient aware of my assumptions about these two aspects of therapy. Then Daniel Y had to go on a week-long overseas trip that made him feel apprehensive since he had not flown in the last few years without experiencing a panic attack. In view of the planned flight I decided to make an explanatory comment, which I expected to have a settling effect. I reminded the patient that he had already successfully gone on numerous trips by car and train because he no longer felt at the mercy of things beyond his control and had obviously regained his capacity to assert himself. My intention was to make the patient aware of this enlarged sphere of action and to reinforce his own self-confidence. The patient was moved by my statement. We were hardly able to talk any more because of his sudden and intense outburst of crying. In view of the experience that it is rather unfavorable to conclude a session leaving a strong affect undiscussed, I was not entirely happy when he left. Yet I also had the impression that Daniel Y had gained self-assurance and could therefore handle his emotions.

Daniel Y came back in the best of moods. He had not, against all his expectations, experienced any anxiety during either of the flights. Since he was familiar with psychoanalytic rules from hearsay, he had in the meantime wondered whether my support was permissable. At the same time the patient was amazed that I had undertaken such a venture and taken the risk of making a kind of prediction. He wondered, furthermore, whether his confidence in my ability would not have suffered seriously if he had had a relapse. I now tried to explain to the patient that I had taken a calculated risk and thus had not acted arbitrarily or made a chance suggestion. Daniel Y had in fact forgotten that I had grounded my assumption that he *might* be able to travel free of anxiety in a reference to his increased self-assurance.

This patient, who was a successful scientist, became increasingly interested in learning more about the curative factors. In a later session we had an exchange of thoughts that again ended in a violent affective outburst, which I will now describe.

Daniel Y was disturbed that he was not able, despite his intelligence, to grasp the reasons for the extent he had become free of anxiety. It was an obvious wish of his to learn something about the conditions of his improvement. It was his approach, as he practiced in his profession, to gain assurance – or correct mistakes – by learning the causes of something. The patient seemed relieved that I considered his curiosity about which factors are of consequence therapeutically as something natural and that I said it was his good right to know. He had expected me to skip over the implicit question or simply reject it. He suddenly became very aroused and anxious. I was now able to explain to him the momentary manifestation of anxiety. He had wanted to know more from me but had been afraid to come any closer. He was very ambivalent, hoping that I was not groping in the dark, but also envying me because of my knowledge and the calm manner in which I took his comment about being afraid that I was perhaps really just stumbling around in the dark.

The inequality between us and the fact that I knew so much about him reminded him of his childhood feelings of powerlessness and being excluded. Daniel Y was encouraged by the fact that I made a few comments about the genesis of his anxiety and did not belittle the intensity of his feelings. Suddenly the patient was overcome by an outburst of hate against an "uncle," who had taken his father's place and whom, at his mother's behest, he had had to obey. He was severely shaken by the intensity of his hate and the anxiety associated with it, and convinced by my references to the connections to his experiencing during the session. From his restrained criticism of me and my reaction to it, the patient thus gained sufficient self-assurance to be able to deal with his strong affects.

The oedipal source of tension had now become so immediate that the conditions were favorable for attempting to revise it. It is noteworthy that although at that time he had won against his "uncle" – his other's lover after her divorce – he nonetheless had retained a deep feeling of inability, even of having a physical defect and hypochondriac anxieties that centered on his heart. Somewhat later he was able to overcome his shame and say that until the late assertion of his sexuality he had felt very depressed about never having ejaculated during masturbation. His anxiety about his pleasurable oedipal aggressions had resulted in inhibition and a functional disturbance that accompanied it. This, in turn, had strengthened his feeling of inferiority despite all his successes in professional matters.

2.1.3 Common Ground and Independence

Gill and Hoffman's (1982) systematic studies have made us aware of the significance of actual cues in transference. Their suggestion is that we should proceed from the plausibility of the patient's perceptions. It often suffices to acknowledge that an observation regarding the analyst or his office is plausible. Frequently, however, a further-reaching explanation is required which cannot be related only to the patient's fantasies. We have dealt with the general problems of treatment technique in this regard in Sects. 2.7 and 8.4 in Vol.1. The following example illustrates the corresponding steps in technique.

We refer to an exchange of thoughts in the 61st and 62nd sessions in the analysis of Arthur Y and occasionally quote from it, in order to show what it means to acknowledge actual truths in the here and now. The metaphors used by the patient are especially well suited to characterize his mood.

The two sessions preceded a longer vacation break. The topic was the patient's curiosity; in my interpretations I had indirectly encouraged him to be more curious. My encouragement led the patient to remember having suppressed his curiosity toward me on an earlier occasion. "At the time I didn't dare ask, and even today it's not easy for me," and the patient immediately said what the reason was, "I wouldn't have received an answer from my previous therapist, just the counterquestion, 'Yes, why does it interest you?' And after you have been asked such counterquestions often enough, you don't feel like asking any more."

Arthur Y was interested in knowing where I was spending my vacation. On an earlier occasion I had given him my address.

Arthur Y talked about a large and well-known ski run, which I am also familiar with. He did not restrict his curiosity and risked asking the question he had previously avoided. Decisive was that I gave him an evasive answer, leaving open whether I had already gone down this ski run. I only made a general, noncommittal statement, "Everybody in Ulm knows this part of the Alps, those mountains in Allgäu."

It was not until the next session that the consequences of my refusal became clear and, what is more important, could be corrected. At first Arthur Y had seemed to be entirely satisfied with my answer, but his momentary subliminal frustration was reflected in the examples he mentioned from his previous therapies. He recalled an important metaphor: the image of a snail that puts out its feelers; you only have to touch the feelers and it withdraws into her shell. "I acted in just the same way with them [the other therapists]." And then he recalled, at the opposite extreme to the snail, a large dog showing its teeth. "You don't go around touching him, otherwise he might bite your finger off."

It seemed obvious that the patient was describing himself as the snail and the analyst as the vicious dog that should not be provoked by asking questions. The patient corrected this assumption in the next session. In the first third of it a good atmosphere was created because I was able to calm him; he had anxieties because of the issue of discretion - information passed on to the insurance company etc. The patient now had sufficient assurance to again return to specific points. In connection with the dog, he complained, "If I had only once been the dog and barked . . . ." I mentioned the consideration that, according to this comment, he was not bitten, but bites. He admitted that my opinion was not entirely wrong. After disarming the criticism in this way and putting me in a friendly mood, so to speak, he remembered the rejection he experienced from my evasive generalization regarding the ski run. He experienced my evasiveness, as he said, as a red light - "Better not ask any further" - whereupon I made an allusion to finger, bite, the object's rage, and retreat (the snail). The patient made it clear that for him such an inner retreat was a defeat that provoked revengeful feelings.

I confirmed that I had been evasive and that this had altered the relationship between the snail and dog at the expense of intense curiosity. My interpretation was, "It's true that I was evasive. I did not say that I know the ski run, but generalized. Perhaps you experienced this as a strong rejection because you were not only curious, but because intrusiveness is linked to curiosity - the vicious dog." Thus, I did not say, "You were afraid of hurting me then," as if he had only imagined this anxiety and I had not been irritated. I instead ackowledged the *plausibility* of his perceptions. Such acknowledgment probably leads to a corrective emotional experience by letting patients test in the next few steps they take whether they remain welcome with their recently acquired new patterns of thought and action.

I later - after explicitly answering his direct question about the ski run - commented that it can sometimes make sense not to answer a question immediately. Responding to my explanation, the patient summarized, "Yes, if you answer questions immediately, the thought process may stop prematurely." The patient thus confirmed that it sometimes makes sense to leave questions open in order not to terminate the thought process.

Upon closer examination of his choice of words, it turned out that he attributed the analyst a cunning form of behavior that he knew from himself and that he sometimes employed to reach goals or just to make ends meet, according to the saying that the end justifies the means.

The patient's curiosity had now become more intense, after we had previously used associations to establish multifacited connections to words such as "drill" and "penetrate." The patient remembered, "People say, 'He's drilling me with questions.'" We talked about the upcoming vacation break. Arthur Y knew that it would not be easy to reach me, which provoked him into being *penetratingly curious*. We reached a compromise that did justice to the different aspects of the technical problem. On the one hand I did not say where I would be staying, and on the other I assured him that in an emergency he could reach me through my office.

In view of the vacation break, it was important to me at the end of the session to emphasize the things we had in common. Since we were familiar with the same region, I used metaphors such as that we are already on good footing.

The acknowledgment of actual truths acquires special significance in situations where the helping relationship is put to a special test, for example by an interruption for a vacation. The analyst should handle questions in a manner that provides the patient both satisfactory answers and the assurance he requires for the period of the separation. Our stance can generally be characterized by the phrase, "As much common ground as necessary, as much independence as possible."

The course of the sessions discussed here makes it clear that the therapeutic process can facilitate the correction of the side effects of analytic interventions, since, obviously, in addition to favorable effects, interventions can have unintended negative side effects that may not be immediately visible.

2.2 Positive and Negative Transference

The spectrum of positive transference is very wide, ranging from mild forms of sympathy and esteem to ardent love. One speaks of erotized transference if it reaches such a degree that it constitutes a lasting obstacle to the working alliance. Transference love often turns into hate. Negative aggressive transference can therefore often be understood as the consequence of an experience of being rejected. The following examples illustrate this spectrum.

2.2.1 Mild Positive Transference

The patient Erna X came to talk about Tilmann Moser's autobiographical account *Lehrjahre auf der Couch* (My Apprenticeship on the Couch), in which he described his strong and aggressive attacks on his analyst (see also Chap.7). She had previously thought it inconceivable that she could become so infuriated. In the meantime she had become skeptical about the absence of negative affects in view of an approaching interruption in treatment, which she was disappointed at.

P: Well, I was unhappy that you didn't tell me where you're going on vacation. But I said to myself that I didn't have a right to know and that you certainly knew what you should tell me or not.

I assumed that the patient suspected that an answer was being withheld from her in order to make her mad. It would then have been consistent for her not to let herself be provoked or manipulated any more. I pointed out that this might be the first sign of a struggle for power or that one might be implied by this topic. I denied having any manipulative intent in not telling her something.

Erna X emphasized that she had not imagined that I wanted to make her angry. She thought that I wanted to do something to make her think, which I confirmed.

The patient added more to this theme and in the dialogue extended and deepened it. At first Erna X was concerned with my 3-week absence. Her ambivalence was connected with two opposing chains of motivation. On the one hand she expected a rigorous professional sense of duty and selfless effort. On the other hand she was looking for a role model in order to transform her life with her husband. In her opinion it was probably fairly hopeless to expect her husband to delegate some of his business obligations and to show more interest in family life and vacation. If I were really to go on vacation for 3 weeks, I would correspond to her ideal. As much as she herself wanted this lifestyle, she was just as afraid that further complications might result from the discrepancy between this ideal and her reality. This was probably the reason that she held tight to the idea that I was not going on vacation.

After some silence the patient related a dream about me.

P: In the second dream I was lying with you on a couch, not here, but in another room. The couch was much larger. I can't remember any details, just a feeling, namely the feeling of security. There was also a feeling of pride and amazement that you allowed it, that you allowed me this intimate closeness, that you didn't run away or shove me away. A telephone call disrupted us. Now it was a room like your office after all. It was a call from a woman, who said that you should pick up your car at the garage. I wanted to know which woman had called. You didn't answer. I thought it was your mother or another woman. Then we went through town together.

It's difficult to describe the feeling that you have in a dream. I was somehow completely at ease with you. When I am here, then I always think that I have to do everything right. In the dream everything was different.

A: Yes, in a dream you can take all the liberties you want.

P: Most of all I would have liked to call you right the next morning. After waking up, I thought about it and was pleased. At first I had the thought, no, I can't tell you that I dreamed we were on the couch together. On the other hand, I didn't dare to not tell you about the dream. Otherwise I like to talk with you about dreams.

A: You were worried because of the intimacy in the dream.

P: Yes, I was embarrassed.

I then referred to natural human desires and emphasized that hers were stimulated by our talks.

A: It's natural for you to include me in your world of dreams and wishes, just as you do other people with whom you discuss personal things.

The patient had had similar thoughts before the session began. I now drew attention to the other woman's intervention.

P: Yes, it was jealousy. Yes, this other woman took you away from me.

I reminded the patient of an earlier dream.

P: Yes, in the dream you cancelled a session. Your car turns up over and over again. Yes, even in the dream you came in the car to visit me. An important factor in my choice of a friend was the fact that he had a big car. That must be the reason that the car plays a special role. We went down the street downtown almost dancing. Why shouldn't I admit to having this desire? But I can't tell my husband this dream.

A: The question is whether you can awaken your husband's understanding for the subject of the dream, namely your desire for more gentleness.

I intentionally used the word "desire," which implies all kinds of erotic feelings, pointing out that therapy wakens more desires and that it would not be simple for her to transform her life and to get her husband's support for doing so. Her husband was involved in his family in a way that was comparable to how she was linked to her parents.

The patient wondered why she had thought of me and not her husband.

A: Probably because you speak with me about it more than with your husband.

I interpreted that the patient was seeking relief via her question.

P: Yes, I could have answered the question myself, but I don't know how things can continue. Yes, I don't want to accept the fact that you meet my wishes in every respect. The feeling of being understood and of security that I had in the dream, I will never have this feeling toward my husband. I have been married long enough that I can predict my husband's reactions. The fact is that I stand there alone and he doesn't help me.

The patient mentioned an example from her everyday activities with her children to show her husband's lack of willingness to help take care of the children.

P: And that's the way it is at home. If I defend myself against my mother and refuse to take on another task, then she gets indignant and complains about my useless and time-consuming therapy.

A few days later the patient's desire for a baby became more intense. Although all reasonable considerations still spoke against it, and although she just recently, at a gynecological consultation, was relieved to hear that she had had only imagined she was pregnant, she still wanted a fourth child. Concerned about the ambivalent nature of her attitude, she tried to clarify her thoughts in the sessions.

In order to make the following interpretation of her desire for a baby more comprehensible to the reader, I must summarize a vivid description the patient gave of children playing, both her own and other boys and girls from the neighborhood. With disbelieving surprise she had noticed the carefree and natural way the 3- to 5-year-olds acted, who made no secret of their pleasure in showing themselves and in touching and looking. In these children's sexual games one of the boys showed his penis, which triggered reactions of penis envy in one girl. This girl held a large crocodile where her penis would be and said it would gobble up the boy, who had already developed a phobia. This girl triumphantly used the crocodile – as a much larger penis – to frighten the boy. It was only with great effort that the patient was able to let the children go on until they, on their own, had satisfied their curiosity and their interests had turned to something else. It would have been more natural for her, like her mother, to intervene and forbid such games, or, like her grandmother, to distract them by telling them about something more beautiful or decent. The patient had drawn conclusions about how her mother probably had acted toward her during her own childhood from the educational measures her mother used toward her children during visits. She was infuriated to observe how her mother made up stories to avoid answering important questions.

Although she knew that having a fourth child would substantially increase the burdens on her and that she would not be able to count on any support from her husband, she was nonetheless filled by a deep feeling of happiness when she thought of the moments of closeness and intimate contact during nursing. Her wish receded completely when she felt understood and when she continued our dialogue by herself after a good hour. Her very busy husband had hardly any time for her, and their sexual relations were unsatisfactory and so infrequent that it was improbable that conception would take place.

Erna X was strongly moved and reflected briefly before responding to my interpretation that she wanted another child in order to repeat her own development under more favorable conditions. I interpreted her further associations that she never had the wish for another pregnancy during the sessions as an expression of her satisfaction at feeling understood, and not as a defense against oedipal wishes.

My interpretation, which I intentionally couched in very general terms, that she was seeking her own unlived life in another child fell on fertile ground and precipitated a wealth of ideas. The patient assumed that the function of her desire for another child was to help her avoid restructuring her everyday life at home and work. The restrictions that a fourth child would impose on her would make most of the professional things impossible that she now - freed of some neurotic inhibitions - felt confident enough to attempt. She told me about a dream that was triggered by the children's games and by my previous interpretations. In it she saw a number of photographs of *me* in various shots on the beach of a lake.

Her sexual curiosity had been stimulated in transference. She herself had been in embarrassing situations at a beach. As a girl she had been laughed out because she wore a padded bra in a bathing suit that was much too large. Although she had caught her uncle's eye, he acted as if he was not at all interested in her.

Finally I interpreted her unconscious wish to have a child with me and from me. She said that this made sense to her although she had never consciously had such a wish. Now I referred to a statement by her uncle that he did like to *make* children even though he did not want to have anything to do with them otherwise.

The topics changed over the next few sessions. Other aspects of this focus became visible. Referring to the last session, the patient remarked that it was easy to start today. She could not forget something I had said in the last session: "Today you are not in the same situation as you were then as a child. Today you have something to offer."

P: What do I have to offer? I am not ugly, and I am not dumb. I sometimes think I am too demanding. I'm never satisfied. But then I also asked myself why you told me this toward the end of the last session? Was I lost? Did you want to give me moral support? Tell me what I have to offer.

A: I didn't say it to give you moral support, although that is one aspect. I wanted to refer to the fact that you are no longer as helpless and ashamed as you were as a child. That you don't have any more associations and ask me seems to me less a consequence of your increased demands than a phenomenon accompanying the fact that you are disturbed here by your spontaneity and associations.

P: That is just how I feel, ashamed and helpless and padded. Today I am almost the same as then. But after the last session I was satisfied.

The course of this exchange differed from that on the beach. The patient told me that she was thinking about the meaning of the words "helpless," "ashamed," and "padded." After a long silence, I encouraged her to tell me her thoughts.

P: It's difficult. I sometimes feel terribly helpless. Then my condition is just the opposite. It's the extremes, the middle is missing. Just like after the last session. I left and was exceptionally pleased, but as I got to my car I had the thought, "Just don't imagine anything; it was probably just a move to give you some self-confidence."

A: And therefore not sincere.

P: Yes, sincere, but with the ulterior motive of helping me.

A: What is wrong with this helpful ulterior motive that makes you aware of something? There is an ulterior motive involved, namely that you can use your body. From time immemorial you have thought that you don't have anything. Today you have something that you can show. [The patient suffers from a fear of blushing.]

P: Yes, but it's nothing I have achieved. It's a stage of development. It came all by itself. I didn't earn it, and then it is obviously nothing for me. [Long pause] I wonder why it is so difficult for me to believe that I have something to offer.

A: Because then you would think about something that is forbidden, and that could have specific consequences, for example, that you could be more seductive than you are supposed to be. And that your uncle then would make or have made even more advances.

P: But who tells me how I could be?

I implied that the patient was so much under outside control as a result of her upbringing that she was not able to test her own sphere of action. Everything was clear when her mother decided what was to be done. At the same time she saw in her own children how pleasing it was for them to try to do something when she left them scope for acting on their own.

P: The whole affair refers to something emotional as well as something physical. I'm insecure in both. Yes, it's part of the nature of thinking and feeling that there are always other sides to things. There is security as long as something is completely determined. When there is more openness, then there are also more ulterior motives.

Thus the fact that I had ulterior motives disturbed the patient.

P: I often believe you have ulterior motives because you're thinking about something and have a goal.

I emphasized that while this was true, it was also possible to speak about it. The patient, in contrast, assumed that you cannot speak about it. Erna X emphasized that she actually did not dare asking about it. She admitted that she sometimes liked to be guided, but added that if you did not take the chance to ask, then you risked the danger of being manipulated, something she certainly did not want. It was nice to let yourself be guided, but on the other hand it was disagreeable.

A: But if you can't know about all of this and can't ask, then you can be manipulated. You have been pushed around and influenced a lot. You would like to have something that suits your needs, and it can't be achieved without more reflection or questioning.

P: Because I don't want to be obtrusive and to ask stupid questions, your ulterior motives remain unclear, but I naturally often wonder what your intentions are. This was especially strong in the last session, because I really would like to offer you something and yet am immensely insecure. The word "padded" moved me very deeply. People think of something that I don't have at all, just like in that moment of undressing on the beach. With the uncovering comes the shame, and I turn red, and the helplessness comes. There are exactly three stages, not from helplessness to being ashamed to being padded, but the opposite.

I confirmed that the sequence appeared to be the one the patient described. Material things were agreeable, and money and a nice car were important to the patient. I reminded her that she had had too little to show at that traumatic experience. She had been padded with something artificial.

P: I can see the image of a balloon, and when you poke it, everything is gone. Yes, that's the exact sequence: padded, ashamed, and helpless. That's exactly the situation in which I turn red. Yet behind the padding there is a lot of life.

A: Yes, it was there too. The bra was padded, but behind it there was something. A nipple, a growing breast, your knowledge of growth from the sensations in your own body and from the comparison with other women.

P: But it wasn't enough, and it was too small, and I was dissatisfied. Nobody told me that my breasts would get larger. It's more likely someone would have said, "Well, what do you want at your age. You're still a child." I couldn't talk with anyone about it. I was on my own. True, I did learn some things because my mother forced me to do them. She gave me exact instructions, and it worked. Commands were given. I had to do something and to learn it by heart, such as going to a government office. But it was more my mother's action than my own. I didn't have a choice. I was forced, and it wasn't really me, and that is probably why I don't have the feeling that I got any further. It's between the extremes - "I can't do anything at all, I can do a lot" - that the middle part of my own doing is missing.

I referred once again to the ulterior motives. Which hidden thoughts were guiding her?

A: You suspected that something was being planned again. Something was being manipulated, and it was very serious because you weren't informed. This is the reason that you were shy to ask what I meant. You followed the reasoning, "They are only thinking of my own good. Then I don't have to ask."

P: I was used. I wasn't told, "Please do it. I don't have any time." No, it was arranged; you do it, there's no alternative, and then I felt the ulterior motives without daring to ask anything. It was dishonest. I knew about the dishonesty but wasn't able to talk about it.

Commentary. The encouraging interpretation of the patient's reluctance in transference had a positive influence on the cooperation. Such observations are exceptionally important for evaluating the therapeutic process.

2.2.2 *Strong Positive Transference*

Strong positive transference remains within the framework of the working alliance, in contrast to erotized transference, which temporarily makes it difficult to uphold the psychoanalytic situation (see Sect. 2.2.4). Because of the complications that occur in erotized transference, it would be important to have criteria that would permit predictions to be made while the indications are still being determined in the early phases of treatment and of course to find interpretive means to avoid it. Can we currently specify a group of patients who will fall so in love with their analysts that therapy comes to a stop? Does this group still consist of women who refuse to cooperate in the work of interpretation, and who only desire material satisfaction and are "accessible only to 'the logic of soup, with dumplings for arguments'" (Freud 1915a, p. 167)? Too much has changed since the discovery of transference love for us to attribute this quality to the class of "women of elemental passionateness who tolerate no surrogates . . . who refuse to accept the psychical in place of the material" (Freud 1915a, pp.166–167).

First it must be pointed out that this complication has traditionally manifested itself in the analysis of woman who are being treated by a male analyst, for a whole range of psychological, historical, sociological, and nosological reasons. After all, the largest group of women who initially went to psychoanalysts for treatment suffered from hysteria. Since then the sexual revolution has made women's emancipation possible, and this can be seen not least of all in liberal sexual behavior. This late achievement has not changed anything in the fact that sexual attacks and transgressions are much more frequent between men and girls than between women and boys. The same is true for the ratio of father-daughter incest to mother-son incest. The predominant form of sexual behavior between the sexes continues to be heterosexuality in which the males dominate. The expectation of everything that could happen at the analyst's is motivated by the experiences that female patients have previously had with men, whether fathers, brothers, and other relatives or teachers, supervisors, and doctors, to name a few. Seduction and the willingness to be seduced are two phenomena linked by a complicated relationship of attraction and repulsion. The disquieting feeling that is emitted by the phrase "If that were possible back then, now anything is possible..." is very strongly dependent on how real the sexual transgressions in tabooed spheres of life were.

Sexual self-determination is one thing. It is quite another that social taboos are being broken increasingly frequently, causing the binding nature of traditional rules of social behavior to disappear. The number of children and juveniles who are abused seems to be increasing, and the number of unreported cases of father-daughter incest is considerable. Transference after abuse, used in a wider sense of the term, is complicated, for traumatized patients put themselves and analysts to demanding tests (see Sect. 8.5.1).

In Sect. 1.7 of Vol.1 we pointed to the fact that the speeds at which changes take place in family traditions and in historical and sociocultural processes are particularly asynchronous. Thus the type of hysterical female patients who not only fall in love with the analyst but who also seek in treatment a substitute for an unsatisfying life and who hold on to the illusion of finding fulfillment from the analyst can still be found in the offices of psychoanalysts today.

With regard to the prediction, i. e., the probability, that an unresolvable erotized transference will develop or not, what is diagnostically relevant is the kind of complaints that a patient makes about her love life. The danger that irresolvable transference love will develop is minor if the factors making it difficult or impossible for a patient to have satisfactory sexual relationships within existing friendships or in long-term ties are primarily the result of neuroses. The prognosis of illusionary transference love is least favorable if a serious neurotic development has led to the patient's isolation and the patient has reached an age at which her chances of finding a suitable partner are small. Despite all the achievements in women's emancipation, social circumstances have an unfavorable effect on such women, in contrast to the comparable group of men, because, as is well known, neurotic and lonely bachelors have less difficulty making contacts with unmarried women. The different natures of male and female *psychosexuality* play a part in this system, in which for example men looking for partners by means of announcements are less subject to traumatizing experiences than women who are "tested" in a short affair and afterwards found to be not attractive enough.

The reader may ask what these general comments have to do with the spectrum of positive transference. One consequence is that it becomes clear why it is less usual for male patients being treated by female analysts to develop erotized transference than vise versa under otherwise similar conditions. We do not shy from referring to another general factor, which can be derived from our previous remarks and which according to our experience should be taken very seriously when considering indications. If the combination of biographical, occupational, and social factors described above and that predispose to the development of regressive erotized transference is present, then a male analyst should critically reconsider his previous experience with erotized transference before deciding to accept a case. If in doubt, it is in the female patient's interest for the male analyst to recommend that she see a female colleague. In spite of our emphasis on the dyadic character of transference neurosis, of which transference love is a part, the neurosis also contains an independent dynamic rooted in the patient's unconscious schema. If the analyst's age and personal situation coincides with the expectations in the patient's unconscious dispositon like the key to a lock, it contributes more to creating emotional confusion. Erotized transference is the term used to describe such a situation.

But what do confusion and even chaos mean? Are the feelings, affects, and perceptions experienced in transference genuine or not? Even Freud did not dispute their genuineness, although transference implies that it is not the analyst who is really meant, but that the wishes and sexual longing are actually directed to the wrong address. The complete manifestation of a feeling doubtlessly includes reaching the intended goal and, in human interaction, getting the other person to answer and, if possible, to cooperate (Dahl 1978). For this reason the patient is also always referring to the person of the analyst. The latter stays in the background, in order to more easily fulfill his function and also be able to take on the role - whether of mother, father, brother, or sister - enabling the patient to experience the manifestations of unconscious clichés, templates, or schemata. (Freud used these terms to describe a disposition regulating affective and cognitive processes.) The interpretation of resistance to transference helps the patient to weaken his repression; in the process the analyst's catalytic function takes effect and enables a new enactment to take place according to our enlarged stage model (see Sect. 3.4 in Vol.1). This is the reason it is so essential to proceed from the plausibility of the patient's perceptions instead of from their distortion. We therefore speak of a reenactment with changing roles instead of a new edition. The analyst, insofar as he temporarily has the role of a director, ensures that the patient tests the reperatoire of roles available to him - unconsciously, that is - and gains confidence to test the trial actions outside of analysis.

In addition to the above-mentioned group of female patients, there is probably also a considerably smaller group of patients who are only able to complete the transition from rehearsal to real life to a limited extent; this occurs for external and internal reasons and despite the use of the modified technique we have recommended. The less a patient is able to achieve an intense interaction with a partner, the greater the fascination with the empathic and understanding attitude of the analyst, if for no other reason than it is not saddled with the everyday disappointments from actually living together.

A few turns in the following case demonstrate something more general in nature. Much of it culminates in the question of how the analyst can provide confirmation while refusing immediate sexual gratification. In the case of a pathogenic condition caused by repression, the oedipal temptations and frustrations have disappeared to such an extent that the existence of unconscious desires can only be ascertained either from the recurrence of repressed material in symptoms or from the conflicting and unsatisfactory relations to the partner. Finding an access to the patient's world of unconscious desires is a precondition for change, in the process of which the patient increases his capacity for finding new ways to solve problems. For example, the *acknowledgment* of desires that are stimulated and encouraged in the analytic situation by the setting and interpretations is not tied to the *satisfaction* of these desires. Yet it is in the nature of desires and intentional acts to strive toward a goal, and it is common knowledge that reaching the goal is accompanied by a feeling of relief and satisfaction. On the other hand, from the very beginning it is a fact of life that many attempts to attain a goal fail (as in trial and error). If intense, vital needs are frustrated, defects occur in an individual's self-assurance and sexual role that have multifaceted consequences on his behavior. The technical problems of handling intense emotions continue to be a major test for therapists, who must navigate between the Scylla of subliminal seduction and the Charybdis of rejection.

The patient described below sought security and confirmation in transference love.

A 26-year-old woman, Franziska X, came for treatment because she suffered from intense attacks of anxiety, which occurred especially in situations in which she was supposed to demonstrate her professional ability. She had brilliantly completed her training in a male-dominated profession and could count on having a successful carreer if she could overcome her anxieties. The latter had developed after she had completed her training, so to speak when things became serious and the rivalry with men no longer had the playful character of her student days. Franziska X had met her husband during her training and they were united by satisfying intellectual and emotional ties. However, she did not get much satisfaction from sexual intercourse in her marriage; it took a lot of concentration and work for her to have an orgasm, which she could have on her own much faster and simpler.

She quickly reacted to the initiation of treatment by falling in love, the first signs of which were already apparent in a dream she recalled in the fourth session. It described, first, a scene between an exhibitionistic girl at a police station and a man who was reacting sexually. The second part of the dream depicted a medical examination in which the patient was observed by someone with X-ray eyes; only a naked skeleton was visible.

The patient's dreams contained repeated permutations of the subject of forbidden love with subsequent punishment or separation. She vacillated greatly between her desire to please me, like a schoolgirl doing her homework, and her disturbing desires, which she also mentioned in her associations.

By the eleventh hour I had already become a "really good friend," who was all her own and who also satisfied the condition that "it" could never become reality. What "it" meant was clarified by her next association, when she asked me, "Did you see the movie late night about the priest who had an affair with a woman convert?" In the fourteenth session Franziska X told me about a dream.

P: You told me that you were in love and then you kissed me, when I am in love it only goes to kissing, that's the most beautiful part, then the rest comes whether you like it or not. Then you said that we had better stop the analysis. I was satisfied with your decision because I got more this way.

The purpose of this intensive manifestation of eroticism seemed to be to fight her experience that analysis is a phase of "hard times" (17th session). At a weekend seminar she was finally able to get the confirmation, from numerous flirts, that was lacking in the sessions.

P: Yes, what you tell me is really very important to me. I sometimes think that I should try to limit the expectations I place on you or overcome them entirely, because I can never have the hope that you will confirm them. Everything would be so much simpler if I could keep these emotional aspects out of here and have an intelligent conversation with you.

In order to enable the patient to obtain some relief I pointed out to her that the setting (her lying on the couch etc.) and the nature of our talks awakened intense feelings and that it was quite natural that I should acknowledge them. Yet because of the special nature of our relationship and the tasks assigned to me, I could not respond to her desires in the way she wished. I saw an analogy between the patient's insecurity toward me and her (previously disappointed) expectations about being completely accepted by a man, and therefore asked about the source of her insecurity as a woman. In doing so I was guided by the idea that the patient was seeking her mother more than her father in transference love and in her friendships.

This topic moved the patient. For the first time she now talked about her impressions of her mother. In the initial interview she had only stated, "There's nothing to say about her." The patient said she had no image of herself as a woman. She came to speak of childhood memories and described her mother and father as they went to communion at church. As a 4-year-old child she had stayed behind and begun to cry because she did not know what her parents were doing. She recalled with photographic precision the moment when her parents came back from the altar, kneed, and held their hands in front of their faces: her mother was an attractive young woman wearing a scarf over her long brown hair, like a maid on a farm who is feeding the chickens, uncomplicated and happy.

Then there was a change in the patient's associations. The mother had entered a hospital when the daughter was aged 6; she suffered from eclampsia, which was severe during the birth of another girl. Her mother never recovered. The image of her mother that now appeared in the patient's associations was the one she had when her mother returned home: swollen, ugly, and arms and legs in some fluid to stimulate her muscles. Since then her mother grumbled nonstop in a language that could hardly be understood. In short, she presented the picture of frightening decay, which might suggest more than just oedipal fantasies associated with pregnancy and rivalry.

The patient avoided these impressions and, rapidly changing her mood, turned to another subject and talked about the lovely weather that made it possible for her to come to analysis in a light summer dress.

Being in love became the motor of the treatment. The patient could only bring herself to talk about disturbing and shameful topics when she was in this mood. She felt that she was in a stalemate because her wishes could never become reality.

This greenhouse atmosphere might be described as "transference yes, working alliance no." This constellation pointed to a lack of underlying security, for which the patient had to compensate by showing and offering herself in a seemingly oedipal way.

In one of the following sessions (the 23rd) the patient was concerned with the question of why the analyst did not wear a white coat. "In a white coat you would be much more neutral and anonymous, one doctor among many." During the session this comment turned out to have two sides, one a wish, the other resistance. It became obvious in connection with her short summer dresses that she desired a stronger separation of roles. The analyst had to remain anonymous, and then she could show herself without being embarrassed. The more she experienced me as a specific individual, the less she could stretch and slide around on the couch. In summer she therefore felt much more like a woman than in winter, when everything is hidden and packed away.

The patient sensed that her erotic attempts to attract me were not succeeding, and she reacted by developing depressive ill will and feeling disappointed.

The development of the transference in the first few weeks and months stabilized itself more and more in one direction. The patient's first attempts to attract my interest were replaced by her anxieties that I would not take a single step toward her. The entire story of her relationship to her father, who had had to take on numerous responsibilities after her mother's paralysis, is too long to be told here. Her father's opinion of her at that time was then, just as it was during analysis, annihilating; "Nobody ever knows where they are with you." This corresponded to the patient's feeling that her father was unpredictable; as a child she had always trembled and been afraid of him.

The development in the first few months made it possible for me to verbalize a growing complaint for the patient. I interpreted that she had tried to win me over and had not reached her aim. Thus frustrated, she simply resigned and became complaining and reproachful.

P: [After a pause] I didn't know who that was supposed to refer to. But, a few minutes ago I thought that the only one that it can really fit is my father. [Silence] Now I recall our church; in it there's a ceiling fresco with a large Lord God, and now I remember our priest and that I was terribly afraid of him.

A: When you think of something else, then the danger quickly appears that I am upset, and then in your experiencing I become similar to your father. You get in a situation in which you have to wait for me to take you back into good favor, as if you were a sinful girl, but this act of mercy will take a long time and really can never be reached.

P: As a 15-year-old I had contact with a young man who had a bad reputation. It was my first love affair, and then he went and got a girl pregnant who was working in the seminary kitchen. My father scolded me as if I had been the one.

A: In your experience that won't have made much difference.

P: Because of such things our contact never did become very good again. I believe that I am still waiting for the sign of a cross that a father marks on your forehead when you leave home. He didn't do it for me in a way that I can genuinely believe.

In the following sessions the patient continued to be preoccupied with her Catholic past. She had seen a movie in which a woman was also named Franziska and acted the way her father thought she should. She recalled that her father had brought her a church booklet on sexual development at the beginning of her puberty and had pressed it into her hand. Its cover showed just such a young girl: a decent Catholic. It was completely impossible for the patient to imagine that her father had ever been interested in women. She was therefore very astonished when I pointed out that she had had to go into a children's hospital while her mother had been pregnant.

The patient continued to be preoccupied with her particular relationships to older men.

P: Actually I've always dreamed about falling in love with such men, and for a long time I dreamed about sleeping with them. But in reality I wanted a patron who understood me and left me completely alone. Sex isn't a part of it. Funny, since I started analysis these dreams have disappeared.

A: That was also your original idea of analysis, to find in me a patron in whom you can place your unlimited trust and who never gets mad regardless what you might say or do.

P: Yes, that's how it was, but I don't have that feeling any more. I simply think that you can always withdraw, and you're outside the situation; I can't pin you down. You are really more like a computer that organizes ideas and makes suggestions, not a human being, you aren't allowed to be like one. Whenever I think about you I come to a deadend. On the one hand it starts with my feeling that I find the warmth in your eyes, the intimacy, and then nothing goes any further and I feel as if I were abruptly awoken, pushed from my dream into reality, as if you were sitting next to my bed in the morning and would wake me up when I dreamed about you at night. And actually I don't want to return to this reality from the dream at all.

I understood her last sentence as an expression of the difficulty of facing reality and discriminating between wishful thinking and a realistic appraisal of my therapeutic role.

2.2.3 Fusion Desires

In a certain context Arthur Y asked me whether I was satisfied with the treatment so far. I said yes but qualified my answer by saying that he, the patient, would probably be even more satisfied if the confirmation would take the form of cash, an allusion to a raise he expected. The patient responded to the analogy by describing the relief he felt after my positive statement. But then he began to feel upset, which he traced back to the fact that I might be critical of him after all. He thought to himself that he might not be contributing enough toward making progress. At the scene of an accident he had recently done everything he could and yet afterwards he had still asked himself if he had really done enough.

In the patient's experience the size of his raise in salary became the symbol of or equivalent to being held in high regard and well liked. He had lost sight of the fact that it would be wonderful to be liked without having to earn it. He referred to this now by surprisingly drawing a parallel to a (homosexual) boarding school teacher he had had in puberty. (He avoided using the disturbing adjective.)

At first the topic of how much affection he could get without taking a very large risk was dealt with by going through the options he had in a forthcoming talk with his boss.

P: Well, I'm willing to do considerably more than is usual but I want to be compensated for it, and the problem is how much I can risk without being turned down. I feel very clearly that I am afraid of two things: that he might reject my wish, and that I might miss a chance if I abstained from asking. That would make me very worried, and something similar is happening here. On Friday, when I asked the question that I brought up again today, I said that my previous analyst would not have answered it but would have slammed it back at me, just like in table tennis. It wasn't easy for me to ask this question because I was simply afraid of being rejected and of the disgrace and humiliation that go with it.

A: Yet there was one hour when it seemed clear to me that although being rejected is bad, it also reestablishes a distance. The authorities keep their distance.

P: This point seems very important. The distance was supposed to ensure that they don't suddenly act like the [homosexual] teacher at the boarding school. I have to think of the question of who guarantees me that this won't happen if I lose too much of my reserve and I'm no longer myself and you're no longer yourself, but like two pieces of butter in a pan . . . .

A: Yes.

P: . . .that melt in a pan.

A: Hmm.

P: Then they flow into one another.

A: You guarantee it and so do I, for you are yourself and I am myself.

P: Yes, yes, but . . . .

A: Hmm.

P: Now I very clearly feel you've hit me, which tells me, "What do you think you're doing making such a comment?"

A: Yes. Yes, yes, you probably experienced it as a blow, as a rejection, precisely because there is this longing for this flowing together, like with the butter. It's a wonderful image of blending that contains something very profound. Blending, exchange, things in common.

P: And because this cannot be achieved, which is why Dr. A. [one of the analysts who had treated him previously] might have said somewhat sarcastically and with razor sharp logic that what cannot be, may not be. This is a part of it although I wanted to stick to the subject, as I said, it's so typical, the words "razor sharp" . . . .

These expressions were made popular in German by a poem by Christian Morgenstern, "Die Unmögliche Tatsache," that closes with the lines, "And he reaches the conclusion: The experience was only a dream. Because, he concludes with razor-sharp logic, that which cannot be may not be."

A: Razor sharp.

P: Razor sharp, I thought again of a girl I could do something to with a knife. So I have to repeat the word "razor sharp" as often as possible and try to think about something else.

The patient continued in another vein. I thought that I could maintain the connection by referring to something both topics had in common.

A: The point was the mixing, and when the knife enters something an intimate connection is created between the knife and . . . .

P: But a destructive one.

A: Destructive, yes.

P: Outrageous.

A: Yes, an outrageous presumption. No flowing together of butter in the pan.

P: No, no, an outrageous presumption by the one who has the knife, with regard to the other person, who is threatened or injured.

A: Yes, yes, hum, the knife, yes.

P: And the teacher [who had also taken care of the patient when he was ill at the boarding school] had such a knife - not the object, but his behavior.

A: In many regards, in his general behavior and in specific things, with his teeth.

P: And when taking my fever, for example.

A: When taking your fever with his thermometer, which he pushed in, and his penis, which you could somehow feel when he put you on his lap.

P: Well, that I can't . . . . [the patient suppressed the phrase "remember any more."] I've asked myself the same thing. But I don't think so. At least I can't remember.

A: It's possible that this has been lost and that he . . .

P: he understood . . .

A: how to hide the fact that his penis was presumably stiff.

P: Yes, we can assume that. Well, I mean I can't remember. Thank God that it didn't get that far, but I still felt threatened and very much in danger. Yes, similar to here. On the one hand, the feeling of being helplessly exposed. I was sick after all and didn't have a chance to say that I would like to have someone else take care of me. No trust. Well, here it isn't always that way, only if I try very hard to think about it. Then somewhere I feel a reservation about going so far because I wouldn't be able to defend myself. Of course, my personality and yours are guarantees, but simply by your saying it I make it into a rejection.

A: Yes, because the flowing together expresses a longing, namely to get enrichment by taking as much of my fat as possible, thus if at all possible not only a raise but a million's worth of affection, as an expression of strength and potency.

P: Yes, all of what you just said gives security. But I have to think of the following: Okay, what should I do with this longing for affection if it's impossible for them to merge to the same degree as two pieces of butter? So, get rid of it.

In a later session the patient described the mixing by referring to two bars of chocolate, thus revealing the anal origin of the reference and its different unconscious aspects.

A: Why get rid of it? Who says that it can't become reality and you can't retain something from here?
P: Yes, yes, either everything or nothing.
A: And you cut a piece of fat off my ribs with the knife.
P: [Laughing] Because I always have the tendency, everything or nothing.
A: Well, you've also discovered that you can be very curious in order to get more, everything if possible.
P: What kind of concrete example are you thinking of?
A: Hmm.
P: Because I wanted to know where you are vacationing . . . .
A: Yes, that is the example I was just thinking of, because that was also a matter of burning curiosity. And then you would like to have a steadfast man you can't disparage, who asserts his independence, because otherwise he would be a weakling.

It is always especially impressive and convincing when the patient's and analyst's thoughts coincide. Then, after a pause, the patient spoke about his boss.

P: You used the words "longing for affection." There was another word. "Longing for agreement."
A: Things in common.
P: Yes, yes.
A: Hm.
P: That is something that has worried me my entire life, when I had my first experiences with girls. It was with my wife that it happened for the first time, that I didn't lose all interest the moment my affection was reciprocated. If they became weak, then they lost almost all value.
A: Yes, yes, weak.
P: Or vice versa, if I showed a feeling of affection to someone, whoever it was, and if it weren't reciprocated immediately, I became aggressive. I not only withdrew my exposed feelers but became more withdrawn. It was an incredible humiliation for me. Just like the fact that the two of us can't simply and completely blend together, like the butter.
A: You mentioned that you used to be more aggressive. At some point there must have been a reversal, to being self-deprecating and self-critical about not being able to finish anything, when you started making yourself the object of accusations.
P: I can now see these two pieces of butter. In religion and in communion you find just the same thing.
A: In communion.
P: In communion, in union, in eating the body, I'm not the only one to have this wish; there are millions. It's simply a part of me because I'm human.
A: Yes.
P: And not because I once knew this teacher.
A: Yes.
P: So it's nothing that I have to continuously struggle against or disparage, nothing that robs me of my value as an individual, it's rather something that belongs to me because I'm just like the rest.
A: Yes.
P: And now you'll say right away that you are also an individual, have feelings just like I do, and it must be possible to make the thing with the butter come true.

A: Yes.

P: On the other hand, ha ha, but just a second, otherwise this will go too far. Of course, you are right. This is so contradictory, just as my mood can sometimes swing within seconds, like a scale trying to get into balance. But my mood doesn't stay in balance. And now I think that if I really manage to go to my boss and talk about money, then maybe he will also think, "Maybe he could do something for nothing once." He will somehow feel disappointed if I demand something from him for what I do, since he's only human. I would have to manage to sacrifice a part of this all-or-nothing standpoint that a hundred minus one is simply equal to zero, but rather that one hundred minus one is still ninety-nine and one hundred minus fifty is still half. Can you understand me? This is so hard for me.

A: Well, yes, a hundred percent is in fact nicer, hm.

P: Yes, but one hundred minus one is still . . .

A: Ninety-nine.

P: And for me ninety-nine turns into one. I'm much more interested in this one part of a hundred than in the other ninety-nine.

A: And everything is invested in this one part, and then you yourself are nothing.

P: Yes, if I can't have everything, then I don't want anything at all. But emotionally I'm still waiting for the bang that happens when I learn something like I have today. Dr. B. used to say, "Then your anxieties will explode like a balloon. Boom, boom. And they're gone." I'm still not finished with it, but it would be lovely if it were possible.

A: I have the feeling that you are happy about the discoveries you've made today, but that you don't really dare to express your pleasure and thus to belittle your discoveries right away. Perhaps you're also disappointed that I'm not dancing with joy at the profound connections you've discovered.

I later thought about the missing explosion prophesized by his earlier analyst. That such an exaggeration, which made the analyst into a magician performing wonders, unconsciously had to lead to the patient's anal disparagement, which in turn prevented both the explosion and a stepwise improvement from occurring, was shown by the history of this patient's illness.

2.2.4 Erotized Transference

Gertrud X, a 33-year-old woman, was referred to me by her family physician because of frequent depressive episodes, which had already led her to make several attempts to commit suicide. The patient complained also about frequent headaches. In numerous talks her physician had attempted to give her support, but in the meantime her relationship to him had become so tense that he did not feel he was in a position to look after her any longer.

The conflict situation was as follows. The patient was an only child, and she had lost her father in the war when she was 3 years old. Her parents' marriage must have been marked by tension, and her mother had not established any close ties to anyone since then. At first she established contact with her brother's family. The patient also greatly admired her mother's brother, who died in the war when the patient was 5 years old. Her mother's father also played an important role; he was an dominating authoritarian who, just like the rest of the family, was staunchly devout. She portrayed her mother as someone who was rather infantile and dependent on the opinions of others and who attempted to tie the patient to her.

A positive development had taken place about 6 years before the beginning of therapy after the patient had established a friendship with a younger (female) colleague, which made it possible for Gertrud X to put some distance between herself and her mother. Now this colleague was planning to get married and move to another location. The patient felt herself exposed to increasing attempts by her mother to cling to her, and reacted by provoking aggressive clashes. The patient had never entered into closer heterosexual friendships. Her relationships to men were characterized by her effort to find confirmation, yet her frequent provocations put their goodwill to a serious test.

In the initial interview the patient appealed especially to my willingness to help, and in particular knew how to describe in a convincing way a long chain of experiences in which she had lost someone. I offered her therapy, whose goals were to reduce conflict, both in her separation from her mother and in her attitude toward men.

Although Gertud X accepted my offer, to my surprise she expressed doubt from the very beginning about the success of analysis. She expressed skepticism especially regarding my age. She said that she was only able to establish a trusting relationship to older men; I was about the same age as the patient. In view of her aloof reservation I paid especially careful attention in our interaction for signs of a flickering of friendship, a desire for confirmation, or erotic interest. The patient rejected interpretations in this vein in a standard way, constantly emphasizing that there was no point in me concerning myself with her in this manner. My interpretations only caused the patient to become more cautious. My attempt to break the ice by interpreting deeper unconscious wishes only had the effect of offending the patient, who reacted by becoming depressed, thinking of suicide, and retreating. These alarm signals led me to be very cautious.

Yet despite all the patient's recalcitrant reservation it became impossible to overlook the fact that her interest in me was growing. She was overpunctual in coming to her sessions, concerned herself increasingly with their contents (even though primarily in a critical way), and started using a perfume that made her "present" in my rooms for hours after her appointment.

These changes were indicative of a new topic in our interaction. With the increasing length of therapy the patient's mother became increasingly jealous, in particular because, according to the patient's reports, I frequently functioned as the star witness in their disputes. Her mother called me twice, attempting to gain my support by complaining about her daughter; I rejected this attempt from the very beginning. On the contrary, the patient's independence became a preferred topic. The patient explained in great detail about her mother's countless attempts to interfere and about her infantile nature and jealousy, and came to me for support in her struggle for more independence. In this phase of therapy our interaction was largely free of outright tension.

The first summer break, which lasted several weeks, was a turning point. There was little indication of this change in the period immediately preceding it; the patient's conflicts with her mother had instead been the prime topic. It was not until the last hour before the vacation break that the patient appeared alarmingly depressive and skeptical. Without wanting to, I adopted the role defending the therapy while the patient continued, without interruption, to deny the value of every positive sign. On the evening of the same day the patient phoned me and spoke openly about her intention to commit suicide. She got me involved in a long telephone conversation, in which we went through the contents of the last session once again.

During my vacation Gertrud X turned to her family doctor again and sought support. An intense dispute developed very quickly, whereupon she took an overdose of sleeping pills and had to be admitted. I detected a trace of triumph in her description of these events. Our interaction after the summer break had resembled that at the beginning: the patient had been skeptical and pessimistic with regard to the success of the therapy. Proceeding from her experience in the summer break, she emphasized over and over that there was no point to her having any hope. Sooner or later she would again be alone and without any human support. Invisaging her next attempt to commit suicide, I tried to show the patient my sympathy and explain to her that it would extend to her beyond the end of therapy. Although I recognized the aspect of extortion in her statements, I did not make it a topic because of my fear of further complications.

My own private situation aggravated these conflicts in this phase of therapy. The patient did not have any difficulty finding out that I was in the process of getting a divorce and that my family had moved to another location. This fact was only very briefly mentioned in the therapy, but I noticed that the patient tried to find out more about my private life by following me in her car. I transformed this fact into the interpretation that the patient had become curious and fantasized about sharing the future with me. As a result of this interpretation, she again attempted to commit suicide by taking sleeping pills; hospital treatment was not necessary, but this event increased my vulnerability to being blackmailed. The patient began to call more frequently after the sessions. Although I regularly referred to the necessity of discussing these things in the next session, I no longer dared to force them to a conclusion and thus over and over again let myself get involved in long disputes on the telephone. This constellation remained stabile for a very long period of time. In the sessions the patient was silent and rejecting and emphasized the hopelessness of the entire situation. I attempted both to encourage her and to confront her latent rejection; in general she reacted by becoming offended and frequently called me after the sessions "in order to get over the weekend." Although I noted that the patient's social conflicts with the outside world settled a litte and that she had fewer conflicts with her supervisor in particular, this had little significance for the therapeutic process. In view of this stalemate I did not dare steer toward ending therapy because there was a very large danger that each announcement of an end would be answered with an attempted suicide.

The culmination and end of this tormentous clash was a call in which the patient said that she had just taken a dose of sleeping pills that was probably lethal. She called me from a telephone booth not far from my office. Rapid action was indicated in this emergency situation. I immediately picked her up with my car and took her to the hospital. This joint trip in my car and handing her over to the emergency care doctor on duty etc. naturally provided her with a large amount of transference satisfaction. For a brief moment it was as if the patient and I were a pair, even if an estranged one. Yet our relationship reached a point here where I had to tell her after her release from the hospital that she could force me into an active act of providing medical help, but that she had thus also lost me as analyst because I could no longer help her in that capacity. Subsequently she tried to make me alter my decision by threatening to commit suicide. Yet my steadfastness at the end of treatment made it possible to find a halfway conciliatory conclusion.

Commentary. The treatment described here resulted from a series of mistakes that are typical for beginners. Yet a beginner's mistakes often reflect an understanding of treatment characteristic of the school of analysis he adheres to. In retrospect it is possible to identify the following undesirable developments:

1. Attempts to master the ongoing crisis situations solely by working with transference and resistance is insufficient if it is not linked to an improvement in the patient's real life situation. The patient had to be reconciled to the possiblity, in fact the probability, that she would never marry; the fact that the analyst wak-

ened unrealistic hopes therefore had to have antitherapeutic consequences. Unreflected rescue fantasies on the part of the therapist had an unfavorable influence in this case.

2. Since the patient had no partner, focussing on unconscious transference wishes had to have an antitherapeutic effect because, once again, the forced reference to transference wishes aroused unrealistic hopes. In the initial phase the therapist fell into the role of seducer, and this role had harmful effects on the rest of the analysis.
3. A topic that went untreated, especially in the first third, was that the patient employed the therapy as a weapon against her mother and that the therapist was led into taking sides. As a consequence, the patient's aggressive impulses, whose development was inevitable after her hopes had been disappointed, were directed onto someone outside therapy, which paved the way for the later, unfavorable collusion.
4. Following her serious threats of committing suicide, the analyst gave the patient more sympathy than can be maintained in an analytic setting. This obstructed the interpretation of her aggressive impulses, especially her using the threat to commit suicide to coerce the analyst. The patient's preexisting tendency to treat the analyst as a real partner was strengthened precisely in this phase of therapy, without patient and analyst jointly reflecting on the role transference played in maintaining her self-esteem. The therapist's family situation, which the patient was somehow aware of, increased her illusory hopes. If an unmarried patient who cannot cope with being alone happens to have a therapist who is the right age, alone, and possibly even unhappy, then the social reality of this constellation is so strong that it is probably extremely unusual for them to be able to focus on the neurotic components of a patient's hopes. Expectations and disappointments that have antitherapeutic consequences are almost inevitably the result.
5. It was almost inevitable that the therapist, under the burden of the disappointments and complications that he at least in part caused, would not be able to resist the pressure of his own feelings of guilt and let himself get tied up in telephone conversations justifying his procedure. In trying to justify himself it was almost a matter of course that the therapist's arguments were dictated by his own interests and not by the patient's needs, which in turn promoted the patient's secret hopes of overcoming the limitations of the therapeutic setting. Indicative of this was the fact that the therapeutic frame only regained its importance the moment the therapist admitted his failure and announced that it meant the termination of therapy.

2.2.5 *Negative Transference*

Negative transference is a special form of resistance that can destroy the analyst's ability to function. Has therapy reached a standstill? Is the patient one of those people who somewhere in their mind desire change - otherwise they would not come - but who at the same time deny that the analyst has any therapeutic influence? How do the patient and the analyst each cope with a chronic impasse?

The analyst can maintain his interest by attempting to recognize the reasons for the negative attitude that eludes his influence. This can be linked with the analyst's hope of interrupting the repetition and at least transforming the rigid front into a mobile war and outright hostilities. It is not difficult to recognize in this martial metaphor that the analyst suffers from such a paralyzing balance of power. One means of making it easier to bear this powerlessness is to detect the secret satisfactions that the patient derives from being able to maintain and regulate the balance of power. This is linked with the hope that knowledge of the destructive consequences of this pleasurable ability to exercise control can also lead the patient to finding new paths to gain pleasure. Abandoning the usual track and seeking free space is tied to a renunciation of security that no one gladly accepts as long as no new and promising sources of pleasure are apparent and, what is even more important, as long as these new sources do not flow precisely in those moments when people thirst for them.

In the last session I had plainly pointed out to Clara X, a patient with anorexia nervosa, that there was a deep and wide gap separating what she said here and how she acted outside - and in general between her thinking and her actions - and that she separated both spheres of her life from one another. I attempted to impress on her that although she suffered from this dichotomy, she also maintained the power embodied in it and that I could not do anything about it. The sense of what I said was, "You are powerful and I am helpless, and I can feel that your power is a strong force." Outwardly she seemed peaceful, she was a peaceful dictator, and she was not even aware of her awesome strength that made me helpless.

In her first utterance in the following session the patient referred to the blow I had given her when she, referring to the fly swat that was lying around, asked, "Do you kill flies in the winter?" And immediately added, "Do you use it to hit patients?" To my interpretation, "You are thinking about the last session," she immediately responded in a reflective manner, "Yes, it hurt me very much."

P: I understood your *criticism* to mean that although I regret not being able to do anything, I do it willfully, that I insist on my habits in order to keep you from interfering, in order to maintain my independence.

A: But not maliciously. It's difficult not to immediately take my thoughts to be criticism. Otherwise you could view your habits self-critically and perhaps see and sense that there might be other and larger opportunites for satisfaction. But by closing your eyes and retaining something that has become very established, you have very little space left to change something and go your way.

P: My perseverance can be much worse. You should inquire about the question of my weight.

The patient then spoke about the only item that might motivate her to sacrifice her perseverance, namely her desire to have another child, but this desire was immediately blocked by the thought that she would then be the prisoner of motherhood again. I picked up this line of thought:

A: Not to persevere would lead to an ambiguous goal, to becoming a mother again, which you experience to be a prison.

P: But then I would have to deny several characteristics even more fiercely. Then I would have to be feminine and patient, wait at home for my husband, be in a good mood and try to please him, try to be as nice as possible and speak with a gentle, soft voice. But beware! This doesn't include having pleasure from physical movement, and social contacts have to be largely abandoned, and I would have to forget any ambitions to have a carreer. One ambiguous situation takes the place of the other. My deepest longing is [pause] to be accepted all around and to be able to accept myself.

A: In other words, to overcome these contradictions.

P: To overcome them by having a second child is an illusion, I would get just as much negative feedback about not being a good mother and doing everything wrong.

A: I believe that you have a deep longing to overcome these contradictions, but that this feeling is unsettling. You refer to these examples in order to wipe away the shame from your demand for instantaneous nursing. You do everything to avoid this shame, which also prevents you from having more happy moments.

After this interpretation the patient replied that she simply could not see how anything could be changed by talking.

Consideration. I had the feeling I was acting as if I wanted to make something especially appealing for her, as if an angel strengthened my powers of persuasion. I surely had this fantasy because the patient some time ago had copied a painting by the pre-Raphaelite Rosetti, "The Annunciation," and brought it along with the comment that the fragile Maria in the painting, showing signs of cachexia, was probably an "anorexa."

I alluded to this in my next interpretation.

A: I am just like the angel proclaiming the Annunciation, and you are the anorexa Maria who is an unbeliever. An angel helps me be persuasive, but I turn into a devil who deceives, and you are intelligent enough to know, and you do know, that such persuasion lies because the salvation that it promises doesn't last.

Then the patient - as if in prayer and after a longer period of silence - made the following statement:

P: Hum, who took You, oh Virgin, to heaven, praised be the Virgin Mary, blessed art thou, naturally I don't believe, after all I have a heretic as father who is sitting on a cloud in heaven, but not because St. Peter let him in, but because hell was overfilled. You also said, however, that he was too much a heretic and what he said was much too unbelievable.

A: You could give me a chance to let my words resound in your ears as if they were sent by an angel, and above all you could give yourself a chance.

P: But Dear Lord, do I need a second child to get rid of this feeling of being torn apart?

A: No, I don't believe that you need another child to do it. In your own mind you already doubt whether it is worthwhile to have a second child. And then you've got the ambivalence again. The second child is a prison for you. Do you want to get started on your way to prison? Nobody wants to do that. The point is thus to give the persuasion and your own hearing more of a chance when you make a decision that could land you in prison. The point is pleasure, pleasure for its own sake, but you will always be more likely to find it where you find it now, for example, when you eat something at night.

P: [After a pause lasting about 4 minutes] The thought of gaining weight and eating doesn't have anything to do with pleasure or with the feeling of being able to accept myself or of having accepted myself or of being accepted. I can only do it because of the insight that it might be necessary for another child, but not otherwise. When I'm well armed, then I enjoy my inner contradiction as undivided pleasure.

A: That is the goal, the undivided, the unambiguous pleasure, not a divided pleasure.

P: I'm sorry, that is something that does happen, but just for seconds and hardly when the object is bread or food or the classical ways of having a good time. Now I can see a funny image. If the Anorexic lets herself get involved and starts to extend her finger, this unusual hermaphroditic figure there, Gabriel or whoever it is supposed to be on the picture, is left hanging, whether the angel is masculine or feminine? In one hand it has a bough of lillies, in the other the fly swat, and if it extends its finger out too far, then the finger gets swatted one. Think of the fact that being a mother is a large responsibility.

A: Just don't stretch out your finger too far and hold the lillies under the angel's nose to smell, and then there is the ugly word "anorexic," not very nice, *Hexe* [witch], *anorexe*. What you give yourself, so to speak, in anticipation of the fly swat, of being hit by the fly swat. You used the ugly word.

P: I always do that. I use all the words to describe myself that others have ever used to describe me and that have been offensive. It makes my condition bearable, the age-old technique of anticipating the attack by inflicting it on yourself. A very helpful invention.

The reader should not overlook the fact that Clara X just provided an accurate definition of "identification with the aggressor." Therapeutically it was a disadvantage for this process to repeat itself after my aggressive interpretations and thus to become stronger.

The last part of the hour was concerned with immediate statements.

A: You asked me to be direct and blunt in telling you what is important and not just to say everything indirectly. I believe this is something you're demanding of me and of you yourself too. You want to hear loud and clear what is frank and unambiguous and undivided. You want out of the ambivalence. That is the problem over and over and is especially true today. I almost would like to thank you for giving me the opportunity.

After a long period of silence in the next session the patient said in retrospect, "Yes, after the last session I really had a feeling of unity and satisfaction. If I say anything, it could get broken again."

A: Yes, the topic was permission. And I had the same feeling you do, I even thanked you for it.

P: Although I don't know what you want to thank me for.

A: Yes, it's an expression of my happiness. I had the feeling, yes, . . .[falteringly] that the wide gap separating us, it seemed to me, got smaller.

P: Yes, do you think there's a wide gap?

A: Yes, I see a wide gap between action and behavior, action, behavior and speaking, and talking and thinking.

P: Don't you also have the feeling that when you start talking it starts getting controversial right away again?

A: Yes, that might be, but there are also points of agreement. There were also some in the last session. Thinking, acting, and speaking are not the same, but these spheres don't have to be as far apart as they are at times in your case. There are optimistic signs that more things are converging.

P: [After a two minute pause] Oh well, that's why I don't dare say what's on my mind. I think it might disappoint you again. And now you can say, "But I'm used to it."

A: No, I wouldn't say that - although it's true - I would rather say that it is a hard path, one filled with disappointments. You know that's how it is.

P: What I was thinking about is why I have new disappointments, more than is normal.

A: Perhaps it's related to the fact that things get too hot when they get closer, and that you become unsettled and retreat when you get closer to somebody.

Clara X again turned to the subject of her role as housewife and mother and to the question of a second pregnancy and whether she should, in this regard, force herself to gain weight. She told the story of an infertile woman, and considered herself a failure if she didn't "make" a second child. In the process it became clear that her body feeling had changed in the last few months, probably as a result of the therapy. I agreed with her that I also supported the goal of reaching a changed body feeling and, as a consequence, of her reaching a normal weight. The patient's anorexia had begun soon after her menarche, so that she had become amenorrheic very early. She had conceived her healthy son following a hormone treatment. The patient knew, after I had explained it to her, that her cycle could not set in before she had at least approximately reached a certain weight. The hormonal regulation of the menstrual cycle is so closely correlated to the amount of body fat that the absence or reoccurrence of menstruation can be predicted from a woman's weight. Psychogenic factors play only a minor role in the disappearance and reappearance of the period.

Clara X refused to fulfill the necessary preconditions for having a period, i. e., to return to a normal weight. She said that this held no promise for the future, it didn't motivate her.

A: Why is this way of reaching a new body feeling only sensible if you have another child? In my opinion you would reach normal weight if you had a different feeling toward life, one that you could develop with more pleasure, and maybe here and there with more disappointment. I see other things in addition to a child. I am an advocate of normal weight, but you put me in the wrong category. I'm convinced that you would feel better. If you think you would disappoint me, it's because you've come close to some very hot feelings, to the hot oven itself.

Commentary. The struggle over the symptoms and goal of changing her weight took up too much space. The negative transference was not traced back to the disappointment of the patient's oedipal wish for a child in transference. One allusion in this direction was not developed. The analyst's remark about approaching the hot oven was an allusion to the patient's sexual feelings; she had frequently used this phrase to refer to her sensations and her genitals. Of course, there was another, deeper aspect, so that the analyst's failure might also have been the result of insecurity. The patient's longing for her mother and to become a mother again might have been behind the topic of having a second child and the talk about her body feeling. The patient incorporated this longing in a simile about a good fairy, in whose lap she could bury her head. The patient used the negative transference and negativism to protect herself from the disturbing fusing and, ultimately, also from separation as well as from simple disappointments and rejections.

After reading this report, Clara X supplemented it with the following dialogue with a fictive reader:

Reader: I was very interested to read what your analyst wrote and thought it was fairly reasonable. What do you have to say about it from your point of view?
Clara X: When I glanced through the text for the first time, very quickly and feverishly, I asked myself whom he was talking about. Am I supposed to be Mrs. X? Did he ever tell me that? I found some expressions and details that could only stem from my own analysis, but I had simply forgotten many things.

Reader: Well, forgotten?
Clara X: The passage from my analysis that it refers to was a long time ago. Besides, I think this Mrs. X is most unpleasant, even repulsive. I can see her in front of me on the couch – I am sitting behind her – like a fat black dung beetle incessantly paddling in the air with her legs and rasping, "I can't get any where, oh, I can't, I can't!"

Reader: A dung beetle on its back is really helpless.
Clara X: Yes, but I'm afraid that if beetle Mrs. X is offered a straw to climb in order to turn over, she would only growl, "I don't like straw! Either I get an orchid or I stay where I am!"
Reader: By using this image - it comes from Kafka, doesn't it - you repeat what your analyst referred to as "negativism beyond my influence." You have even taken his seat. Is what he said about you really correct?
Clara X: I have the feeling it is. It's probably much too true, and it makes me feel ashamed. According to my idea of what I would like to be like, I move forward on my own two legs. Just why was I that stubborn in analysis?
Reader: You don't want any help, not even a straw.
Clara X: That's nothing new to me! I want to justify myself; I want to pluck apart what disturbed me, why I acted this way and accepted so little of the help that was offered to me. But it doesn't lead to anything but a repetition of the moaning that I've already gone through in therapy.
Reader: Tell me anyway what you have to moan about.
Clara X: I've always felt deeply disappointed. I longed for something closer, more direct, for aggressive physical contact, as it were. I'm much too experienced in throwing words around. Despite my own longing, I can use language to perfection to keep my partner at a distance. I was raised with words. My parents talked more than touched. My mother said herself that she wasn't able to really enjoy her children until she was able to talk to them: "I can't and couldn't do very much with little children who crawl on the floor, babble, slobber, smear their food, whom you let ride on your knees, and with whom you cuddle and be silly." The climate in our home was not cold, but cool, like the days in early spring. You could smell the promise of sunshine and violets in the air, but you still shivered and needed a sweater . . . .
Reader: And this promise naturally wakens an immense longing.
Clara X: Precisely. The merry month should come finally. And instead, the next cloud, the next hail storm. Parents demand that a child be reasonable, control himself, be understanding. They appeal to his pride that he is already big . . . .I recreated this state in therapy. And suffered from it. Incidentally, I've acted the same way toward my son. He was able to talk very early. When he would come into the kitchen when he was nearly two, to be close to me, I had the urge to interrupt my work and pick him up. And what did I do instead? I *told* him that he could play with the pots.
Reader: Can't you also overcome this distance by speaking?
Clara X: Fortunately I know I can. Sometimes. I distinguish between language and talk. For example, you can say "the language of anger" or "the language of love," but not "the talk of love." At the most we talk *about* love. But it's worthless straw, while language . . . .
Reader: is the grain that bread is made of.
Clara X: You understand me. When two people speak with one another, something really happens. During therapy I lost much valuable time talking *about* facts, going in circles, about some symptoms. I'm afraid I sometimes led the analyst around by the nose, unconsciously, and he trotted around behind me, going in the same circles.
Reader: Do you think so? At least he must have had a lot of patience.
Clara X: Yes. And I could hardly imagine when the talks were so unproductive that he might also be paralyzed. I admit that I was happy that I was able to affect him, hurt him. But a child only perceives its own - presumed - helplessness. He once even called me a tyrant, while trying to clarify a resistance. *That* hurt, and I'll never forget it. I was outraged, and while going home I recited to myself the opening lines of Schiller's *Die Bürgschaft*, "To Dionysus, the tyrant, crept the demon, carrying a dagger . . . ."

Reader: Something like that can get things moving again, can't it?
Clara X: Moving - yes! I was hoping just that would happen when I tried to arrange situations in which he and I would do something together. I'm disappointed that I didn't learn to be more spontaneous. For example, I suggested that we spend one session walking.
Reader: What came of the walk?
Clara X: We didn't get beyond discussing it. He didn't think the suggestion was entirely absurd, unacceptable, or childish. He left it open - then I gave up the idea myself. My motivation was gone. The motivation and the pleasure. I'm disappointed that I didn't learn to be more spontaneous.
Reader: But despite everything, you liked going to therapy?
Clara X: Yes. After all, I felt I was being given more attention and understanding than by the people allegedly close to me, the ones I had ties to in everyday life. My resistance was more; it was a sign of my constant devotion, if not to say a declaration of love to my analyst. Unconsciously I was saying, "Look, I'm retaining a couple of defects so that I need you. Because I know that it's good for you, like for everyone, to be wanted. I bring my sorrows, my inner images (and sometimes even real pictures), and my money to you regularly and punctually. I do my part that you have a task to do and can earn a livelihood. And at the same time I watch out that I don't claim too much of you, don't take too much of your time and strength, because I only make limited use of your advice on the outside."
Reader: Hum. Sounds a little megalomaniac, but seems convincing to me.
Clara X: That's why I find the expression "negative transference" insufficient. My attitude was fed in part by feelings that I felt to be positive. When my mother used to say, "I don't have to worry about my daughter; she just runs along, she is stable, thank God," then my little ears took it to be strong praise. I thought that my analyst would also have to positively acknowledge my inclination to only accept a very limited degree of help.
Reader: I just had a thought. If somebody prejudiced against psychoanalytic treatment is listening to us and collecting counterarguments, then this is a real treat. The therapeutic relationship that maintains itself. The client conserves her symptoms because the couch is so nice and familiar to her!
Clara X: Sure. I know such people. Let them listen until their ears ring. They only hear what they want to. But I know that I have changed. There's been a radical change in the circumstances of my life, as a result of my own action. With the emotional support I had in therapy, I was able to untie the knot, something that seemed impossible years ago and that I tried to escape from by dissolving into nothingness. It's possible that that untying this knot was the only task I saw throughout all the years of analysis. The other kinds of problems were also important, but ultimately maybe secondary.
Reader: That sounds positive. But may I nevertheless make a critical comment?
Clara X: I know that you're just as crazy as I am.
Reader: Huh?
Clara X: Somebody who tacks a "but" onto every positive statement! Shoot!
Reader: Among the other, allegedly secondary kinds of problems are your eating habits, weight, looks, health, body feeling, ability to tolerate the closeness of others, no, to perceive this closeness as satisfactory and not to always run away . . . .Aren't you cheating yourself tremendously when you refer to everything as secondary?
Clara X: Heavens. I don't consider myself cured. But I don't blame it on my therapy, and it doesn't make me feel inferior. I know that I'm in danger, and I like to balance my way along the edge. But maybe I will be able to handle it better in the future. In the meantime I'm having enough fun in life not to "beat it" voluntarily.

Consideration. It was impossible, retrospectively, to overcome the deficiency that Clara X complained about, and the question whether the therapy would have been more successful if . . . must therefore remain unanswered. This "if" can be tied to many conditional clauses. Should I have stood up immediately and gone for a walk with the patient? And what would have to have happened during the walk to create the new beginning in the sense of the spontaneity that Clara X was longing for? Once, without any previous announcement, Clara X invited me to breakfast, which she had brought along and spread out on the table in my office. I was naturally surprised but not irritated, and behaved, at least according to my perception, completely naturally. I had already had breakfast, and so I drank a cup of coffee. Clara X had fruit and a whole grain cereal. What she had expected of this arrangement stayed unclear, and in retrospect it was not a success.

Commentary. Since subsequent reflection about which real or symbolic wish fulfillment would have facilitated a new beginning for Clara X is idle speculation, we will mention a few of the general points that guided the analytic strategies. It is advisable to take complaints and accusations seriously in a comprehensive sense. This widens the scope of psychoanalysis without leading to transgressions that are ethically dubious and technically fatal. In the standard technique the limits were surely drawn too tightly, a fact which was partly a side-effect of Ferenczi's alarming experiments. Aside from flexibility, however, the analyst must be aware that a patient's complaints and accusations about deprivations and deficits in his relationship to the analyst fulfill a function that originates in neurotic dissatisfaction. If the analyst assumes that defects and deficits definitely result from what happens to someone in childhood and in the course of their life, then there is little chance for change. Strictly speaking, these events cannot be put right in retrospect. The professional means of psychotherapists, whatever their provenance, would in any case be subject to narrow limits. Anna Freud (1976, p. 263) took this position, that namely an individual can only change what it itself has done, but not what was done to it. This argument pays too little consideration to the fact that the incapacity to act constitutes neurotic suffering. A patient's accusations about not being offered enough in therapy are assertions that also serve to protect himself against not having to take the risk of fulfilling the potential for his own thoughts and actions. The analyst was obviously not successful in sufficiently freeing Clara X from her self-induced limitations to enable her to reduce her complaints about deficits in present and previous interpersonal relationships. Although individuals with anorexia nervosa deny that they suffer from self-induced hunger, the condition continues to maintain and reinforce a deficit state. Kafka's *Hunger Artist* complained that a fundamental deficit in maternal love was the cause of his fatal illness. After the artist died of starvation, Kafka has a panther take his place in the cage. The short story concludes with the panther being shown to the audience in place of the artist. It is not an easy task to reconcile a patient with the pantherlike components of his own self.

2.3 Significance of the Life History

2.3.1 Rediscovery of the Father

Twenty years ago Friedrich Y suffered numerous periods of serious depression; the symptoms were so serious at that time that psychotherapy was not even considered. After an initial outpatient therapy with an antidepressive, lithium was administered as prophylactic medication, which has continued until the present day. Although psychotic mood swings had not become manifest in the meantime, Friedrich Y reported that he fell from states of high spirits into black holes.

He had postponed his desire to seek psychoanalytic treatment for a long time, and could now for the first time take the liberty of having one and was also willing to wait a long time for it. He sought therapeutic help because he had felt "walled in" for years. He described his condition with the image that he lived under a layer of concrete that he has to break through every morning after waking up; he reasoned that this condition stemmed from the years of treatment with the lithium medication. The indications for psychoanalysis were the depressive disturbances of the patient's ability to work and of his interpersonal relationships, which were very comprehensible psychodynamically and were probably due to neurotic conflicts.

After one and one-half years of analysis the patient had made great progress, particularly in his capacity to assert himself at work. As a consequnce of these changes, which made a great impression on him, he wanted to make the attempt to get along without taking the prophylactic medication of lithium. The question of the medication's somatic and psychological side effects had to be taken into consideration in making this decision. Schou (1986) reported that patients occasionally describe a modification of their personality as a result of lithium treatment. After considering the entire course of Friedrich Y's illness, his psychiatrist and I made the decision that the lithium medication could be gradually reduced and eventually discontinued.

The following sequence describes a phase from this period of time in which my worries and anxieties in view of the responsibility I had nolens volens accepted can also be seen.

Friedrich Y demonstrated again today very clearly that he had made great progress. Yet I was preoccupied by how little he knew about his father, a fact we had already spoken about several times. His memories of his father, who had died when the patient was 13 years old, hardly went further back than to the age of 7 or 8. This period of his childhood development appeared blurred. Although he knew a lot about the time he had spent with his mother, with regard to his father he could only remember a few Sunday walks and that his father had worked in his workshop "as if he were crazy." The shop was in their house, and his father, a Swabian craftsman, retreated there to avoid his wife, whose ideals of order and obedience ruled upstairs.

As a boy the patient had usually not been allowed into the shop and had been very distant to his father. He got all the more under the thumb of his pious mother, under whose upbringing two older sisters were already becoming depressive. The same thing happened to him; he experienced states of severe depression when he left home to begin studying at the university.

With this previous history in mind, I attempted to make him aware of the distance between us by telling him that he described exciting developments taking place outside and I could watch with great pleasure how he was unfolding, but that I noticed, alluding to transference, that he hardly perceived my workshop. He would barge into the room, lie down on the couch, take his glasses off, and not see anything else of the momentary situation.

He confirmed this, laughing. Just today he had noticed this as he took his glasses off. Moreover, there had been a time when he had trained himself to look out of focus, in order to be able to concentrate fully on his inner images and thoughts. When I emphasized his pretending to be blind, he interrupted me.

P: This is like being in front of a pane of frosted glass, glass like that in the door to father's workshop.

A: Yes, that's a remarkable parallel. But it is also surprising that we still know so little about you and your father after more than two years, as if his death had completely obliterated him, and that we know little about what you perceive here.

P: [A short period of silence] That's true. I'm very happy about the good progress I'm making, but I really don't exactly know how it takes place, how it functions, I don't know, it's pretty nebulous.

A: It probably has to be kept nebulous in order to avoid conflicts with me.

In one of the following sessions he spent more time talking about his father and the remarkable phenomenon that he had such a limited picture of him even though his father had worked at home as a craftsman for 10 years. He had grown up with the feeling of always standing outside the door. He had probably been disappointed that his father could never get his way against his mother. This time he mentioned not only his mother, but his father's mother, his grandmother. She was a woman in love with life and apparently enjoyed retirement; she came to them every day for her meals and spoiled the children with chocolate - which his father approved of but his mother criticized. His father apparently enjoyed the fact that the children were happy and being spoiled by their grandmother, who had grown mild in old age.

The patient had had a daydream after his father's death. In it he had seen an image of his father sitting in heaven and observed him masturbating. When he mentioned this image for the first time, it seemed as if his father had had a stern and evil look on his face. In today's session he attempted to differentiate, saying that it could be that the stern and evil aspects had been his mother and that his father had looked at him in a different way - as if he had felt a bond to him that was rooted in what his mother would never have accepted.

A: So it's conceivable that this image of your father in heaven portrays a connection, that something has stayed alive between the two of you and that you have bridged death in this way.

P: Yes, I wasn't able to mourn at all, I wasn't able to cry. Somehow it was as if I didn't have any use for it. I stood there in front of the door to the workshop and imagined that he was very far away.

The patient continued this line of thought, saying that this daydream might portray the wish to have received more encouragement from his father. He linked this to the fact that his mother had not permitted him to get a driver's license and that he had not had his way until he was away at the university.

At this juncture I pointed out to the patient that he had recently begun to furtively look around my room more and more, but had avoided me. I also pointed out that the treatment would be concluded sometime and that he then would again be in a situation like that when things between him and his father had not been out in the open. At this the patient became disturbed.

P: That's something I'd rather not think about yet; there are a few things I have to find out before I can go.

A: So that you won't only have stood outside the workshop door.

He then started to cry. I was surprised by his strong outburst of feelings because he had not been able to mourn. He is one of those people who rarely cry. Such moments of loosening up provide great relief, particularly in depressive personalities.

After the patient's crying had subsided somewhat, he said, "Those are moments when I have the feeling that there is never enough time. I can sense it: Our time is up again today." Although this was true, I had the impression that the patient also used the time limit to restrict himself and to keep from having any pleasurable fantasies about uniting with me. Therefore I said, "Well, I always have ten seconds time for a bold thought if you dare to tell me one." At this he laughed in a very relaxed way, sat up, and enjoyed staying seated for a moment before he stood up and left the room.

While entering the room for the next session, the patient said, "Today I'm going to be very demanding." It was two minutes before the beginning of the session. The door was ajar, and I was sitting at my desk. He did not want to lie down immediately and sat on the couch, his legs spread apart. I found it strange to sit at my desk while he was sitting on the couch, and said, pointing to the two armchairs, "Then it might be more comfortable to sit over there." "Yes," he said, "today I want to take a good look at you. I have the feeling I don't know you well enough. I realized it recently when we met in town."

We continued on the topic of observing something, of looking very carefully. He didn't pick it up himself, but left it to me to say, "In that regard you have been very restrained." Yes, he said, he had never exactly asked himself whether this was a Freudian or a Jungian analysis. He mentioned that a friend of his had gone to a Jungian. The therapy was over now, and they were going sailing together. The question of whether something similar could happen to us was in the air.

A: And now you had to take a good look. Isn't that so? You think if I were a Freudian, then something of the sort probably could not happen.

P: No, I don't know enough about it at all. At the university I did read *The Interpretation of Dreams* once, but since then I haven't wanted to know anything about it. It's always bothered me when my friends turn to theoretical writings during a personal crisis. Yet, after all, [laughing] you probably have written something at some time, and I could go look for it.

A: Yes, you could.

Then he recalled that he had driven to his home town last Sunday and visited an old friend of his father. He had asked the old man, who was 80 years old, to tell him something about his father. He hadn't spoken to the man for 25 years. He learned once again that his father had been injured in an accident and that he had gone about his work despite having great pain. The pain was caused by cancer, which was diagnosed when Friedrich Y was 6-7 years old; his father died when he was 13. Friedrich Y mentioned further that the Sunday walks had ceased when he was 6 or 7. After that his father had worked all the time, even on Sundays.

Subsequently he remembered a dream about an acquaintance with whom he had business contacts. This man had recently fallen from a fruit tree and was now tied to a wheelchair. In the dream he had thrown the man out of his wheelchair and rolled around with him on the ground, developing a feeling of tenderness in the process.

He was amazed at this because he otherwise had always had arguments and disagreements with this acquaintance. But he had the feeling that it had somehow done him good to reach out once. I linked this to his father and to the feeling that he had brought to this session, namely of being demanding. He laughed. He recalled that he currently did not need much sleep, that he woke up at 5:30 but did not dare to get up because his wife might wake up.

A: Yes, then your mother is sitting there in the room again and watching that you don't demand anything of your father, that means, that you don't go out jogging in the woods early in the morning when you wake up so early.

He thought about whether it had anything to do with the fact that his dose of lithium was already reduced to one tablet a day. Although he still needed a midday nap, he had the feeling that he needed less sleep at night and was strong enough to uproot trees.

Considering the responsibility that I shared for discontinuing the lithium medication, I inquired about his psychiatric consultations and the nature of his high spirits. On further reflection I came to view my concern in the framework of a countertransference reaction. I had sensed in this way that the patient was worried about whether he might act destructively when in closer contact, whether he might develop too much aggressiveness, whether he, in the cheerful mood accompanying his progress, might turn everything topsy-turvy. Not only his wife would be a victim of this expansiveness, but I as well. I therefore made the interpretation that he was on the lookout for limits and restrictions.

From the beginning of the following session Friedrich Y was busy telling me that he had had a celebration on the weekend and was very satisfied with it, as he had been able to develop his professional role. The next night he had had a dream in which he saw himself hiking with his father and going into a shower room in a youth hostel, and that naked women had also been there, which came as a surprise to him. While he was still telling me about it, it became clear that he had enjoyed the view in the dream. Without directly associating to elements of the dream, he continued that he thought over and over again about his father being married twice although he hardly knew anything about his first wife. He had never been able to imagine that, in his father's second marriage, his father and mother ever had anything to do with one another. At his birth his father had already been 40. Laughing, he noted that this "already 40" was an unusual way of expressing premature aging and, in matter of fact hardly justified.

He continued thinking about his father, and now he also recalled that he had learned something from his father, specifically how to look at trees, to look at them like people. In contrast, his mother had insisted that he learn the names of plants and that he know the exact details of all the flowers. This was his mother's world. His father was much more alive when they walked through the woods. He said that his father had also shown him how to make small water wheels out of bark and twigs and that he could still do it, which he did with great enthusiasm.

After the image of his father had been blurred by the pane of frosted glass for a long time, it now seemed to brighten. This happened in direct correspondence to the increasing normalization of his interest in me (i. e., as an individual) and to the revitalization of childhood memories that now surfaced and became accessible to him.

I ended the session with the interpretation that in the dream he had apparently been able to express his wish that his father open his world of women to him. He might, as a boy, have felt that his father did not want to let him into it.

The patient started the following session by saying that he had finally been able to discuss various problems with a colleague. He had expressed his complaints and reservations and dissociated himself, although he had noticed over and over again that he was concerned not to cause the colleague very much suffering.

He then remembered that while coming to the session he had thought about the title he would give his biography if he were to write one. The first detail he recalled was that as a child he had once released the hand brake of a hay wagon, which landed in a pile of manure. "Thus at some time," he said, "I must have been more able to do something like that, until I pulled the brake again. For twenty years I've been braking all the time."

I picked up his comment about being braked and his cautious attempt to release the hand brake and said, "Yes, you've recently made various attempts to release your brake, as well as to make some critical remarks here." This was a reference to the various attempts he had made to take a close look at me, and I had both many positive aspects and some critical ones in mind. To my surprise the patient picked up this line of thought:

P: Yes, for a long time now I've noticed out of the corner of my eye a microphone on the chair in front of you. I've asked myself whether you were planning to make a recording or whether you were even making a recording now. [Tape recordings were not made of this patient; this report is based on detailed notes taken during the sessions.]

A: Even though reason tells you that I wouldn't make any recordings here without your express approval, there seems to be a latent possibility now, a pleasurable idea that you could criticize me very intensely if I did such a thing behind your back.

P: Even though I don't believe you're capable of doing it, it would give me the opportunity here to start a real attack on you.

A: To become fierce.

P: Yes, to take the offensive. Incidentally, I wouldn't mind at all if you made tape recordings here. I can imagine that it's interesting for you.

Proceeding from this brief exchange, the patient returned to the topic of his profession and clearly indicated that he could be more outgoing in some gatherings. He could risk saying things in groups that he otherwise would only have secretly said to the colleague sitting next to him.

A: Yes, you're taking the initiative. You would like to open yourself to others.

P: Yes, I've probably kept many things to myself for too long. And even when I told my wife something, it wasn't enough. Something was incomplete.

The dialogue then returned to the therapeutic situation. The patient said once again, "Looking around in this room and perceiving personal things, it's a very difficult process for me."

Commentary. The course of this therapy raises a number of questions that deserve brief mention. The reader will have noticed the lack of speculation regarding the psychogenesis of the patient's illness as it manifested itself twenty years ago. It can nevertheless be clearly seen in the analyst's countertransference that he was nagged by substantial concerns about whether, after working through the clearly neurotic depressive conflicts, the anticipated release of expansive energy might lead to a destabilization of those sectors of the patient's personality that in psychoanalytic theories are associated with the genesis of psychotic conditions, in particular with manic ones (Abraham 1924; M. Klein 1935; Jacobson 1953, 1971). To understand the dynamics of this case, other components, especially the effects of the long-term adminstration of lithium on the patient's personality, a subject that has previously received little study, have to be taken into consideration (Rüger 1976, 1986; Danckwardt 1978; Schou 1986). Medication that works psychotropically inevitably has a psychodynamic effect in addition to its pharmacologic one. Lithium became, for this patient, the epitome of the prohibitive maternal principle. He plunged from typical adolescent hypomanic experiences, which for him were overpowering, and the medication provided the protective shield that he did not dare to question. With regard to technique, it was therefore important for the analyst, together with the patient, not to focus primarily on discontinuing the lithium treatment, but rather to initially focus on working on the factors disturbing the patient's capacity to work that were linked to his difficulties with his father.

2.3.2 Brother Envy

The psychoanalytic situation stimulates a patient's needs that are rooted in the mother-infant relationship. This relationship, i. e., the mother-child template, constitutes the silent background that makes it inevitable that third parties - e.g., other patients - will at some time be experienced as trouble makers and rivals.

For Käthe X an unexpected pregnancy precipitated intense feelings, which may have stemmed from earlier moments when she had experienced envy and jealousy. Since the patient had a negative attitude toward being pregnant, the first signs of a pregnancy led her to pay increased attention to her own body and to show more interest in women who were pregnant or had just given birth. In the session of analysis described here a presumed childhood experience, which might have only been based on a single fictive memory, was linked to an stress situation she had experienced and to an antagonistic constellation in the therapeutic relationship.

At the beginning of the hour Käthe X described a visit she had paid to a colleague who had just given birth to a son. During the visit she had suddenly noticed her period had come. In her words, "I visit her in the hospital, and then this starts." When the young mother was supposed to nurse her child, Käthe X prodded a colleague who had come along into watching with her,

P: "Let's watch, I want to see this." I simply overpowered her.

A: Take a close look, just like you like to do.

Commentary. This remark was directed at one of the patient's strengths, which she had acquired in her defensive struggle against closeness and desires to fuse. She was particularly gifted in perceiving the personal details that create distance.

P: The colleague I visited is otherwise relatively thin. Now she's got real breasts. Makes her look good. I told my other colleagues about it. The baby is nice and has blue eyes. The others said, "Now it's your turn to have one."

The patient hesitated and became unsettled, so I said:

A: It makes you feel funny, completely different.

P: Yes, I'm all confused. That it starts bleeding now, funny, just like in menstruation.

Then she remembered an acquaintance who had had a miscarriage in the third month. I commented that the impressions she had had during the visit had confused her.

P: I've been to the hospital quite often. Actually, it didn't seem strange to me.

A: This time the situation was different, and you believe you're pregnant. It touches you very personally. The bleeding would mean that you aren't pregnant after all, a kind of negative decision.

Consideration. I hypothesized that there were psychic reasons that the patient had not become preganant previously, yet she herself did not raise the topic.

P: Could be that I've deceived myself. The situation in the hospital room, the solemn mood. It was a dear child. [Pause] The father was also nice. The mother was a little pale. That's not really an impression that scares me.

Since the patient withdrew affectively from the current scene–which made a strong impression on me, inasmuch as I was familiar with the patient's life history - I decided to take an active step to tackle her avoidance and affective reattribution ("solemn mood") and asked a question linking the situation in the hospital with an experience in her past when the birth of her brother had forced her out of her parents' apartment when she was just 2 years old.

A: When Karl, your brother, was born, how must it have been then?

P: It happened at home. I heard it. It wasn't a difficult birth.

A: What does a 2-year-old hear?

P: No idea. I can't remember Karl until we had to go to the children's hospital a few months after he was born. That's the first thing I recall. I can still remember exactly how father pulled me on my sled to the hospital. Karl was in the hospital at the time.

Commentary. This early memory can be considered a relationship paradigm, in the sense described by Mayman and Faris (1960). This paradigm, on which Stiemerling (1974) has published a quantitative study of 500 people, represents the loss of the mother and an intimate relationship to the father.

A: Why was Karl in the hospital?

P: Don't know. Never interested me.

A: This time you were interested in your colleague and her baby. Why now?

P: Yes, I wanted to see the baby. Yes, what was the reason? I don't even have close contact to the colleague. I was interested in the baby and how the mother looks, how she has changed.

A: Just like we're interested in the changes that have recently begun to take place in your body.

P: Yes, yes. How she holds the baby in her arms. She is usually so unfeminine.

A: Well, if she manages to change, then . . . .

The patient interrupted me and continued my own line of thought.

P: Don't know what's wrong now. [Paused about one minute] Now I remember that I talked with colleagues yesterday about cats. We used to have cats. And a pregnant cat is always coming to me now. She's bound to have her kittens at our house. What should I do? A colleague killed a young cat once, simply flushed it down the toilette. And now I'm beginning to feel very funny.

She was freezing, something that always happened when she had to confront stressful subjects that overwhelmed her resistance.

P: I recall that my mother once used the expression for a miscarriage, to flush it down the toilette.

A: It's hard to bear the thought.

P: Yes, my mother had her miscarriage when a letter made it impossible for her to overlook father's adultery. When mother told me, I thought to myself that she had killed the baby.

Commentary. Although this statement by the patient contains a highly ambivalent identification with her mother as her father's lover (inasmuch as the father involved the patient in allusions of an incestuous relationship), it also contains an identification with the aborted baby. She experienced herself to be the aborted baby, which also represented her wish that her brother had been aborted.

A: And something similar is in the offing for you, as if viewing the nursing mother made you aware of something that is completely unthinkable. The sight of Karl at your mother's breast, "If I could just get rid of him!" And your first association corresponds nicely. Karl was gone again and you were satisfied.

P: [Laughing] Yes, yes, that was the right place for him.

After thinking for a moment she again began to speak about her mother's miscarriage.

P: I regretted it. I would have liked to have seen it.

A: Since you couldn't prevent it, you could at least have seen it. What did the intruder look like? How did your mother look? Looking has become one of your strong points.

P: Has it? Do you think so?

The patient was touched by my reference to the fact that her "looking" was rooted in conflict. In my next intervention I therefore referred to a characteristic habit that the patient had often mentioned. She customarily arrived early, in order to see the previous patient leaving my office.

A: The way you look around my office, to see if everything is still in the same place or if I've changed something or removed anything.

P: [Correcting me] Yes, but I don't do it any more, it's different now. Today I've only looked at the potted plant.

The plant, a hibiscus, is on a toy box that I only use occasionally. In the subsequent long period of silence I felt I could sense how she gazed around the office. Innerly I agreed with the patient that what she had said was very accurate, namely that she no longer felt the need, out of mistrust, to inspect the room and its contents for changes; in the meantime she had come to feel comfortable. Then she said matter of factly, "Interesting, the things a toy box can be used for!" Then she recalled a television film in which a boy was featured in two scenes playing with such a toy box: in one he flushed a baby down the toilette, in the other he let a crocodile eat it.

The thought of it made her shiver. She thought it was very bad, the poor baby. I chose, in contrast, to emphasize the aggressive element: "It upsets you to have to observe how this boy can openly give in to his impulses. That he simply eliminates the bothersome baby." The patient responded, "The boy was entirely aware of his rage at his mother, which was very intense." At the same time she made a powerful gesture, clasping her hands and rubbing them together.

P: I'm actually not as angry at my mother as I used to be, and have noticed that my husband and I almost rival for my mother's attention - which really amazes me.

She said this slightly mockingly, surprised because it used to seem completely inconceivable to her, although she had always clearly recognized that she envied her brother at how he managed to gain mother's favor. Mother gave him beautiful things, while she herself only got some money. She always gave Karl the things he had wished. But with her? She could tell her mother for days what she wanted, but it was of no use; her mother never remembered anything. "It's clear," she said, "Joseph [her husband] has taken Karl's place. I notice that I become envious of my husband and how my mother likes him."

Käthe X now summarized how her mother and husband agreed that she should be very happy to have managed to get somebody like him. Her mother simply had not given her enough attention.

A: Yes, we are concerned about whether the same feeling always returns, the feeling namely that somebody else gets my full support, and not you, and you have to make do with money.

P: I was already well on my way to seeing things here just like with my mother, to have just the same experiences.

She seemed to turn cold from inside and began to shiver.

P: When I imagine that the woman who's here before me always marches out with a happy look on her face, that would bother me very much. Then I would think that things are much better between you and her than between us.

Käthe X attributed, in transference, different roles to the previous patient, which were expressions of sibling rivalry. The conflict culminated in the patient identifying the other patient with her brother, which meant that the other patient would have to leave as soon as she felt better. The following interpretation picked up this line of thought: Her envy of the other patient, who should be sent away, would also be directed at herself if she openly displayed something positive.

A: This idea is a great burden on you. You can't permit yourself to be happy here, to make any progress, or at least only in a disguised way. I'm not supposed to notice that you're improving.

P: Yes, that's correct. My progress, I show it ouside. You can't see it then, and I can still be happy about it.

A: There's no danger in showing it to others.

P: But I also show it here. Because I'm happy when things change. But perhaps a little more carefully, cautiously.

In conclusion we will now discuss the patient's feeling of *envy for her brother* in more detail. If we raise the question as to why the patient envied her brother, we strike upon the feeling she repeatedly had as a child, of being excluded from the primary family, a feeling she had in connection with the birth of her brother. Because she had cried and whined a lot even as an infant, after the birth of her brother when she was two she was quartered out of her parents' apartment to her grandparents, who lived in the same house. The family's circumstances lead one to assume that she was an unwanted child and that the birth of her brother was linked to some extent with a normalization. It was thus natural to assume that the patient had received too little motherly attention instead of that she had a hypothetical envy for the "breast," and to assume that in the following years she had identified with this deficit in a way that made her angry and stubborn, as justified by her mother's behavior. There are, in fact, deficit experiences that can be strengthened or weakened by subsequent fantasies. This tension also characterizes the basic pattern of envy and jealousy that M. Klein studied retrospectively and linked to a two- or three-person relationship.

Envy is basically directed at the productive strength: that which the envied breast has to offer is unconsciously taken as the prototype of the capacity to produce, because the breast and the milk that it provides are viewed as the source of life. (M. Klein 1962, p. 185)

As a result of infant research, the chronology of the manifestation of envy and jealousy is a matter of more controversy today, although in a different sense, than at the time of the great controversies between A. Freud and M. Klein (Steiner 1985). Micropsychological studies of the interaction between mother and child make it dubious that the process of splitting, which was linked to the handy metaphors of the "good" and "bad" breast, can be considered the cause of envy.

In contrast to the assumption that splitting involves very early intrapsychic processes, Stern's (1985, p. 252) results indicate that splitting is tied to later symbolic operations. Stern's criticism emphasizes the clinical relevance of splitting processes but severs them from their hypothetical anchoring in early infancy.

The frequently recurring experiences that occurred throughout the childhood of Käthe X led to an extension of the basic pattern: "If I am kind and good, they will keep me; if I am bad and stubborn, then they will drop me." Although a large number of such splitting processes - into good and bad - can be demonstrated in the case of this patient, they must be viewed as the outcome of a development in the course of which recurrent experiences led to the stabilization of this early fundamental experience. The modification of this unconscious schema in the transference situation - as the patient's reaction to another patient she considered in even greater need of assistance and with whom she could unconsciously identify - was an indication of the increase in underlying security that she had already gained in analysis. Rosenfeld (1987, p. 266) emphasized in a posthumously published work that envy is gradually reduced when the patient feels accepted by the analyst. He criticized, in hindsight, the typical Kleinian interpretations of envy, which lead to a dead end. Stereotype interpretations of envy make the patient feel humiliated, resulting in an antitherapeutic *circulus vitiosus.* If, in contrast, the patient feels that he has room for thinking and developing, his envy gradually decreases. Since Rosenfeld was a leading representative of the Kleinian approach, his late change of opinion might be of consequence for all of psychoanalysis.

2.4 Transference and Identification

2.4.1 The Analyst As Object and As Subject

Freud's demand that "the patient should be educated to liberate and fulfil his own nature, not to resemble ourselves" (1919a, p.165) seems to contradict the large, decisive therapeutic significance of the patient's identification with the analyst. At a symposium on the termination of analyses, Hoffer (1950) declared the patient's capacity to identify with the psychoanalyst's functions to be the essential component of the therapeutic process and its success. This topic is thus of fundamental importance for an understanding of the therapeutic process and for the tension between the poles characterized in the following quotations:

> We serve the patient in various functions, as an authority and as substitute for his parents, as a teacher and educator . . . .However much that analyst may be tempted to become a teacher, model and ideal for other people and to create men in his own image, he should not forget that that is not his task in the analytic relationship, and indeed that he will be disloyal to his task if he allows himself to be led on by his inclincations. (Freud 1940a, pp.175, 181)

Yet this raises a number of questions. What does the patient identify with? What are the consequences of the psychoanalytic theory of identification for the optimization of therapy in the sense of facilitating the patient's task of grasping the analyst's functions? What does the psychoanalyst contribute, and how? Is it possible, with regard to the patient's experiencing, to distinguish the functions from the person embodying them? What is the relationship between identification and the demand that the transference neurosis be resolved at the end of analysis?

Identifications with persons from the patient's past are repeated with the object of transference. For various reasons it is useful to distinguish between the analyst's roles as transference object and as a subject. Significant persons from the past become inner "object representations" and ally themselves with "self representations." These inner images and the effects they have on experiencing and behavior form the starting point of the process that Freud (1900a) referred to as the reestablishment of "perceptual identity." This affective-cognitive process leads to the rearrangement of current relations according to old patterns. It follows from this that the patient, on the basis of his unconscious disposition, also attributes roles to the doctor. In the constellation of transference neurosis the analyst can feel the strong pressure that the patient exerts to compel the analyst to accept a role. The patient would like to get to know the psychoanalyst in order to be able to identify himself with him, e.g., as an idealized object. The other person's subjectivity is not taken into consideration in these unconsciously governed and powerful attempts to reestablish a perceptual identity; the other person is made into an "object." By going along with this, the psychoanalyst can recognize the discrepancy between what is attributed to him and what he is. In this way he acquires the knowledge that makes it easier for him to make transference interpretations, as described particularly by F. Morgenthaler (1978). As a result of transference interpretations the past becomes present, opening new opportunities and perspectives.

Qualifying the psychoanalyst as a "new object" thus in our view does not go far enough (Loewald 1960). Although, according to psychoanalytic theory and terminology, the "object" comprehends the "subject," the development of a psychoanalytic "personology" (a two- or more-person psychology) requires that the subjective nature of individuals be fully acknowledged. The analyst fulfills his therapeutic function as a genuine subject and only in part by letting himself be made into an object.

The attempt to avoid directly influencing the patient has, in connection with Freud's mirror metaphor, contributed to the fact that the role identificatory processes play in therapy has been neglected although they have great significance for a cure. We want to modify rigidified and sedimented "object identifications" by helping the patient make new experiences. The subject pursuing this goal, i.e., the analyst, must be acceptable to the patient; he should not stand out among the "average expected environments" in the sense described by Hartmann (1939), in order not to precipitate xenophobic reactions. However since the special status of the psychoanalytic dyad differs substantially from routinized communication, in which only clichés are exchanged and which is itself a kind of mirroring of a rigidified state, the situation is novel, characterized by a quality of strangeness.

Although the transference neurotic repetition – itself strongly dependent on the situative conditions created by the psychoanalyst – determines the form and content of observable phenomena, the identification with the psychoanalyst's functions provides insight into previously unknown, unconscious connections and new experiences. Sterba (1940, originally published in 1929) emphasized the therapeutic significance of identification in an early article which, in contrast to his later publication (1934) on therapeutic ego splitting, has remained relatively unknown.

The analyst assists the ego, attacked by the id, offering it the possibility of an identification which satisfies the reality testing needs of the ego. This identification of the reality testing parts of the patient's ego is made possible by the fact that the analyst continuously observes and interprets to the patient the psychological situation without prejudice.

The invitation to this identification comes from the analyst. From the beginning of treatment, comments are made by the analyst about the work they will have to accomplish in common during the cure. Many phrases such as, "Let us recall what you dreamed, or thought, or did there," used by the analyst contain this invitation to identification with him as it is implied every time the analyst uses "we" to refer to the patient and himself. This identification with the analyst is based first on the patient's wish for recovery and second on the positive transference.... This identification is based finally on a narcissistic satisfaction resulting from *his participation in the intellectual work of gaining insight* during the analysis. (Sterba 1940, p. 371, emphasis added)

In this passage Sterba came close to recognizing the important fact that the identification can also be directed at the joint work and not just at an object. Thus the form of communication that can lead the patient out of the neurosis is itself one of the major issues.

Although the intensified formation of "we-bonds" is to a certain extent not unproblematic, because it can have a seductive effect or make contradiction and independence more difficult, we nevertheless believe that the "standard technique's" understanding of psychoanalytic rules has impeded the identification with the psychoanalyst's functions and the formation of we-bonds as called for by Sterba. The primary unity of person and function is associated with complications, which in our opinion can be resolved in the course of treatment, e.g., in identification leading to the adoption of self-reflection. The opposite attempt, namely to carry the incognito to an extreme and provide the therapeutic functions impersonally, fails for anthropological and psychoanalytic-psychogenetic reasons.

The fact that we put things in a new context and thus give them a new meaning always implies that we inform the patient of our views and divulge ourselves personally. Since, from a psychoanalytic perspective, an individual's personal identity develops both from within to without and from without to within, there are often limits on how much external influence can be exerted, and not only for practical reasons. Although we reject a purely social psychological explanation of identity development (from without to within), its theses, as argued for example by Luckmann, have serious consequences for our understanding of interpersonal mirroring.

An individual does not experience himself in an unmediated way. Only the environment can experience an individual in an unmediated way, only the environment gives itself to consciousness directly. An individual experiences others in social relationships. These others are given, unmediated, by their physical presence. The physical presence of fellow humans (or more generally, of others) is taken as a field for expressing their conscious processes. Yet insofar as the other's experiences are directed back at him, "the individual is mirrored in his fellow humans." In social relationships, which take place in a common environment, the individual experiences himself via his fellow humans. The capacity for interactive mirroring is the fundamental condition for the individual human being to form a personal identity. (Luckmann 1979, p. 299)

This understanding of mirroring makes it possible to grasp Freud's mirror metaphor in the sense of mediated self-reflection (see Vol.1, Sect. 8.4).

Yet there are a number of questions regarding the modified mirror metaphor that cannot go unmentioned even if answering them goes beyond the framework of the cases discussed in the following sections. The form of communication – therapeutically helpful and leading to changes – that is conceptualized as "mediated self-reflection" is inadequate both theoretically and practically because more is involved than the perception of previously unconscious "contents" and the emotions linked with them that are conveyed to the patient. Discovery and rediscovery take place within the framework of a special form of communication that makes it possible for the patient to find a new relationship to himself. The nature of the relationship that the psychoanalyst exhibits toward unconscious material - and this implies *his* relationship to himself, as elaborated by Tugendhat (1979) - becomes the model for the process of transformation that also changes the patient's relationship to himself.

2.4.2 Identification with the Analyst's Functions

Amalie X came to psychoanalysis because the severe restrictions she felt on her self-esteem had reached the level of depression in the last few years. Her entire life history since puberty and her social role as a woman had suffered from the severe strain resulting from her hirsutism. Although it had been possible for her to hide her stigma - the virile growth of hair all over her body - from others, the cosmetic aids she used had not raised her self-esteem or eliminated her extreme social insecurity (Goffman 1974). Her feeling of being stigmatized and her neurotic symptoms, which had already been manifest before puberty, strengthened each other in a vicious circle; scruples from compulsion neurosis and different symptoms of anxiety neurosis impeded her personal relationships and, most importantly, kept the patient from forming closer heterosexual friendships.

The analyst offered this woman, who was hard working in her career, cultivated, single, and quite feminine despite her stigma, treatment because he was relatively sure and confident that it would be possible to change the significations she attributed to her stigma. In general terms, he proceeded from the position that our body is not our only destiny and that the attitude which significant others and we ourselves have to our bodies can also be decisive. Freud's (1912d, p. 189) paraphrase of Napolean's expression to the effect that our anatomy is our destiny must be modified as a consequence of psychoanalytic insights into the psychogenesis of sexual identity. Sexual role and core identity originate under the influence of psychosocial factors on the basis of one's somatic sex (see Lichtenstein 1961; Stoller 1968, 1975; Kubie 1974).

Clinical experience justified the following assumptions. A virile stigma strengthens penis envy and reactivates oedipal conflicts. If the patient's wish to be a man had materialized, her hermaphroditic body scheme would have become free of conflict. The question "Am I a man or a woman?" would then have been answered; her insecurity regarding her identity, which was continuously reinforced by her stigma, would have been eliminated; and self image and physical reality would then have been in agreement. It was impossible for her to maintain her unconscious fantasy, however, in view of physical reality. A virile stigma does not make a man of a woman. Regressive solutions such as reaching an inner security despite her masculine stigma by identifiying herself with her mother revitalized old mother-daughter conflicts and led to a variety of defensive processes. All of her affective and cognitive processes were marked by ambivalence, so that she had difficulty, for example, deciding between different colors when shopping because she linked them with the qualitites of masculine or feminine.

When structuring the psychoanalytic situation and dealing with such problems, the analyst must pay extra attention to not letting the asymmetry of the relationship excessively strengthen the patient's feeling of being different. This is important because the idea of being different - that is, the question of similarity and difference, of identity and nonidentitiy - forms the general framework within which unconscious problems appear. In this case the analyst and patient succeeded relatively quickly in establishing a good working relationship, creating the preconditions for recognizing the internalization of earlier forms of interaction with primary reference persons - parents and teachers - during the development of the transference neurosis. The correction that was achieved can be seen in the changes in her self-esteem, in her increased security, and in the disappearance of her symptoms (see Neudert et al. 1987).

The two excerpts of treatment given below are linked, despite the time that elapsed between them, by the fact that each is concerned with enabling the patient to make new identifications as a result of the analysis of transference. The analyst's "head" became the surrogate of old, unconscious "objects," and its contents the representative of new opportunities. The representation on the "object," which is simultaneously self-representation, made it possible to establish a distance because the analyst made his head available and kept it too. Thus he became a model for closeness and distance. This example clearly demonstrates the therapeutic effect that insight into the connections between the analyst's perceptions and thoughts can have.

We have selected this case because in our opinion it is suited to provide several lines of support to our argument. Although the head acquired sexual importance as a result of the process of unconscious displacement, this displacement did not alter anything regarding the primacy of intellectual communication between the patient and the analyst about what was sought hidden inside the head. The search for knowledge was directed at sexuality. This secret and well-guarded (repressed) treasure was assumed to be in the head (as the object of transference) because of the unconscious displacement. The rediscovery of "displacement" brought something to light that was "new" to the patient.

The ideas that formed the background for my interpretations are given in addition to the abridged verbatim dialogue. These "Considerations" were subsequently added to the interpretations and the patient's responses. It is obvious that I was led not only by the ideas described here when I arrived at my interpretations. However interpretations may be created, any interpretation actually made to the patient must be aligned along "cognitive" criteria, as demanded by Arlow (1979). My comments refer to the "cognitively" and "rationally" groundable "end products" - my interpretations - and neglect their genesis and the intuitive, unconscious components in their genesis. The source of each of my analytic thoughts thus remains open. If we assume that the analyst's perceptive apparatus is steered by his theoretical knowledge, which may have become preconscious, then it is very difficult to trace the genesis of interpretations back to their "beginnings." For example, theoretical knowledge about displacement also facilitates preconscious perception; it pervades the analyst's intuition and blends with the countertransference (in a wider sense).

The patient suffered from severe feelings of guilt, which were actualized in her relationship to me. The Biblical law of an eye for an eye and a tooth for a tooth was reinforced in her experiencing because of her sexual desires. Her life historical role model for the contents of her transference neurosis was a fantasized incestuous relationship to her brother. The increase in inner tension led the patient to reconsider the idea of dedicating her life to the church as a missionary or to contemplate committing suicide. (As a young girl she had wanted to become a nun and nurse but given up this idea after a trial period because the pious confinement became too much for her. Leaving also helped her establish some distance to the strict Biblical commandments.) Now she wielded her "old" Bible against me, "in a fight to the finish." This fight took place at different levels, and the patient invented a series of similes for them. She had the feeling that the analyst's dogma, the "Freud Bible," could not be reconciled with her Christian Bible. Both bibles, however, contained a prohibition of sexual relations with the anaylst.

The patient struggled for her independence and needs, which she defended against both of these bibles. She developed an intense defense against my interpretations, and she had the feeling that I knew in advance exactly "what's going to happen." She felt humiliated because her detours and distractions had been detected. She had the intense desire to mean something to me and to live in me; she thought about giving me an old, lovely, and wonderful clock that would strike every hour for me (and for her).

In this phase of treatment one topic took on special significance and intensity; this was her interest for my head. What had she learned from measuring my head? In a similar situation Amalie X had once said that for a long time she had thought that I was looking for confirmation of what was already there - in books, in my thoughts, in my head. She wished that something completely new would come out. She herself looked for interpretations and made an effort to understand my ideas.

The patient mentioned her strict boss, who had unjustly criticized her and for whom she was no match.

A: You presume that I'm sitting behind you and saying "wrong, wrong."

Consideration. This transference interpretation was based on the following assumption. The patient attributed me a "superego function." This interpretation took the burden off her and gave her the courage to rebel (the patient had recognized long before that I was different and would not criticize her, but she was not sure and could not believe it because she still had considerable unconscious aggressions against old objects). I assumed that she had much more intense transference feelings and that both the patient and I could tolerate an increase in tension. I repeated her concern that I could not bear it and finally formulated the following statement: "Thus it's a kind of a fight to the finish, with a knife" (not specifying who has the knife). I meant for this allusion to phallic symbolism to stimulate her unconscious desires. It was an overdose! The patient reacted by withdrawing. Assumption: self-punishment.

P: Sometimes I have the feeling that I would like to rush at you, grab your neck, and hold you tight. Then I think, "He can't take it and will suddenly fall over dead.

A: That I can't take it.

The patient varied this topic, expressing her overall concern about asking too much of me and of my not being able to take the struggle.

A: It's a kind of a fight to the finish, with a knife.

P: Probably.

She then reflected that she had always, throughout the years, given up prematurely, before the struggle had really begun, and withdrawn.

P: And I don't doubt any more that it was right for me to withdraw. After such a long time I have the urge to give up again.

A: Withdrawal and self-sacrafice in the service of the mission instead of struggling to the end.

P: Exactly, nerve racking.

Consideration. She was very anxious about losing her object.

A: Then I would have the guarantee of being preserved. Then you would have broken off my test prematurely.

We continued on the topic of what I can take and whether I let myself be carried along by her "delusion." The patient had previously made comparisons to a tree, asking whether she could could take anything from it, and what it would be. I returned to this image and raised the question of what she wanted to take along by breaking off branches.

Consideration. Tree of knowledge - aggression.

P: It's your neck, it's your head. I'm often preoccupied with your head.

A: Does it stay on? You're often preoccupied with my head?

P: Yes, yes, incredibly often. From the beginning I've measured it in every direction.

A: Hum, it is ....

P: It's peculiar, from the back to the front and from the bottom. I believe I'm practicing a real cult with your head. This is just too funny. With other people I'm more likely to see what they have on, just instinctively, without having to study them.

Consideration. Create shared things as primary identification. [This topic was discussed for a long period of time, with some pauses and "hums" by the analyst.]

P: It's simply too much for me. I sometimes ask myself afterwards why I didn't see it, it's such a simple connection. I am incredibly interested in your head. Naturally, what's inside too. No, not just to take it along, but to get inside your head, yes above all, to get inside.

Consideration. The partial withdrawal of the object increased her unconscious phallic aggressiveness.

The patient spoke so softly that I did not even understand "get inside" at first, mistaking it for "put inside." The patient corrected me and added a peculiar image, "Yes, it's so hard to say in front of 100 eyes."

P: Get inside, the point is to get inside and to get something out.

I saw this getting inside and taking something out in connection with the subject of fighting. It was possible to put the sexual symbolism resulting from the displacement from the bottom to the top to therapeutic use by referring to a story that the patient had told in an earlier session. A woman she knew had prevented her boyfriend from having intercourse with her and had masturbated him, which she had described by analogy to head hunter jargon as "head shrinking." The unconscious castration intention dictated by her penis envy created profound sexual anxiety and was paralleled by general and specific defloration anxieties. These anxieties led in turn to frustration, but one which she herself had instinctively caused, as a neurotic self-perpetuating cycle. The rejection of her sexual and erotic desires that now occurred unconsciously strengthened the aggressive components of her wanting to have and possess (penis desire and penis envy).

A: That you want to have the knife in order to be able to force your way in, in order to get more out.

After we exchanged a few more thoughts, I gave an explanation, saying that there was something very concrete behind our concern with the topics of getting inside, head, and the fight to the end with a knife.

A: The woman you mentioned didn't speak of head shrinkers for nothing.

P: That's just the reason I broke off this line of thought. [For about ten minutes the patient had switched to a completely different subject.]

After expressing her insight into her resistance to an intensification of transference, she again evaded the topic. She interrupted the intensification, making numerous critical comments.

P: Because at the moment it can be so stupid, so distant. Yes, my wishes and desires are the point, but it's tricky, and I get real mad, and when head and head shrinking are now ....

She laughed, immediately expressed her regret, and was silent. I attempted to encourage her.

A: You know what's in your head.

P: Right now I'm not at all at home in mine. How do I know what will happen tomorrow. I have to think back. I was just on dogma and your head, and if you want to go down . . .[to a shrunken head]. It's really grotesque.

Consideration. I first mentioned the shrunken heads because I assumed that the patient would be more cooperative if the envious object relationship could be replaced by a pleasurable one.

Then the patient came to speak of external things. She decribed how she saw me and how she saw herself, independent of the head, which then again became the focus of attention in a general sense.

A: By thinking about the head you're attempting to find out what you are and what I am.

P: I sometimes measure your head as if I wanted to bend your brain.

The patient then described the associations she had once had when she had seen my picture printed somewhere.

P: I discovered something completely different at the time. There was an incredible amount of envy of your head. An incredible amount. Now I'm getting somewhere at any rate. Whenever I think of the dagger and of some lovely dream.

Consideration. The patient obviously felt caught. She felt humiliated by her own association, as if she had guessed my assumption as to what the envy might refer to. In this case I would have rushed ahead of her, so to speak.

A: Humiliating, apparently to you, as if I already knew which category to put it in when you express envy, as if I already knew what you are envious of.

P: That came just now because you had referred to the shrunken heads, which I didn't even make. But what fascinated me is this fight to the finish, for the knife, to get to the hard part . . . . Yes, I was afraid that you couldn't take it. My fear that you can't take it is very old. My father could never take anything. You wouldn't believe how bland I think my father is. He couldn't take anything.

Consideration. A surprising turn. The patient's insecurity and her anxiety about taking hold developed "unspecifically" on her father.

A: It's all the more important whether my head is hard. That increases the hardness when you take hold.

P: Yes, you can take hold harder . . .and can – simply – fight better.

The patient then made numerous comments to the effect of how important it was that I did not let myself be capsized, and she returned to her envy. Then she mentioned her university studies again, and how she used to "measure" the heads of the others. Then she introduced a new thought.

P: I want to cut a little hole in your head and put in some of my thoughts.

Consideration. An objectivistic image of "intellectual" exchange as a displacement?

The patient's idea about the two-sided nature of the exchange led me to recognize another aspect of this fight. It was also an expression of how important it was to me that she remain a part of the world (and in contact with me), and digress neither into masochistic self-sacrifice nor into suicide.

P: That came to me recently. Couldn't I exchange a little of your dogma for mine. The thought of such an exchange made it easier for me to say all of this about your head.

A: That you continue coming here so that you can continue filling my head with your thoughts.

Consideration. Fertilization in numerous senses - balance and acknowledgment of reciprocity.

P: Oh yes, and mentioning really productive ideas.

The patient returned to the thoughts and fantasies she had had before the session, about how she had been torn back and forth. Whether she had a future at all, and whether she shouldn't withdraw in some way or other and put an end to it all.

At the beginning I had attempted to relieve her intense feelings of guilt with regard to her destructiveness. I picked up the idea once again that her thoughts about my stability were in proportion to her degree of aggressiveness. The patient could only gain security and further unfold her destructiveness if she found strong, unshakable stability. The topic of dogmatism probably belonged in this context. Although she criticized it - both her own Bible and my presumed belief in the Freud bible - it also provided her security, and for this reason the dogmatism could not be too rigorous or pronounced.

A: Naturally you wouldn't like a small hole; you would like to put in a lot, not a little. The idea of a small or large hole was your shy attempt to test my head's stability.

My subsequent interpretation was that the patient could also see more through a larger hole and could touch it. She picked up this idea:

P: I would even like to be able to go for a walk in your head.

She elaborated on this idea and emphasized that even earlier, i.e., before that day's session, she had often thought to herself how nice it would be to relax in me, to have a bench in my head. Very peacefully she mentioned that I could say, when looking back on my life when I die, that I had had a lovely, quiet, and peaceful place to work.

Consideration. Quiet and peacefulness clearly had a regressive quality, namely of completely avoiding the struggle for life.

The patient now viewed her entering the motherhouse as if a door had been wide open and she had turned away from life. She then drew a parallel to the beginning of the session, when the door was open.

P: I really didn't have to drill my way in. Yes, there I could leave the stuggle outside, I could also leave you outside, and you could keep your dogmas.

A: Hum.

P: And then I wouldn't fight with you.

A: Yes, but then you and your dogma would not be afraid of mine. In that setting of peace and quiet everything would remain unchanged, but the fact that you interfere in my thoughts and enter my head shows that you do want to change something, that you can and want to change something.

About five minutes into the next session, the patient returned to my head and measuring it and to the fact that it had disturbed her that I had started talking about the shrunken heads.

P: I told you so. Why do you simply want to slip down from the head?

She then described how she had hardly arrived at home before she recalled the thoughts she had had when she had said hello but then had completely forgotten during the session.

P: To me, he [the analyst] looks as if he is in his prime, and then I thought about the genitals and the shrunken heads. [But she quickly pushed this thought aside, and it was completely gone.] When you started with the shrunken heads, I thought, "Where has he got that again?"

The next topic was the question of my security and my dogmatism, and it was clear that the patient had taken a comment I had once completely undogmatically made about Freud and Jung (I have forgotten what it was) to be dogmatic. She then thought about living a full life, about the moment when everything stopped for her and she became "ascetic," and about whether everything could be revived. Then she again mentioned fighting and my head.

P: I was really afraid of tearing it off. And today I think that it's so stiff and straight, and I think to myself, "I somehow can't really get into my head. I'm not at home. Then how should I get into yours?"

The patient then began to speak about an aunt who was sometimes so very hard that you might think you were facing a wall. She then continued about how hard and how soft she would like her head to be. Her fantasies revolved, on the one hand, around quiet and security; on the other hand, she was concerned about what might be hidden in her head and the danger of it consuming her.

Consideration. This obviously involved a regressive movement. The patient could not find any quiet and relaxation because her sexual desires were linked with pregenital fantasies, which returned in projected form because they were in danger of being consumed. These components were given their clearest, and in a certain sense also their ultimate, expression in an Indian story the patient later associated, in which mothers gave pleasure to their little sons by sucking on their penises but bit them off in the process.

The comparisons of the heads and their contents always revolved around the question of whether they went together or not.

P: The question of how you have your thoughts and how I have mine . . . .Thoughts stand for many things . . . .

A: How they meet, how they rub off on one another, how far they penetrate, how friendly or unfriendly they are.

P: Yes, exactly.

A: Hum, well.

P: You said that a little too smooth.

The patient thought about all the things that scared her and returned again to the shrunken heads.

P: There I feel too tied to sexuality. The jump was too big.

The topic was continued in the question of her speed and of the consideration I pay to her and her speed.

P: But it is true; naturally it wasn't just your head but your penis too.

Amalie X was now in a position, with phases of increasing and receding anxiety, to distinguish between pleasure from discovering intellectual connections and sexual pleasure. The couch became her mental location of sexual union, and her resting in my head the symbol of pregenital harmony and ultimately the location of shared elements and insight. This aspect became even clearer a little later.

With regard to the patient's symptoms, the topic of the sessions was characterized by her anxiety about having injured herself, which was a reaction to a harmless cystitis. The patient suffered from a constant urge to urinate, which she assumed might be the result of having injured herself while masturbating. With the aid of anatomy books, she had tried to imagine her genital region. She localized her complaints to her entire abdomen. She imagined that she had destroyed a muscle by pushing and rubbing it, similar to how the sphincter muscle of the bladder can be damaged during difficult births. The patient was greatly disturbed by this anxiety, and her sleep and capacity to work were also disturbed. She was afraid that someone might notice a wet spot on her pants. Destructive fantasies predominated in her masturbation.

Despite her growing complaints the patient showed trust. She expected a clear answer about whether it was anatomically possible for her to have injured herself while masturbating. My assurance that this was not the case reduced her anxiety and temporarily provided her with great relief but also with the feeling of having blackmailed me or of having "somehow seduced me." This was to be a source of "new dangers." Blackmail, confession, and seduction became mixed. She was afraid that I would "lead her somewhere where everything was permitted," as if there were no place for guilt in my point of view. The patient alternated between two images; in one she viewed me as the seducer, in the other as the judge of public morals. Retreating to pious religiosity seemed to her the way to escape the threatening boundlessness in herself, which would muddle and destroy everything. Yet her religiosity still meant little to her, especially since she had loosened her ties to the church prior to analysis because she had not felt any relief of her distress but repeatedly felt new stress from the commandments.

In this phase there was a decisive turn in the relation between transference and doctor-patient relationship, which resulted from the fact that I had offered an explanation for my technique. Amalie X took this as a sign of my trust. This facilitated her identification with my function as analyst of providing insights. My willingness to inform her of my thoughts, which appeared to her as a special treasure, raised both the relationship and the transference to a new level. Having a view and being able to gain insights, i. e., being less excluded, made her aggressive intruding into my "head," her drilling a hole, superfluous, or in other words brought us closer together and let her participate at a friendly, pleasurable, playful level.

It is nothing special for me to offer a patient insight into my psychoanalytic thinking. In my view it is a completely banal situation, which however might provide the patient an entirely new experience. In a displaced transference to her supervisor she exhibited an "immense respect," as shown by her boss' lack of time, which did not permit her to clarify a small dispute in another talk.

The patient apparently experienced the trust I showed as an sign of great freedom, as if I had freed myself from some inhibition. Then we worked through the fact that she had known for a long time what my opinion about important items in her experiencing was and that she was in fact entitled to intrude and know.

The patient mentioned a problem with her boss and made it clear that she felt freer toward him. She attributed her success in an exaggerted way to psychoanalysis and to me. Then we turned to the question of encouragement and I said that the wish she expressed for encouragement deprived her of being able to enjoy her own success. The session continued about the excessive respect she still had.

A: That is getting quite a bit smaller by itself.

P: I still have a terrible fear of being thrown out.

(For a long period of time the patient had regularly left my office a few minutes before the end of the session, creating a minisymptom. The numerous determinants of this behavior were never a particular topic of concern. The patient's behavior changed by itself step by step. Among other things, the patient wanted to avoid being sent away, which could "annul" an entire meeting.)

To my surprise the patient asked, "Have you noticed that you've just given me an explanation for your technique, something you rarely do?" In response to a question, I find out that the patient was impressed by my statement that something decreases of its own accord. (In retrospect, I thus did give her encouragement, namely that many things happen on their own and not everything has to be fought for.) The patient then spoke for a long time about how unusually positive she had experienced my statement to be and that she viewed it as an sign of my freedom.

P: Don't you like the freedom that I attribute to you?

I showed my surprise at her belief that she was not supposed to intrude in my thoughts and learn the reasons for my statements and ideas, although she had known this for a long time.

P: But that I could say it, that is what I found incredibly new.

A: Then it is almost as if my saying that you may know something that is completely natural and that you have known for a long time was a sign of approval.

P: There was more to it, namely the image you've always had for me, simply that you protect your treasure. [She laughed.] I've always had the feeling . . .head, book, and all the things, and when you open your own head, then I don't have to drill, and that is simply something completely different. It's just an openness or freedom that exudes from you. A proof of trust, I think, when you say, "I do it for this and that reason . . . .I think it is this or that." It seems to be different if you say it or if I say it to you.

With regard to the open book it must be added that the patient in the meantime had read a publication of mine and a second one I had jointly authored with my wife. The patient had somehow attributed commandments prohibiting the acquisition of knowledge to the "Freud bible," and she was apparently surprised that I viewed her curiosity as something natural, just like her gathering of information about my family background. And with regard to my Christian Bible, even before beginning analysis she had had a vague idea about my far-reaching family ties.

New and more intense transference fantasies developed with the increase in the patient's trust and her identification with my function as analyst in helping her achieve insights. A continuous working relationship was thus assured, which was symbolized by the "stable, reliable face," by the "I-am-there-face" of the psychoanalyst, and by his "warm hands."

3 Countertransference

Introduction

As we explained in the first volume (Chap. 3), the history of countertransference exemplifies the rediscovery of complementarity as the fundamental principle of social interaction in psychoanalysis. If we acknowledge that Heimann (1950) explicitly grounded the positive value of countertransference, then we may consider the introduction of the concept of interaction into the discussion of psychoanalytic theories as characteristic of the next stage.

> The effects of each psychotherapeutic interaction, regardless of its provenance, are doubtlessly reciprocal. Yet the doing of the one is not the action of the other; ... the therapist's reactions in particular are partially balanced by his reflection, i. e., by his consideration of the intended, desired, expected, and feared reactions that the patient would like to precipitate. This is the case because, first, according to Freud thinking and reflecting in the psychotherapeutic situation comprise a trial action and, second, the affective precipitants *inevitably* have some effect within the professional relationship. (Thomä 1981, p. 391)

Of the various theories of interaction, the ones that Blumer (1973) used the fortunate term "symbolic interactionism" to refer to are particularly useful in psychoanalysis. According to Weiss (1988), this term refers to an approach to research whose primary premise is that individuals act toward subjects and objects on the basis of what these subjects and objects mean to them. Knowledge of the theories of *intersubjectivity*, for example as they have been summarized by Joas (1985), make countertransference phenomena more comprehensible. Mead, one of the leading representatives of symbolic interactionism, wrote in his study *Mind, Self, and Society* (1934):

> We are more or less unconsciously seeing ourselves as others see us. We are unconsciously addressing ourselves as others address us .... We are calling out in the other person something we are calling out in ourselves, so that unconsciously we take over these attitudes. We are unconsciously putting ourselves in the place of others and acting as others act. I want simply to isolate the general mechanism here, because it is of very fundamental importance in the development of what we call self-consciousness and the appearance of the self. We are, especially through the use of the vocal gestures, continually arousing in ourselves those responses which we call out in other persons, so that we are taking the attitudes of the other persons into our own conduct. The critical importance of language in the development of human experience lies in this fact that the stimulus is one that can react upon the speaking individual as it reacts upon the other. (Mead 1934, p. 69)

Role theory has enriched our conceptual repertoire for a new understanding of the processes of transference and countertransference by introducing the inseparably linked concepts of role and self:

Playing a role is related, in colloquial language, to the theater, and many of us would not like to see our professional activity and its serious implications for human beings classified on the basis of this understanding of role [although the concept of role was borrowed there]. Yet we acknowledge and appreciate the fact that Habermas drew on the stage model to interpret the psychoanalytic situation. In fact, in the clinical situation we often speak very naively about the role the psychoanalyst must now be playing in a patient's transference. (Thomä 1981, p. 392)

In Sect. 3.4 of Vol. 1, after fully acknowledging Mead's contribution, we described an extension of the stage model. One aspect of the psychoanalyst's professional role is that he is sensitive to both the patient's emotions and his own affects but - and this is the crucial point in what is called controlling countertransference - without transforming them into action. In providing interpretations the psychoanalyst fulfills his professional role as well as goes beyond it. The language he uses in an interpretative comment reveals his thoughts - and his self as well - even if the comment is restricted to a patient's minute, detailed problem and although he may believe he has completely withdrawn his personal views.

Role and self thus take on concrete form in social interaction, which provides a basis for understanding them. Sandler et al. have accordingly pointed out "that transference need not be restricted to the illusory apperception of another person ..., but can be taken to include the unconsciuous (and often subtle) attempts to manipulate or to provoke situations with others which are a concealed repetition of earlier experiences and relationships" (1973, p. 48).

Beckmann (1974) systematically investigated the phenomena of symmetry and asymmetry in the assignment of roles in the transference-countertransference configuration during the process of diagnostic evaluation, but his study has not attracted the attention of clinicians. He refers to the significance of repetition compulsion; it is the means by which complementarity becomes the rigidified role relationship that the analyst personally experiences as an actor on the stage of the analytic situation. Unconscious role relationships lead to "cyclical psychodynamic patterns," to use Strupp and Binder's (1984, pp. 72ff.) description. In this explanation, the psychodynamic patterns are understood to consist of repeated interpersonal transactions that perpetuate themselves, as in vicious circles. This is also the fundamental aspect of psychoanalytic interaction diagnoses; according to Sandler (1976), the analyst must demonstrate the willingness to adopt the particular role in order to gain knowledge and in turn to make such diagnoses.

The relatively constant situation offered in therapy makes it possible to actualize the rigid structures that have molded the patient's experiencing. The analyst's special function facilitates both his complementary and concordant identification with the patient. Both of these positions have the features of an object-reference relationship, in which sometimes the one side seems to be emphasized and sometimes the other.

Transference and countertransference reactions can be understood in this context as communicative and interactive processes in which unconscious dispositions selectively affect the perception of external precipitating factors, i. e., affect the status of situative stimuli. Numerous variations of the well-known simile of how lock and key fit together could be mentioned. The more a patient is bound in his relationships to a specific pattern, the stronger the pressure on the analyst to adopt the corresponding complementary or concordant role. Lock and key depend on one another. Wittgenstein coined the following aphorism for Freud's "idea": "The lock is not destroyed in insanity, just altered; the old key cannot unlock it any longer, just a different key can" (Wittgenstein 1984, p. 496). Instead of further extending this metaphorical description, we prefer to draw on the available knowledge about regulatory processes in affective and cognitive microinteraction (Krause 1983; U.Moser 1984; Zeppelin 1987; see also Vol.1, Sect. 9.3). This knowledge is corroborated by the results of research in modern developmental psychology, which has discovered convincing evidence on mother-child intersubjectivity (Lichtenberg 1983a; see Vol.1, Sect. 1.8).

In the first two sections of this chapter (Sects. 3.1 and 3.2) we give examples of concordant and complementary countertransference. We follow Racker's statement that the analyst's identification with the object with which the patient identifies him and the accompanying pathological process must be so brief and so moderate that they do not interfere with the analytic work (see Racker 1978, p. 78).

The subject of retrospective attribution and retrospective fantasy acquires fundamental significance. In Sects. 3.4 and 3.5 we discuss, with reference to specific examples, the controversial questions of how the anaylst lets his patient share in the countertransference or how he inadvertantly attempts to protect himself by employing irony. A critical commentary to the example we give in Sect. 3.6 deepens the self-psychological understanding of countertransference. Finally, in Sect. 3.7, in our explanation of countertransference we arrive at the topic of projective identification. The burdensome side of countertransference is very accurately described by Racker when he, in an easily comprehensible statement based on a verse by Nestroy, writes:

> We thus admit that we sometimes lose our understanding, but not completely, just enough that we notice our pathological countertransference and can diagnose it, in order to use this perception later, when we have control of the countertransference, for the analysis of the patient's transference processes. (Racker 1978, p. 76)

Whatever the patient precipitates in the analyst, it is the analyst's business and duty to fulfill his therapeutic tasks in the patient's interest. It is not easy for the analyst to make his role in this "impossible profession" harmonize with his personal ego and private life. We take part in a double, a multifaceted life; this is what one of the philosophical fathers of the stage model, Schopenhauer, had in mind when he wrote:

> Here in the realm of quiet reflection that which completely preoccupies and moves man appears cold, colorless, and for the moment foreign; here is is merely an onlooker and observer. In this withdrawal into reflection he resembles an actor who played his role and takes a place among the audience until it is his turn again. From his seat he calmly watches whatever may be happening, even if it were the preparation for his death (in the play), and then returns and acts and suffers as he has to. Human calmness proceeds from this double life and is so different from the lack of contemplation of the animal realm, the calmness after contemplation and a conscious decision or acknowledged necessity to do what is most important and often most terrible, the calmness with which someone coldbloodedly lets something be done to himself or commits a deed: suicide, execution, duel, dangers of every kind. (Schopenhauer 1973, p. 139)

3.1 Concordant Countertransference

In Sect. 3.4 of the first volume we described, following Racker (1957), that in concordant transference the analyst experiences feelings similar to those of the patient, which is a consequence of his identification with the patient. In classifying jointly experienced emotions within the framework of psychoanalytic theory, according to Racker there are concordant identifications that refer to the superego, the ego, and the id personality components. We now report about concordant countertransference from two sessions of treatment.

Ignaz Y was in a difficult situation following his divorce. He was constantly having problems arranging the legal aspects of his debts, which he had acquired as a result of the life style that his former wife had forced him into. His desperate internal and external situation intensified his longing for a caring father and the corresponding transference. The patient, who had grown up in Switzerland, felt homeless again and sought more support in analysis. On numerous occasions we considered increasing the frequency from three to four sessions a week. Ignaz Y paid the fee himself. He did not display any of the symptoms of illness that would have justified psychotherapy under the framework of the health insurance system. Since increasing the frequency would have led to further burdens, it was necessary to carefully weigh the investment and the gain.

He said that he was confronted by new financial demands and that it was urgent for him to see his lawyer. He also said he had to put up firm resistance against always being burdened with new financial demands, saying literally, "There has to be a limit somewhere." Hearing the word "limit," I asked myself how much strain the patient could bear. Could he stand the pressure? Would he cross the border to start over again in Switzerland?

At this point the patient actually began to speak about his family. His sister had sent him a letter: "Well, at least one positive sign." She had also left the family home - just like he had when he went to the university - moving to a larger city closer to the German border and thus making it easier for him to visit her.

I was concerned by the fact that he had previously said little about his sister. I knew that their parents had given her, their legitimate child, preferential treatment. The patient had been born out of wedlock, his parents not marrying until he started school.

Ignaz Y continued his story before I could say anything about this. One of his supervisors, who was also Swiss, had been made an attractive offer to work on a development project; he would be the right-hand man of a ministry official. I could sense a trace of displeasure and resentment, to which I attached the feeling, "Aha, he wants to go back to Switzerland." I developed my first intervention out of this, along the lines that he saw no end to his burdens and that life had been kinder to the others. He sighed and again started to talk about the problems linked to the sale of his house, which he was trying to solve by working extra hours. On the one hand, he needed the additional income; on the other, the fact that his nighttime work was getting out of hand was also an indication of his overestimation of himself. His subsequent neglect of his profession took its revenge, causing him to have conflicts with colleagues and supervisors at his regular employment.

I was not convinced by his ideas on how to solve these problems since in my opinion they also involved unresolved conflicts about potency and creativity. Before I decided whether I should follow this line of thought, the patient began to speak about his father, who was not supposed to know anything about the renewed debacle concerning the sold house; otherwise he would have just rubbed his hands and said, "See what a mess you've made of things over there after all." The patient became very animated, having a fictive exchange with his father that was fierce and marked by disappointments.

A: Maybe you have the wish to return home to find a father who would push aside all of the mess you've made here.

P: Yes, I've always wanted to have such a father, but I never have.

He recalled that as a child or young boy he had never felt close to his father; this was exemplified by the fact that his father had never given five franks. He had instead stayed near his mother, who had tied him to her by giving him money. Ultimately he had left home because he had had enough of being tied down in this way, of being his mother's prisoner. He had not found a way to get to his father. Recently it had become clear to him that his father was an old man who had become peaceful and longed to find his son again.

The patient's comments rounded off my image: he longed to be welcomed at home as the prodigal son. I recalled that Ignaz Y had for a while had the wish in puberty to become a priest. I reminded him of the story of the prodigal son. The patient, very vibrant and happy, imagined a festive meal: "Maybe I should read more in the Bible again."

This was the first session in which there was a religious mood and a feeling of trust in the power of old images. He had previously never mentioned the remnants of his religiosity, except to say that he now had an image of God that was based in a philosophy of nature.

His tenseness dissipated and our contact became noticeably more harmonious. The patient seemed to get heavier and heavier lying on the couch, and I became sleepier and sleepier. I had the feeling of a pleasant warmness and withdrew into it. The patient continued imagining the welcoming scene; when he included his sister in his daydream, the atmosphere changed again. This was an opportunity to return home.

I recalled a poem by the Israeli poet David Rokeach, especially the concluding line: ". . . and at the end of all the paths is the return to Jerusalem." By not interpreting anything to the patient, but just leaving him to his fantasies about returning home, I experienced my sleepiness as a pleasent mood and as a moment of relaxation. In pursuing my thoughts further I remembered a passage from the beginning of treatment. In a fantasy the patient had described me as a strict analyst who would never permit him to stand up and walk around. I now developed the following interpretation: "You imagine a welcoming home scene in which you arrange your relationship to your father the way you have always wanted it to be. Yet here you are in stress and desire more support to balance your deficiencies: the temporal distance to the last session, the reference to the missing fourth hour. Aren't they an appeal to a caring father, who should prepare a home in which you can feel well and to which you can return whenever you want?"

The patient was touched. In doubt, he said, "It's hard for me to even think about it. I have never had such a father or the feeling that I could feel at home."

A period of silence followed, which the patient ended by pointing out that the session had already ended a few minutes ago. Without noticing it, I had apparently made the patient's wish for a lengthening of the session come true and acted accordingly.

The idea of returning home continued to be a topic in the following sessions and for the patient became connected with the thought of wanting to put more order into his life. He would have liked to change the present location of his burdensome situation in life or at least to atone to the location of his evil deeds.

He then reported about a dream in which a man who was left unidentified cleaned up a church filled with junk. In the process he discovered a toy, which he laid on the altar.

For a while in his youth the patient had sought in the church the security he had not found at home, and in the comforting idea of becoming a priest. He had frequently accused himself of filling my office with disarray. It thus seemed natural to view the church as a metaphor for therapy. We then returned to the role I played in his life, as portrayed by the unidentified man in the dream. In the first year of therapy Ignaz Y had used the sessions primarily, together with my help, to put some order into his chaotic life. At times I had largely had the function of providing support. To keep from sinking into chaos, Ignaz Y had frequently gained orientation with the aid of my perspective and judgment. Because of his narcissistic self-overestimation he was rather blind in many private and professional spheres of his life and was flabbergasted when he appeared to suddenly be at a dead end. In fact we were each busy with cleaning up, just in different ways. In this process we had discovered a valuable childhood toy, which he himself had already made inaccessible from the outside. As a child the patient had invented a private language [see Sect. 7.3]. The patient's references to his dream made me think of seeing a mixture of the two of us in the unidentified man. Amazed at these thoughts, I recalled that I had read a book a few days before whose title, *The Pronouns of Power and Solidarity*, had appealed to me. It seemed possible to me that I had sensed in the tension between power and solidarity the patient's ambivalent mood that he gave a lot and I took it without his knowing for sure what he would get for it. Before I reached an interpretation based on these ideas, the patient recalled a television program in which the picture of A.S., a wanted terrorist, was shown; he commented, "If we were liberated by her, that would be a relief."

At the same time Ignaz Y had started therapy he had freed himself - outwardly - from his dominating wife and her family, yet he was afraid of getting in a similar situation again sometime. As the next step I made the following interpretation: "When you have completely freed yourself from the wreckage of your unsuccessful marriage . . . ." The patient interrupted me, saying, "Then I would donate a picture for you to the pilgrimage church in my home town." He then compared the therapy with the Way of the Cross, a way full of thorns. I pointed out that this process was very painful for him, one-sided, and completely unclear with regard to what awaited him at the end. The patient thought of his father, who had seldom done anything good for him; his father had never let him forget that he was a bastard and not really wanted. Just once, when the patient was still small and was sick, had his father carried him around. I concluded this passage by indicating that he might have felt like a bastard during his difficult search for an offer of therapy, since several therapists he had consulted had led him to understand that he should first straighten out his life outwardly before it would be possible to think of analysis.

3.2 Complementary Countertransference

In Sect. 3.4 of Vol.1 we gave the following summary: H. Deutsch (1926) used the expression "complementary identification" to describe the analyst's identification with the patient's objects of transference. The analyst then experiences feelings in the same way as the patient's mother or father, while the patient reexperiences feelings like those he had earlier in his relationship to each of his parents.

Erich Y came to the 249th session in a light-hearted mood. To him, life was again worth living. With great sensitivity he described a pleasant dream:

P: I was at work and had a very good relationship with my boss. It went so far that we took turns on the telephone. I talked first, then he took over; and then the department head, and I can't remember exactly whether it was ice cream or something else, he ate some more.

A: While on the phone in your presence, or how?

P: Yes, when he took the receiver he took the chewing gum or whatever it was.

A: Yes, did he eat your chewing gum or ice cream, creating a very intimate exchange?

P: Precisely.

Consideration. The harmonious and intimate nature of the dream colored our relationship. I focussed on this mood, and as if by itself I absorbed the patient's transference wishes. I was also interested in doing justice verbally to the unconscious longing and in making it possible for the intimacy of the exchange to be felt. That was my intention, which was also expressed in later interpretations. But I unintentionally attributed the chewing gum primarily to the patient, as if he had had it in his mouth first. I noticed that the patient had hesitated in describing the intimate exchange, and he himself had switched from ice cream to chewing gum. But it was because of my unconsciously guided *mishearing* that I put the *chewing gum* into his mouth. In which way my countertransference had led me to mishear this item was inaccessible to me consciously. I experienced the patient's transference, portrayed in the dream, at different levels. His longing for his father was expressed as an oral relationship. Interruptions or inclarity in his recollection could indicate resistance to latent phallic tendencies. Apparently my emotional resonance had encouraged the patient to give up his resistance. Everything proceeded in such a natural way that I did not notice my lapse until I read the transcript. The fact that the patient immediately approvingly adopted my interpretation of the sequence of events by saying "precisely" might have contributed to my lapse.

Following the patient's "precisely" I added:

A: You became pals through this intimate exchange.

P: It's a special human attraction. Something is created, being attracted and not repelled, and also being equal. In such a mood it doesn't bother me at all if our little son is in a bad mood, which hurts me otherwise.

The patient then turned to his change in mood. Before the session he had also had a brief negative phase when a colleague of mine appeared in the waiting room. Although where he had been sitting he could hardly be seen, he had been torn back and forth about whether he should greet him or not, whether the doctor would respond in a friendly way or not, etc. He had immediately become tense and cramped, and the symptoms had come immediately.

Consideration. The patient's associations confirmed to me that I had accurately guessed his longing for harmonious unity and togetherness. The appearance of the doctor ended the patient's harmony because he was then torn back and forth about whether he would be seen, whether he should greet him, whether he had to stand up, etc. In brief, he described the nascent tension, which developed because the comparing had set in: large-small, important-unimportant. The analyst who had come in does in fact have an impressive figure.

Erich Y described that the tension declined when he put himself mentally at the same level, in human terms, as the doctor. Then he mentioned how he shifted back and forth between the two extremes.

Consideration. My goal was to make, by referring to intimate exchange processes, the patient's unconscious longing even clearer. I therefore referred back to genetically early exchange patterns and to his dream.

A: Yes, there the dream is the opposite image. There you are the best of friends. There isn't any tension there. He takes your chewing gum and you take his. Whatever he has in his mouth, you have in yours. It's like between father and child or between mother and child, namely when the mother puts something into her mouth and says, "Oh, that's good." and then puts it into the child's mouth.

P: Even in the dream I stopped at this moment and couldn't believe it. I took a step back and looked at it once again, to see whether it was true, whether it was really true that he continued to chew the same chewing gum.

A: Yes, and interestingly, probably because you were ashamed, you said at first that you couldn't remember exactly any more. It could also have been ice cream, which melts. You can't put it into your mouth twice. It wasn't until then that you mentioned the chewing gum, as if you first had to tell me that it was really very hygienic. With the chewing gum it's more intimate, so to speak. You put something into your mouth that somebody else has already had in theirs. Or how do you see it?

P: Right, just right.

The patient then described his own resistance, which had already started during the dream. Even if Erich Y was only obliging in order to please me, his associations still indicated that I had guessed his unconscious wishes. In my next interpretations I tried to strengthen the oral object relationship and focused on orality in order to enrich him emotionally.

For a while Erich Y attempted to reduce his longing again:

P: I thought to myself again, "Oh, dear me, such feelings, something like that awakened in me, what must you think about it?"

A: Yes, that this doesn't simply happen to you, but that you yourself are looking for something that the head of the department has. You share in it when we trade words here back and forth. Then it isn't any chewing gum, but it has to do with your mouth and with the relationship, with words that fly back and forth and link. What else can you think of? Perhaps there are even more fantasies, if you have a little more confidence in yourself and if you aren't as scared, for God's sake.

P: At the moment I'm a little distracted.

A: By what?

P: I'm fidgety again. [He was trembling.]

A: Yes, I just included myself. What was the distraction like emotionally?

Erich Y now began speaking about his dream again, and I seemed to form a unit with his department head. He said, "Even in the dream I stopped at this moment and couldn't believe it. I took a step back and looked at it once again, to see whether it was true, whether it was really true that he continued to chew the same chewing gum." My reference to his being ashamed, which had led to an interruption, encouraged him to give more space to his deep longing for his father. For some time I had thought that the patient had been homosexually seduced in puberty, and I assumed that he was disturbed in transference by the contents of his dream. I therefore pointed out that the unusual and indecent exchange in the dream is customary and natural between child and mother or father and that this naturalness is continued in an adult's sexuality. I intentionally described orality in very general terms.

P: See, when you say such things, I become uneasy again, as if something resisted it.

A: Yes, with these words it almost seems as if my tongue entered your mouth, and my chewing gum too, which is then an intermediate member.

P: Yes, I believe that the thoughts you exude could be my own and that you discover the evil in me and portray it as perverse.

A: Yes, it is almost a fear that you are being perverse when you sense your longing for your father.

P: I've already told you that another boy showed me everything there is.

A: Who fiddled with your anus.

P: Yes.

A: And who also wanted you to put his member into your mouth, or what do you mean?

Oral practices had not taken place at the time, and there had not been any reciprocal masturbation, as the patient now added.

The patient's hesitation led me to assume that he felt insecure because intimacy was unconsciously linked with perversion, which was the reason I mentioned the word. It was important to me to weaken his anxiety that his oral longings, which he elaborated on in the further course of the session, could be perverse. I therefore made a reference to the naturalness of these wishes in the child-parent relationship. Here it was again shown that it had been the real behavior of his wife that had strengthened his guilt feelings and the instances inhibiting his libidinal impulses.

From his recollection of his needs during puberty Erich Y now returned to the present, which provided the day residue for the dream work. Yesterday evening he had been gripped by a sex scene in a television film, in which a man looking through a key hole observed a woman undressing. He was afraid that his wife, who was somewhere in the apartment, would catch him.

Consideration. Here his wife, as was frequently the case, was the representative of inhibiting superego figures. This attribution, which was eased by her actual behavior, resulted in inevitable disappointments and real conflicts. I assumed that his wife's rejection strengthened his longing for his father, or in other words, that a regression from the heterosexual to a homosexual relationship was initiated by the day residue and the later, real rejection by his wife. At the same time, the man adopted a maternal function. Oral intercourse was depicted at the latent dream level. In keeping with my countertransference feelings and the considerations I just described, I interpreted this connection by saying, "Yes, that could be. You weren't allowed to take a closer look and therefore sought consolation in a dream.

Commentary. We would like to draw attention to the fact that this session not only illustrates *complementary countertransference* but is also instructive because of the fact that physical symptoms also played a role. Such observations of actual genesis enable us to take a look at the psychodynamic connections of the immediate development of somatic symptoms. The analyst attempted to come as close as possible to the physical needs by creating analogies between the verbal and the material exchange. Thus although we cannot examine the body as the object of somatic medicine, the psychoanalytic method permits us to study the body image, i. e., the experiencing that is linked to an individual's body.

3.3 Retrospective Attribution and Fantasizing

The following example from Erich Y's therapy is part of the comprehensive topic referred to by the above heading. We obviously cannot familiarize the readers with all the problems included in this topic in a short report on an individual case, but in order to be able to comprehend the exchange between Erich Y and his analyst, it is necessary to be familiar with several aspects of the theory that provides the context of *retrospective fantasy* and *retrospective attribution.* The excurse following the report on this session informs the reader about the significance of retrospective attribution in Freud's vocabulary, which can hardly be overestimated.

Erich Y's 254th hour of treatment began outside my office on the parking lot. We had arrived at the same time and parked our cars some distance apart. As I observed from a distance, the bumper of his car touched that of a parked car. At first he did not mention this event. He began the session by reporting about a dream, at the center of which was a defect in a water line and its consequences. After the water had been turned off, examination of the problem showed that the pipe in the wall had been partially or completely sawn off over a length of about 8 inches. The surrounding masonry had hid the defect from view.

The patient emphasized that in the dream he had evaluated the damage soberly and objectively. After all, it was not in his house; if it had been, he would have made the little affair real big and attributed an immense significance to the damage.

I immediately saw a self-representation in the dream. In reality the patient was terribly busy renovating his house at the time. He had laid new water pipes and made repairs to others. I fantasized about the patient's body image and saw in the water pipes a description of his urogenital system and of an injury to it, which manifested itself in the patient's deformation phobias, i. e., in his ideas of having too small a chin etc. At first I stayed at the level the patient offered, and commented on how he still experienced small damages as if they were immensely magnified (because of the self-reference and the unconscious accompanying fantasies).

I limited myself to repeating in dramatic form the size of the damage as he had experienced it: "Since you were small, if you were offended or hurt, it was immediately a question of to be or not to be and of your body as a whole, crooked nose, small member, and attacks, damages, and injury." Erich Y mentioned some analogies extending my allusions, which finally brought him to the incident that occurred on the parking lot: "My bumper just touched the other one, just pushed it. Only the dust was gone. I could see that while I was getting out, which is why I didn't go any closer. I just had the thought that you may have seen it, and the inkling of a bad conscience because I walked away."

The damage worsened in his experience in front of my eyes. It can be assumed that such harmless encounters unconsciously signalized serious collisions to the patient because he had a high potential for aggression. For this reason he also immediately felt that he was being observed and punished.

We spoke about his own capacity to judge and that he nevertheless needed the assurance and wanted to hear that everything was alright. The serious damage in his dream and its unconscious background were related to his harmless behavior and his bad conscience.

Erich Y extended the topic by giving a long description of his dependence on confirmation. But there was also another aspect, namely his originality and perfectionism in carrying out tasks and in not letting anyone else take part in planning and completing them. He did not even inform his wife.

<u>Consideration.</u> His drive for perfectionism should be seen as an ongoing compensation for existing damage, whether it be the damage that he experienced on his own body as a victim, or whether it be damage that he inflicted on himself. Even if unconscious intentions do not reach their mark because resistance processes intervene and inhibit them, thoughts and unconscious fantasies still suffice to make a bad conscience and to demand compensation. The patient's numerous reaction formations – just like his occasional outbursts of rage – were signs that a high potential for aggression had to be held in check.

In the next interpretation I focussed on the word "scratch" and related it to the patient's body feeling (see Sect. 5.2).

A: If there's a scratch anywhere, then it's as if you had been scratched; you are the victim and you can't do anything about it. The larger the injury that you experience on yourself, the more you are enraged. This rocks itself up to a higher level, like the time I scratched you by demanding you pay a part of my fee yourself .... Everything that has happened in your dreams .... Everything has to be compensated.

P: Yes, this perfection. I thought the same thing this morning. But why are these external injuries, or if something happens, why are they immediately related to me and my body and have such drastic consequences without my initially being able to perceive and sense them?

A: Yes, look at the damage in the dream. The body's water line is urination, and people are very sensitive if you meet them there. All of this has to do with the water line, with the house that each of us is, and that somebody maliciously sawed on it, and in the dream cut through it.

P: It had already been damaged when it was installed.

A: Already damaged when installed, aha.

Consideration. Between the patient's statement that the pipe had already been damaged when it was installed and my reinforcing repetition of his thought, I had an idea inspired by my theoretical understanding, namely that the patient lived with the unconscious fantasy that he had already been damaged in his mother's womb and that something had gone wrong when he was produced. I was not very surprised that the patient now remembered something that had been *retrospectively* kept alive through his mother's repetitions. This was that his head had been deformed at birth. Thus he fantasized his disturbed body image, especially the deformation of his head, back to the beginning of his life. I viewed this regressive fantasy as an attempt to create a status quo ante, i. e., to reattain the pretraumatic state described by Balint. And in fact the patient mentioned other associations that were explicitly related to his first injury.

The patient picked up my the phrase "already damaged when installed," adding:

P: As I said, the mistake was built in during the construction; it is deeper, and the comparison to birth is straightforward. I am reminded that my mother said to me that it had been a very difficult birth. They had to get me with the forceps, and it was so difficult that they deformed my head.

A: That means that it was already deformed when it was created and produced.

P: Being created .... [long pause] It's very funny, as if I were lying in my mother's belly, in this cavern. There everything is so clean, pure, uniform. And then there is the immediate jump to a few years later, to kindergarten, before the war broke out. This was the first injury. I don't know whether I have mentioned this before. My brother and I, we were playing behind the house, in the farmyard. The field was on the side of a hill and there were some motor vehicles around. I released the brakes of a hand cart. It started rolling and rolled over my brother, but since he was playing in a large chicken hole, the car just rolled over him without hitting him.

A: Hum, just scratched. The cart ....

The patient then described how the cart had rolled down the hill and was stopped by a barn, and the collision had caused considerable damage.

The patient's vivid recollection rekindled fairly similar memories in me about my childhood. The intensity of my retrospective fantasy was so strong that I did not limit myself to the material damage mentioned by the patient or to the uproar that he caused. The interpretation I made was dependent on my countertransference and was a direct continuation of the patient's description.

A: Because you nearly killed your brother. You nearly committed fratricide, Cain and Abel.

After a longer pause the patient discovered still another aspect:

P: I was also something like a small hero, who had already accomplished something.

A: Yes, you can set a lot of things rolling. And then people are blissful and happy if everything turns out alright, and say that it wasn't so bad. And that is the way it was this morning, where you would have liked to use me as a witness to verify that no damage had been done, that nothing had happened, that the damage that had been done would be compensated - the damage you caused and that which you in fact did not cause, although you assume you are the culprit and have it on your conscience.

From his description that he apparently also was a small hero I gathered that my countertransference-dependent Cain-Abel interpretation had asked too much of the patient. The patient had obviously had enough for today with regard to affective intensity because he dedicated the rest of the session to superficial injuries from his adult world.

Looking Back. [Dictated immediately after the session.] My fantasy about the origin of the "imagined" injury was countered by the idea his mother kept alive, namely that the damage to his head went back to his birth. I fortunately did not say anything. I was very surprised that the patient stopped talking about his difficult birth and turned to describe the harmonious situation in the womb. In this session we thus have the opportunity to see different features, the new beginning and the transferral of the harmonious state to the period prior to the first trauma, which the patient described as the birth trauma. His experience and my surprise coincide. The question is who initiated the fantasizing, the patient or I? Very important is also the fact that the recent event on the parking lot before the session precipitated his associations. Finally I put myself in the patient's place and in my retrospective fantasies revived my own memories, which motivated me to make a Cain-Abel interpretation that was dependent on countertransference.

Comment. In the summary that the analyst dictated immediately after the session and in the accompanying commentaries that he wrote later, the anaylst made it clear that he let himself enter into a concordant countertransference. He participated in the patient's retrospective fantasies and remembered analgous childhood experiences. Also impressive is the fact that this mutual induction was molded by ideas that belong to psychoanalytic heuristics and clearly originated in the analyst's head as well as in his warm-hearted empathy.

Comments on Retrospective Attribution. The term "retrospective" (*nachträglich*) and its noun form "retrospective attribution" (*Nachträglichkeit*) were frequently used by Freud in connection with his conception of temporality and psychic causality. As early as in a letter to Fliess dated Dec.6, 1986, Freud wrote: "I am working on the assumption that our psychical mechanism has come about by a process of stratification: the material present in the shape of memory-traces is from time to time subjected to a rearrangement in accordance with fresh circumstances - is, as it were, transcribed" (1950a, p. 173). Laplanche and Pontalis (1973, p. 112) consider the view "that all phenomena met with in psycho-analysis are placed under the sign of retroactivity, or even of retroactive *illusion*. This is what Jung means when he talks of retrospective phantasies (*Zurückphantasieren*): according to Jung, the adult reinterprets his past in his phantasies, which constitute so many symbolic expressions of his current problems. On this view reinterpretation is a way for the subject to escape from the present 'demands of reality' into an imaginary past." Without rejecting this view, Laplanche and Pontalis emphasize that Freud's conception of retrospective attribution was much more precise. According to them, it is not the lived experience itself that undergoes a deferred revision but specifically that which was not completely integrated into a *meaningful constellation* the moment it was experienced. The *traumatic event* is for them a model of such experience. Freud adopted the idea of retrospective fantasy, and the expression appears in the context of retrospective attribution numerous times:

I admit that this is the most delicate question in the whole domain of psycho-analysis. I did not require the contributions of Adler or Jung to induce me to consider the matter with a critical eye, and to bear in mind the possibility that what analysis puts forward as being forgotten experiences of childhood (and of an improbably early childhood) may on the contrary be based upon phantasies created on occasions occurring late in life.... No doubt has troubled me more; no other uncertainty has been more decisive in holding me back from publishing my conclusions. I was the first - a point to which none of my opponents have referred - to recognize both the part played by phantasies in symptom-formation and also the "retrospective phantasying" of late impressions into childhood and their sexualization after the event. (Freud 1918b, p. 103)

We assume that this quotation suffices and will make a very deep impression on the reader. At least we are able to comprehend the analyst's enthusiasm about his retrospective fantasies and his rediscovery of retrospective attribution, which was one of Freud's grandest guiding ideas. The fact that Strachey translated this expression as "deferred action" therefore certainly had many consequences. With reference to our comments in Sect. 1.4 of Vol. 1, we would like to emphasize, in agreement with Wilson's (1987) recently published argumentation, that Strachey did not invent Freud and that the present crisis of psychoanalysis cannot be traced back to the fact that Freud's work was transformed in the *Standard Edition* into Strachey's Anglo-American scientific language. That Strachey translated *Nachträglichkeit* as deferred action is more than simply a trivial error, as recently pointed out by Thomä and Cheshire (1991). The Freudian concept of *nachträglich* cannot be reduced to the concept of a deferred action. Disregarding for the moment the consequences that Strachey's translation may have had on the understanding of Freud's works in the Anglo-American countries, even in countries where the original (German) text was used the understanding of retrospective fantasying has inexorably led analysts to trace the etiological conditions of psychic and psychosomatic illnesses back to the very first hour and even earlier. The very concept *Nachträglichkeit* in fact forbids reducing the history of the subject to a monocausal determinism that only pays attention to the influence of the very early past on the present. The tendency to trace the causes of psychic illnesses further and further back into the past has become stronger over the decades, as if an individual's fate were determined in the first months of life or even in the intrauterine phase - and this not as a result of his genetic code or of inheritance but of presumed environmental influences. This development has been universal, i.e., independent of language or translation, and can also be found where the significance of *Nachträglichkeit* has been fully recognized, for example in the works of Lacan, who linked Freud's idea with Heidegger's philosophy of temporality. Retrospective fantasying back to the beginning of one's own life and beyond in self discovery is a fascinating subject in the fairy tales and myths that live in us.

This excurse shows that simple concordant retrospective fantasying has a meaningful context. The psychoanalyst's cognitive process is borne by many preconditions even though he may not be aware of them in the session itself. This may well have been the case in the session described above, which was full of feeling and by no means overly intellectual (on deferred action, see also Thomä and Cheshire 1991).

3.4 Making the Patient Aware of Countertransference

One consequence of innate biological patterns is that vivid erotic or aggressive scenes quite naturally have psychophysiological resonance, especially when the analyst is involved in the transference. By empathizing with the scenes described by the patient, the analyst is put in moods that can lie anywhere within a broad spectrum. In his book *Zur Phänomenologie und Theorie der Sympathiegefühle and von Liebe und Hass* from 1913, Scheler pointed to the primary object relatedness and the bipersonal nature of these processes that reach deep into the sphere of the body (see Scheidt 1986). From psychoanalytic perspectives, our view is directed at the unconscious preliminary forms of these phenomena. Data from physiological measurements are not necessary for the analyst to feel that his partial identification with the patient's experience in countertransference has an animating effect. This effect is dependent on, on the one hand, the nature of the scene, and on the other hand, on the analyst's general disposition and specific resonance capacity. The analyst in effect displays all the affective reactions that belong to the nature of mankind and that Darwin, Freud, Cannon, and Lorenz attempted to explain with their theories about affects and emotions.

A consequence of the professional tasks and duties is that feelings of sympathy and love and hate become manifest in weakened form. The analyst has, so to speak, only one leg in the particular scene; his standing leg and, most importantly, his head ensure that he stays, to refer to Schopenhauer's words that were quoted above, "in the realm of calm consideration" in order to be able to jump in full of knowledge and ready to help. Although it is impossible here to discuss man's nature - which is an inexhaustible interdisciplinary topic - no side doubts that psychoanalysts are also subject to this nature. They are even more receptive for sexual or aggressive fantasies because they train themselves to perceive the smallest microsignals, which are even entirely unconscious to the patient sending them.

All patients obviously know, without saying so, that their analyst is subject to biological facts of life. The technical problems begin with the question of the way in which the analyst acknowledges that he is affected by the sexual or aggressive fantasies of his patient in the same manner as all other people. Not acknowledging the bipersonal nature of emotions confuses the patient. His common sense was oriented until then on experiences he now sees cast into doubt. Given that some sort of relationship exists between two people, the emotions of the one do not leave the other cold. At least in a vague way the patient feels something of his analyst's countertransferences, and requires his analyst's emotional resonance just like he does his clear head. Acknowledging this tension keeps the patient from landing in one of the numerous deadend streets that end in an impasse or the breaking off of treatment. The failure of more than a few therapies has resulted, in our opinion, from the fact that the patient who is secretly convinced of the lack of credibility of his apparently untouched analyst repeatedly puts his analyst to the test, which he intensifies until he obtains his proof. There is a wide variety in what patients consider proof in their attempts to convict analysts. Spontaneous nonverbal reactions or interpretations that permit the patient to draw conclusions about the analyst's own curiosity serve the patient as indications that the analyst was aggressive or sexually stimulated. This was the proof, and the analyst discredited himself. Thus the intensification of aggressive and erotic or sexual transference fantasies results in part from the analyst's denials. It is not easy to find one's way out of this deadend. It is therefore advisable for the analyst to acknowledge his own emotions from the beginning and to clarify the professional tasks that enable him to have milder forms of affective reactions. The patient's curiosity for personal matters (e.g., the analyst's private life) weakens if the analyst makes him aware of his thoughts about him, for example, the context in which his interpretations are grounded. In our experience it is then not difficult for the patient to respect the analyst's private life and to limit his curiosity about the personal and private sides of the analyst's moods and thoughts. It is a tremendous relief to the patient that the analyst does not answer in kind and does not react as intensively as the people with whom the patient was or is in an emotional clinch. The analyst's milder reactions, rooted in his professional knowledge, enable the patient to have new experiences. In this way the analyst can pass the patient's test in a therapeutically productive way instead of losing all credibility as a result of a misunderstood and unnatural abstinence and anonymity, and of precipitating the vicious circle outlined above.

Let us now look at a few details. What does it mean when Ferenczi (1950, p. 189) sees the mastery of countertransference in the "constant oscillation between the free play of fantasy and critical scrutiny"? What do analysts mean when they talk of their dealing with countertransference? There is definitely a difference between retrospectively talking about this or that feeling that arose as a reaction in the therapeutic session and having this feeling while sitting opposite the patient. Obviously the point is precisely how the analyst copes with being exposed to a multitude of stimuli. The analyst's profession would in fact be impossible if every sexual and aggressive wish would reach its goal unbroken and carried the analyst from one peak to the next trough. Regardless of how intense the emotional involvement and the exchange may be, one consequence of the analyst's reflective thoughtfulness is that the patient's emotions only reach him in weakened form. He is certainly the goal of the patient's dispairing cries for help, his sexual longing, and his disparaging manner; he is meant and touched, but for various reasons the intensity of his experiencing is weaker. The analyst's knowledge of the processes of transference offers a certain degree of protection. Love, hate, dispair, and powerlessness were originally distributed among numerous people. By empathizing with the patient, the analyst ceases being the passive victim of the patient's cynical criticsm; on the contrary, he can participate in the patient's pleasurable sadism and find intellectual satisfaction in understanding such patterns of behavior. The calm thoughtfulness, which may coincide with great intellectual satisfaction from identifying the roles the patient attributes, creates a completely natural distance to the proximity of the moment.

The reader may be surprised that we view this as a natural process that is in no way characterized by splitting, but that also does not force constant sublimation. No further proof is required of the fact that countertransference problems can be solved in the manner we have outlined and not, in contrast, by sublimations. It would not take long for analysts to become exhausted and incapacitated if they had to expend their strength on ego splitting or sublimation.

Our view clarifies why it is one of the most natural things in the world that the patient in certain circumstances may experience - or even must know - what countertransference he has precipitated in the analyst. The analyst should not have a bad conscience about admitting something, and it definitely cannot be the point for the analyst to burden the patient with his own conflicts or to give him examples by telling him stories from his own life. For a great variety of reasons, counselling sessions in which the parties act like good friends frequently take such a turn, with both parties finally pouring out their hearts. Many doctors also believe they can provide consolation in their office by describing examples of how they have coped with illness and the other burdens of life. However important identifications and learning from models are in every form of psychotherapy, it is just as decisive to help the patient himself find acceptable solutions to his problems. If a patient denies his genuine knowledge that the analyst is also subject to fate, then there are more helpful ways of informing him than admissions that hurt more than they help even when they are made with the best of intentions.

Helplessness, at least in the sphere of symptoms, is a characteristic of all suffering. The patient (the sufferer) complains about disturbances against which he is powerless and which impose themselves psychically or are caused by his body. Complaints often turn into indirect accusations. This is particularly true in all psychic and psychosomatic illnesses, where complaints soon become accusations directed against parents and family. In order not to be misunderstood, we would like to emphasize that an individual's complaints and accusations about what has happened to him or was done to him must be taken seriously. A child's long period of dependence is accompanied by a one-sided distribution of power and powerlessness. Yet even in the struggle for survival the powerless victim finds ways and means to assert himself. Psychoanalytic theory offers a wealth of explanatory models that facilitate the therapeutic understanding at those points, in particular, that are unconscious to the patient himself. The common element linking these points together is the unconscious influence that the patient himself exerts, regardless of what was done to him.

Our exposition justifies letting the patient share in countertransference under certain circumstances. Theoretically this necessity derives from the further development of object relationship theory into two-person psychology. The great therapeutic significance of letting patients share in countertransference becomes visible everywhere patients are blind to the consequences that their verbal and nonverbal statements and their affects and actions have on the people around them and on the analyst. It is probably even the case that some transference interpretations which create a distance to the patient stimulate him into attributing human qualities to the object and in the process into testing the limits of his own power. By deliberately speaking of the patient's sharing in the *analyst's* countertransference we mean that the countertransference only in part belongs to the patient's sphere of functioning and organizing. Precisely because the analyst does not cooperate fully, but in all seriousness plays along as described above, the patient discovers the unconscious aspects of his intentions. Intuitive psychoanalysts who have also had the courage to describe their experiences in public have always known that this kind of sharing has nothing to do with confessions from their private lives. It is completely inappropriate to speak of personal confessions in connection with countertransference. Such a term is a burden on dealing with countertransference in a natural way, because the analyst does not make confessions to his colleagues just as we are not concerned here with confessions of a personal nature that an analyst has made to a patient, as we pointed out in Sect. 3.5 in Vol.1. Letting the patient under certain circumstances share in countertransference is an accurate description of an emminently significant process, which opens up new therapeutic opportunities and also deepens our knowledge.

Our explanations may contribute to lessening the shock that is still evoked by the frankness with which Winnicott (1949), Little (1951), and Searles (1965) wrote about their countertransference. Winnicott (1949, p. 72) wrote, unmisunderstandably:

> In certain stages of certain analyses the analyst's hate is acutally sought by the patient, and what is then needed is hate that is objective. If the patient seeks objective or justified hate he must be able to reach it, else he cannot feel he can reach objective love.

We now refer to two examples demonstrating that letting the patient share in countertransference can have a beneficial effect.

3.4.1 Erotized Countertransference

Toward the end of Rose X's analysis, which lasted several years, she surprised me by directly asking, after hesitating a moment, about my reaction to her sexuality. Sexual fantasies and experiences had always played a large role. It had been "transference at first sight"; a strongly erotized quality and the inhibitions and aversions linked to it had characterized long periods of her analysis. The disappointments, separation anxieties, and aggressive tensions that surfaced were so interwoven with sexual desires that the separate components were often difficult to identify.

Periods of intense anxiety neurosis and anorexia had existed since she was 10 years old. As a girl, especially in puberty and adolescence, she had often felt alone with her sexual feelings and thoughts. My reserved behavior and the analytic situation had fostered her feelings of being left alone in treatment, especially with regard to aspects of her relationship to her father. He had been very affectionate to her for a long time while she was a little girl but had withdrawn at the beginning of her puberty and had avoided her questions about the meaning of life. On the one hand his change in behavior was incomprehensible to her, on the other she related his turning away to her sexual development.

The transference and the realistic aspects of the analytic relationship were consequently particularly full of tension. Rose X was frequently moved to ask questions about the ways I personally reacted and experienced, yet she primarily expressed her questions indirectly. I had unconsciously contributed to this avoidance, as I could recognize in looking back from the late phase of analysis. Precisely because of her strong positive, often erotized transference I had been relieved in the sense that the patient observed the given framework and the limits, the justification of which ultimately lies in the incest taboo. My retrospective transference interpretations were related, accordingly, to her oedipal and preoedipal disappointments and their reappearance after the withdrawl of her father, who had evaded all kinds of questions about life and did not answer them in a personal way. This change in behavior formed an inconceivable contrast to how he had spoiled her and to the intimacies they had shared until her prepuberty. As an only child, she had been exposed to her parent's peculiarities to a very strong degree. Further, she had taken in her father's care in a rather passive manner. In many ways her father had also taken over a maternal role and provided compensation for the traumas she had suffered as a result of numerous severe illnesses during childhood. Her mother, who was superstitous and suffered from anxiety hysteria, remained dependent on her own father for her entire life, which complicated both her marriage and the care she gave her daughter. The disappointments that Rose X had suffered at the hands of her mother reinforced her inner contradictions and the associated tension between her aggressiveness, which had become unconscious, and her manifest feelings of guilt, which were of unknown origin. Some of her symptoms were a typical continuation of her ambivalent relationship to her mother.

From this psychodynamic summary it is easy to see that, given an interruption of the analysis or imagined separations, recent disappointments could form the point of departure for retrospective transference interpretations and it was only in passing that a hint of personal, specific questions were detected. The latter were probably avoided in order not to burden the relationship. Sometimes Rose X would cast a short but insistent glance at the expression on my face and at my expressive behavior, and occasionally she made allusions about, for example, her concern about the serious face I made. We then racked our brains about the genesis of her feelings of anxiety and guilt.

We then approached the envisaged termination of treatment. In this phase the patient increasingly mentioned sexual ideas, in addition to aggressive ones, the majority of which referred back to fantasies (e.g., from dreams and daydreams) that she had previously not been able to talk about.

After criticizing my professional role as an "impersonal analytic apparatus," Rose X asked me directly how I handle her hundreds of thousands of sexual fantasies and allusions, i.e., whether I sometimes got excited or whether I had imagined something similar for several seconds. She referred particularly to sexual desires and experiences that she herself felt to be pleasurable - scenes in which she animated men into aggressive sexual behavior by her own exhibitionism. The patient now wanted to know what I desired or imagined and whether I had the same feelings as other men.

When sexual ideas had previously been hinted at, especially if they had had any link to me, I had asked for clarification and finally made retrospective transference interpretations or interpretations of their latent aggressive, momentary contents. During the final phase of this treatment I had, on the basis of earlier experience, come to the conclusion that it was possible and sensible to let patients share in the countertransference without getting involved in complications and without confusing my the professional and personal roles. On the contrary, letting patients share contributed to clarification and relief. At first I had in fact really behaved in a reserved way, like her real father, who had become impersonal and drawn limits where there really had been room for a more personal exchange. In other words, possibly because of his own fear of transgressing limits, the patient's father had abruptly switched to anonymity, just as I myself had adopted an impersonal attitude at just the first hint of possible sexual actions. In this case the patient's real experience with me and her traumatic experience with her father coincided in the therapeutic relationship so that for her the character of transference was not distinguished from that of real experience.

Against the background of such considerations I gave her the following answer, which became part of a longer exchange of thoughts. I said, truthfully, that I was not left cold by her thoughts and fantasies, which she herself referred to as provocative and exciting, and that otherwise even her own perception told her that I was not significantly different from other men. I added that although a certain amount of resonance and emotional reactions were also necessary because I otherwise would not be able to put myself into her emotional situation well enough to draw my conclusions and formulate interpretations, a certain distance from my own desires and fantasies was necessary for therapy. I drew pleasure and satisfaction not from letting my fantasies turn into desires or actions but from using them to make helpful interpretations that I hoped would be of use to her and could ultimately bring her therapy to a good conclusion. The most important item, however, was the statement that I felt something and even had some sexual thoughts in reaction to her fantasies. I concluded that we had just discovered something that we had not mentioned before although each of us had perceived it during a long phase of the therapy, namely that we stimulated each other and that I was occasionally moved by her erotic attraction.

Rose X was surprised and relieved by this answer. She immediately added something to the description of a dream she had given at the beginning of the session, which was one of many with sexual and aggressive elements and which was about meeting a man who resembled her father and an unknown woman and about the danger of poisoning. Her first associations were about the poisoning and the evil stepmother in Snow White. After I had let her share in my countertransference, other associations followed, as did the patient's own interpretations. She said that she was immensely relieved and was able to speak more frankly about sexual contents that had gone unmentioned - with the consequence that there was less tension and more interpretive work. It was possible to comprehend the significance of the dream as the symbol of her traumatic situation as an only child, with her erotically seductive but also very reserved father and with her mother who was filled with anxiety and feelings of guilt. The patient had felt emotionally very dependent on her mother and in her childhood and adolescence had often thought about her mother's inner emotions and thoughts. Her mother had died from cancer while the analysis was in progress, about 18 months before it ended.

This was the first interpretation that really seemed clear to the patient. The component that was related to the past was not at all new, and included aspects of her relationships both to her father and to her mother and was most importantly also a confirmation of her concrete interest in gaining some insight into the other person's feelings and ideas. It seemed clear to her because it happened against the backdrop of a new experience: learning about my psychological self and my opportunities for processing material. The patient could see in my statement *confirmation* of her own sexuality, sensualness, and physical self. Her doubts about what her exciting fantasies precipitated in me lost all connection to reality. My interpretations that human sensations were the basis liberated the patient from the feeling of being powerless and excluded or of having been guilty. In the course of the following session, the climate improved visibly. The traumatic affects in transference were discussed more frankly in the relationship and resolved so that the analysis came to a good conclusion.

3.4.2 *Aggressive Countertransference*

We will first present a summary of Linda X's specific problems and then describe the intensification of the transference-countertransference constellation that occurred in a session preceding a longer interruption.

One unusual feature of this case was the fact that her appointment was made by the company doctor of the firm at which Linda X, who was 23 years old at the time, was being trained as a technical assistant in a pharmaceutical laboratory. She would not have managed this step on her own; for this reason the worried colleague not only made the appointment but also insisted on bringing the patient to my office.

Linda X placed great value on getting an appointment with me since she had recently heard me present a speech. She was shy, anxious, and depressive and expected me to send her away after just a few sessions, as she told me immediately after we greeted each other. Her behavior and statements displayed a depressive and anxious attitude, which had been stable for about ten years. She had grown up as the youngest child in a family with a prude sexual morality and suffered from anorexia in puberty, which had been precipitated by comments that offended her. She had reacted to a doctor's statement that her dangerous loss of weight would have to be treated by tube feeding by overeating and rapidly gaining 36 kg (79 lb), reaching a weight of 80 kg (176 lb). When she was 16 she suppressed her craving for food by taking appetite suppressants. These were later replaced by psychopharmaceuticals, and Linda X had been dependent on them for years. She alternately took various benzodiazepin derivatives and other tranquilizers, without which she would have been paralyzed by her anxieties.

To escape from her loneliness and to overcome her anxiety about making contacts, Linda X satisfied her great longing for tenderness by turning to brief sexual escapades; her choice of partners was relatively arbitrary and hence dangerous. These frequently changing relationships did not provide her anything else than to help her momentarily overcome her loneliness and give her a vague feeling of taking revenge on her parents for some neglect. Her inner emptiness and dispair had increased in the last few years, creating a chronic danger of suicide.

Because of her intelligence Linda X had managed, despite her serious symptoms, to successfully finish school and to find an apprenticeship. Her achievement in these courses brought her recognition and satisfaction.

This short description of this woman's rather difficult situation raises a number of questions concerning the adaptive evaluation of the indications for psychoanalysis. This evaluation was on shaky ground in this case if for no other reason than because it was impossible at the beginning to estimate the severity of her habituation and dependence on the benzodiazepines and the resulting vicious circle. It was impossible to exclude the possibility that the patient's anxieties would increase even without discrete withdrawal symptoms, compelling her to take more and more tranquilizers. Despite her at least psychic dependence on benzodizepine and chronic suicidial tendency, the analyst suggested that outpatient treatment be attempted. Long-term inpatient therapy would have interrupted her apprenticeship and led to additional stress because the patient actually feared being committed and thus losing her place in her course. It would have hardly been possible during inpatient treatment to compensate for the loss of self-esteem that she would have incurred from the loss of the recognition she drew from her good work. Furthermore, the possibilities for controlling any drug abuse and protecting against attempted suicide are limited, even in institutions.

With regard to the prescription of psychopharmaceuticals, agreement was reached that the analyst would continue them. This approach proved completely successful in this case. The complications that arose in transference and countertransference were solved in constructive fashion. Starting from the situative worsening of her condition, it proved possible for the analyst to penetrate to the depths of her anxieties; in the process the contemplative patient gained security step by step.

Just as prior to the beginning of treatment, suicidal crises recurred during the several-year course of therapy when the patient had to endure being offended by her parents or friends; they were usually linked to separations. Interruptions of treatment for vacations were, similarly, accompanied by crises and made various emergency measures necessary, such as temporary admission to a rehabilitation center and, later, substitute appointments with a colleague.

Just prior to a relatively long interruption of treatment that had been announced long in advance, the patient again entered a chronic suicidal state and indirectly made me (the analyst) responsible for it. Her refusal to use the preceding time as effectively as possible and to accept temporary help during my absence made me increasingly helpless; my powerlessness was accompanied by aggressive feelings toward her negative attitude. My attempts at interpretation, in which I used all my knowledge about narcissistic rage (Henseler 1981), failed. The patient clamored to the idea that the entire world had left her and that therefore she would now kill herself.

In one of the last sessions prior to the break, she put a farewell letter on the table, which I was supposed to read. Since the patient then remained silent, I had much time to reflect about it. I noticed her black clothing and thought of mourning and death.

A: If I were to read this letter now, then I would accept your departure. You hate me because I'm going away.

The patient's lack of reactions and her silence were a burden on me. It did not seem to be at all clear to her how much I was affected by the aggressiveness contained in her threat to commit suicide. She also often hardly realized that she seriously offended and injured those who were friendly to her. Various possibilities went through my mind. Should I send her to a hospital, for her own protection and my safety, or should I, thinking about Winnicott's recommendation (see Sect. 3.4), let her share in my countertransference? I decided on the latter, because I also feared that she could otherwise take my refusal to read her letter as indifference. Furthermore, it was important to me to argue the continuity of the relationship after the break. I therefore made a relatively long interpretation in which I also expressed my concern by telling the patient that I was in such a dilemma that I was furious with her.

A: I am really very dismayed by the fact that by making your threat you want to make it more difficult for me to leave and put a burden on my return. I will return and our work will continue. That's why I'm not going to read your farewell letter.

In this way I wanted to express the fact that I did not accept her suicide as a departure. After a very long period of silence I continued:

A: You give me the responsibility for your life or death and ask very much of me, too much, more than I can bear. I don't share your view that you should invest your power in such an indirect way in suicide. You are testing how much power you have over me.

I pointed out the very disguised pleasure contained in self-destruction. Although the patient was still silent, I could feel that she was very touched. I therefore reminded her that her therapy had had a personal quality from the very beginning because of her wish to come specifically to me. To provide her relief, I referred to the fact that confronting me directly with her threat to commit suicide, instead of relating it to events outside, was an indication of progress. As I spoke of progress the patient looked up and awoke from her rigidity; she stared at me disbelievingly. I summarized for her where I saw progress.

A: Perhaps we can find out after all which of your desires and needs is contained in this accusation, so that you can know more precisely what's on the other side of the scale.

P: Yes, that's it, because you can go far away, because you're successful and people in other places want to have you, that makes me terribly aggitated. I don't have any hope or any perspective for ever really being able to work, being as independent as you, I'll always be just the little nuisance that you have to take care of materially although you could use the money much better somewhere else. It's a bit of a problem with my friend too, you know it; my friend only tolerates me, rejecting me when I turn to him for support, he wants me to be different, more self-secure, independent, beautiful, and more feminine, he doesn't like me this way, and you don't like me this way either. You only drag me through. My parents want to enjoy their old age and don't want to always have to be worried about me, as my father once said, and then he added, "Your Mr. Analyst can't always be with you."

A: Yes, and now your analyst goes on a trip, far away, he packs his caravan, so to speak [An allusion to her parents, who intended to take a long trip through Europe in the summer]. Your father was right: Those who have it, security and money, they pack their things, and this has come between us because in the meantime you yourself have felt these desires inside you. That is the difference to earlier. Do you still know that at the beginning here you once said: "I'll never let go of my parents. They shouldn't think that they've already done enough for me." Now you would like to be a woman who enjoys travelling, just like your colleague from work, like the analyst who enjoys travelling, who just travels far away and doesn't have a bad conscience about what those staying behind do.

This interpretation of her envy, which the patient had given a self-destructive turn, provided the patient relief, as her subsequent reaction showed:

P: Yes, this summer we can only manage 14 days vacation in a small house belonging to his [her partner's] parents, and they carp around again. If this goes on forever, I won't take it, I can't come to terms with my averageness in this way, and all the years of my illness have ruined all my chances of studying something proper, and that's the state I'm in.

A: The final good-bye is at least something special, nothing ordinary, it will break at least one jewel out of the analyst's crown, yes, it really would.

The acknowledgment of her desire to be and achieve something special - even if it were by means of a self-destructive act - did her good. It was true that the severe disturbance of her development, which had set in very early, had also destroyed a lot that could not be replaced. Her insecure self-esteem, which in childhood was obscured by her dependence on her parents, had obstructed her ability to have many experiences of other of her age since the beginning of puberty. She had instead had a wealth of disparaging experiences, in regard to her body and to relationships that damaged her self-esteem, which could only gradually be balanced by new experiencing. She was now able to ask with a strong voice:

P: Would you have come back to my funeral?

A: No, because you would have already destroyed our relationship, but I will be glad to come back to continue working with you. That I will be happy to return is perhaps also a sign of power and strength that you have. I know how much effort it takes for you to overcome your numerous difficulties.

By overcoming this critical phase it became possible for us to together think about ways and means that would be available to her should she need help to tide her over during my absence. The further course of the therapy was interrupted by relapses over and over again, but the patient was able to draw the experience from the situation described here that we would be able to get through and survive her conflicts. The patient has been able to stabilize her partnership and further improve her professional qualifications during the four years that have elapsed since the end of therapy.

3.5 Irony

As welcome as it is to us for therapeutic reasons when submissive, masochistic, or depressive patients reach a natural self-assertiveness and the ability to criticize, it is often just as difficult to bear an exaggerated amount of devaluation that characterizes the sudden transition from submission to rebellion that is hoped for and desired. Some of the affective burdens that arise can be controlled by analytic knowledge. Further protection is offered by irony (Stein 1985).

Konrad Lorenz is supposed to have once said of his especially beloved objects of ethnologic study, "But geese are only human." In our opinion it does not suffice to refer to the fact that psychoanalysts are only human and that it belongs to human nature to respond to attacks by running away, playing dead, or counterattacking. Psychoanalytic knowledge can filter and weaken these and similar spontaneous reactions. While the analyst is nevertheless not immune to his patient's criticism, he should not be so seriously affected that he becomes unable to provide treatment or pays it back to the patient in one way or another. In the latter case the reestablishment of a productive form of cooperation would be much more difficult or impossible. We consider the phrase "affected yes, but not seriously enough that countertransference cannot be made productive in interpretations" to express a good solution to a fundamental problem of psychoanalytic therapeutic technique.

Negative countertransference is often expressed indirectly. This was the case in the treatment of Arthur Y, which we will now describe by referring to the analyst's summary protocol.

One session was a complete failure, in particular because my interpretations were boring. I had tried, among other things, to help the patient comprehend a statement he had made a long time ago, for he had repeatedly enquired about his chances for improvement or a cure. This topic had already been frequently discussed at all possible levels.

A particularly difficult situation arises if the desired criticism a patient makes becomes mixed with a destructive doubt that does not unfold freely. In an earlier dramatic session Arthur Y had let his fantasies have free run, with my support, and admitted that he would not believe me unless I gave him the names of patients who had been successfully treated, which I refused to do for reasons of discretion. It was thus a hopeless situation.

The patient's pronounced ambivalence together with the corresponding splitting processes led him to want to make me bankrupt - in reversal of the fate that almost overtook him. On the other hand, he put all his hope in the expectation that I would withstand his destructiveness and would not lose faith in him, in myself, and in psychoanalysis. Although I was aware of the unfavorable effect of irony, my affect led me to make an ironic interpretation that the patient had, understandably, completely forgotten and that months later led me to give the boring explanations in the session referred to above. At the time I had, referring to the patient's penetrating curiosity about my success, told him that my longest therapy had lasted 100 000 hours and had been unsuccessful. It was understandable that this interpretation had disturbed him so much that he had completely repressed it.

My subsequent comments did not lead any further; the patient remained confused. I did not succeed in making him aware of his omnipotent aggressiveness, which was the assumption behind that interpretation. This was probably connected with the fact that the patient immediately mobilized counterforces. Failure would have sealed both his omnipotence and his hopelessness. He did not want to undermine me so completely that I could no longer be a object-subject providing help. It was noteworthy that it was still difficult for the patient to approach this problem although just a few days previously he had fantasized how he would punish me in public and, by committing suicide, expose me to be a bungler. He said he kept all the invoices in order to denounce me as the one responsible for his suicide. He also had fantasies that I would have to treat him for another 300 hours without payment after his health insurance organization refused to make further payments, and that he would then decide at the end whether and what he would pay me - a fantasy that with the help of an interpretation was intensified to the form that he could, in addition, demand repayment of previous fees by complaining that I had done poor work. He had already secretly imagined suing me for a long time.

This session ended with his remembering that he felt the same as in mathematics class. The teacher would stand up front and write clever equations on the board, and he would not understand anything. The patient added that everything I had said today seemed to him to be nonsense. Disturbed by his criticism, he raised the question of what he could do and what might happen during the rest of the day. The sense of the interpretation was: A lot depended on whether he punished himself immediately for his statement or whether he managed to assert himself against his teacher without letting the word "nonsense" destroy their relationship and without letting everything be destroyed when he put up some resistance.

I was not satisfied with myself in this session and felt at odds with myself and the patient. I was irritated that I had let myself be driven into a corner, and the long interpretations also constituted a kind of compensation for my provoked aggressiveness. I noted that I had made rather gruff comments to his boring questions, to my own relief. This was confirmed by another sign, i. e., after the session I thought I would have to find a way to stop prescribing Valium. The fact that I had not given the patient a prescription before the summer break had had unfavorable consequences. At the time he had viewed this as mistrust, but had subsequently punished himself for having had this feeling by not taking anything despite the progressive deterioration of his condition, which was connected with his displaced anger at me. In the meantime the patient had found a doctor who had quickly prescribed him 50 tablets of Valium during a consultation for something else. The patient still had most of these 50 tablets, but since we were approaching a break and he had already announced that he wanted these 14 days to be different and less fraught with anxiety than the summer vacation, I expected another conflict before the break. Thus after this session I was in a state of negative countertransference.

The next session was less tense and more productive. Good and evil were divided, with me the representive of evil and the doctor who had given him the prescription, whom the patient called the "obscure" person, the representative of a carefree lust for life. Arthur Y vividly described how the other doctor took prescribing Valium lightly and gave him the feeling that he was still very far from being dependent.

Arthur Y associated man's fall from paradise and the pleasure from eating the apple with the prescription of Valium. By strongly cautioning him when I had given him the prescription, I had ruined his pleasure; my threatening gesture had made him afraid. Arthur Y emphasized that the prescription and my gesturing with my index finger had created more problems for him that the prescription had solved. Arthur Y now fantasized putting the other doctor in my place; he imagined he visited this doctor, who prescribed the medication with the quieting comment: "Come back in 4 months, everything will be over, and then we can reduce the medication." In this fantasy he sought the doctor who accepted the entire responsibility and who assured him that everything would be fine. Although I had already told the patient some time before, in reply to an unjustified accusation, that by giving him a prescription I had taken and demonstrated partial responsibility for him, it now became apparent again that partial responsibility was not enough. He was looking for total responsibility and a valid assessment of what would be reached by a certain date. I had, in contrast, left it up to him to take Valium as he needed it, so that the dosage and any possible dependence were his own responsibility.

Now the other side came into play. After having made these accusations, he expected that I would stop the therapy and throw him out. He compared me with his earlier therapists, especially with Dr.X, who had reacted in a cold manner when asked about a prescription and some form of help other than psychoanalysis. I had shown myself to be uncommonly generous, had given him a prescription, and now he was so ungrateful although I had gone far beyond everything he had ever experienced with psychotherapists. The ingratitude which he felt and whose consequences he feared was emphasized by his description of the very generous doctor who had given him a prescription for 50 tablets of Valium without any ado. This doctor had only laughed when the patient asked questions about the danger of dependence.

After giving this description the patient thought about the rest of the day and returned to the question of what he could still do and whether he felt better because he had told me everything. I pointed out to him that his condition probably depended, just like after the session the day before, on whether he punished himself now or not. The patient was again concerned with the question of what he could do in order to utilize the insights he had gained.

The interpretive work had provided such relief that no relapse occurred and Arthur Y hardly used the prescribed medication.

3.6 Narcissistic Mirroring and Selfobject

There is more to the myth of Narcissus than the mirroring surface of a pond in which the young man, losing control of himself and enchanted by the strange beauty, discovers another self. Not only are mirrors nowadays almost everywhere, so that we can reassure ourselves of our appearance, but cameras also have delayed action shutters that enable us to take self portraits and compare our real selves with our ideal selves, i. e., our various body images. Rehberg (1985), following McDougall (1978), showed that an individual's mirror image provides support for the consolidation of his perception of his body.

After the following description of a case, we will make some comments on the mirror metaphor. The analyst in this case was familiar with Kohut's theory but did not follow its specific recommendations about therapeutic technique. We discussed the reasons for this in Vol.1. We emphasize, of course, the significance of self-experience and man's lifelong dependence on confirmation by significant others even though we do not put them in the framework of Kohut's selfobjects. We are pleased to provide the readers a detailed selfpsychologycal commentary at the end of this report.

Arthur Y had taken an unusual step to gain reassurance about his body image, namely by viewing himself. This action, together with his fantasies, provoked a wide variety of countertransference reactions in the analyst. One question the patient raised temporarily elicited insecurity, following which the analyst became aware of something therapeutically productive.

Arthur Y had finally decided to carry through a plan he had had in mind for a long time. He had struggled with himself to speak about it here without demanding that the tape recorder be turned off. He said he had finally done what he had planned to do for a long time, namely to take pictures of his genitals with a camera that he had kept for just that purpose for a long time. One of the pictures turned out very good, and he did not get any better pictures when he later repeated his plan.

I was surprised and pleased by the decisiveness with which Arthur Y finally fulfilled a long held plan without letting himself be inhibited by me or the tape recorder. The patient gave a rather sober report at the very beginning of the session, which left everything open. Neither did the patient describe why the especially good picture was so good, nor did he indicate his motives or what he was looking for in taking nude photographs. I stayed completely reserved because I had the feeling that I was not supposed to disturb his narcissistic satisfaction in any way, although I was very tempted to find out what this objectification meant to him. My guess was that he had photographed his penis in an erect state during masturbation, but I suppressed my curiosity. I reflected that it made a difference whether you look at yourself and always have an incomplete view of your genitals and from a different perspective than when you look at the genitals of other men. I thought that the resulting cognitive difference might play a role in such comparisons, which are very important, especially in puberty and for men who lack self-security.

My fantasies led me to make my own comparisons and ultimately ended in thoughts about the fact that female genitals are hidden and that their position keeps women from viewing their genitals without using a mirror. Finally, in a matter of seconds I thought of Jones' (1927) theory of *aphanisis*, which has always held a special fascination for me, specifically *disappearance* as the factor precipitating elementary anxieties.

It did not surprise me that Arthur Y, as he then told me, had suffered a serious worsening of his symptoms since he had taken the photographs. This worsening may with certainty be traced back to his self-punishment for the nude photopgraphs, but also to the feeling he was a spendthrift and ruining his family because he had gone to an expensive restaurant with a customer and spent, in my opinion, a relatively modest sum for an evening meal. Arthur Y looked almost desparately for further reasons to torment and belittle himself. Thus in one session it sufficed for me to use the word "self-punishment" to reinforce these tendencies in him. He also criticized himself for having found the sight of a young and attractively dressed girl a real treat for the eyes. This occurred after he had taken the nude photos. I therefore related the one viewing to the other and pointed out the pleasure and self-punishment that they had in common. I said this found its culmination in his fear that he could end in complete isolation after all and that his symptoms could become so tormenting that he would not be able to speak another word. It was clear to the patient that he apparently had to pay a high price for his pleasurable actions.

In rather strong terms the patient again demanded that I provide him assistance in transforming the insights he had gained here into action outside - what he could do to behave differently outside, in real life? I explained to him why I do not give any instructions on how to act, and he reluctantly accepted my explanation. He added that he really understood why I refused to answer. The patient was obviously waiting for me to forbid something.

In the following session my conjecture about the nude photos was confirmed. Since the last session the patient had continued his self-observation and photographed his penis in an erect state. During the subsequent masturbation he had once more and with great anxiety observed the discharge of a secretion from his urethra before ejaculating. He was not aware that this was secretion from the prostrate gland. He wanted to ask an expert whether his long-standing fear that this drop of liquid might contain semen was true and thus whether it would be possible for his wife to become pregnant in this way. At first I offered him some of the information he wanted and in response to a question told him that this question belonged to the responsibility of dermatologists, specifically the subspecialty andrology. At this moment I knew that he would request that I recommend a competent specialist, and I thus had a little time to think about how to react.

As a result of the experiences he had had in life, the patient already knew that doctors hardly ever attest something with 100% certainty in such tricky questions. After he had recalled this and laughed about his idea of obtaining - in the manner of a compulsive neurotic - absolute accuracy even down to the last uncertain decimal number, I decided to answer his question myself: "I don't believe that an andrologist would give you any different information than I would. It is highly improbable that semen is contained in the secretion and that conception is possible in this way."

Now he spoke about his anxiety about being abnormal or having venereal disease. The information that the prostatic secretion is discharged prior to ejaculation in all men calmed him. There was a difficult situation because I was unsure whether answering the patient's question as to whether this secretion also appeared in my case could be reconciled with analytic neutrality.

Personally I was not irritated by Arthur Y's question, but rather surprised by his lack of logic, which I pointed out to him. As far as I belonged to the category of men, I also had this prostate secretion. In retrospect, I attributed great significance to the amusement we both had subsequently felt. If Arthur Y had not had unconscious doubts about his (and my) sexual roles, he would have been logical and the question would never have crossed his mind or he would have rejected it immediately. A lack of self-confidence is always accompanied by insecurity toward others. The patient's anxiety about his own bodily products was connected to many frightening questions that the patient had not dared to raise in his childhood.

What had happened at the level of the unconscious? A shared quality was created. From Gadamer's (1965) philosophical perspective, every successful discussion involves a transformation to something shared, leaving nobody as they had been. One factor in the psychoanalytic dialogue that leads to transformation is the discovery of vital items that the analyst and patient have in common. It was logical to assume that Arthur Y experienced himself as a man by imagining the biological events that occur during ejaculation, which gave him increased self-confidence. The prostate secretion was transformed from a disturbing sign to a common denominator linking pleasure in men. Now the patient had acquired enough security to speak about other unconscious causes of his anxieties and doubts.

It is therapeutically decisive that at this moment each party senses the *similarity* in human nature. This similarity in human nature "consists of instincutal impulses which are of an elementary nature, which are similar in all men and which aim at the *satisfaction* of certain primal "*needs*" (Freud 1915b, p. 281, emphasis added). Of course the pleasure linked with sexual function, which Bühler attributed an overall importance as functional pleasure, is experienced individually so that distinctiveness is discovered along with the shared features, the difference along with identity. This is the reason that both in and outside of analyses the question is raised whether, because of their different bodily bases of experience, it is at all possible for the different sexes to understand each other. In Orwell's *Animal Farm* comparisons are made that start from equality and end in disparaging contrasts: "All men are equal, but some are more equal than others."

Returning to the therapeutic discussion of sexual function, which touched on many levels of transference and countertransference, no one should underestimate the fact that sex education provides knowledge in personal form. That was the point in this exchange, which led to a reduction in anxiety and an increase in security. With this protection the patient was able to give more room to his pleasurable curiosity and study new objects.

What impact did the discovery of common biological features have on the analyst's neutrality? His answer did not divulge anything personal, remaining, so to speak, simply one in an anonymous group with the same biological functions. Yet it was apparently essential that the patient first had to find something in common with him, as a member of the same sex, in order to be able to reach the pleasures of life blocked by his anxieties.

This subject formed the background for his observation of his genitals in the photograph. He came closer to understanding the unconscious reasons for his anxieties about the secretion. It now became clear that all of his products had an unconscious anal component. In order to keep his wife from becoming filthy, he often started a fight in the evening, to avoid intercourse; in the process he frequently rejected his wife and hurt her feelings very much. Surprisingly he recalled a dream that had previously seemed strange to him and whose meaning suddenly seemed clear to him. He had viewed an extensive sewage system in a region where he enjoyed vacationing and where he felt very happy. In connection with his self inspection and anxieties about filth, the scales fell from his eyes that he was looking for something down there that exerted a pleasurable attraction on him but that had remained sinister and strange because of his fear of punishment. His associations led him to discover important preconditions of these anxieties.

3.6.1 Mirror Image and Selfobject

The mirror image exerts a fascination that touches on topics as divergent as magic and the idea of having a double (Rank 1914; Roheim 1917; Freud 1919h).

With regard to the question of the nature and background of the mirror image contained in the myth of Narcissus, which Pfandl (1935, pp. 279–310) described in an early psychoanalytic interpretation that has been nearly forgotten, there are two different kinds of answers. In the one group the nature of the object relations and the fellow humans is narcissistic. In the other group the answers are influenced by the idea that the dialogue with the other in the mirror image is more than a continuation in the sense of a comparison with one's self. Both of these psychoanalytic traditions of understanding narcissism can be traced back to Freud, who doubtlessly preferred the derivation from primary narcissism. Two influential representatives of the first type of explanation are, despite all their differences in detail, Kohut and Lacan. Lacan is included here inasmuch as he emphasizes primary narcissism in his original anthropological conception of the mirror image; for him primary narcissism is the term with which "the doctrine refers to the libidinal cathexis suited to this moment" (Lacan 1975, p. 68).

Although Kohut gave up drive theory and narcissism after 1976, all of his descriptions of selfobjects are constructed according to the pattern of primary narcissism, which biases the descriptions of selfobjects. In our opinion, Kohut (1959) paid much too little attention to the high degree to which the empathic-introspective method is dominated by theory. In his attempt to make emphathy an independent cognitive tool, he did not distinguish between the *genesis* of hypotheses and their *validation.* Kohut's selfobjects are constructed entirely according to the libido theory he alledgedly had given up. Analysts who, like Erikson, are oriented toward social psychology can in contrast be characterized by Cooley's beautiful verse, "Each to each a looking glass, reflects the other that does pass."

Freud discovered the dialogic nature of preverbal mirror images from an experience with his approximately 18-month-old grandson:

> One day the child's mother had been away for several hours and on her return was met with the words "Baby o-o-o-o!" which was at first incomprehensible. It soon turned out, however, that during this long period of solitude the child had found a method of making *himself* disappear. He had discovered his reflection in a full-length mirror which did not quite reach to the ground, so that by crouching down he could make his mirror-image "gone". (Freud 1920g, p. 15)

The discovery of the mirror image took place here through the imitation of the motoric action of somebody else (the mother). The interaction was continued via identification; in this way the person who was absent remained present in the other's imagination. At the same time it was an act of self-discovery, at least in the sense of the self-perception of a moving object. Since then a wealth of observations have been published that, by referring to reactions to mirror images, have deepened our awareness of the development of self-perception and self-consciousness. Amsterdam and Levitt (1980) have reported the results of informative experimental investigations; in their interpretations they also take into consideration the phenomenological studies of Merleau-Ponty (1965) and Straus (1952) on the significance of upright posture and shame. We can realistically expect that the results of these and other studies will have substantial effects on the therapeutic understanding of disturbances of self-esteem such as have previously been described in metaphors.

The mirror phase should be understood, "according to Jacques Lacan, [as] a phase in the constitution of the human individual located between the ages of six and eighteen months. Though still in a state of powerlessness and motor incoordination, the infant anticipates on an imaginary plane the apprehension and mastery of its bodily unity. This imaginary unification comes about by means of identification with the image of the counterpart as total *gestalt*" (Laplanche and Pontalis 1973, pp. 250-251). Lacan referred to this moment of jubilant assumption of the image as an exemplary situation representing the symbolic matrix on which the original form of the ego is expressed. "This form could be referred to as the alter ego, to place it in a well-known conceptual frame of reference" (1975, p. 64). But the experience of anticipated unity is threatened by the continuous invasion of fantasies of bodily fragmentation. From this perspective Lacan spoke of the mirror phase as a drama that constantly exerts a compulsion to new repetitions (1975, p. 67).

Because the orientation on the familiar is especially important for Lacan, whose own texts are very difficult to understand, we quote once again from Laplanche and Pontalis (1973, pp. 251-252), who also took the clinical aspect into account. They compared Lacan's conception of the mirror phase with

> Freud's own views on the transition from auto-eroticism - which precedes the formation of an ego - to narcissism proper: what Lacan calls the phantasy of the "body-in-pieces" would thus correspond to the former stage, while the mirror stage would correspond to the onset of primary narcissism. There is one important difference, however: Lacan sees the mirror phase as responsible, retroactively, for the emergence of the phantasy of the body-in-pieces. This type of dialectical relation may be observed in the course of psycho-analytic treatment, where anxiety about fragmentation can at times be seen to arise as a consequence of loss of narcissistic identification, and vice versa.

Kohut traced mirror transference back to needs directed at "selfobjects" (see Vol. 1, Sects. 2.5 and 9.3). Selfobjects are objects that we experience as a part of our self. There are two types of selfobjects: those that react to the child's innate feelings of vitality, size, and completeness and confirm them, and those which the child can look up to and whose fantasized calmness, infallibility, and omnipotence it can fuse with. The first kind is referred to as a mirror selfobject, the second as an idealized parental imago. Deficient interaction between the child and its selfobjects leads to a defective self. By coming to psychoanalytic treatment, a patient whose self has suffered an injury reactivates the needs that remained unsatisfied because of the deficient interaction between his nascent self and his selfobjects earlier in life - selfobject transference develops.

Regarding therapeutic technique, it is essential that the selfobjects and the corresponding transference be attributed a comfirming function. Disregarding all the secondary features, acknowledgment and confirmation by the other person constitute the common denominator linking the different schools in psychoanalysis.

The object relationship psychologies, aside from the Kleinian school, had good reasons for separating the therapeutic factors of agreement and approval from their ties to instinctual satisfaction or to simple suggestion. These corrections have deepened our understanding of what the patient wants from the analyst. They have also thrown a new light on the development of regressive dependence. If the analyst views the exchange from the perspective of instinctual discharge and satisfaction, then he will insist on frustration or make half-hearted concessions, which could be objectionable for reasons of principle or for ethical or technical reasons. If, in contrast, dependence is viewed as a phenomenon of human interaction that is not closely linked to oedipal or preoedipal satisfactions, it is possible to provide genuine confirmation that does not lead into the dilemma of choosing between satisfaction and frustration. Thus, according to Winnicott, if the analyst fails to provide the patient adequate confirmatory support and primarily directs his interpretations at unconscious sexual wishes, the patient uses the latter as a substitute for confirmation. A vicious circle might then develop: sexualized transference wishes increase because the analyst fails to communicate his personal appreciation to the patient, which would strengthen his self-security. Although Kohut's interpretation of the desire for a confirming mirror image satisfies the rule of abstinence, it remains within the narcissistic circle - even if it appears to depart from the circle en route to a selfobject - and does not provide the real confirmation actually needed in certain cases.

According to Winnicott's observations a mother's face does *not* work like a mirror. The child's affective condition is communicated unconsciuslv to the mother, which she answers independently. Winnicott described this continuous process in the language of object relationship psychology: the mother reflects unlike a mirror because she is a person, i.e., a *subject*, and not an inanimate object. Finally, Loewald has attributed the mirror metaphor the function of pointing to the future. He gave it a prospective dimension by emphasizing that the analyst reflects what the patient *seeks* as his unconscious image of himself. This searching is tied to a style of dialogue that makes restraint necessary in order to prevent the patient from being overloaded by strange images. The remaining positive meaning of the "mirroring analyst" lies in the fact that the analyst enables the patient to achieve a self-presentation as free from disturbances as possible. The patient is to be provided an ideal, i.e., unlimited, space for playing with his thoughts, so that self-recognition is not limited from without. We agree with Habermas (1981) that this, of course, cannot be seen as the result of self-observations in which one part of the person, as the object, faces the other, the observer. On the contrary, self-recognition must be understood as a communicative process enabling the patient to discover his self in the other ego, in other individuals, and in his alter ego, or in analytic terms, to refind unconscious self-components or even to recreate them. In our opinion, acknowledgment by a significant other - in the person of the analyst - is fundamental (see Sect. 9.4.3).

Now we can consider countertransference from the perspective of selfobject theory, which is easier to grasp if we refer to Wolf's (1983) description of it. He took selfobjects to be functions that the developing self (the growing child) attributes to objects. An infant expects maternal caretakers in particular to provide the confirmation that Kohut expressed in the beautiful image of the glance in the mother's eye. The selfobjects stand for functions that significant others have to fulfill from the very beginning and for their entire life, in order to develop and maintain the narcissistic balance, which Kohut distinguished from homeostasis. We intentionally refer to Mead's concept of significant others in order to indicate that our understanding of selfobjects is located at the level of general social psychology.

The expression "selfobject" is an unfortunate neologism containing a fragmentary interpersonal theory. The development of identity in an comprehensive sense is accompanied by the integration of numerous social roles. Self-esteem is very dependent on, among other things, confirmation during the acquisition of ego competence (White 1963). Kohut correctly emphasized the significance of such confirmation, thus removing the perjorative quality from narcissism. On the other hand, the numerous psychosocial processes during self development are reduced to the metaphor of mirroring, which does not adequately accomodate the diversity of significant others in an individual's development. It is therefore logical that Köhler's (1982) description of various selfobject countertransferences proceeds from intersubjectivity and interdependence, which have been confirmed by many detailed studies of the mother-child relationship in the last decade (Stern 1985). Köhler followed Kohut's description of selfobject transferences in describing countertransferences. This typology is oriented around the analyst's unconscious expectations, which he applies to the patient and which are considered in the sense of Kohut's theory. It seems logical that the emphasis Kohut placed on empathy led him to give countertransference a reciprocal or complementary function (Wolf 1983; Köhler 1985).

The therapeutic function that the anaylst fulfilled in this session can be described in different languages. Although the analyst had not seen or admired the photograph, his indirect participation did give the patient confirmation that enabled him to master deeper anxieties and feel more secure.

3.6.2 Self-Psychological Perspective

It is instructive to see what can be drawn from this text, or what is missing from it, when criteria taken specifically from self-psychology are applied. One's understanding of the course of the described excerpt of analysis and the subequent choice of technical actions differ depending on whether this vignette is considered from the perspective in which the drives constitute the primary motive or that in which self experience does. The statements contained in an evaluation based only on knowledge of the two hours described above, i. e., an abridged excerpt from a long process, and lacking awareness of the patient's life history and of the rest of the analysis can only have limited validity. In addition, each analyst-patient pair develops its own structure and dynamic, determined by their specific personalities. Comparisons with the procedures used in other cases therefore always suffer from the inability to obtain conclusive proof. Our sole intention in this section is to describe different accents that can be set given different theoretical perspectives.

If self experience is considered the primary motive, the question will be asked if the fact that the patient photographed his genitals does not indicate that early objects and selfobjects provided insufficient active and happy mirroring. Although the photograph may provide a certain answer to the question "How do I look?", what is significant is that the question "How do I look?" was raised at all and posed to the camera.

Nothing was said about why the patient photographed his genitals at precisely this time, so that we can only make assumptions, which are in turn dependent on particular theories. Perhaps it is a perverse act – the satisfaction of voyeuristic and exhibitionistic impulses – in view of a threatening fragmentation of his self. The apparently good transference-countertransference relationship (the patient can speak about the event, the analyst is surprised and pleased) speaks against this, however; thus, it seems probable that the patient sought self-reassurance, given his lack of self-security, particularly regarding his genitals.

In the description of the session it was remarkable that the patient "had to force himself" to say that he had realized a long-held intention, namely to photograph his penis, without demanding that the tape recorder be turned off. He apparently had to give himself a push. In a certain sense, in this session he stepped out of himself and made himself an object of perception. It therefore is not amazing that his report was "relatively" objective.

The analyst reacted innerly by having many different feelings and associations, and was pleased and surprised by the decisiveness with which the patient had forced himself to take this step. We ask: Why? Because his patient dared take a step forwards, be active, be phallic? This might be the result of a specific countertransference, namely a mirror countertransference, which we will discuss later. Furthermore, the analyst reacted with curiosity; he would have liked to know more. Then he identified himself with the patient. He imagined that it makes a difference if a man looks down at his own penis or if he compares it with those of other men, remarking that such comparisons "play a large role, especially in puberty and in men who lack self-security."

Further associations by the analyst followed. He no longer thought of men's genitals, but of women's, i. e., he made comparisons between the sexes. But then his associations led him in "a matter of seconds" to Jones' (1928) theory of aphanisis and to castration anxiety. In this way the analyst put the event in a theoretical framework. Was he perhaps protecting himself? What's more, he employed in this very emotionally laden situation (the patient reported a perverse act!) he employed an objectifying expression in his description, i. e., "nude photo." He stayed reserved although he was tempted to find out what this objectification meant for the patient.

Yet objectification is precisely the factor that, from the perspective of a theory of self-experiencing and its disturbances, must be viewed as what is actually pathological. Pathological is that the patient seeks mirroring with objective methods, which he reports on soberly in a session objectified by a tape recording. From the perspective of self-psychology, one would probably have first looked at the transference aspect: What does it mean for the patient to tell this embarrassing story? One would have probably picked up the patient's sober form of presentation and would have turned to his defensive posture toward the feelings that were involved, and to the effort it took the patient to report what an unusual thing he had done. *Here*, namely, the patient's desire for mirroring lies at the surface: How will the analyst react to the terrible things being told? Did the patient perhaps turn to the mechanical means of photography for his self-presentation because he was afraid of the object's undesired reaction and then very tensely wait for the reaction of his analyst? The latter was, as the frank presentation of his countertransference associations indicates, very involved innerly, but remained "completely reserved" because he did not want to disturb the patient's narcissistic satisfaction. This shows the differing views. From a self-psychological perspective the narcissistic satisfaction is less in the forefront than the anxiety and expectation of the analyst's reaction in the transference situation, which represents a repetition of earlier experiences. Picking up what it means to the patient to talk about this event - which feelings, specifically of shame, are connected with it - would not be a violation of the appropriate neutrality and abstinence, and would have made it easier for the patient to come closer to the feelings he warded off, e. g., his lack of self-security, anxiety, and shame.

Superficially the problem was guilt. The patient told of the worsening of his symptoms, which for the analyst can "with certainty be traced back to self-punishment." The analyst became even more convinced of his opinion by the patient's additional associations, in which he accused himself of being a spendthrift and ruining his family. The analyst mentioned the word "self-punishment," and the patient - grateful for it, because the analyst thus gave up his reserved behavior and said something - continued criticizing himself because he had found the sight of an attractively dressed girl a treat for the eyes. Now the analyst created a connection: Both the nude photo and the girl created *pleasure*, and he therefore had to punish himself. Feelings of guilt are again referred to, but do the patient's self-accusations not possibly serve to ward off much more delicate feelings of guilt that have arisen in him as a result of the fact that his primary objects did not mirroring his vital male pleasurable sensations?

It would namely be possible to see both the nude photo and the girl as representing pleasure in something alive, but the patient did not receive any mirroring in return, so that it is not surprising that he fears of "ending in complete isolation." Yet because of his great insecurity, the patient was dependent on the analyst. The frustrated yet not analyzed mirroring wish was replaced by a view of guilt feelings that was shared by the analyst and the patient. The patient "accepted the fact that he had had to pay a large price for his pleasure." They create something shared, but on a side track; on it the patient continued with the secondary material. Primarily he did not receive any reaction. Now he wanted to have suggestions. (It can be assumed that he did not receive any emotional mirroring in childhood, but that he did get advice about how to get ahead.) The anaylst refused to give the advice, and the patient experienced once again the denial of a request, now in the form of a confirmation. Now he had both a rejection and a narcissistic satisfaction. He had known the answer.

In the next session he again spoke about the photos, this time with anxiety and no longer shy. He was afraid because of his prostate secretion. Well, since this was anxiety and not narcissistic satisfaction (for instance), the analyst answered and made a reference to dermatology. Now the patient's concerns were whether the drop from the prostate gland could cause a pregnancy or not. Again the discussion was more concerned with reality than the patient's insecurity: "Am I normal, am I dangerous, am I like all the others or am I different?" The expected question appeared, "What is it like with you, analyst?" who answered with the comment that as far as he belongs to the category "men," the prostate secretion also appears in him. The tension that had developed was released and there was cheerfulness that had something of the unconscious relief following a joke. Unconsciously both know that they are the same, they are both men. Now they have created something shared in this important sphere. The patient was relieved because he heard that he was the same as all men.

In conclusion, the question might be asked why the patient had such doubts about what he produced (the prostate secretion) and why he required a nude photograph for his self-reassurance - this was presumably because the selfobjects of his childhood, mother *and* father, did not mirror him in a active way. His mother might have mirrored the patient's anality positively or aversively, for one dream finally led him to the conditions in his life history that were behind the development of his anxieties.

The theory that the self constitutes the primary motive - in contrast to drives - underlying these self-psychological considerations requires some theoretical clarification.

A patient with a damaged self, with a narcissistic personality disturbance, directs his reactivated selfobject needs in regressive transference at the analyst, while according to the view based on drive theory the analyst becomes the object of the patient's instinctual desires. Selfobject transference develops, a mirror transference or an idealizing transference. When these forms of transference are present, the patient takes it for granted that the analyst will fulfill those functions for him that he himself cannot fulfill because of the failures made by those around him in the phase-dependent execution of these functions during his childhood. Thus in technically handling such transferences the question foremost to the analyst is, "What *am* I now for the patient? For what purpose does he need me?" (In a transference of instinctual needs he asks what the patient is *doing* with him now.) He will attempt to empathize with the patient and show his *understanding* my making corresponding statements. This kind of understanding is an optimal form of frustration because the existing mirroring and idealization wishes are not satisfied. The analyst only lets the patient know how he recorded his inner feeling and experiencing. In a certain sense this empathic step may mirror the bahavior of a mother grasping the condition of her child. Sander (1962) spoke of "shared awareness," Stern (1985) of "affect attunement," and Loewald (1980) of "recognizing validation," without which psychic development is arrested or impaired. In analysis the first step, that of understanding, is immediately followed by the second, that of *explanation* or interpretation, which through reconstruction unites transference and cure.

The position we took in Vol.1 - namely that the patient cannot be considered alone, but that the analyst's involvement must be included when studying the analytic process - is in full agreement with the conception of the self-selfobject unit constituted by the patient and analyst. However, it is also important to pay attention to the specific countertransferences that can arise in this context.

Selfobject transferences can give rise to countertransferences in the analyst because it is often not easy to bear the patient experiencing you as a part of his self instead of as the center of one's own initiatives. Kohut (1971) described the ways in which an analyst can react to such challenges if he is not conscious of them, possibly disturbing or destroying the course of transference. Wolf (1979) pointed out that selfobject countertransferences are also possible. Through them the analyst can experience, for example, the patient as part of his self and interpret to him (in the sense of a projective identification) what seems important to himself, without correctly grasping the patient. It is also possible for selfobject needs directed at the patient to be mobilized in the analyst and for them to remain unconscious (Köhler 1985, 1988). These selfobject countertransferences constitute a parallel to those countertransferences in which the analyst falls in love with his patient or becomes his rival. In a mirror countertransference, for instance, the analyst would require a mirroring confirmation of his self feeling from the patient; this would take the form that the patient shows improvement, testifying to the fact that his therapist is a good analyst. The analyst gets into the situation of parents who want to be good parents and see their child prosper. An analyst's unconscious expectation that the patient should show improvement can be an important cause of the chronic negative therapeutic reaction, because for the patient improvement would be a repetition of earlier patterns of adjusting to parental expectations and not the liberation sought from analysis.

The countertransference in this case did not lie in the analyst's resistance to the fact that the patient needed him as a selfobject. He reacted with curiosity and interest to the patient's descriptions, not by being completely bored. Yet mirror countertransference may well have been involved, for the analyst said, "I am surprised and pleased by the decisiveness with which Arthur Y realized his long-held plan, without letting me restrict him." Did the patient perhaps fulfill the analyst's expectations and thus a selfobject function? The patient for his part had a mirror transference. The analyst fulfilled the selfobject function by participating and confirming the sexual role they held in common. From the perspective of the theory of self-psychology, it is possible that the analyst, despite his neutral attitude, acted more in transference than he analyzed through interpretation.

3.7 Projective Identification

During the resolution of symptoms in analysis, the inner dialogue that a patient previously conducted with himself is transformed into a two-person dialogue by the analyst who is trying to help him. Substantial burdens are put on the countertransference, in particular when the patient has a narcissistic personality structure. Because of the perversion that the patient described below suffered from, there was very limited space for therapeutic intervention. The countertransferences that this patient precipitated were closely tied to his symptoms, which were also reflected in the specific form that his transference took. The patient wanted to keep all the reins of therapy and be the director, letting the analyst dance like a puppet on a string. Such control is an important element of the theory of projective identification, which we discuss after presenting two cases. The summary and case reports demonstrate that several general aspects of this theory of projective identification were helpful to the analyst conducting the therapy; his interpretive technique itself did not follow Melanie Klein's assumptions.

For didactic reasons it would be appealing to simulate school-specific dialogues. We can conceive of different variations that make it possible to play through interpretive actions at a fictive level, such as at a seminar on therapeutic technique. The absence of the patient sets limits on the substantive reality of such thought experiments. The same is true of the customary clinical discussions, where participants offer alternative interpretations of certain situations, because in the patient's absence these theoretical games are necessarily one-sided. The enactment could be made complete by including the *expectations* that the analyst making the interpretation had regarding the patient's reactions.

Theoretical considerations have an outstanding heuristic function. It might therefore be helpful for the reader to first turn to our comments on projective identification before examining the two descriptions of cases for possible applications.

3.7.1 Case 1

Johann Y gave his analyst a notebook containing a description of his symptoms, which he was very ashamed of, at the beginning of his first session; he did not want to speak about them yet. I learned from the notes that he suffered from a perversion. As a 7-year-old he had stolen a pair of rubber pants that his mother had gotten ready for his 2-year-old sister. He took them to the toilette, put them on, and defecated in them. At the beginning of puberty he began making his own rubber pants from plastic bags. His very strong social isolation was accompanied by the fact that his feelings were seriously hurt, which precipitated several attempts to commit suicide. His fetter rituals, which went back to early adolescence, enabled him to overcome states of extreme powerlessness and control tension by himself. The patient was not able to indicate the connection with masturbation until in an advanced phase of therapy. He sought treatment after the fetters came to pose a much more serious danger to himself because he had used electrical wiring; a temporary paralysis once caused him to panic, when he feared for several hours that he would be unable to free himself.

The patient himself related his illness to anxieties about being left alone and disintegration, which went far back into early childhood and which had became substantially stronger since puberty, in part as a result of a psychotic illness afflicting a younger sister.

Despite the danger that the bondage posed, the patient did not want to initiate treatment unless he was permitted to determine conditions such as the frequency and setting (lying or sitting); an earlier attempt at treatment had failed because the analyst had insisted on observing the standard technique.

The analyst who agrees to "flexible" arrangements with such patients puts himself in a special situation. He conforms to the patients wishes and deviates from the rules characteristic of psychoanalytic technique. In our opinion the meaning the deviation has to the analyst when he adjusts the setting to the patient's demands is very significant. Is it extortion? No, the analyst will not feel as if he is the victim of extortion if he lets a seriously ill patient determine which therapeutic conditions are still tolerable. Inasmuch as the altered setting permits the analyst to acquire psychoanalytic knowledge and to exert therapeutic influence, this is not a one-sided act, or more correctly, the analyst's agreement means that he can work within the given framework even though the opportunity to establish a therapeutic alliance may be very minimal. At least agreement is reached that is satisfactory to each participant.

Naturally the question is immediately raised as to why a patient has to pursue his autonomy so rigorously that he reacts to each intervention that does not suit him by stopping the session or making chronic accusations and criticism. Prescribing the analyst what he may say and when he had better keep his mouth shut precipitates powerlessness and the feeling of being "in bondage" in the analyst's countertransference. The analyst is then obviously no longer the master in his own house, but lets himself get into a manipulative relationship that he hopes to escape from in time with the help of his interpretations.

The "bondage" resulting from the "dictatorship" of the patient inevitably leads to affective problems that, according to the patient's rigid regulation of the relationship, are always in danger of becoming a analogously rigid "projective counteridentification" in the sense described by Grinberg (1962, 1979). We would also like to refer to a case report by McDougall and Lebovici (1969, p. 1), who describe the 9-year-old Sammy, who for a long time only spoke when the analyst wrote down each word. The boy frequently screamed, "Now write what I dictate; I am your dictator."

The affective problem consists in not becoming angry or apathetic during the imposed passivity and even powerlessness. With patients whose potential for change is very slight it is especially important that the analyst maintain his interest by gaining insights into psychodynamic connections, i. e., by acquiring knowledge. This is a source of satisfaction for us in difficult psychoanalyses, without which desolate periods could hardly be borne. In our opinion it is important for each anaylst to find out how he can maintain a positive attitude in difficult situations and have at least a minimal amount of satisfaction despite the substantial burdens.

The following session took place at the end of the third year of treatment.

The patient, who was usually punctual, arrived late and immediately went to the armchair, commenting that his tardiness was an expression of his inner conflict; he did not have a plan for today, no map for how he should proceed. He stated that his previous manner of working with me was not functioning quite right.

To clarify his position, Johann Y used expressive and metaphoric descriptions, which to him were orientations providing support; I was not permitted to analyze their metaphoric meaning.

P: I believe that I have to tell you about the thoughts I have been having, about how I believe that the therapy and, incidentally, my life too are functioning. There are two processes, one of *compensation* and one of *development*. Because of the many troublesome experiences I had in my childhood, my developmental process came to a standstill, and I became involved in compensatory processes; women play a special role in them. Last night I saw an image, maybe it was a dream or a vision, that isn't clear to me.

This description was characteristic of his difficulty to maintain a stable border between the outer and inner worlds. He had great difficulty identifying inner visions as such.

P: In the valley of memories I met four women who accused me of having stolen things from them and they wanted them back. I couldn't give them back; they were simply used up. That was the image; I think the four women were the first four girls before Maria.

The patient had not yet had a closer heterosexual relationship, but he was always able to find women for whom he was a platonic friend without any touching ever occurring. They were usually women who were experiencing conflicts in another relationship and who found consolation and help in talking with the patient. The patient found satisfactions to disguised fantasies in each of these relationships, regularly experiencing the disappointment of the woman leaving him to return to her "real friend." The acquaintance with Maria differed from his previous relationships to women primarily in the fact that it had already existed for several years. The fact that she was not a part of his everyday life played a large role. She lived several hundred kilometers away, so that only sporadic visits were possible. At this distance he was able to develop a stable relationsip to her, in which Maria functioned as an externalized ego ideal.

P: I believe that a new era started with Maria, which is why I can't walk through the valley of memories yet, but have to study it more closely; but at the moment I am in the desert again.

The primary purpose of his statements was to master inner tensions; superficially they were typical intellectual games. Yet this was how he maintained his balance. I often had difficulty grasping, even at the manifest level, where in his complicated network of ideas the patient wanted to lead me. The patient had referred to the phase preceding the valley of memories as the march through the desert. I therefore attempted to establish a tie to his decision not to lie on the couch and to seek a secure spot in the armchair instead.

A: Presumably it is therefore both more secure and more reasonable for you not to lie on the couch because you are still in the desert, and nobody goes into the desert without a route.

I adopted the patient's language although I knew that this maintained the distance created by this language.

P: Where am I? In which part of the process? I think I am in the compensatory world, but the valley of memories would reopen the world of development. I wish you would go down this route first, letting me watch from a great distance.

A: Our previous excursions into the valley of memories were always accompanied by very many painful memories that were a burden to you, and if I am the one who goes first, then I determine the pace and not your. This is where I see a risk.

The patient confirmed this; he said he now had to learn to set the pace together with me. This was definitely true, and at the same time it would give him the assurance that he could regulate the work. (At the beginning of the analysis I had often gone far beyond the patient in different attempts to reach him in his schizoid isolation.)

In the next sesson he brought me a written statement and demanded that I simply read it. *Not* to read this note and to request that the patient tell me its contents directly would have led him, according to my previous experiences with him, to immediately stop the session. I therefore read his note:

In the previous session we made a decisive step toward clarifying the question of what I want reach with you. I now have the confidence to give you a description that means something to you.

The point is "nails without heads." In clarification, nails without heads are analytic (i. e., in the theoretical sense of categorizing) approaches to problem solving without their concrete implementation. (The head would be the form of realizing or further developing the approach that is possible at any particular moment.)

It is my intention to alter this pattern of behavior. In principle there are three goals, described as follows:

1. I alone make "nails with heads" and don't talk about it.
2. You make "nails with heads," but then they are your nails and I can't use them.
3. You help me here to find "nails" and leave the making of "heads" to me.

After reading this note I did not interpret its formal nature but turned to the image it offered.

A: The task you give us is not easy but probably very important: that you have the opportunity to get nails here - the ideas I can give you - and that you in turn have the assurance that the implementation is really only your business.

The patient was satisfied at first and told me about numerous activities where in the last few months he had created fields in which he could move relatively safely.

P: I believe that I am looking for freedom of self-determination. My kind of freedom. Last year your big mistake was that you followed me too closely during my positive, active development and that you even forced the pace. That is why I reduced the number of sessions. Now you are just accompanying me.

The patient was referring to an episode in which I had attempted to interpretatively break through his restrictions, with the result that he fell into a suicidal mood and entered a psychiatric hospital for a few days. My feeling that developed in that particular situation of being bound by him - restricted and tied down, not fascinated - had led me to make the interpretation that he was not letting me participate in his development in the way I would wish. This attempt by means of an interpretation of our interaction to give him a perspective of how he handled our relationship presumably reactivated an experience in which his mother had interfered.

The schizoid component of the patient's disturbances could be traced back to traumatic experiences he had had in early childhood. In his memories the patient saw himself as the infant who cried for hours and who was neglected by his mother. After the birth of his sister, when he was 5 years old, he became increasingly difficult and his mother did not want to leave him alone with his little sister, so she used the curtain to tie him down in the next room. The patient was still able to recall how ashamed he was when he defecated in his pants again, although he had been clean at an early age.

The strategy behind my interpretations was directed primarily at clarifying the current genesis of the connections between rejections, feeling hurt, women's temptations that caused him anxiety, each of which initiated a narcissistic retreat. His increasingly improved mastery of these situations led, correspondingly, to a clear decrease in the frequency of his perverse acts.

After 3 years of treatment the patient was able to write down the following thoughts about his fetters:

The meaning of my fetters is now clear to me. It is a self-experience of elementary importance to me. Here it is true that I can only escape if I concentrate on it and push aside other aspects such as pain or anxiety. If the anxiety predominates, I have hardly a chance. This corresponds precisely to my real situation; if the anxiety predominates, if I don't have any room left to think and act "freely," then my illness is acute. My bondage is just as dangerous as the danger to me from the particular situation. Simple fetters without any additional restraints leave me more time, namely until I die of dehydration, or about 3 days. I have never needed longer than a good hour under these conditions. When electricity or too little air, possible even overheated surroundings, play a role, then I have correspondingly less time and my concentration has to increase by the same amount. This increases the value of "self-experience." Depending on the combination, I have needed up to 3 hours, but given "fortunate circumstances" I have been free after only 2 minutes. The meaning of being bound is thus to hinder the acute state of the illness because it takes the place of the experience of myself or my identity that is necessary during a particular period of time and that cannot be guaranteed in any other manner.

What the patient described as an acute illness consists of massive anxieties, which appear during too direct interaction. In the act of binding himself he mastered the fantasized dangers by himself carrying out the humiliations inflicted on him and thus controlling his own destructiveness. The anxious loss of control over defecation he described was an intended and willful bowel movement and was somehow linked in the perverse act with ejaculation. This was the end of his pleasurable triumph over his mother and all women after her who disturbed him and made him feel hurt. The disparagement of women - which also contained an aspect of identification with his father, who said he held little of his wife - can also be seen outside the perversion and in the accompanying transformation into compensation, admiration, and idealization. At the same time the patient was forced to maintain a distance to protect women from his attacks and retain his mother's fantasized love, as Stoller (1968, p. 4) has emphasized:

Perversion, the erotic form of hatred, is a fantasy, usually acted out but occasionally restricted to a daydream .... It is a habitual, preferred aberration necessary from one's full satisfaction, primarily motivated by hostility .... The hostility in perversion takes form in a fantasy of revenge hidden in the actions that make up the perversion and serves to convert childhood trauma to adult truimph.

In the unconscious exchange of roles, the patient himself was the mother, even more powerful than she was, and controlled everything. The patient linked a superficial motivation of his controlling - identifiable as anal autonomy - with the fact that he moved frequently, which kept him from being able to develop a feeling of being safe and at home anywhere.

3.7.2 Case 2

In the following example the phenomena are traced back to reconstructed processes whose diagnosis was grounded in an understanding of countertransference of the kind made possible by the theory of projective identification. The analyst in this case stood, on the basis of his training, in the Kleinian tradition. He was not only familiar with its theory but also trained in the application of its therapeutic technique. Of course, in judging a therapy it is irrelevant whether some authority has declared it to be characteristic of a particular school. It is necessary, however, to reach agreement about specific criteria in order to compare therapies from different schools or approaches. This is not the point in this example, although we do consider comparative elements in our commentaries. The purpose is to explain problems, and we only touch on the question of differences in effectiveness. The independence of the metaphorical therapeutic language mentioned above imposes reservations on us in this regard.

Veronika X started psychoanalytic treatment at the age of 24 because of spastic corticollis. Her wryneck came in attacks that only occurred during emotional stress and especially during examinations in her professional training. The psychogenic factor precipitating her peculiar involuntary twisting of her head and/or the fact that emotional influences reinforced the symptoms of her neurological illness were confirmed by carefull observation and had even been noted by the patient herself. What resulted was a vicious circle, which we describe in Sects. 5.2 and 5.5, in the context of another case of wryneck, as being typical for many illnesses, regardless of whether their primary causes are more in the psychic or more in the somatic sphere.

In Veronika X's therapy the neurologic syndrome receded into the background in comparison with a severe borderline structure. The working alliance was continuously undermined by the fact that the transference was strongly erotized, which put a considerable burden on the countertransference in many sessions.

In the first year of treatment the patient was seldom able to lie on the couch for the entire hour. Most frequently she would walk through the room anxiously, from time to time throwing angry and evil looks at me and at the same time expressing a deep helplessness. Veronika X often sat cowered at my feet, while I sat in my armchair. My toleration of this form of behavior was accompanied by my attempts to interpret the patient's feelings and her anxieties about a further loss of control. Once it had been necessary to draw a clear line. When the patient refused to tolerate that I took a few notes during the session and she jumped off the couch to grap the pen out of my hand, I reacted very firmly: "If you don't give me my pen back immediately, you will force me to end the treatment."

Commentary. The analyst pulled the emergency brakes to prevent further incursions, which pose a burden for the analyst and can be highly traumatizing for the patient. The loss of control strengthens deep-seated anxieties and leads to a feeling of shame. Having a tantrum is a means by which children seek support from adults.

Yet despite everything Veronika X was capable of productive therapeutic work. She reported dreams that were accessible to analytic work despite their strong fragmentation and the predominance of a world of partial objects and body language. This enabled each of us to maintain the hope that the treatment would be worthwhile, which was confirmed by the progress she made in everyday life and the reduction in her psychic symptoms. My ability to stay calm, keep an overview, and recognize connections aroused great admiration from the patient. She often expressed the view that she would not have any more difficulties if she could think like I did. This admiration raised questions about how I came to understand something in this or that way, and she often reacted by becoming very angry at answers. She did not change her opinion that my answers were evasive and incomplete or expressed my desire not to indicate the "source" of my knowledge.

Commentary. As we explained in Sect. 7.4 of Vol.1, it is important precisely in borderline cases to give realistic answers. Furthermore, it is helpful in all psychoanalyses to let the patient participate in the context of the analyst's knowledge, as we described in Sect. 2.2. This does not eliminate all the patient's complaints or accusations about being excluded from the source of knowledge, but they often become mild enough that the tension between power and powerlessness shifts slightly to the patient's favor. We are making this commentary for didactic reasons and without being able to know whether the analyst in this case could have given any more information about the background of this interpretations at all.

The negative therapeutic reactions became more frequent during the course of analysis, with one component, envy, gradually becoming clearer and clearer. Every time the patient had the impression that I remained able, despite all the difficulties which she was completely aware of, to continue my work and to recognize her extreme need for help, she reacted in a very ambivalent manner, combining her tantrums and acknowledging that the therapy was really advantageous for her.

In the third year of analysis and at the beginning of the second session in one week, Veronika X looked me in the eyes with a long and rigid, even penetrating glance, before she laid down on the couch; this glance had an important effect on my countertransference, and I was unable to really understand its origin. A long moment of silence followed, and in response to the question of what she was thinking about, she gave the same answer she had given numerous times before: her sexual desire for me. In contrast to previous occasions, her direct, sexual statement had the effect of arousing sexual fantasies in me. I began to imagine a sexual relationship with the patient in very concrete terms, which made me feel very insecure. My first reaction was that I felt provoked, not through her direct sexual statement but in a way which was hard to define. During a long period of silence I struggled to understand what had happened this time and had led me to become so emotionally involved. I asked the patient again what was on her mind in this moment. She answered that she remembered an experience she had had a few years earlier in Spain. On a very hot day she went down into a crypt in a medievel castle together with a group of tourists. There it was cool and there was a very pleasant atmosphere. In the crypt there was a stone sarcophagus with a beautiful reclining figure, picturing a prince. She was fascinated by the beautiful figure and felt at that moment a strong longing to possess it, together with rage at the fact that it was available to the many stupid tourists. In response to this association and on the basis of my sexual fantasies (in which the patient approached me and stroked me), I made the following interpretation:

A: I believe that you would like to have my body and my spirit, which are one and the same thing to you, all to yourself. Just for you, without having to share me with the other stupid patients. To have me to yourself and to study me somehow, examine, palpate, learn to know very precisely, and to read my thoughts to find out what's in me.

Extending and confirming my interpretation, the patient added that in her fantasies she had entered the sarcophagus. Inside the sarcophagus she felt very well and had the illusion that the prince belonged to her alone.

A: Yes, for you alone, but transformed into a corpse. You have the idea that you can only possess me completely if you sleep with me. It should be my initiative, my wish to possess your body. At the same time it is clear to you, however, that in the moment you succeed in tempting me into a sexual relationship, I will be transformed into a dead analyst, that as an analyst I will die.

After this interpretation I sensed very dramatically how my arousal subsided. Later in the session I expanded on this interpretation.

A: I believe that you can hardly bear your intense wish to have a complete relationship and that the only possibility for making this state more bearable is to attempt to give me the same feelings, namely the desire that paralyzes you and keeps you bound to the couch like the reclining figure on the sarcophagus. This is your only chance to give me this intense feeling.

At the beginning of the next session the patient said that my interpretation in the preceding session had made her "yellow with rage." I replied that "yellow with envy" was the correct expression and that red was the color of rage. After a few minutes of silence Veronika X told me about a dream from the preceding night. She had been a very little child and huddled at the feet of an old man who was very good at telling fairy tales. She was enthusiastic about the stories, yet at the same time she was enraged that this old man possessed this ability. Then she began to climb up his body, up to his eyes, and attempted to poke out his eyeballs by sticking her finger inside. The old man evaded her very adroitly, without openly rejecting her, and she did not succeed in blinding him.

Because of the dream I was able to understand the patient's negative therapeutic reactions and her use of projective identification. On the one hand, she was enthusiastic about my ability to tell her stories about her own psychic reality, but on the other, this enthusiasm awoke greed and envy in her, together with the feeling of being very small and helpless. As a result of this feeling of helplessness the need grew in her to get rid of this dangerous difference by destroying its source, i. e., my ability to look into the patient. The patient defended herself against this difference by trying to "inject" in me sexual desires that could have confused me. When Veronika X noticed that I had retained my capacity for insight despite her efforts, she felt eased on the one hand, but on the other the vicious circle was reinforced. The fact that the patient did not show any negative therapeutic reactions this time but, entirely to the contrary, was able to relate a dream explaining the previous negative therapeutic reactions was probably a sign that the vicious circle was interrupted in this session, which was confirmed in the later course of the treatment. Veronika X now had the confidence that the working alliance could bear her aggressiveness, which she herself was most afraid of; her attacks of envy were instances of this aggressiveness. She knew from experience that I was in a position to bear stronger emotions and to descend with her into the depths of a crypt without losing my capacity for insight.

Commentary. The vicious circle was perhaps initially strengthened because the analyst had seen something new in her. This was the reason she wanted to blind him. Why was it impossible for her to identify with the pleasure of seeing and being seen? And what could be done to interrupt the vicious circle? The analyst's imperturbability was unnatural to a degree that it exerted an immense attraction to make her become confused and lose her way. The purpose of the introjection was to attain a balance between top and bottom, between right and left, between those possessing and those without.

3.7.3 Notes on Projective Identification

As we explained in Sect. 3.2 of Vol.1, the purpose of the theory of projective (and introjective) identification in M. Klein's school is to explain and ground the holistic understanding of countertransference. The concept of projective (and introjective) identification was originally based on assumptions about the importance of early "persecutory fear and schizoid mechanisms," which M. Klein referred to as assertions and hypotheses deduced from material she had gained from her analyses of children and adults (Klein 1946, p. 102). The direction in which the deduction was stronger - from the material to the theory or vice versa - is irrelevant. The latter is probable since Melanie Klein was one of those analysts whose interpretive technique is extremely strongly colored by her theory, as can be seen in her case description of little Richard (Sect. 1.3). However the case may be, the theory of projective and introjective identification refers to early and primitive fantasies.

The core of this implied interactional system consisted of fantasies of entering the mother and projecting parts of oneself that had been split off into her body or, vice versa, of being penetrated. Klein initially considered this as the "prototype of an *aggressive object relation*" (1946, p. 102, emphasis added). Later Bion (1959) and Rosenfeld (1971) described a special form of *projective identification serving communication*, in which the projecting of a feeling into the mother (or analyst) had the purpose of precipitating a certain feeling in order to indicate a psychic state that could not be verbalized and possibly get mother (the analyst) started in some direction.

If it were possible to understand and explain the analyst's capacity for empathy and the important part of the patient-analyst exchange according to the pattern of projective and introjective identification, then psychoanalysis would have its own and original theory of communication. These elements would be largely beyond the critical examination of other sciences because it would be possible in doubtful cases to always return to the argument that these are unconscious processes originating at an early preverbal stage of development. This argument would apparently make it possible to push aside the results of direct mother-child observation. Even well-founded scientific criticism does not convince many analysts, probably because the clinical language associated with this theory can evoke a strong resonance from the patient. The metaphors that are used to lend color to the intellectual exchange are derived from body experience. To name just two examples, "That gets under my skin," and "I'll tell on you." A favorite verb in the language of Kleinian therapy is "to put into" which awakens both oral and phallic connotations. The therapeutic language linked with projective identification is thus an accentuated "action language" emphasizing aggressiveness (see Thomä 1981, p. 105).

The key verb "to put into" presumably goes back to metaphors that Klein used in her attempt to describe the process of projection:

> The description of such primitive processes suffers from a great handicap, for these phantasies arise at a time when the infant has not yet begun to think in words. In this paper, for instance, I am using the expression "to project *into* another person" because this seems to me the only way of conveying the unconscious process I am trying to describe. (Klein 1946, p. 102)

For these reasons analysts can put the concept of projective identification to wide use, all the more so precisely because it is defined vaguely and is one of the least understood concepts in psychoanalysis, as one of its proponents stated (Ogden 1979).

We now come to the difference between *projection* and *projective identification*, which allegedly can be seen in if and how the projecting person remains tied to the projected contents and at which level of consciousness. Yet it is doubtful whether it is possible to see the difference between projection and projective identification in the fact of whether the person projecting remains tied to the expelled and denied self-components or not. According to Freud (1937d, p. 268), such ties also characterize the paranoid systems that developed by means of projection and then maintain them circularly. We must emphatically point out that the process of projection, in which unconscious identifications are at play, can be linked with numerous contents. Thus it is misleading to only think of the projection of homosexual contents during paranoid developments, as Freud described for delusions of jealousy. Since Freud was especially concerned with the projection of homosexual desires, the fact was largely overlooked that the theory of projection refers to *formal* processes, which can be linked to many unconscious *contents*. Significant differences between it and projective identification can apparently only be created in an abridged description of the theory of projection.

Our knowledge of projection is age-old. According to the *Bible* (Luke 6:42), you see the *mote* in the eye of the other but not the *beam* in your own. This fits in with Freud's explanation of paranoid systems, which are maintained by the "beam carrier" who looks for and finds little motes everywhere, which confirm to him how evil fellow humans are to him. In this way he keeps from recognizing that his own "beams" form the basis for his raised sensitivity to the evil in others, and from recognizing what he does to them. This describes the fact that projective processes are anchored in intersubjectivity (Freud 1922b, p. 226).

Kernberg (1965, p. 45) described the process in the following way:

> Projective identification may be considered an early form of the mechanism of projection. In terms of structural aspects of the ego, projective identification differs from projection in that the impusle projected onto an external object does not appear as something alien and distant from the ego because the connection of the ego with the projected impulse still continues, and thus the ego "*empathizes*" with the object. The anxiety which provoked the projection of the impulse onto an object in the first place now becomes fear of that object, accompanied by the need to control the object in order to prevent it from attacking the ego when under the influence of that impulse. A consequence or parallel development of the operation of the mechanism of projective identification is the blurring of the limits between the ego and the object (a loss of ego boundaries), since part of the projected impulse is still recognized within the ego, and thus ego and object fuse in a rather chaotic way. (1965, p. 46, emphasis added)

We emphasize the empathic contact because this statement clashes with the assertion that the "ego and object fuse in a rather chaotic way." It seems that the micropsychology of these processes has largely been metaphorical.

Projective identification, like other unconscious mechanisms, is not directly observable and must be deduced. It consists of assumptions about fantasies, not the fantasies themselves. In deductions of this kind the plausibility of the theoretical assumptions on which the interpretations are based must be examined particularly carefully. In the case of projective identification and its twin, introjective identification, the extent to which these assumed processes and positions are dependent on the hypothesized psychotic core in infancy must be clarified. Many analysts probably presume the validity of the paranoid schizoid and the depressive postions, keeping any doubt from arising about whether the psychotic core actually constitutes a universal transitional phase whose consequences are almost timeless.

In Vol. 1 (Sect. 1.8) we considered the different mythologies of the infant. The myth of the psychotic core makes it necessary to find an explanation for every *healthy* development. Many premises that served as the foundation for typical Kleinian interpretations can no longer be upheld (see for example Lichtenberg 1983a). Thus clinical interpretations derived from the assumption that there is a psychotic core are wrong. This does not impress analysts who are firmly tied to this tradition. They point to the clinical evidence, claiming that it shows that Melanie Klein's ideas have proved themselves to be exceptionally productive. Is it possible to act correctly despite false premises? What is logically impossible seems to function in practice because therapeutic activity can find a foundation of its own and its direction is thus not at all determined by the false theoretical premises. In this regard there is no fundamental difference between the different schools of psychoanalysis.

Separating the concept of projective identification from its untenable premises creates a new perspective. Entirely aside from the fact that Klein established a counterposition to Freud in the psychoanalytic movement, fulfilling a historically significant function, her ideas must be seen as the precursors of the social psychological foundation of psychoanalysis. Projective and introjective identification refer to exchange processes in which individuals exert influence on each other.

Exchange processes determine human life starting at birth. It is to be expected that projective identification and other psychoanalytic concepts will be integrated in a scientifically grounded theory and practice of intersubjectivity. The language of therapy, which is rich in metaphors, is affected by this transformation. Several problems appear in the use of metaphors. Since projective identifications are defined as unconscious fantasies, they can even be interpreted if the analyst does not feel any countertransference that can be associated with this patient's particular fantasy. For instance, the patient can report a dream, and the analyst may draw inferences as to a projective identification. Here the problem consists in putting the contents of unconscious fantasies in a causal relationship with the patient's experiencing or behavior; this relationship must be with regard to the *specific intentionality* of the fantasies, e. g., the desire to project something into the body of the other. It is not sufficient to proceed from the *principle of intentionality*, i. e., the primary object relatedness, of all desires and fantasies.

The first step is for the analyst to recognize that a certain experience in his countertransference was actually precipitated by the patient. Then he has to find an access to the patient's presumed fantasies and relate them to the means (expressions, gestures, patterns of behavior etc.) the patient uses in their interaction to precipitate the analyst's corresponding experience. Finally the analyst must clarify whether the purpose of the projection is to attack the patient's ties to the analyst and paralyze his mental capacity, or is communicate an averbal inner state. In this regard the fate of a specific projective identification is ultimately *dyadic in nature*. This means that the character of a specific projective identification is not determined by the patient's presumed "intention," but depends on the analyst's ability to understand his countertransference feelings and to "digest" them in this way, i. e., to decode them and to give them back in interpretations. Bion described this process as the capacity for *rèverie*. According to Bion, if the analyst's ability to daydream fails him, then he will be flooded by the precipitated feeling, will not be able to think, and will feel confused. His communication with the patient will be interrupted and the analyst will tend to assume that the patient has "projected" his own confusion into him.

In the same situation another analyst might not get confused by the same projective identification and is in a position to understand the message it contains; his interpretation can then reach the contents of the unconscious fantasy. In these two cases the analysts react in opposite ways. In the first case the satisfaction gained from destruction might be the object of interpretation, in the second the libidinal need to maintain the tie. The result is that the function of the projective identification depends on the interpretation.

Although Klein's original description did not dictate that only negative self-representations can be projected into other persons (the mother) in this way, its clinical applications primarily emphasize, as Hamilton (1986, p. 493) showed in Bion's case, the destructive aspects of projective identification in psychotic patients. Hamilton therefore rightly pleads for analysts to also consider the clinical uses of "positive projective identification," in which good and loving self-representations are projected. By reintrojection it is possible to promote the development of positive object relations through the empathic connection to the receiver (see in this regard our discussion of Kohut's selfobjects in Sect. 3.6).

We can now return to a concluding evaluation of the concept of projective identification by adopting one of Meissner's arguments. He states that assuming the existence of a "basically psychotic mechanism" is a precondition for making the concept clinically valid (1980, p. 55). The diffusion of the self-borders is then the same as the loss of self-object differentiation. In particular Bion's (1967) later extension of the concept in his use of the metaphor "container" contributed to a change. In a very critical manner Meissner thought this through to its logical conclusion:

In Bion's terms, then, projective identification is a form of symbiotic relationship taking place in reciprocally beneficial ways between two persons, between a container and a contained. Consequently, projective identification becomes a metaphor, translated loosely into the terms of container and contained, which applies to almost any form of relational or cognitional phenomenon in which the common notes of relation, containment, or implication can be appealed to. (1980, p. 59)

The nonpsychotic form of projective identification and, correspondingly, that of projective counteridentification (Grinberg 1979) can presumably be better and more economically understood by referring to the conception of reciprocally elicited roles from the repertoire of cue behavior. We agree with Grey and Fiscalini that the talk of "putting into" vividly describes subjective experiences:

Perhaps, "putting into" may be understood as cue behavior expressed by one participant to elicit a reciprocal response by the other; if so, the initiator does "put into" the situation an invitation to a defensive interaction, as does any transference activity. Otherwise, such *metaphoric evocation of psychic possession* is potentially misleading. (1987, p. 134, emphasis added)

Our case descriptions permit an interpretation that agrees well with the following statement by Porder:

I believe that projective identification can best be understood as a compromise formation that includes as its major component an "identification with the aggressor" or a "turning of passive into active," in which the patient unconsciously *acts out* in the transference the role of the major pathological parent or both parents and, via this re-enactment, induces feelings in the analyst similar to those that the patient experienced as a child. I suggest that the replay of this drama, with the roles reversed from the ones that took place in childhood, is the crucial unconscious transference/countertransference interaction observed in patients who demonstrate what has been called projective identification. (1987, p. 432)

In similar fashion Heimann also put the exchange in rolls at the center of this concept:

"Projective identification" appears as a countertransference reaction when the analyst fails in his process of perception; instead of perceiving the transference in time, he unconsciously introjects the patient who is at this moment acting on the basis of his identification with his rejecting and overpowering mother, what ultimately results in a reenactment of his own experiences in an exchange of roles. (1966, p. 257)

In our opinion the function of projective identification is determined by its interpretation. What is involved is above all that the patient recognizes his own positive and negative self-components that he attributed to the analyst. Analysis of these processes should begin by examining the real events in the interaction. The patient's behavior forces an interaction that the analyst cannot understand until he has let it happen for some time. The "empathic contact" with the projected self-components emphasized by many authors originates in their unconscious awareness of the script of this interaction. With the help of the analyst involved in the interaction and of his interpretations, it is possible for the patient to recognize his own transposed self-components. This self-recognition precedes their reintegration. As long as an individual is alienated from his self-components, it is impossible for them to be accepted and incorporated.

4 Resistance

Introduction

In the corresponding chapter in Vol. 1 we described the classification of different forms of resistance; in this chapter, from the perspective of analytic technique, we focus on the *regulatory function* that resistance fulfills in the *relationship.*

The extension of the theory of transference that we described in Vol. 1 (Sect. 2.5), has obviously had a significant impact on the theory of resistance that corresponds to it. Although the differing views of well-known contemporary analysts remind us of the controversies between A. Freud, Fenichel, M. Klein, and Reich in the 1930s, at least in their wording, there are nevertheless numerous signs that resistance phenomena are today increasingly being viewed in terms of the relationship. This change was made explicit in a public discussion between Sandler and Rangell, held at the Madrid psychoanalytic congress in 1983. The following passage contains the essential points of Sandler's arguments:

> It seems clear that the introduction and description of these object-related processes, particularly the *object-related defences,* reflected a major *new dimension* in the analytic work and in the concept of transference. The analysis of the here-and-now of the analytic interaction began to take precedence, in terms of the timing of interpretations, over reconstruction of the infantile past. If the patient used defences within the analytic situation which involved both him and the analyst, this was seen as transference, and increasingly became a primary focus of attention for the analyst. The question "What is going on now?" came to be asked before the question "What does the patient's material reveal about his past?"
>
> In other words, the analytic work became more and more focused, in Britain certainly, on the patient's use of the analyst in his unconscious wishful fantasies and thoughts as they appeared in the present - i. e. in the transference as it is explicitly or implicitly understood by most analysts, in spite of the limited official definition of the term. (Sandler 1983, p. 41, emphasis added)

Rangell commented on this passage by raising the critical question:

> Is it still resistance and defences first, as it has been with Freud, Anna Freud, Fenichel and others? Or have we moved to what is promulgated by many as transference first, or even transference only?

Everything seems to boil down to a new polarization: many psychoanalysts give the here and now precedence over reconstruction and insight. Rangell demanded that a decision be made:

> Ultimately we may have to decide between two different concepts of transference, intrapsychic versus interactional or transactional. The same choice may need to be made between the intrapsychic and interactional models of the therapeutic process. (Rangell 1984, p. 133)

In the long run the questions raised by Sandler and Rangell will be answered by research on the course and outcome of psychoanalytic treatment. We do not expect new polarizations to develop because it is impossible to establish a hierarchy of interpretations concerning resistance and transference in the manner that Reich and M. Klein claimed in their extreme positions. Reich systematized defense theory in terms of therapeutic technique in his rigorous analysis of resistance, which ultimately resulted in his strict theory of *character analysis.*

Reich made the rule of proceeding from the manifest a firm principle and applied it rigidly: "*No interpretation of meaning when a resistance interpretation is needed*" (Reich 1949, p. 27). By describing transference resistance specifically with regard to a patient's behavior, both in general and in particular actions, and to the way in which he follows the basic rule, Reich introduced a useful distinction between form and content. In his words:

> The character resistance expresses itself not in the content of the material, but in the formal aspects of the general behavior, the manner of talking, of the gait, facial expression and typical attitudes such as smiling, deriding, haughtiness, over-correctness, the *manner* of the politeness or of the aggression, etc. (Reich 1949, p. 47)

He used the terms "armor" and "character armor" to refer to neurotic character traits, regardless of how much they differed, in order to describe the fact that certain manners of behavior function like compact defense mechanisms, which operate by regulating the distribution of libidinal energy between the outside and the interior.

The consequence of Reich's recommendations is that analysts should initially limit their interpretations to the resistance *to* transference and avoid interpretations of meaning, especially all deep-reaching, genetic interpretations. Reich formalized the following general rule: "*One cannot act too early in analyzing resistances, and one cannot be too reserved in the interpretation of the unconscious, apart from resistances*" (Reich 1949, p. 38).

Reich also forced the analysis of resistance in the here and now. In the first few sessions of a therapy Reich would establish a connection between resistance and transference by saying at some opportune moment that the patient had something against him but did not dare to mention it (Reich 1949, p. 55). Ferenczi (1950), taking up a similar suggestion that Rank had made, also recommended that each dream, gesture, parapraxis, and deterioration or improvement be considered first of all as an expression of transference and resistance. According to Ferenczi, Groddeck deserves the credit for this principle; at any sign of a deterioration in the patient's condition he asked the stereotype question, "What do you have against me? What have I done to you?" The similarity between Reich and Ferenczi in emphasizing that the here and now is a reaction to the phase of technique that Ferenczi and Rank (1924) criticized as *interpretation fanaticism* is just as significant as their differences with regard to technique (i. e., Reich's character and resistance analyses versus Ferenczi's technique). The term "interpretation fanaticism" was used to refer to interpretations that reconstructed events, making the patient an intellectual expert on the genesis of his illness yet without leading to any therapeutic gain.

Emphasizing the current significance of resistance and transference is thus nothing new. The here and now is the starting point in many otherwise very different psychoanalytic techniques, whose conceptions of it differ accordingly. Ferenczi's understanding of a resistance to transference was presumably very different from Reich's although both followed the same rule and in their interpretations may have proceeded from manifest events.

The discussion between Sandler and Rangell may be considered a belated renewal of the earlier discussion about superficial and deep interpretations that was the basis of the controversies between the adherents of ego psychology and the Kleinian school. Fenichel's commentary on the earlier discussion, although written long ago, is still instructive:

> Taken correctly, this can only mean that it makes no sense to give "deep interpretations" (however correct they might be as to content) as long as superficial matters are in the way. For this reason one cannot, as Melanie Klein wants, "get into direct contact with the unconscious of the patient," because to analyze means precisely to come to terms with the patient's *ego*, to compel the patient's ego to face its own conflicts.... The defensive attitudes of the ego are *always* more superficial than the instinctual attitudes of the id. Therefore, before throwing the patient's instincts at his head we have first to interpret to him that he is afraid of them and is defending himself against them, and why he does so. (Fenichel 1953, p. 334)

By emphasizing the *object-related defenses*, Sandler is apparently situated between the traditional ego psychological analysis of resistance and the interpretive technique of the Kleinian school. We too proceed from the assumption that human beings strive toward objects and are characterized by a primary intentionality. One consequence of this assumption is that all unconscious fantasies are *object related*, which is the reason that the fundamental human anxieties manifest themselves on points of interpersonal contact. In Vol. 1 (Sect. 2.5), we emphasize the positive nature of the fact that M. Klein brought movement into the rigidified fronts of resistance analysis. Subsequently, however, new polarizations and one-sided positions arose once again. The connection between unconscious fantasies, anxiety, and defense became the focus of the typical Kleinian transference interpretations. Projection replaced repression as the prototype of defense mechanisms, and repression resistance lost its importance. In the Kleinian therapeutic technique, the analyst operates behind the back of the resistance, as it were, because the anxieties appear to offer a means of direct access to the presumed unconscious fantasies. For both theoretical and technical reasons it was therefore possible for the term "resistance" to disappear from the terminology of the Kleinian school. In fact, the term "resistance" does not even appear as an entry in the indexes in representative books by Kleinian authors (M. Klein et al. 1952; M. Klein 1962; Segal 1964; Etchegoyen 1986), or there is only a note referring, for example, to the negative therapeutic reaction, as in Rosenfeld's (1987) book.

The atemporal nature of the Kleinian unconscious seems to let the here and now merge with the past. The Kleinian understanding of the relationship in the momentary analytic situation is thus completely different from Gill's although both attribute equal significance to the actuality of transference. By proceeding from ahistorical repetitions, which are manifest as object-related wishes and anxieties, a Kleinian analyst seems to acknowledge that everything of importance takes place in the therapeutic relationship, yet he nevertheless neglects the reality of the therapeutic relationship (i. e., the realistic aspects of the patient's relationship to the analyst). The analyst's contribution to the patient's resistance appears negligible from the point of view that unconscious fantasies and anxieties manifest themselves in transference almost independent of time. In contrast to the Kleinian school, Kohut (1977) emphasized the *dependence* of the resistance on the analyst's current *behavior* and especially on his lack of empathy. It is obvious that we, in this regard, are in complete agreement with Kohut.

It is now time to focus on the regulatory function of resistance in connection with the security principle. Misunderstandings are bound to occur in this regard since Groddeck, Ferenczi, Rank, and Reich all considered the forced linkages we have referred to above to constitute the analyst's contribution to resistance and transference. This type of intervention seems to be expressed by the questions "What about me?" and "Aren't you really talking about me?" In any case, Reed (1987) referred to an example of a female patient's initial interview with an analyst-in-training to indicate how this analyst directly related the patient's description of a traumatic tonsillectomy to himself by suggesting that she was really speaking about him. Although one objective of analysis is to discover similarities, this is only possible if dissimilarities are also recognized. Using the above-mentioned questions to force the creation of transferences makes it nearly impossible to recognize the analyst's influence on the patient's resistance to experiencing transference, in the sense described by Gill. The erroneous use of the here and now, i. e., the actual genesis, is widespread. Such forced transference interpretations have a deterrent effect in the introductory phase, and can lead the patient to doubt the analyst's normality and to not begin treatment at all. In later phases this type of interpretation makes it more difficult to distinguish the different levels of the relationship and of the transference, i. e., the "realistic" and "new" versus the transferred, old aspects.

In contrast to this method of stimulating resistance or transference, we recommend, together with Gill, that the analyst thoroughly investigate and eventually interpret the *realistic* aspects of the patient's affective and cognitive processes in order to determine his own contribution to transference and resistance - in other words, that he examine the situational genesis of the resistance. This is the common denominator linking us in this regard with Gill, Klauber, Kohut, and Sandler.

The point is to gain the patient's confidence that he need *not* fear a repetition of his previous failures in the new relationship. He can then give up his habitual self-defenses, as Weiss and Sampson (1986) have convincingly shown. This approach is particularly helpful for dealing with superego resistance. If the analyst orients his actions toward the goal of increasing the patient's feeling of security, it is possible for him to test different kinds of interventions, taking advantage of the entire scope offered by a therapeutically helpful dialogue.

An illustration of the regulatory function of resistance is provided by the following passage from Cremerius' reflections about the correct technique for dealing with patients who cannot freely associate:

> The analyst only has to think what effort and struggle his patient had to go through in childhood to successfully manage to socialize his instincts while preserving portions of them, in order to be able to understand his behavior in therapy.... And when this point has become clear to him, then he will also understand that the patient cannot simply permit something to happen that his

own survival may once have required him to repress. He understands that his patient has in the meantime made his arrangements and has become accustomed to living in this way, and he will therefore be able to empathize with what it means to expose oneself to a process whose goal is the return of what was repressed. (Cremerius 1984, p. 79)

Because of the ubiquity of the phenomena of resistance, the reader can find examples of it in every chapter of this book. We would like to emphasize the instances of resistance to transference; it is especially important therapeutically that this form of resistance be recognized as early as possible. In Sect. 4.6 we discuss identity resistance and its relationship to the security principle, which is beset by unusual technical difficulties.

The phase of an exaggerated focussing on the analysis of resistance (and the polarizations related to it) has been overcome. Our understanding of resistance is based on viewing the mechanisms of defense within an interpersonal matrix. In this sense we adhere to the idealist utopia that the limitations on experiencing and behavior caused by resistance are in prinicple accessible to analysis. We therefore recommend that the following examples be read from the primary perspective of this textbook, namely that the exchange between the patient and the analyst be examined with regard to what the latter contributes to the development and overcoming of repetition in the various forms of resistance and transference.

4.1 Disavowal of Affects

Nora X arrived late for her 413th session - an unusual event. During the 5 minutes I was waiting for her, I thought about her very intensely. On the one hand, I was worried; on the other, I detected a growing inner tension that was tinged with aggression. I was worried because the patient was inclined to inflict harm on herself, e. g., she was a reckless driver. When she finally arrived, I was surprised to see her smiling and beaming with happiness; upon entering the room, she looked at me longer than customary and in an inquisitive manner. Her happiness and my displeasure created a very discordant contrast.

P: I'm all out of breath, and I'm late too. [Short pause] But I can tell that somehow something is wrong. And I don't know right now if I'm happy because I'm late and made you wait, or because of what happened before.

She described how she had been together with her boyfriend. They had been sitting in a cafe and so engrossed in conversation that she had forgotten the time. At the end she had had to pay, and the patient recalled that this had also been the topic of the last few sessions. In the previous session she had been concerned with the fact that she frequently waited for longer periods of time before paying the bills for her analysis.

P: Yes, what really concerns me, I believe, was the last comment I made before I left, about paying, which was also the topic of the previous hour, and I thought it was simply indicative that precisely the same topic was the last point in my conversation with my friend, although we had talked about something entirely different.

She had talked with her boyfriend about the difficulties she was having with her superior. She felt that these conflicts were like the "back and forth in a ball game." She experienced the same back and forth with her boyfriend when, while paying for the coffee, they played a "funny game of give and take." For me, the aggressive aspect was in the forefront. With regard to her being late and my unease about it, I created an analogy between the outside situation and the one in analysis.

P: Now today . . . I play it where the point is to say what I think, hold it back, then with the bills and . . . I wonder whether there is a connection with my being late.

A: Hum, I think so.

P: You think so. Ok, I take some time away. But I actually divide it up differently, and my friend and I were together a little longer.

A: We recently spoke about you wanting to give it to your friend, and today it's my turn.

P: Yes, it's fun.

A: And that's why you were beaming when you came in.

I shared my impression with the patient to make it clear to her how much she enjoyed coming late and how much pleasure she had acting out aggressive impulses.

P: [Laughing] That honestly gives me a feeling of "illicit pleasure."

Affect and behavior were linked together in this illicit or forbidden pleasure; the patient's repelled aggression was expressed both in her pleasure and in the fact that her behavior was at the expense of the relationship.

A: Yes, that's clear, and you let yourself have this pleasure. But I'm not very sure whether you also see the consequences of your pleasure.

P: Yes, well, the question as to "What does it give me?" is one I haven't asked myself before. But when I raise it now, then I think that acting this way I gain your attention, because you might think "What's keeping her?" or something of the sort, and then I also think of how I react if someone else is late. It makes me pretty upset.

A: Hum, you're pretty sure of that.

P: That it makes me upset. But that it upsets others, I don't want to know that.

A: That is just the source of your pleasure, that you can make people upset in a seemingly unguilty manner.

This would have been an opportunity to refer to the patient's feelings of guilt as the reason that she felt compelled to ward off affects, but the moment did not seem ripe for this step, and the patient continued talking about being angry.

P: I recall that my boyfriend kept me waiting three times last weekend. The first time I didn't say anything, although he mentioned the subject. The second time I didn't say anything either, not until the third time. So I've just experienced what it is. And yet, just as I said before, I recently let him have it . . . . Now what was the reason?

While in the act of speaking the patient forgot the way in which she had innerly turned away from her boyfriend. Although this momentary forgetting (see Luborsky 1967) was an interesting detail of the patient's distancing, in my next interpretation I reconstructed everything that had happened with regard to her being late in order to interpret the change she had undergone from being passive (as the victim of the tardiness of others) to active (by being late herself).

A: On the weekend you were the one who had to wait, and you were angry, specifically you were passive and the victim. Now you just did something that we've seen before a number of times, namely you turned the tables and let me wait. You tell yourself, "I don't want something to be done to me, so I'll do it to someone else." That is how you deal with being disturbed or hurt in this way. And so the real issues in your being late are provoking anger and being angered.

P: Hum. [Short pause] Maybe provoking anger and being angered are the point.

In the following passage the patient made it clear that she had indeed spoken with her boyfriend about his being late, but it had taken a long time before she had been able to overcome her inhibitions and express her feelings. After her reflection on how she acted to her boyfriend had made it clear to her how she dealt with aggressive impulses and how she transformed these impulses into acts, I directed her attention to her behavior during the analysis.

A: You've talked about giving and taking, but the subject is actually provoking anger and being angered. Of course they're closely related, because you know that you get angry when you don't get what you expect, whether it has to do with being on time or with money. And you assume that I react, think, and feel just the same way, namely that I get angry when I don't get what I expect. And your desire to provoke anger is reflected by your actions, and your laughing and the happy look on your face reveal what a forbidden pleasure you get from making me angry. And you can be so happy about it because you don't really perceive the anger, just as you don't with your boyfriend either.

The patient responded to this interpretation by once again describing the interaction between her and her boyfriend, this time putting more emphasis on the aggressive character of the back and forth. At the same time her gaity and laughing increased.

P: [Laughing, she quoted her friend] "Okay, before you say it again you're going to get it" [and she added very forcefully] smack!

A: But that sounds as if you slapped each other. The one goes smack, and then the other goes smack. [The patient confirmed this in a reserved way.] And I've also got my smack! [The patient laughed.] And you're happy about it.

P: Yes, even very much so. Somehow I don't want to let you take this pleasure away from me. It's a feeling as if it is finally out in the open and can come out.

After the patient had become aware of the previously preconscious pleasure she obtained from acting aggressively, both with regard to her most important current relationship outside of analysis and to her transference, the next step was to establish the connection to her main disturbance (breaking off relationships).

A: Yes, your pleasure comes from using the one person to give it to another. Today you used your discussion with your boyfriend to let me have it. It's hard for you to stay with one person and to tell that one person what's moving you. You look for a second person, who then gets what the other deserved. This is what characterizes your relationships; instead of concentrating on one person, you take your feelings and go to the next.

P: [Softly] Because it's fun.

A: Yes, it gives you pleasure, but it also makes you unhappy.

P: I have the feeling I've never found pleasure. That's why I said that it's also important that I finally let the laughing come out, because I hide it otherwise. I don't feel any pleasure and happiness, I just always feel sad. Sadness is always there first, but it doesn't help me get any further.

A: Both are important. The pain is one thing, and it's closer to you; and your forbidden pleasure from this form of revenge or rage or anger wasn't a topic before.

In the following exchange I referred to the patient's earlier friendships. She had not been conscious of her own aggression in them, but had only perceived it mirrored in the behavior of others.

A: And we can now see how much pleasure you get, expressed in simple terms, from treating men badly. You treat me badly when you enjoy letting me wait, and you're overcome by laughter when it becomes apparent.

P: Yes, but that's something new. I used to always fall into sadness, and then it was over.

In the following sequence of comments I made a longer, summarizing interpretation in which I connected, on the one hand, the patient's development from her wishes to her disappointment and then to her transition from being passive to active as her means of warding off feared traumas and, on the other, the aggression that resulted. The individual links of this chain that were not discussed in this session were the result of prior work. I concluded this summarizing interpretation by referring to the aspect of transference in this behavior.

A: And to avoid this disappointment and the anticipated pain, you turn the whole story around and don't give me what you think I expect. In doing so you inflicted something on me that you feared would be painful to you.

P: Funny, I had to think about how the sessions end. My anger at the fact that you say, "Now our time is up."

A: Yes, I hurt you by doing that, and now you turn to counterattack. But the consequence is not that the situation gets better, but that the fact that you feel angry makes the hour even shorter. And this is the fatal aspect of this pattern - namely that your reaction does not make the situation better, only worse.

P: Innerly I take more and more measures to make the time seem shorter, because even when I start to feel that the end of the session might be approaching I think: "When are you going to say it, when are you going to say it?" And recently I realized that my thoughts were already somewhere else. As if I wanted to simply ignore this pain. And now I just had the thought that in this way I at least have a little pleasure, namely in leaving mentally, and then it isn't as painful.

A: You become active, which on the one hand gives you the nice feeling that you are in control, but on the other has the disadvantage that you get even less.

P: Then I can't concentrate either, and I'm not intensely involved, and on the one hand it is pleasurable, leaving, but on the other hand it is also a loss because of the loss of intensity.

A: Right, and what we see here in miniature is a pattern of how you organize your relationships, because when your friendships could have become intense, you've always taken some action to end them prematurely. For the same reasons that you innerly prematurely end our sessions, namely out of fear of the pain that someone else could inflict on you by saying, "Now it's over." In doing so, you actively cause something to happen that might have happened sometime.

P: Yes, here for example, here I know that it's coming. And in a relationship I would always be afraid it would happen.

A: And that's your problem. It's hard for you to let it end either way; you always cause the separation when it starts to become intense.

P: A moment ago I wasn't actually thinking as much about the separation from my father, as about how my mother and I acted toward one another.

The patient provided details about this point for the rest of the session and related it to her mother's typical forms of behavior.

Triggered by the patient's late arrival, it was possible for us to clarify her masochistic reactions regarding rejection and separation and to elaborate on them in transference. The course of the session led from her desire to her disappointment to her transition from being passive to active, and ultimately to her defensive aggression. It was possible to trace this sequence of topics back biographically to her relationship to her mother.

If we, following Klauber (1966), formulate the guiding elements in the session in terms of anxiety, defense, and enactment, we can give the following summary. The patient's primary anxiety was that her affects could gain control of her. It was therefore necessary for her to deny them. Giving and taking, as part of this, were a pleasurable game, but also one that was invested with anxiety and that necessarily ended in pain for the patient because she had internalized the expectation that her wishes (e.g., for attention) would not be fulfilled. Her primary defense was the disavowal of affects and acting out of aggressive impulses. In this way she enacted an anticipated disappointment, which she brought about in an unconscious yet active manner.

4.2 Pseudoautonomy

Although we would prefer to analyze patients who are independent, we are aware of the possible difficulties with those who desire to do everything alone.

A marked tendency prevails to regard independence as something frankly positive and dependence as something frankly negative, from the point of view of psychological cure or evolution. The positive aspect of independence seems to lead one to overlook the negative one and thus is apt to mask neurotic ends. In the same way, the negative aspect of dependence seems to lead to a concealment of the positive one and the criticism of dependence may equally serve to cover pathological tendencies or defences. (Racker 1968, p. 181)

The issue of independence also has implications for how the analytic interview is handled. A very early feature of the clinical description of the forms of resistance was that the degree of deviation from an ideal dialogue was subsumed under the category of resistance; this was true regardless of how the ideal form was determined and of the direction of the deviation. Cremerius has correctly emphasized that we must specify the criteria according to which we judge that a patient speaks too much:

The answer is that this too much is not something quantitative, but rather something qualitative, namely that in this case speaking - and specifically, speaking too much - supports the defense and resistance. (Cremerius 1984, p. 58)

We would like to use the following example to illustrate how to deal in a calm and composed manner with a patient who talks too much. In doing so the analyst gives "the patient time to become more conversant with this resistance with which he has not become acquainted, to *work through* it, to overcome it..." (Freud 1914g, p. 155). The example is taken from a session of an advanced analysis of a 35-year-old man named Gustav Y, whose disturbed ability to work manifested itself as a transference resistance that took the form of stubborn silence (see also Moser 1962). After warded off aggressive impulses had been worked through, the patient developed the pseudoindependence described below, which manifested itself in statements that - although expressing reflection - were in fact monologues.

The patient first told me, in a comment phrased as a question, that he would have to end the session "a little early" in order to pick up his children on time. He explained this by referring to the heavy traffic and a dangerous encounter he had had while driving to that day's session.

P: While driving here I was in a pretty precarious situation. Someone was driving behind me, then passed me and pulled to the right... and then on the other lane someone else, a wide semi, was coming toward me, and I wouldn't have had a chance to get out of the way. And it would have been hard to brake because there were puddles of water on the road... and it was really just a matter of inches, he just managed to pull over in front of me, and well, I don't really want to risk anything. It's clear; if I drive and think that there isn't much time, then you just drive a little, a little faster than may be sensible.

The patient has a 35–40 minute drive. He requested that we stop 5 minutes early.

P: [After a pause] Yes, and there's something else, something that I read in the newspaper just before I left home today, that yesterday there was . . . I don't know, was it . . . just a . . . the B30 just before the . . . before the exit to this . . . the wider stretch of road over there . . . that there was a serious accident there yesterday, and a woman died at the hospital and there were three or four seriously injured . . . hum . . . so I thought about it as well, that's how it is on our roads today, they were even . . . dry, by and large, so that I somehow thought, "Now you can drive normal again" and although I had enough time I did drive pretty fast . . . I mean on that stretch later, where you can drive 80 mph, I mean I know that my speedometer is slow so I mean 90 . . . but just before I . . . when I realized I had to be where it had happened and looked out and didn't see anything, and then I realized then . . . and then the thought just passed through my mind what that just . . . . what kind of a feeling that has to be, isn't it, and it said that this . . . this car that caused the accident, that it's from Heilbronn, it traveled at a . . . it skidded in the corner, turned around and was standing broadside on the road, and the other one hit it from the side and the . . . well, the mother-in-law of that driver, she was injured so severely that she later . . . that she later died. And so I wondered, when I was driving past the spot, what kind of a feeling that had to be if you have an accident and somebody in your car, they're killed, or if I cause the accident myself and then other people, I mean, from a different car, are killed, yes.

The patient continued his "free associations" in this manner for quite a while. He remembered that while driving to the session yesterday he had become so tired that he had had to stop for a break.

P: I mean that this itself . . . I mean that really . . . here too, in our conversation just this . . . the question played a role, right, it . . . that just because of the road conditions there is a danger and I didn't really talk about it here.

A: Hum.

Commentary. The patient mentioned other associations to demonstrate the risks connected with his driving to treatment. Then the patient found a link to the previous session, in which the indirect dangers of the treatment, i. e., from the analyst, had been a topic.

P: Maybe also because I then somehow immediately . . . this . . . somehow retreat into this role and something . . . well why not . . . I mean, I . . . or in the sense that this . . . this stress or other, I have to . . . simply to take it upon myself, right.

A: What do you avoid by bearing it all by yourself?

P: [After a pause] Yes, perhaps it is somehow the other side of these unpleasurable and . . . and . . . and burdensome . . . and definitely also a certain enjoyable side of the treatment, that I then namely have the feeling, hum, right here really being able to decide by myself what I want to do and whether I want to do something, that is, that I . . . uh . . . although it isn't quite right, isn't entirely clear, well, would like to avoid it, now somehow . . . let's say . . . that now . . . expressed a little pathetically . . . uh . . . somehow now, somehow like pity or something . . . for example, that you now show your understanding somehow that it simply is a difficult situation or is dangerous or so.

A: Hum.

Commentary. The patient was able to gain something from the analyst's reference to the purpose of his behavior, namely that he would like the analyst not to come too close by talking about the danger – as he had in the previous session.

P: And that is somehow . . . and somehow there is . . . I mean, but I . . . but it simply isn't . . . very clear yet what the . . . uh . . . primary thing is, if I . . . uh . . . if I don't really want it, if I just . . . if I really would like to do it alone or if it is also just this . . . this shyness toward any . . . well . . . any personal nearness or so that is somehow expressed. That is . . . uh . . . it just is not . . . not so clear . . . to, and I think that my [cleared his throat] now viewed from this aspect, the idea that I have is that I myself . . . that I would like to decide it myself, and also the other possibility, let's say, that I would not make up my mind now, would simply now say, "No, I won't do it, it's too risky for me" or so, yes, and this . . . and somehow I would then like to . . . hum . . . to make this decision by myself, without now . . . for example . . . without somehow here . . . uh . . . getting permission. Yes, that's . . . that's also part of it.

A: Yes, that means that independence is something very important to you, and you yourself raise the question, "Is it really primary, or could it be that this independence is the consequence?" Perhaps you have given up expectations, and that the act of giving them up proved to be a gain in independence. You are independent of me now, regardless of whether I say something helpful, understanding, or not. You are – and this is an image that we have been following for a long time – you are now the hero who is mastering his dangerous path alone.

One of his frequent daydreams in this phase of treatment was about a Western hero, who comes to the aid of widows and orphans, only to reject the offer of a rescued woman at the end and travel on.

P: Yes, that actually . . . a few minutes ago that . . . let's say . . . entered my mind, and precisely now the . . . the way in which I . . . hum . . . how I act toward my wife right now, that I withdraw and only keep up a formal politeness.

He then described how his wife complained about his rejection of her wishes for nearness and intimacy.

P: But from my point of view, I really don't have any need for it, so that right now sexually . . . I actually don't miss anything and don't have any needs.

Gustav Y then formulated his wish that he would only like to sleep with his wife if she would not place any demands on his autarchy.

P: Not, and this is really the truth, that at the moment I'm particularly strong . . . hum . . . yes . . . how should I say it . . . I simply want to have my peace and quiet. People shouldn't bother me with with such things. And that's really how it is, perhaps I have arranged things that way, that I actually somehow feel quite well . . . hum . . . in the situation, or at least . . . or perhaps have . . . by and large repressed my other wishes and needs . . . uh.

A: Hum.

Commentary. The concrete form that his heroic dream took in everyday life provided confirmation that the patient preferred to suppress his sexual wishes in order not to get in a position of uncomfortable nearness to his wife. Since his childhood had been overshadowed by the long absence of his father (who had been held a prisoner of war until Gustav was 10 years old), he – "the only surviving man in the family" – was spoiled and constrained by the dominant feminine environment. His childhood was constantly accompanied, understandably, by the worried complaints that nothing should happen to him. It was precisely this that he did not want to hear from the analyst. His understanding about the dangers on the street and about the dangers of pleasurable phallicism could only cover up accusations.

P: Not, and it's naturally the case now too, that when . . . not when I . . . when my wife then somehow makes . . . the . . . the accusations and . . . says to me that she hates me or whatever, really, then my reaction is, "Yes, alright then, yes, what do you want after all, it would be best if . . . uh . . . we restrict our contact to practical things and otherwise each of us can do what what we want."

A: The decisive point is contained in the feeling you express as "What's the point," that you shrug your shoulders and think to yourself, "What should I say about it, what's really the point?" Almost as if you put yourself into the situation you had in your fantasies about what happened the day before and then hit the gas pedal and then - what happens then - what is really expressed in your "What's the point?" You almost killed yourself. By letting somebody else do it, but it's also possible that you could have seen the other car . . . uh . . . just a few seconds earlier and then it would have been a little less dangerous.

P: [After a pause] Yes, yet . . . yes, of course, as far as the overall situation is concerned, yet I . . . yet I don't . . . yet it isn't entirely clear, I mean, what I just described about yesterday. I said it happened while driving here, naturally . . . but it therefore can't . . . hum . . . let's say . . . have been a direct reaction to what we talked about.

Commentary. The patient was immediately unsettled by the interpretation the analyst offered, and he therefore had to, first of all, make a denial. In contrast to earlier phases of the analysis he was able, however, subsequently to permit himself to have a productive association.

P: Yes. Yes, but . . . it . . . now I can think of something that makes that even clearer. Such fantasies occur precisely at the moment when it's possible to dose them accordingly, right, that I could get out of everyday life in a small accident, but of course the stress at work also plays a role, right, to get put up in a hospital with some injury or other and there somehow get some peace and quiet to come to your senses. Right? It's therefore also . . . I mean that . . . this also indicates that some . . . uh . . . some wish or so played a role.

Commentary. In the course of treatment the patient was able to overcome the regressive idea of having a serious case of tuberculosis, at least to the extent that he could limit himself to a "small accident" in order to get himself "out of everyday life."

The patient then described an important observation he had made about himself, about how he had calmly accomplished a task he had been assigned, "with substantially less nervous energy than earlier," and that he was startled by his own generosity. There had always been a critical element in the patient's fictive conversations with others: "My God, when people read that, they'll think, 'What a planner you are.'" Yet to some extent he was able to escape these expectations.

P: I said to myself, "Why burden yourself with such work. It doesn't matter after all, and if it doesn't work, then there isn't anybody around to fix it again," right, and so now I'm going to work with this kind of an attitude. I prepare even less than normal, but without punishing myself afterwards in such a terrible way.

A: You reject certain expectations that you've placed on yourself, and in doing so you have simplified your situation.

P: Well, yes, I mean, it's also contradictory, of course. If I really relativize it and tell myself that it doesn't matter, then on the other hand, this doesn't fit with the wish to avoid everything right now. At least I still see some contradiction in this at the moment, but I think that it naturally could also be that I just didn't immediately think that these problems at home might even play a bigger role, problems that I then wouldn't have to face, right?

A: You have to realize that a certain question was obviously implied when you talked about your additional tasks at work the first time, namely, "Why did the boss only give them to *me*, why me of all people?" And there was a small implication about whether he would really say it. It may really have been your expectation to be praised. And this "It doesn't matter" could be a reaction to your disappointment, a withdrawal into not caring, and analogously the "It doesn't matter" here could also be a reaction to a disappointment. In this way - by saying "it doesn't matter" - you make yourself independent.

Commentary. In the previous interpretation the analyst attempted to indicate to the patient one reason for his pseudoautonomy. The patient avoided disappointing the wish that he was looking for acknowledgment and instead only met concern. At home good grades at school had been a matter of course, because his mother had only had him to care for, but she had not fostered the development of his motor ability. In adolescence he had run his laps as a long-distance runner, where nobody watched; his daydreams, however, were about victories in the 100 meter dash that took place in front of the main grandstand.

A central aspect in this transference relationship was the patient's attempt to avoid his wish for confirmation of his dangerous journey through "life." In retrospect, this aspect does not seem to have become very clear. The analyst's interventions were directed at the resistance that concealed his desire for dependence.

4.3 Unpleasure As Id Resistance

To gain a better understanding of this section we recommend that the reader first turn to Sect. 9.3, where we summarize the case history of Christian Y and report about the external and temporal circumstances of his analysis. After he had overcome his separation anxieties - in Sect. 9.3.1 we give an example of them from the 203rd session - it was possible for his treatment to be continued on an outpatient basis, starting with the 320th session. His unpleasure and incapacity reached their low point in the 503rd session. He was just barely able to walk to my office. Several fanciful activities did not provide him any satisfaction at all or increase his self-confidence.

In this phase of treatment his symptoms consisted in an extreme lack of vitality, which manifested itself in an incapacity to work and in laziness. For a long time his laziness, which at this point was a source of serious distress, was overlaid by severe attacks of anxiety that prevented him from being active and working.

From a descriptive point of view we attribute the patient's all-encompassing unpleasure to id resistance, which we however do not trace back to "inertia" or "sluggishness" of the libido (Freud 1918b, p. 116, 1940, p. 181; see also Vol.1, Sect. 4.4). In fact, there does not seem to be any movement in the two sessions reproduced here, which were typical for a longer period of treatment. The analyst dispairingly attempted to make some sense of the patient's monotonous complaints about his complete lack of ability to accomplish anything. He viewed the patient's listlessness as the manifestation of an almost insurmountable resistance that contained concealed and completely unconscious satisfactions of anal spite and of the regressive self-assertion that accompanied it. Of course, the patient was far from recognizing the power of his passivity and from enjoying his triumph. His moods alternated from one extreme to the other, yet his anxiety signal was unchanged and independent of whether Christian Y openly expressed his rage or it receded behind his passivity or self-destructiveness. His anxiety also protected him, however, from breaking off the treatment or committing suicide. He secretly prepared circuit diagrams and programs, overshadowing his father, yet his visions of omnipotence were deflated when he took a realistic look at his achievements. The more he achieved in life step by step, the more obvious it became that his central problem in analysis was the discrepancy to his subjective view of himself.

As the following excerpt from the 503rd session shows, Christian Y insisted on the idea that he could only become a hard worker if the analyst made him one. He expected the analyst's interventions to provide him vitality or to result in activity.

P: I'm always afraid of getting on someone's nerves or of being too impudent. I'm usually already nervous when I get here, so I can't bear any additional stress, however minor. I can start with whatever I want, but you always lead me to spite. What are you trying to get at? I'm bored about talking about spite because I'm interested now in how to become hard working, and I can't see any connection between spite and laziness, and I don't think it's necessary to talk about spite because it includes rage, and rage is something different, it still doesn't go away. There must be some reason that you keep coming back to spite. What's wrong? Why don't you say anything?

A: [After a pause] One important aspect is to block direct pleasure and to incapacitate the other person. That was something you were able to follow yesterday.

P: No, I don't understand anything. Getting pleasure from spite isn't interesting, because I really don't want to slow things down. I try to talk about something. That I'm happy at those moments when you don't say anything, as if I had gained control, isn't interesting at all. What is important is being aware that I haven't drawn the conclusion that you can't help me. Otherwise there's nothing else to it. I think we've lost time again, and that makes me upset; I want to get ahead, for example, become a hard worker. Why isn't anything said about that, nothing at all? I don't want to exert myself; I'm afraid of doing something silly. Why don't you help me then? I can't have any thoughts of my own, have an opinion of my own; I've always been dependent on what others think. Why am I afraid of being criticized? In my opinion everything I do is full of crap. I talk, think, do something – crap, nothing else. I wonder why I wouldn't be satisfied with your approval. But it isn't any more important than getting the approval of other people. And besides, I don't want to do anything in order to get your approval in exchange, because that's precisely what I want to be independent of. It doesn't help me at all for you to give me your general consent; that's too watered down. It's no help to me; I'm still afraid that everything is full of crap, whatever I do, however I walk and stand, whatever I touch, whatever I think; somehow whatever I do is really full of crap. I'm terribly afraid of making a mistake. Afraid of being laughed out, afraid of becoming angry. I'll always be making mistakes, and what I do will never be perfect, and I therefore always have to reckon with something unpleasant. Another thing is that I can never have a conflict with anyone, and it always makes me angry. I can only give in, agree, but I don't want to. If you don't help me to get over it, then things will just stay like they are.

A: So you're afraid that if I don't give you anything, any help, that you won't be able to do anything yourself.

Consideration. This was an attempt to show the patient that he could be independent, although it was very cautiously implied. This caution was connected in part with the fact that almost everything I could say, suggest, or do would be "wrong." On the other hand, from experience I knew that Christian Y could not bear a longer period of silence. He needed the reassurance of my reaction. This can also be seen in how he concluded his opening remarks in this session, "What's wrong? Why don't you say anything?" By remaining silent I might make his feeling of concern become intolerable. At the same time, what I might say exposed me to his biting criticism. For a while the patient had learned my comments by heart, and I had not realized that this provided him support.

P: Yes, that's how it is. I'm not afraid of it being that way; that's how it is. Or can you give me a different interpretation? If nothing were to come from you - if I stayed away, then what about my anxiety? What's the point of all this? I can't understand you. Listen, how can I get over my anxiety in everything I do? I come here afraid, you don't offer me anything, and then I'm unhappy again that I haven't got anything new. For instance, right now I'm really looking forward to my vacation because I won't have to be afraid every day of wasting my time coming here.

A: Yes, you're really looking forward to not having to come here for a while.

P: Just looking at it from the one side.

A: Real pleasure.

P: But there is also a kind of spite. I turn away from you, enraged, and accept the disadvantages.

A: Which is the precondition for the idea that if I don't offer anything, then you can't have anything either. Apparently my silence is turned into your experience that I don't have anything to offer. But why don't you have anything either?

Consideration. This question presumably expressed my helplessness. Indirect encouragements were insufficient, and all that was left was for me to bear the fact that I was doing something wrong.

P: Then let me try asking a question. How would you say that I have profited from today's session? Or how did I profit from yesterday's? Can you tell me that?

A: Yes, to know what a benefit is is a real question.

P: A benefit is when I'm better able to solve a problem, a benefit is when I'm less anxious.

A: Yes, then you would have benefited from today's session if you had learned that you have something that I haven't contributed to.

P: I don't have anything, I'm just afraid, too afraid.

A: You mean there's a connection between my being silent and your fear.

P: You haven't said anything for practically the entire session that is related to any of my fears. If I'm still afraid of making a fool of myself, then I haven't benefited at all.

A: What's taking place here is an example of the disturbance of your ability to work. If I don't immediately refer to something you've said or confirm it indirectly, then you jump to the conclusion that everything that happens here is crap, that it isn't worth anything, and that it won't become anything until I make something out of it, until I've added my two bits to it.

Consideration. Christian Y was extremely dependent on confirmation from others. His mother had spoiled and loved him in excess, as he mentioned in another context, which resulted in a deficit that consisted in his still being incapable of being the person he wanted to be. I nevertheless felt that I could expect him to show initiative. His deficit was an atypical one, caused by too much good. In other words, the good turned into the false self. What the patient wanted to be remained a mysterious idea.

P: Yes, yes.

A: Until the two bits, my two bits, are added. The fact that you quickly become discouraged when you try something new is part of your disturbed ability to work.

P: I still can't agree with it. I haven't done anything else; I've only described some fears of mine. I haven't tried to solve anything because I know that I can't and because I don't have the faintest idea how, and I don't think it's possible to simply go from one to the other. I've raised questions and on the whole haven't found any answers. That's a disappointing experience because whether I continue to be so afraid or whether it decreases depends on the answers to these questions. I'm right, and it would be self-deceiving to act as if I weren't afraid, because I am. Just talking like this cannot be very valuable. I just don't see how I should have benefited from today's session. You haven't said anything about the anxieties I have, and at the one place you said that you had said something, it was a deception.

A: So if I don't say anything, you become afraid?

P: I'm afraid even before then.

A: Yes, I know, but what's important right now is, in simple terms, that you're afraid when I don't say anything.

P: At first I get angry, and maybe I get afraid then.

A: So being angry makes you more afraid?

P: We're losing time, and I don't understand what you're trying to get at.

A: If I don't do anything, then you think that you can't do anything either.

P: Yes, that's how it is; naturally not nothing, but far too little.

A: So if I don't have two bits, then you don't either.

P: Yes, that's how it is. I think that's how it is because it makes me feel so bad.

A: Yes, yes.

P: And as long as I feel bad, then I don't have two bits.

A: This must be taken very seriously. The connection is so close that what you have is only good if you have the same thing I do, when we can mix our bits together. If you do something alone, then it's – how should I say it – crap until I've added my two bits and it can all be put in one pot.

P: But I haven't found anything, so in my experience it's all crap. So I think I'm right, and if I seem stubborn, then maybe I'm just too dumb to grasp it; I can't understand you. I can solve the problem in another way, by not looking for anything here, but then I won't achieve anything in end effect. Where am I making a mistake? Where's the catch? I don't want to block myself in if you know something better and can give it to me.

A: The problem is that you have to have something in common to be able to do something yourself.

P: Yes, and if you don't say anything?

A: Right now we see that you are obviously still very afraid if we don't keep our bits in the same pot, that is, if you produce something yourself. That's why I said it would be a real pleasure for you not to have anything to do with me for a while. Although there is spite and rejection in it, it's also a demonstration of your independence.

Consideration. How could Christian Y overcome the dilemma that he detested being dependent and yet he didn't have the confidence to be independent? The patient's self-deprecation was so hard to bear that presumably I now attempted to emphasize his own ability.

In the following session things continued in the same vein.

P: I get scared shit when I feel the first signs of being tired. So now I'm at the subject of laziness again. You know, I'll never be healthy. I don't have any inclination to work. Doing something is completely alien to me; there's nothing I can do about it. Last Friday I was in dispair again when I looked back at the week. There wasn't anything, nothing at all, that could stimulate me to want to work, nothing, and I reject work altogether. And I don't want to work; there's no point in your exerting yourself. Everything is so boring, life itself is a bore, empty and unexciting, and it won't get better, I'm convinced of that. Why should I get involved in such an unexciting, gray future, absurd ....

A: So, where the issue is that you should do something yourself, that's where my contribution is especially small, nothing or as good as nothing.

P: That's the topic.

A: Where you do something and I don't do anything. Where the point is that you develop more activity without me. So, is it your goal to do more without me?

P: Yes, but I can't because I'm lazy, for example.

A: What does your laziness get you? What do you want to achieve as a result of my intervening?

P: I don't know. Why should you intervene? I want to do it myself, but am afraid, as I've told you over and over, but you don't show any interest in why. I'm afraid to do anything. I'm afraid of tests. Last night I had a dream about something like that. I had to take a test and sat there and didn't know anything and got scared shit and was even punished by somebody. I'm scared. That's where we can get started. What do I want from you? Nothing! I don't want anything personal; I like to live impersonally. I want to be cool and keep my distance; that's nicer.

Commentary. Here the patient referred to his conflicting desires in one breath. The moment the patient wanted to do something himself his paralyzing fear manifested itself. Entirely aside from the fact that the analyst was too restrained in providing confirmation in specific situations, the patient was also ashamed of being dependent; it was therefore hard for him to accept help. His unhappy complaining about the lack of help was not only hard for the analyst to take but also caused the analyst to become concerned that the resulting feelings of guilt might have the effect of increasing the patient's fear.

A: Yes, that's what I mean. You want to do something all by yourself, something objective, and that's the problem. Why isn't it possible? Why?

P: For instance because I'm afraid that I will do something that somebody else will examine closely, for example, because I can't afford to have an opinion of my own, because I can't stand to have a conflict with anyone, what do I know. I'm so imprecise, so in a rush and unable to concentrate that when I do something I'm afraid of being rejected in some way. It's terrible for me when I do something wrong.

A: Yes, and as long as I take some of the burden off you, think for you, and become active, then you're out of the danger of having to do something yourself and I slide into the role of the critic.

P: I can't understand that.

A: As long as somebody else takes all your burdens off you, as long as you can be completely passive and someone else acts for you, holds your opinions, and takes your place, that's how long you will feel secure.

Commentary. The analyst viewed the patient's inactivity in these sessions primarily as anal spite. Consequently, he looked for the pleasure concealed in his passive aggression and his spiteful self-assertiveness. In the session described here the focus of the interpretative strategy was the interactional side of the patient's spite, and the unconscious scheme of anality was discussed, if only by analogy. The analyst attempted to get the patient to understand the (transference) relationship as something in which the patient can openly pull the analyst along into the crap. The patient referred to himself as "somebody full of crap."

Even in this phase it was still possible to identify a component of castration anxiety in the patient's complaints about his physical inability. The roots of this component reach far into deeper levels, as these excerpts demonstrate.

The patient's idea that his "material defects" can only be healed if the analyst supplies him with materials results in a very serious problem of analytic technique. This problem is further increased by the fact that the patient was suspicious and experienced any true closeness as a severe humiliation. His recurrent mood of hopelessness, which was accompanied by his threats to break off analysis and commit suicide, was one consequence of this.

4.4 Stagnation and the Decision to Change Analysts

If stagnation or an impasse happens to occur in an analysis, the analyst can usually find very plausible reasons for it in the patient's psychodynamics. It is logical for him to think of a negative therapeutic reaction (Freud 1923b), and we have discussed the unconscious motives of such reactions in Vol.1, Sect. 4.4.1.

This attitude disregards, however, the analyst's contribution to the stagnation. If therapeutic change is missing, part of the responsibility probably lies in the analyst's personal equation and technique. The results of research emphasize namely that an unsuccessful prior therapy does not necessarily justify a negative prediction about the outcome of a subsequent therapy. This result of statistical studies probably contradicts widely held clinical attitudes (see Kächele and Fiedler 1985).

Because of a protracted standstill in her therapy, Maria X consulted, by mutual agreement with her (female) therapist, another analyst, this one a man. Each side experienced the futility of the therapeutic work, yet drew different conclusions from it. The patient was absolutely against stopping, while the therapist recommended a break and left it to her discretion to later switch to a male analyst. This pessimistic point of view was the result of the fact that all of the analyst's efforts to communicate something good to the patient, who had diffuse anxieties and whose general mood was depressive, had apparently failed. The patient's chronic dissatisfaction with herself and the circumstances of her life, which was caused by a fundamental feeling that she was deficient, had remained inaccessible for a period of almost two years. Since the patient's response to each insight into unconscious conflicts led to a deterioration in her condition, the analyst diagnosed a negative therapeutic reaction.

In unsuccessful therapies analysts ask themselves critical questions, and such situations put them in the position of being the accused, as Wurmser emphasized:

One defensive tactic that is especially popular if not typical of depressives consists in trying *to make the other person feel so guilty and humble* as they themselves feel. How is it achieved? By means of open and disguised accusations. It is a kind of turning the tables that includes the defenses of projection and the turning from passive into active and signifies a transition from the identification with the victim to identification with the prosecutor. This can also turn into a immensely strong kind of transference resistance. I think that a large portion of the *negative therapeutic reactions* can be attributed to precisely this turning the tables of prosecution. (1987, p. 149)

There are, of course, different ways of confronting such prosecution. Wurmser described in an impressive manner how he has learned to wage such onerous struggles for years with such patients, who seem to be beyond treatment. Among other things, he emphasized flexibility, which under certain circumstances can include a change in therapists.

Maria X, a 37-year-old woman, complained bitterly in the consultation that, although she had always made an effort to cooperate during her nearly 2-year-long therapy, there had not been any change in her basic problem of being dissatisfied with herself or in her feeling that she was a failure. I inquired about the patient's view of the nature of the therapeutic relationship, and discovered that there were a large number of questions that the patient had not yet dared to ask, especially those that concerned her female analyst as a person. In summary, my impression was that the patient had not received enough encouragement to deal with her negative transference stemming from her relationship to her mother.

In our opinion a diagnosis of a negative therapeutic reaction one-sidedly made the patient responsible for the previous lack of success. The task should be, instead, to determine which interactional reinforcements have led to a situation in which the patient's difficulties can no longer be favorably dealt with. The goal of a renewed attempt at treatment in this case had to be to transform the patient's negativism into an open negative transference.

The procedure of first offering this patient a focal therapy in which the negative aspects of her relationship to the therapist that had previously not been dealt with are made the center of attention took the skepticism of the previous therapist into account in one regard. In another regard, however, the plan was designed to first tackle, as its predetermined goal, the problem of negative maternal transference that the first analyst had correctly described.

Maria X had originally been referred to a department of internal medicine for examination of her high blood pressure of unknown origin. She had suffered from high blood pressure for 11 years, and the somatic examinations revealed that the hypertension was the result of a stenosis of a renal artery. Surgical correction was not recommended. The patient's "dissatisfaction," as she herself referred to her symptom, had also existed for 11 years. She had furthermore suffered from anxiety since puberty; it manifested itself especially in stress situations or in conflicts with persons in positions of authority. A visit to a psychosomatically oriented consultant regarding her hypertension had led to the initiation of regular analytic psychotherapy. The patient had feared that they might have a negative impact on her relationship to her friend.

The analyst's application for the approval of insurance coverage emphasized, with regard to the psychodynamics of the conflict, the tension that existed between her being closely tied to her mother and the insufficient separation from her, which was accompanied by corresponding reactions of rage and disappointment. Attempts to achieve a separation had led to reactions that were externally inadequate and that in turn were associated with strong feelings of guilt. The patient and therapist agreed upon an analysis of unlimited duration. According to the application, "The fundamental issue of separation and the massive aggressive conflict connected with it make me expect substantial resistance."

After this introductory sketch of the problem we will now reproduce several passages from the therapy in which the behavior that the younger (female) therapist had described manifested itself again, and will try to demonstrate a productive method of dealing with it.

After we had agreed that she would continue treatment with me, I gave her the application form for an extension of insurance payments. The moment the patient picked up the form, she sighed--not loudly, but perceptibly. I drew her attention to this expression of discontent, and she reluctantly answered that she didn't want to fill out such things.

I was impressed by this first demonstration of the behavior that the patient's previous analyst had told me about. In accordance with my understanding of the situation I gave the following interpretation:

A: In your subjective experience it's even too much to fill out a questionnaire you're familiar with. It won't take two minutes, and it's in your own interest; it's worth 6000 marks. The relationship between the real benefit and what it means for your experiencing doesn't coincide, does it? Maybe your sigh contains your wish to be able to stay in paradise, the land of milk and honey.

My attitude toward the patient was not at all unfriendly, rather one of surprise at the paraverbal manner in which she expressed both her dissatisfaction and her listlessness. My comment therefore expressed some sympathy for the patient.

P: Well, I've had to fill in a lot of such forms, starting with the preliminary examinations at the university. At the time I didn't object, although I could have.

A: In this case we're talking about something to your advantage, and you sigh.

While I was saying this, I thought about the fact that her sigh could be a reaction that had become chronic to a feeling that too much was being asked of her, and could reflect a shift in her protests to the level of paraverbal utterances. The sigh would then also fit the distinct feeling she gave me, namely that she dressed tastefully and could act accordingly but that her face nevertheless contained an expression of a gloomy mood, despite her make-up.

P: Yes, I lose control whenever it's a matter of something to my advantage. In the last few days I've become more anxious; at work I have to take over and train a new group.

Proceeding from her comment that her anxieties were stimulated by the increased demands being placed on her knowledge and competence as the person responsible at her firm for further training, I concluded that the patient had a fundamentally self-critical attitude.

A: You may be able to comprehend your anxieties when we deal with the questions of what you are confident you can do and what is expected of you.

The patient then described her school career, which had been disappointing to her. She had failed twice and had to leave high school (*Gymnasium*); she did not explain why she had failed. She had obtained her secondary school degree in an adult education program after she had realized that she was not satisfied with her simple work.

At the next session she sighed as she gave the application back to me. Referring to it, I said, "It's just too much." That was her opinion too. She looked at me, slightly startled that I had made such a direct comment about her mood, grinned a little, but there was no change in her bad mood.

P: Simply the feeling of having to come to therapy, of having to be here and talk, everything is just too much for me.

A: Then I would like to better understand what *everything* means. Can you mention any examples of how everything changes from being pleasurable to an obligation?

P: Yes, for example, I have to play tennis when the weather is good, or I have to go for a walk. Everything that I want turns into a "You have to do it." When I tell myself today that I want to go to an educational event tomorrow, then tomorrow I'm bound to remember, while I'm in the process of going to it, that it's become another must.

Her pained description made me think of an infant that sometimes wants to say ha and sometimes ho, that doesn't want to (or have to) enter into any obligations. Then I verbalized part of this idea.

A: Your wishes turn into musts, compulsions, the moment you have the feeling that they have become independent, that you have to obey your own wish. You want to be able to say ha or ho at any moment, and without having to fear the consequences.

We then began to speak about her mother, who had had to work a lot, and had talked to herself while she worked, saying "I still have to do this, I have to do that." Her father had tried in vain to tell her mother that she didn't have to keep busy all the time.

I made the interpretation that the patient carried her mother around inside her and acted toward herself as her mother had acted toward herself. She had two sides: one of wishes and one of her conscience, which was very strong. While I was making this detailed interpretation, which I attempted to make emotionally accessible to her, she began to cry. She soon managed to regain her composure. It became clear to me that she was always surprised by her longings to be spoiled and to have her wishes fulfilled, which she otherwise effectively kept under control. After imagining her fantasies and since she had already had a longer therapy, I told her that this soft, crying side would prefer to be bundled in a blanket on the couch, but that her other side would not permit it.

P: I can't at all imagine lying here and not having to say anything. It's impossible for it to be successful. I wouldn't consider it. I'd feel as if I were even more helpless, I'd feel even more like a patient and inferior to you.

A: Even the idea disturbs you; then it's better to stay in the middle, like Buridan's mule - do you know it? It stood halfway between two bundles of hay and starved. You stay in the middle, in the stagnation that you discovered during your therapy with Dr. B [her previous therapist]. I think the first issue is whether it's at all possible for you to accept the idea that you can turn around if you have the feeling while you're driving here that you have to come.

After a break of a few days, when the patient had a few days off from work, she was furious when she came in because she had not been able in the meantime to free herself of the feeling that she had to do something and that even relaxing had become a must, a bothersome task. The patient gave an example of how it should be. She had gone to bed with a case of the flu and dozed the entire afternoon, and the feeling of being compelled to visit friends in the evening had disappeared completely. She said that this was how it was supposed to be. I emphasized the congruence between her thoughts, feelings, and actions.

The patient then spoke explicitly about a voice inside her that constantly guided and directed her. When she read a book, the voice would tell her that had to read it to the end, ruining all her pleasure. This voice was not a delusion; it was the inexorably impregnated voice of her conscience, which she immediated associated with her mother, who had constantly told her not to do something. At the beginning of school vacation her mother would always say, "Good that you're here; now you can do this or that." The patient's associations clarified why going to bed had been so satisfying; she could just let everything lie where it was, throw her clothes in a corner, and doze.

A: That was a few hours vacation from your watchful and evil conscience.

It soon became clear to me that for her the analyst embodied this internalization. The beginning of the sessions were a regular torment for the patient. The opportunity to speak about what was on her mind her became a demand, a must. She responded to the implication that she could also remain silent if she felt like it by having aggressive doubts.

P: It's just a matter of time until you feel the same way that Dr. B did. In the course of our second year she raised the question of whether I would really benefit from the sessions.

The patient's dilemma consisted in the fact that her own intentional acts unconsciously always had to correspond to her mother's ideas. In this sense, the analytic situation inevitably became a repetition that she countered with a hostile lack of enthusiasm. The primary purpose of her talking in therapy was to satisfy the analyst, which corresponded to the patient's accusation that she had worked hard in the previous therapy, i. e., had fulfilled her mother's expectations. At least her mother had shown her appreciation when she had done something successfully. Yet her deeper, unconscious desire was to receive confirmation *without* having to accomplish something. This was in turn concealed by her strong rivalry to her brother, who was four years older and earned good money as a tax advisor. The consequences of this could be seen in the patient's relationship to her partner. One point of friction was her friend's self-satisfaction; he seemed to be satisfied with himself although he did not earn much money.

The psychogenic underpinning of the patient's lack of self-esteem was strongly reinforced by her physical illness. She was now really threatened by a condition that could be controlled with medication but that in fact could not be overcome.

I managed to weaken the patient's stubborn resistance by trying to avoid certain situations of conflict. If I waited a little longer to respond, there was usually a revival of her disappointment, and any suggestions I made, usually in reference to her momentarily visible mood, helped her to verbalize her difficulties.

She had so many wishes that she wanted to make come true all at once. In her career she wanted to attain a higher qualification, and privately she hoped to read many books. Just when she was deeply engrossed she would be overcome by panic, jump up, and have to go to a bar. "I want to do so much and don't have any time."

Her pubertal feeling of having lost something subequently became accessible to her. She had felt that her father did not appreciate her any more because of her poor achievement. There were still many layers of feelings of guilt and shame that had to be worked through before the accusations with which the patient had *successfully* obstructed the first attempt at therapy were diminished.

4.5 Closeness and Homosexuality

Arthur Y enjoyed going to a swimming pool, but felt very inhibited about it. Bathing in the nude, in particular, provided him pleasurable physical sensations, which he felt ashamed of. While discussing this topic in the last session it had dawned on him that I also like to go swimming, which is true although it was not explicitly mentioned. Yet the patient acted as if he had to be ashamed of the special sensation that contact with water, i. e., of his skin with water, gave him. I then startled him very much by drawing his attention to the fact that he had noticed something of my positive attitude to bathing, swimming, and water.

P: I hope it doesn't become apparent now that you also like to go swimming without any trunks, because that's what I thought of, and since I spontaneously thought of it I've wondered whether I could dare to mention it here. So, well, so I'll just say it: Then you're the same bitch that I am.

A: When you and I go swimming, both of us in water, then we're connected, one bugger to another. Your unease probably has something to do with contact.

I switched from the word "bitch," which has various connotations, to "bugger" in an effort to relate the patient's pleasurable experience more closely to its unconscious homosexual components.

P: Then there isn't any distance left between us, and that brings me back to my question of why I'm being so cautious.

The patient spoke again about contact and what we have in common when we swim in the same water.

A: The distance isn't entirely gone; each of us has his own skin, his own border.

P: This conversation is very disagreeable. It just amounts to blurring the distance.

Arthur Y mentioned that in earlier therapies he had found that keeping his distance gave him a sense of security:

P: For the simple reason that I told myself, the larger the distance, the greater the superiority of these analysts and their learning and the better my chances of being cured.

A: But that made you even more inferior, leaving you to hope that the stronger your admiration, the better your chances of getting something would be.

P: But they didn't try hard to change this condition, but maybe I'm not being fair to them.

A: And maintaining the familiar balance also provides relief, even though it is connected with much suffering.

This intervention was a reference to the beginning of the session, when the patient had expressed his concern with the fact that it was not easy for him to break out of or change patterns of behavior formed over decades. The purpose of my "bugger" comment was to raise the conflict to a genetically higher level, from the anal to the phallic.

Some time later this topic was raised again in another context. A scheduled meeting with his boss about a reassignment of responsibilities precipitated a completely irrational disturbance and a worsening of the patient's symptoms. Arthur Y was sure of his boss' respect and sympathy, was superior to his competitors, and led in sales.

P: But I experience it as if I would lose my territory or have to accept substantial limitations. I know that my boss values my opinion and that he accepts me as a partner, yet I still have the feeling of being helpless, at the mercy of alien forces.

The patient was even afraid that his boss might fire him if he raised any objections. All of his compulsive symptoms and anxieties had grown stronger.

P: I simply have the feeling that I'm not a subject, just an object.

After the patient had provided a detailed description of the objective problems resulting from the proposed realignment of work, it became clear that the rivalry between him and his colleagues would increase because he wanted to extend his area. He wanted to have some compensation for the increased stress that he expected. He had started waking up early, which tormented him. He would lie in bed sweating and afraid of what would happen that day.

P: There is the fear of failure, the anxiety about these fantasies, these compulsive fantasies, they could become so strong that I wouldn't be able to move around normally any more and you could see that something was wrong .... Although I have always proven myself in the past 25 years, I'm simply afraid of being nothing, just a picture of misery. It makes me sick. For example, I tried to analyze my agitation myself, to get over the problem. I recalled a teacher from boarding school who almost raped me, and I noticed the horrified feeling I had when his face came close to me, his repulsive mouth and his ugly, protruding buck teeth. It was so on my mind - it must mean something - that I repeatedly thought about blood and slaughtering animals, and I'm so fascinated by pigs. Then I thought of this man, who was probably an unhappy bitch, but in my experience he was a repulsive creature. If I had had the power I might have literally butchered him just like a pig in a slaughterhouse.

One anxiety that this patient had was to end up a sex offender. This anxiety was precipitated by a movie and was linked to the role of a specific actor (see Chap. 9). The patient's associations moved from the teacher to the actor to scenes in the movie. I asked about the similarity between the actor and the teacher, to prepare a transference interpretation. The patient confirmed my assumption.

P:Yes, I realized that while thinking about the whole matter, and it calmed me down so much that I fell asleep, and I told myself that my experience with this man wasn't so terrible after all. I had classmates who said that it wasn't that bad. He only meant well, he only wanted to give us some consolation. Yet I was very afraid of him and somehow have suppressed this fear and not really let it out in the last few years.

A: Something important now is prompting your memories. You've entrusted yourself to me. In connection with your desire to go swimming, especially naked, you've had the thought about me: "That bitch might go swimming naked too and tempt me into physical pleasure."

P: Well, yes [laughing].

A: Here you entrust yourself to me. The relationship could be misused and turn into one . . . too close . . . a homoerotic one . . . two bitches.

P: Yes, yes, that's true. I think I sometimes experience you the same way I did this teacher. Right now that's very clear to me, and it's very unpleasant for me to talk about it.

A: The subject is whether you experience it as something good, without any boundaries being transgressed, only good, not misused.

P: I've often thought, like with the teacher Mr. Benignus [the fictive name used in this treatment], that I was on a certain trail that could lead me to gaining control of my anxieties and overcoming them. And such comments, like that I experience you the same way I did him, irritate me. They make me feel insecure and anxious. Because if it were to turn out that you are really like he was, then I would be at your mercy just like I was then.

A: No, you wouldn't, because you're not as dependent on me as you were on your teacher. You're in a completely different situation. It still sounds a little as if you were just as dependent and couldn't bash my teeth down my throat and expose me to be a bitch and lead me to the slaughterhouse.

Arthur Y then described in very vivid and expressive terms the teacher's unshaven face and how it had scratched him. First he developed fantasies about how he could stick a knife into his fat neck and let the air out. The first manifestations of his neurotic anxieties occurred in connection with these experiences, both temporally and thematically, as the patient related at the end of this session.

P: When I was about 12 or 13 years old and read in a detective story that a man died after being stabbed in the back, I was terribly afraid that the same thing could happen to me. I tore up the book, threw it in the toilet, and flushed it down. It must have been around the time when I had the problems with the teacher. Then it went away again, this anxiety. Perhaps I felt I was a bitch as well, and maybe I even had an impulse to, well, how should I say it, to somehow give myself to this man, if not in this way. But all of that was years ago and shouldn't keep me as preoccupied as in the last few days. Well, the feeling was just horrible.

A: Yes, that was a long time ago. The subject was revived by the therapy, by your coming here, namely the subject of, well, how you will come to terms with another man. Are you still the small, dependent boy who can't defend himself? Are you loved only if you subjugate yourself? Or can you express your doubts, your dissatisfaction, or demand something?

Commentary. As the phrasing of the interpretation shows, the analyst emphasized the revival of old problems in transference. The questions he raised contained an indirect encouragement for the patient to critically examine past and present relationships. He suggested answers that enabled the patient to establish some distance and thus to have a new experience in his present interpersonal relationship to the analyst. In this sense many interpretations contain a suggestive component, which however is very different from the obvious attempts at persuasion that gave suggestion such a bad name. The stimuli contained in psychoanalytic interpretations are not at the level of persuasion. As we explain in Vol.1, the patient is encouraged to make his current experiences the starting point for critical reflection.

4.6 Resistance and the Security Principle

In this section in Vol.1 we attribute identity resistance and the security principle a comprehensive function exceeding that in Erikson's definition. At the descriptive level they resemble narcissistic defense. Yet while the latter concept is embedded in the untenable economic principle, the concept of identity resistance belongs in a comprehensive theoretical framework that takes the results of modern social psychological research on the development of the ego and self-esteem into consideration without neglecting the significance of sexual gratification for personal identity. In contrast to Erikson's integrative theory, Kohut viewed the development of the self and the drives as separate processes, and despite his later modification of his self psychology this view leads to inconsistencies within his system and does not do justice to human life. The process of satisfying various kinds of needs leads to the development of security and self-esteem.

A strong identity resistance can be observed in all patients who do not accept the fact that they are ill and, subsequently, do not desire to be treated. The circumstances are then reversed: those near the patient suffer and attempt to convince the recalcitrant relative that something has to be done. Yet how can you convince someone who is apparently satisfied with himself and in fact thinks he is healthy - but is considered by those around him to be ill and crazy - that he should try a therapy that in his view would at the most lead to change he does not desire?

Identity resistance represents the triumph of the human capacity for self-assertion at any price, even at that of negating the principle of biological self-preservation. Perhaps it was rather in passing that Freud (1940a) attributed the ego not only the task of *self-preservation*, as he had previously, but also that of *self-assertion*. (This difference is eliminated in the *Standard Edition* because Strachey translated each of the German words - *Selbsterhaltung* and *Selbstbehauptung* - as self-preservation.) This human capacity is the precondition for anyone assigning a higher value to self-assertion in the achievement of ideals than in the preservation of one's own life and sacrificing oneself for a good cause. This is the result of decisions rooted in the freedom of the individual. The situation is different in the cases of self-assertion found in identity resistance; here there are good reasons for assuming that the individual is unfree even though he rejects the notion that he is ill, unfree, and in need of help.

Identity resistance and the security principle pose numerous ethical and philosophical problems as well as serious questions of analytic technique. Who gives us the right to attempt a therapy of someone who at the most only half-heartedly considers himself a patient? We are faced with the dilemma that treatment is even less possible that it is otherwise, for example, to unintentionally analyze someone with anorexia and to refrain from active interventions if self-preservation has reached its limits and death seems imminent. Particularly the therapy of anorexia nervosa confronts analysts with problems that seem hopeless. This dilemma results in complete paralysis; Kierkegaard referred to it in his religious philosophical interpretation as "illness unto death." From a psychoanalytic perspective it is possible to localize despair, as the manifestation of illness unto death, in the self. In doing so we attribute a psychodynamic meaning to Kierkegaard's (1957, p. 8) sentence: "Dispairing of not wanting to be yourself; dispairing of wanting to be yourself." This contrast characterizes a dilemma that dominates many people. Chronic anorexics especially impress their environment with the decisiveness with which they hold on to their very idiosyncratic selves. The therapist becomes the source of temptation, who attempts to make a self image available that arouses their own resistance. The despair does not transpire between two self images but between the individual and his environment. Thus how can we use psychoanalytic means to intervene in a dilemma and struggle with female patients who for years have made their cachexic body image their second but true nature and who view the analyst as a troublemaker? In these cases identity resistance is literally linked with a balance that has an inertia of its own after years or decades of constancy: this identity has become second nature.

Clara X brought the copy of Rosetti's painting The Annunciation that she had painted to the 427th session; this painting had impressed her for a long time. The Maria is almost cachexic. That the copy is a kind of self image can be seen in the addition to the signature, Maria the Anorexic. Clara described the junction she was at: she was still sitting there (like Maria) and was indecisive.

Her thoughts still revolved aroung the image of a fairy sitting at the junction to point her in the right direction.

A: Give the fairy a chance, all the fairies sitting there–and yourself too.

P: One evening recently I saw the fairy sitting there and myself still burdened with the same habits. The fairy smiled, half amused, half disconcerted, asking "Why are you doing that?" I have to move around to get tired, in order to fall asleep and stay close to the fairy. The fairy said there was a real mountain of mush, like around the land of milk and honey, and that I would have to eat my way through it.

Clara X exhibited all the signs of revulsion.

I considered the picture to be an expression of the struggle we were having at this junction. Clara viewed my allusion to a strugggle as an opponent, without describing it more closely.

Struggle was a subject that had played a important role from the beginning. The fact that I had predicted in the first interview that there would probably be a hard struggle had made Clara X angry. The struggle had become more intense in the last few weeks and months and had taken on the form of the patient's image of a junction. A good fairy was part of this metaphor; it was a maternal transference figure, and the patient wanted to stay at its bosom. Yet it also had the function of leading her away from the anorexia, which had become her second nature.

My interest in her self-representation was thus concerned with her struggle to maintain her previous identity and now, at the junction, with her attempt to make a new beginning. Its immediate relevance could be seen in the fact that the patient first interrupted me when I repeated the sentence "Now that will . . .," saying "Hum," and after I had completed my sentence ending "be a hard struggle" she continued:

P: Yes, I thought of that again this morning too. I'd like to know who is going to struggle against . . . .

A: Hum.

P: And I don't really want to have to struggle with myself. Just against some parts of me. Right now that's funny. I've accepted the idea that I have to try to eat more during the day, and I do. Usually it turns out that I want to eat some cake. I buy something in the bakery, but then I immediately have the feeling that it's not really the right thing. Cake isn't the most nutritional food. And so my wanting to eat cake doesn't make me feel quite right. I used to solve the problem by not even thinking about food during the day. I kept my head free for other things, something that is frequently reported in the literature on anorexia, which I always read with mixed feelings . . . with great interest. I had gotten over the phase in which my thoughts constantly revolved around food, as is the case for many anorexics and which I think is pretty degrading.

It is true that the feeling of being hungry changes in severe and chronic cases, enabling some patients to achieve the condition that the patient just described with the words that she "kept her head free for other things." She had managed to limit the times and places at which she satisfied her feeling of being hungry, restricting it primarily to eating cookies at night.

It seemed natural for me to draw Clara X's attention to the difficulty that arose when she attempted to modify her behavior. She experienced the fact that she now had to concern herself more with food and everything associated with it to be degrading.

P: Then I quickly get to the point that I think too much about my household and shopping. Nonsense. There are other things that are more interesting and more satisfying. Yes, right now I'm asking myself, hm, whether I should take something along from home for a snack or buy something, and what I should eat and what I should give to Fransziska [her daughter] to take along? I can make big decisions out of these questions and let my indecisive anguishing between yes and no and good and evil go unchecked in this small matter. But then I've had enough of it again; yet why shouldn't I attempt to want to eat and to enjoy it? Yesterday morning I was at the point of thinking "Hum, . . ." but then it was gone again.

A: Yes, inner necessity is important in such changes. You know that the feelings of being hungry and wanting to eat can change. You apparently used to be very free, but in contrast to you I think this freedom was only apparent. However, it was an excellent way to get past a lot of things. Getting started is very difficult.

P: Yes, an apparent freedom. I really wonder whether I can get used to simply eating at certain times. Just thinking about it makes me feel bad. I've at least made an effort to eat something during the day. That's why I was really a little baffled to have lost a little weight. Is it the fear of craving something or what? On the other hand, I really have a very positive feeling toward life and feel like doing something again and want to get up in the morning. My condition last year - you're sure to remember it, as I thought that everything around me was dreary and boring - is a thing of the past.

The patient then described her hectic daily routine as housewife and mother. She was very unhappy with these tasks. "Now home to the jail, make something to eat, put the kid to bed, and then I feel jailed in." Her detailed description ended with her telling me about her incredibly hectic manner, which pushed her and made her be unfriendly and impatient.

Then she related a wonderful daydream, which might be viewed as a sign that with the help of a good fairy which she herself had invented she could follow a different path to find a modified identity. At the center of her story was her mother, who had a lot of time, waited for the children to come home, and had harmonious and close ties to them. She described a day with her mother as if it were in a fairy tale. Clara X doubted whether I, as a man, could understand her almost timeless happiness. She was outraged by punctuality and regularity and by the rhythm she had to keep in her household.

P: Bum, bum, bum, my husband would like to have everything done at home just like it is in the factory. His expectations provoke strong feelings of dislike and anxiety in me. I can't express it in words, and I think you don't understand it. It's terrible.

A: I think I can understand it, but it's logical that you are skeptical because I live here close to bum bum. Daily schedule, time. If my schedule says the session is over, then that's how it is; it's a disturbance that doesn't correspond to the daydream. Letting punctuality be imposed from outside is disturbing if we contrast it to this enjoyable image.

P: What, do you think that my fantasies are really only related to the beginning and end of the sessions up here. That is . . . .

A: Yes, that was a little hop, skip, and jump. I wasn't only thinking about the beginning and the end; in between there's a lot that can be done. No, I was only thinking of this one hop, toward the end of the session. I mentioned a parallel to one tiny point, the interruption at the end of the session. Whether it's true is something else.

Excerpts from later sessions show how difficult it was for Clara X to form another image of herself. It wasn't possible for me to be as unintentional as she wanted me to be. In any case, a comparison I drew between another, beautiful picture that the patient had painted and her reality greatly offended her.

She thought her body and appearance were ideal. She was afraid of being like a stuffed goose and not being able to slip "through the bars of her prison."

I raised the question of why she had formed the repulsive image of the stuffed goose. She emphasized that the sore point was the prison. She doubted whether any man could really understand how a woman could experience the role of housewife to be a prison.

A: By staying skinny you're really expressing your aversion to your marriage. And in the process you're also struggling against your chocolate coating.

The patient had introduced this ambiguous term, and ever since it was used to refer to her sweet side, both in a literal and metaphorical sense of the word. Clara X made external circumstances responsible for the fact that it was impossible for her to make her chocolate coating, i. e., her sweet and tender longing, come true, which tied her all the more to her nightly "orgies." The patient satisfied the hunger she suppressed during the day by eating large amounts of candy at night when she was half asleep, and managed in this way to at least keep her substantially reduced weight constant. These typical night-eating binges, to use an expression Stunkard (1986) introduced, can also serve as a substitute satisfaction. And the patient did in fact claim that her husband was partly responsible for the continuance of her illness because he overlooked the tender and feminine side in her Death skeleton.

I explicitly acknowledged the realistic component of her difficulties. Furthermore, I told her that being rejected and offended in the guise of Death had apparently also led her to employ her condition as a weapon. This was a special form of *self-assertion* she had cherished for a long time. Any modification would lead her to look more pleasant and no longer be a skin and bones. She would lose the identity she had developed in the course of decades and be more pleased with herself. She would then be like Sleeping Beauty [in German, thorn rose] but without the thorns, beautiful to look at, because she had also painted the picture. "If you permit me to say so, I like Sleeping Beauty too."

Consideration. I alluded to a very impressive water color that the patient had given me some time earlier. The circular painting shows girls interwoven in the shape of a rose, and the use of color emphasizes their breasts. The cautious manner in which I expressed myself might seem exaggerated, but caution was called for. The patient's sensitivity was demonstrated by events later in the session and by which ones she remembered and retained. I let myself be led into contrasting the rose woman with the repulsive image of Death that Clara X had described, without at the time taking into consideration that it makes a difference whether a patient uses a negative self-image to refer to himself, or whether the analyst employs the same expression. The fact that two people do the same thing does not make it the same.

Clara X referred to her paintings throughout analysis. They were frequently related to topics we had discussed, but frequently also provided insights into unknown aspects of her experiencing. They were self-representations that vividly expressed her inner condition. The following excerpt makes it clear that painting and making presents of her pictures naturally also had a communicative function for her. I attempted to use them as a means to influence her inner life and vivid imaging. We have thus returned to the decisive question: What can the analyst do to facilitate change?

P: I don't even want my husband to see this picture. I painted it when he couldn't see it, and then rolled it up. Because I have the feeling that in his opinion it might be repulsive.

A: But perhaps you were also afraid that he would make some comment. Maybe he would have made some comparisons.

P: He might have said, "Are you completely crazy? Now you've started painting naked women."

I asked in an empathic manner about her fears of being hurt. Maybe that was the reason she had the idea that a female analyst would understand her better - from woman to woman, from Sleeping Beauty to Sleeping Beauty.

The patient began the next session by making the observation that she was upset. "You compared me, the picture of Death, with my own picture of the rose woman." She said she did not like comparisons; they were typical educational tools. "My parents say, 'At your age I was already able to do this and that.' It hurts to be compared."

A:But what is it that hurts? That you are also the rose woman?

P: That you prefer the rose woman.

A: Yes, yes, the comparison reminded you of what's missing, of the deficit.

P: No, the point is that you're posing conditions. I felt your wish, or request or question, and it seemed very ungentlemanly. "Could you bring the picture along once more, so that I can make a copy of it? I don't have one. I gave it to you." Demanding something back like this isn't right. There's a little spite involved: "But it's my picture!"

The patient emphasized this again:

P: There is some spite involved: "But it's my picture!" There's some piggishness involved in saying, "If the oldster uses the picture like that, then I at least want to have something from it."

A: Wonderful, hum. So that it can't be used against you anymore. You experience it as if I used it against you, and now it could be that if you had a copy, then you could also use it for yourself, and it wouldn't be so one-sided. And I didn't experience your giving it to me as a formal cession. I view it as a picture between you and me, not as my possession. I see it as your picture of yourself and also as the ideal you have of yourself.

P: It has both parts, but the moment I gave it to you - it makes me happy if you accept it - it was meant as a present. [Long pause] At the moment I don't have the feeling that the picture could represent an ideal for me.

A: And at the moment you have a strong feeling that people don't like you the way you are, and it's terrible when people set conditions. Yet it wouldn't be rejection if looking different made you more pleasing. And I assume that you like your chocolate side better than your ascetic one, too. I also relate what you said about yourself to me. But I'm powerless.

P: It's not true that you can't do anything. You act as if none of your words fall on fertile ground.

A: Well, I can't do anything unless you accept something. And one thing it depends on is whether I can offer it to you bite size. But when it is too bite size, it gets difficult again. It really is a hard struggle, but I do think that you are enormously fertile ground and could be even more fertile. What would happen if you gave up some of your power and discovered that it wasn't a loss of power but an increase in a different kind of power? You can certainly feel that there is power in your picture, in your Sleeping Beauty. Of course, you'd be more sensitive and more sentimental about having needs and showing them when they aren't noticed, recognized, or satisfied. That's bad.

Consideration. Here I made the patient aware of my countertransference (see Sect. 3.4). Telling the patient about a mood precipitated by his behavior can have a therapeutic function, as can be seen in Clara X's reaction. Letting her participate in my countertransference had the effect of serving as an anchor for both of us. I knew and could somehow sense that precisely my open and honest admission of being powerless would mobilize the opposite attitude in the patient. Clara X was really not looking for a powerless, castrated man, otherwise she would remain infertile too. The therapeutic problem consisted in putting the fertile elements into such bite-size pieces that words and deeds would be equated with life, not with terrible elements and ultimately with death. Transforming the destructive no into a constructive yes to life means acknowledging biological rhythms and temporality. Although being able to say no belongs to human nature, no mortal who says no in a destructive manner has ever fallen from heaven. Regardless of what philosophers and theologists have to say about the constructive significance of negation, arduous psychoanalytic investigations are necessary to be able to understand and explain the development of pathological negativism. It is the self-destructive form of one's own aggression, and also denies that the "object" is affected. This enables anorexics and other pathological nay sayers to deny the mortal danger they are in. The perception of the danger must be rediscovered in transference.

P: [After a long pause] That sounds convincing. But I can't really imagine that it's true.

A: It's nice that it at least sounds convincing. In that moment neither of us has power over the other. It's true that I mentioned it, but by finding it convincing you have annexed it, have incorporated it. For a moment we're in agreement. Of course, it can always be ridiculed; somebody might say that there are nicer things.

P: I wasn't thinking of that just now. It's such a nice feeling that I can't believe it. It just can't be true. There are three buts, five ifs, and five other conditions just waiting around the next corner; they are not mentioned right now, but they're there.

The patient referred to an earlier comparison with porcupines.

A: The feeling of being in agreement contained a barb, as if I weren't satisfied with the agreement itself and wanted to have an immediate success.

P: I cannot imagine that you're satisfied with a momentary agreement.

A: Yes, I think that nobody is entirely satisfied with one. You would also like to have more, but don't dare to make the moments last longer. Your dissatisfaction comes to you from outside then: I want more, not you.

Commentary. The analyst made too great an effort to achieve a change. Just like in the proverb, the result was just to disgruntle the patient. Clara X criticized his "educational" goals, which points to the fact that the analyst apparently did not have much confidence in the patient's other self. Otherwise he would not have given her so much encouragement, even if indirectly. The analyst's admission of powerlessness was apparently also made with the therapeutic intention of motivating Clara X to reflect on her strengths and of helping ease the sacrifice. In short, there is more to an identity resistance that has formed over twenty years than meets the eye.

5 Interpretation of Dreams

Introduction

Readers of this book will frequently encounter the interpretation of dreams as being the *via regia* to the unconscious and, at least as dreamers, they will also have taken this royal path. A dream cannot be equated with the unconscious but it is, in Freud's words, the *via regia* to it, getting lost somewhere in the depths of the unconscious. Dream interpretation enables analysts to get close to unconscious fantasies. The interpretations lead to the latent, i. e., the unconscious meaning of the dream. To be precise, then, the interpretation and not the dream itself is the *via regia* to the unconscious.

The series of dreams described in this chapter were embedded in a course of treatment that formed a significant phase in the life history of a patient and in the course of his illness. In order to be able to follow dream interpretations critically, it is essential to be aware of the patient's biographical background, his illness, and the implications of his illness for his self-esteem. Information and discussion of these points serve several purposes. For example, a patient's dreams are influenced by his neurotic and somatic illness. It therefore seems logical to take this case as a starting point for discussing general problems of psychoanalysis and psychosomatic medicine that go far beyond dream interpretation.

In 1924 Rank published a monograph entitled *Eine Neurosenanalyse in Träumen*, in which he described a therapy that took the form of a pure dream analysis. In interpreting a large number of dreams during a 150 session therapy, which was successful, he did not distinguish between abstract interpretations and individual therapeutic ones. We mention this typical publication from the 1920s because the contrast between it and the present day demonstrates the progress that has been made in analytic technique. We believe it is essential to make the reader aware of the individual steps in an analyst's interpretative work in his dialogue with a patient.

5.1 Self-Representation in Dreams

In Vol.1 (Sect. 5.2) we drew attention to the intricate relationship between word and image in Freud's theory. This relationship is characterized by several transformations that on the one hand led Freud to distinguish between the latent and the manifest contents of dreams and, on the other, are related to the therapeutic task of translating images into words and thoughts. The plastic portrayal of the manifest content of a dream becomes a relatively superficial event of the dream genesis only if the latent *dream thoughts* forming the basis of dream work are taken to constitute the essential content of the dream. Freud spoke, in this sense, of the manifest dream element as being a "concrete portrayal ... taking its *start* from the *wording*." At the same time, Freud also wrote, in this contradictory context, that "we have long since forgotten from what concrete *image* the word originated and consequently fail to recognize it when it is replaced by the image" (Freud 1916/17, p. 121, emphasis added). Bucci (1985) has since replaced Freud's inconsistant "zig-zag theory" of the relationship between word and image, which depended heavily on his untenable economic principle (see Vol.1, Sect. 1.3), with the dual code theory (Paivio 1971). As a result, the distinction between the manifest dream image and the latent dream thoughts in the *dream genesis* is shifted in favor of stages of *dream interpretation*. The significance that images always had in Freud's theory as *symbols* is also reestablished. Erikson (1954), in his configuration analysis of dreams, initated an interpretative technique that in large measure corresponds to the primacy of plastic portrayal.

These introductory comments are meant to prepare the reader for the fact that the self-representations contained in the following series of dreams are variations of the important subject of *body image* (see Sect. 9.2.1). The images that we have of ourselves and that others have of us are not only related to personal characteristics and manners of behavior, but are always also related to our physical existence. The images that we and others have of ourselves comprise both personal identity and body image, whose numerous and discordant layers are important determinants of an individual's sense of self-security. In addition to these general points, the fact that body image plays a special role in specific interpretations in the series of dreams reported here resulted from the nature of the patient's symptoms.

Freud's advice for therapy was to look for the dreamer's ego in the person who succumbs to an affect in the dream. In patients whose conscious experiencing is affected by imagined physical defects, the defects will probably be presented in a scene and possibly be expressed by different individuals. Yet before we, with the help of dreams, start down the royal road to the unconscious in order to reach the dreaming ego's enactments and answers, let us turn to the general and specific problems posed by a typical case.

5.1.1 Dysmorphophobia and Spasmodic Torticollis

Erich Y suffered from a dysmorphophobia since adolescence, i.e., for about 25 years. He was also afflicted by spasmodic torticollis, which first appeared about three years prior to the beginning of treatment. The patient's *wryneck* made him feel so insecure that it precipitated episodes of depression.

Dysmorphophobia is defined as:

> the unfounded fear of a circumscribed physical deformity. The phobic ideas refer to body parts assigned a special aesthetic or communicative function .... The fears of an unaesthetic, ugly, or repulsive appearance are almost exclusively focused on circumscribed body parts and only in exceptional cases on a person's overall appearance. The most frequent objects are facial and sex-specific features. (Strian 1983, pp. 197, 198)

Küchenhoff (1984) has described the history of this concept and assigned the fear of deformity a position of its own in psychiatric terminology and nosology, locating it between hypochondric syndromes and the delusion of reference. From Küchenhoff's review of the literature it can be seen that early psychoanalytic case reports describe dysmorphophobic patients without designating them as such (e. g., Freud's Wolf Man).

In the psychoanalytic literature the predominant view about the relationship between the psychodynamics of body image and psychosexual development is much too one-sided to do justice to the genesis and therapy of the rich diversity of imagined defects or deformities. The earlier tendency to reduce everything to the castration complex has been succeeded by the emphasis placed on narcissism. Finally, the symptoms are often considered to fulfill the function of protecting against psychotic disintegration, similar to the situation in chronic hypochondria (Philippopoulos 1979; Rosenfeld 1981). We believe that an interpersonal approach can clarify many of the puzzles surrounding the genesis of such body images.

According to our experience, dysmorphophobia is gaining in significance because many of those turning to plastic surgeons for, for instance, mammoplasty or rhinoplasty imagine they have a deformity. Yet an operation can hardly alter the attitude of these individuals toward their presumed unaesthetic appearance (Mester 1982).

With the passing of time the anxiety component of the belief that one has a partial deformity often recedes behind a less anxious hypochondric or obsessive preoccupation with the deformity and its correction. Since the belated recognition of the significance of Schilder's works (1933, 1935) by Fisher and Cleveland (1968), the theory of body image has been profitably applied to the analytic understanding and therapy of dysmorphophobia. Of course, Erikson's and Kohut's theories of identity and self have contributed to our improved understanding of this form of insecurity, which is central for these patients and for many others (Cheshire and Thomä 1987). The body, however, is not the focus of these theories, in contrast to the theory of body image, whose interactional development was excellently described by Schilder (1933) (see Sect. 9.2.1).

Erich Y suffered since puberty from a severe case of dysmorphophobia, i. e., from the unfounded idea, which was more hypochondric than phobic, that he had a receding chin, a crooked nose, and a deformed head. He attempted to balance these presumed deformities by, for example, compulsively taking care of his hair and pushing his chin forward. His self-security was further limited by his belief that his penis was too small, with the logical consequences that this had on his capacity for making contacts. The only reason this belief is mentioned here as the last in this series of symptoms is that this patient, like most of those with similar symptoms, did not mention it at first. The hesitancy to mention it is not only the result of a displacement to other parts of the body, as is typical for phobias; the shame anxiety of these patients is so strong that they do not discover the preconscious starting point of their presumed defects until later in analysis.

It was natural that Erich Y's unstable self-feeling was badly shaken when he acquired a symptom that was definitely more than just imagined, namely a typical case of torticollis with his head turned to the right. According to his recollection, it had first appeared during a meditation exercise, i. e., in a situation in which he was trying to find relaxation. He had immediately given it a meaning, seeing a connection to a crisis in his marriage. He observed, above all, that the automatic twisting movement of his head occurred or became more pronounced especially when he felt observed or was supposed to present himself in some way. The shame affect that was already present became very substantial, making his suffering become quite severe. His suffering increased as a result of his depressive reaction to the symptom, i. e., from the way in which he coped with it.

Approximately two years after the successful conclusion of psychoanalytic treatment the patient became impotent during another marital crisis. In this connection he had a recurrence of his torticollis symptoms, which led him to resume his therapy. He overcame his impotence, and his neck condition improved significantly. We will now give a brief description of his case to demonstrate that the causes of the torticollis and the dysmorphophobia were at different levels.

Torticollis is an abnormal twisting or inclination of the head that cannot be willfully suppressed, is frequently accompanied by tremor, and is caused by continuing contractions of the head and neck musculature that are primarily unilateral and spontaneous. The increase in tone of the individual muscles that slowly sets in and does not relax until many seconds later, the hesitant movements, and the stereotypic features of its course and localization must be viewed as dystonic hyperkinesia in conjunction with an extrapyramidal illness. These movements are neither a reflex precipitated by passive expansion nor an increased muscle tone such as in a spasm during a central motor disturbance.

The dystonic movement in torticollis cannot be suppressed by voluntary tensing of antagonistic muscles or by pressure applied externally. It decreases during sleep and under anesthesia, and increases primarily as a result of intentions to move as well as from *affective arousal*, focusing *attention* on it, and *exposure* in public. By using certain grips, which themselves do not require any force, for example placing a finger tip lightly on the contralateral cheek or side of the face, it is possible to reduce or suppress the abnormal movement.

Clinical observations have demonstrated that the momentary manifestation of the symptoms is dependent on situational factors, which have been very impressively described by Bräutigam (1956). Many patients are free of symptoms in the solitude of nature. The involuntary twisting of the head occurs especially when disconcerting eye contact is made.

What is important now is the significance attributed to these precipitating factors, whereby it is important to distinguish between the patient's view and the interpretation the expert makes on the basis of various diagnostic findings. It has been proven that persons suffering from such conspicuous symptoms become insecure and that, when they feel they are being observed, they twist their head all the more and with extreme force; a slight tremor can also occur. Anxieties initiate the manifestation of the symptoms. There are different ways this partial cause can be interpreted. In our opinion, the grave misunderstandings of the psychogenic and somatogenic factors arose because the environmental dependence of this and other somatic illnesses led doctors to misdiagnose torticollis as "hysterical." This fact was emphasized by Bräutigam (1956, p. 97): "The dependence on situational conditions is surely one of the important reasons that extrapyramidal symptoms were long misinterpreted as hysterical."

It was incorrect from the very beginning for the psychogenic element in the genesis of symptoms and the course of an illness to be restricted to the model of the genesis of *hysterical* symptoms. To determine the psychogenic element in extrapyramidal movement disturbances in which the brain is the organic cause, it is necessary to start by establishing correlations, just as in any physical illness (Alexander 1935; Fahrenberg 1979; Meyer 1987). It can be said in summary that the occurrence of wryneck in conjunction with stress does not justify the conclusion that the former is expressive movement, whether in the sense of an emotion or of a unconscious action.

Hypotheses about the psychogenic element in etiology must be compatible with the physical findings in order to escape the either-or dichotomy of somatic-psychogenic. We believe it is then possible for the neurologist to give appropriate consideration to the importance of the emotional disposition of the patient reacting to environmental factors (i. e., precipitating factors).

The analyst can employ his therapeutic means everywhere that certain forms of latent dispositions are activated and reinforced by a *circulus vitiosus*, as in an exaggerated shame anxiety. In such cases there is a chance to achieve change as far as reactions have not become completely determined by somatic causes. Much depends on whether the analyst successfully manages in the first diagnostic interviews to discover together with the patient that the latter's experiencing has influenced the course of his symptoms, as indicated above, and to make the patient's observations the starting point of their joint reflections. One could make the somewhat daring statement that the Oedipus complex never entirely disappears in any man, it just "wanes" and "repeatedly requires ... some forms of mastery, in the course of life" (Loewald 1980a, p. 371). Many clinical and experimental data, as reviewed by Greenberg and Fisher (1983), suggest that men are more insecure than women with regard to their physical integrity. Previous anxieties and mastered insecurities may be revived when a patient encounters new burdens, and they may be strengthened by realistic fears during physical illnesses, making it more difficult for the patient to cope with his illness. These general points apply to both men and women regardless of the differences in body-related anxieties between the two sexes. It is obvious, however, that the unjustified fear of having a physical deformity has a different conscious and unconscious background for women than for men. The genesis of imagined defects in one's self-image (in the comprehensive sense of the term) follows the typology of phases of psychosocial development. All the factors causing insecurity toward one's sense of identity can also have an impact on body image. Why specific deficits are limited in one case to the level of self-consciousness and in another are related to physical appearance is a difficult question that we will not go into here.

5.2 A Dream Sequence

Self-representations in dreams open up a hidden dimension because of the scenic character of "dream language." Deformities of the body image then occur in an interactional context. In comparison with dream language and in contrast to the vividness of hypochondric complaints, the descriptions of imagined deformities are one dimensional. Patients describe the ways they experience their bodies to be defective - such as a small chin, crooked nose, deformed back of the head, overly narrow vagina, and an injured heart - and how this diminishes their self-esteem without the patients themselves being able to understand or to experience the processes in which their frequently abstruse ideas about their body images develop. Self-representations in dreams, in contrast, exhibit latent dimensions lost to conscious experiencing and absent in descriptions of symptoms except for the fixed imagined final product. The scenic context of the dream thus makes it possible for the analyst to have insights into the genesis and meaning of disturbances that in conscious experiencing take the form of psychopathological phenomena, that is of a "damaged body image" to use a brief but appropriate expression.

The following dream sequence provides an insight into the analyst's interpretations. The analyst added the notes about his feelings and thoughts either immediately after the session or soon thereafter upon reading the transcript.

5.2.1 Dream About an Injection

At the beginning of the 37th session Erich Y delightedly told me about his discovery of things that he had in common with his boss. He used to have many disputes with his boss; both had been "blinded by our ambition." Spontaneously and without any apparent transition the patient started telling me about a dream he had had the previous night. "I saw a younger doctor in a hospital. I told him about my illness, and he gave me some hope. He claimed he knew something that would help. He experimented by giving me injections in my back, and while he was giving me a shot - it took a long time - I pulled away because it hurt."

He then came to speak in a vague manner of agreeable experiences, ones he might have had together with his wife. The day before, for instance, he had experienced something good at home. It had become clear to him how important mutual confirmation is. Following his longer statement there was a pause, which I interrupted by pointing out that the patient had received something good in the dream but that it had also caused pain. The topic shifted to the patient's ambivalence to therapy. A few sessions earlier the patient had been at a loss as to what he could answer curious questioners who wanted to know what he got from analysis. The experience that he frequently had not received any concrete support from me could have led the patient in his dream to turn to a young doctor who - as I interjected - knew of a particularly good form of medication.

P: Yes, it took a long time.
A: You mean, the injection.
P: Yes, and I got uneasy. I wanted to get it over with.
A: Hum.
P: It took too long. And then I had to think again about whether it was already working.
A: Yes.
P: While he was still giving me the injection, I tried to move my head again.
A: Hum.
P: Well, it worked right away.
A: Yes, and that is where the treatment situation comes into play, with the worrisome expectation: Yes, does it help? It's taking a long time.

Consideration. The patient's expectation of getting rapid help was disappointed. Although he tried not to become impatient, he looked for concrete help directly related to his symptom.

P: Hum.

A: I'm sitting behind you. In your dream something is happening to you from behind, isn't that right? Behind.

P: Hum. [Long pause]

The patient formed the image of a piece of granite that he himself or someone else was chiseling at. He also had, in contrast, weak impressions that he lost without being able to describe them. To me, the patient seemed a little unhappy, which he confirmed. I viewed the patient's statement that he could not hold on to anything and that he had the impression he were on a turntable as a sign of resistance. At this point the patient mentioned his dream again, including a few key words such as the sudden stop and the departure, which he then summarized.

P: There are so many things going through my mind again today. Lots of weak impressions.

A: You sound a little unhappy, as if you would change your mind too much. Or? Some place you had the feeling that you would not have liked to think it through or fantasize any further, for example as I referred to my view that you're looking for more. In the dream you're given an especially good drug. This went on for a long time, and you had the feeling that you don't want to be concerned about it any more.

P: I just had the thought, again in connection with my impatience and possibly with the dream: stay involved for long enough, don't give up early, so that there's nothing left that's only half done.

Consideration. The disappointment triggered dissatisfaction, which was suppressed. This topic was picked up in the next interpretations.

A: Hum. Yes, that's the one side, the disappointment, but your wish is still there. The wish behind it is, well, to get as much as fast as possible, isn't it?

P: Yes, yes, yes, yes.

A: This is presumably one of the wishes you had in your dream.

P: Right.

A: And as much as possible as fast as possible, and something really special . . . .

P: Hum.

A: . . . being able to get something really special.

P: Effectively. [Short pause]

A: It's a younger doctor who gives you something, younger than I am.

P: Yes, that seems to be the case.

A: Hum.

Commentary. The patient did not grasp at the offer, which was relevant to transference. The analyst realized this without commenting on it.

P: This impatience, it's true that I get impatient. Something has to happen fast. There has to be something effective, something I can grasp. Yes, and if this isn't the case, then I get impatient and would like to forget the whole thing. If I conclude everything correctly, then I have a lot more from it.

A: And then you almost force yourself by being patient, don't you? You suppress your natural striving and make an effort not to become impatient.

Commentary. By emphasizing that impatience is something natural, the analyst encouraged him to experience the aggression contained in his impatience.

P: Yes, yes, yes. I don't want to know about it.
A: Hum, hum, hum.
P: Well, when I think of it, then I have the feeling . . .
A: Hum.
P: . . . that I hope you don't drop me.
A: Hum. Yes, perhaps you're making a big effort not to be impatient because of this concern, as if you would be dropped if you got impatient once.

Commentary. This was a typical kind of a statement offering indirect encouragement: You will not be droppped if you get impatient. It was only the later and unmistakable assurance that made it possible for the patient to open himself more. As-if formulations frequently do not provide sufficient security. This type of interpretation is based on the assumption that the patient really knows that his anxietiy is unfounded. On the one hand this grammatical form creates openness, which stimulates reflection, yet on the other the patient is left in the dark. Reassurances cannot cancel unconscious expectations. As accurate as these observations may be, it should not be overlooked that stereotype as-if interpretations can undermine self-security. We have the impression that such stereotype interpretations can frequently be found in unsuccessful treatments.

P: I've often had the thought that this might be my last chance, and that I probably won't have another one in my life, to see something like that. And afterwards I have the feeling of being able to make even more out of it, to take . . .
A: Hum.
P: . . . even more out of it and to be creative.
A: Hum. Yes, and perhaps the dream is related to the fact that just today you would like to take as much as you can, because there's going to be an break in treatment.

Commentary. This established the connection to the situative factors possibly precipitating the dream: the break and the distance.

P: Hum, yes, it could be.
A: To get as much as possible.
P: Hum.
A: The subject of distance is still there too, in view of today's session, because of the break.
P: Hum.
A: However, you're the one moving away, away from the injection.
P: Hum.
A: Perhaps symbolically there is a little pain portrayed, yes, somewhere it hurts that there is going to be a break, a distance. [Short pause]
P: Yes, I just had a thought. My wife has asked me a couple of times: "What are you going to do when you can't go to your doctor any more, when you're on your own again?"
Consideration. A confirmation of the assumptions contained in the interpretations?
A: Hum, hum.
P: [Taking in a deep breath] And I said I hadn't actually thought about it and don't want to either.

A: Yes, for now you're still here, and I am too.

P: Yes.

A: Yes, hum, hum. [Longer pause]

P: Somehow I suddenly feel so protected and have to think of puppets who get to walk around but who are really on strings, I mean who aren't free. Well, I have some room to move but there is somebody there who's leading me.

Consideration. My pacifying comment that "for now you're still here, and I am too" enabled the patient to have an insightful fantasy and initiated a regression. Maybe the point is not for some substance (which?) to be injected but for the patient's father or mother to take him by the hand.

P: I'm just asking myself, well, room to move, to move, and – without being arrogant – say to myself that I can really try everything, can do everything, because I know that someone is there. [Very long pause] I have to think of this dream from last night over and over again. The doctor is standing there, and I move.

A: Hum, hum.

P: I'm in a certain place and feel my way around.

A: Hum, hum.

P: And this and that come by.

A: Hum.

P: And he stands there watching, watching me. [Breathes very deeply]

A: A while ago you thought about puppets who move, who are led by someone's hand and moved, in other words who aren't merely observed.

P: Hum.

A: That you can feel and can move and turn and move around, can't you?

P: Yes, yes.

A: Hum, yes.

P: Suddenly I have some help. I have somebody who is there. Because of my insecurity I didn't even know whether I was right or wrong. [Long pause]

A: Yes, I have to stop for today. We'll continue on Monday, the 25th.

P: Doctor, I hope you have a good time.

A: Thank you, I hope you do too. Good-bye.

P: Good-bye.

In Retrospect. [Dictated by the analyst immediately after the last session] It's difficult for me to summarize the main topics of this session, which was crammed full of information. At the end there was a sentimental separation. For my part, I too sense a particularly close relationship to the patient in response to efforts to find harmony. I think of the puppet theater, which always impressed me very much, Kleist's puppet theater, then of a mother who takes her child by the hand. In the last few minutes I made an interpretation to decrease the distance the patient referred to and to balance his feeling that was left all alone and being observed from outside. This feeling has to be seen in connection with the dream that was the center of interest in this session and that the patient mentioned toward the beginning. I have the impression that he encountered resistance to continuing where he wanted more from me. He said he would start too many different things, and I agree (because of resistance to passive, receptive, homosexual transference wishes?). Important is his concern that he will be rejected when he demands something impatiently, which is the reason that he forces himself to be patient. I think of his oral and other wishes to get as much as possible as quickly as possible, and then of his anxiety that he would not get enough because he's presumably been rejected frequently when he has raised such demands. I formulated his anxiety. The third topic was the break in treatment. And in reaction to my suggestion that he wanted to take as much as possible from the last session, he actually mentioned comments by his wife, asking what he is going to do when he can't go to the doctor any more. I confirmed the continuity by assuring him that he would not be turned away if he gets impatient.

5.2.2 Dream About the Crane

Erich Y opened the 85th session by telling me about a dream that apparently had made a special impression on him. He only interrupted his comments to make several short pauses.

In the dream a neighbor, whose relationship to the patient was not free of conflict and who talked a lot, was involved in putting a crane together. The patient immediately added that he did not want to disparage the neighbor, but he then had a slip of the tongue, referring to a struggle instead of a dream. In the dream Erich Y was an interested onlooker without any immediate function. An important part of the crane, the boom, was missing.

P: I was completely absorbed in the dream. What could the boom look like? How did it fit? I couldn't tear my thoughts away from this missing part - what kind of a structure was it? What was it like? It seemed to me as if it lasted the entire night. All my thoughts were concentrated on finding the crane's missing part. This morning I don't know what meaning it might have; I don't think it has any special meaning.

The patient did not have any associations. To stimulate the interpretive work I reminded him - thinking of the castration complex - that he had desparately looked for the missing part. The patient repeated that it had tortured him until morning: "What's missing, and why?" In the following description of his mood he mentioned a word that was a first reference to his memories of his traumatic experiences at the end of the war, which he mentioned later.

P: The bad part is that I was as absorbed as if I were involved, as if I were captive. I couldn't get out; there was no way around it. But as an engineer I ought to be able to solve the problem. I ought to have the ability to solve it.

In response to my questions about the missing part the patient described the exact form and function of the crane's boom. The boom, he said, was an important connecting piece, and without it the whole thing would not work. He was outraged by the indifference of the construction crew; at the same time it irritated him that he was upset even though he was only an onlooker. He got more and more involved while the crew responsible for it was indifferent.

Consideration. His affect is a clear sign that he was by no means only an onlooker but that he was very much involved, just like I was. His story reminded me of my own desparate searching for misplaced objects and of exaggerated anxieties about having lost something.

A: You are not merely an onlooker. You are obviously so affected by it because you might be missing something. That would make your intense attempt to use all your means to find the missing part comprehensible.

P: But then I'm not uninvolved.

Consideration. He had formed an ideal of being uninvolved. I therefore pointed to the connection between being affected and disquieted, on the one hand, and distancing as a reaction formation on the other.

Once again Erich Y emphasized how upseting it was not to get away from the narrow confines of this spot, with no chance of getting out of the way. After a short pause he mentioned that he sometimes felt good, but saying this did not help him any further.

He then surprised me by recalling childhood memories, of events when he was 3 or 4 years old. "Prisoners were driven through the village, first Russians by the Germans, then Germans by the Russians. He recalled feeling miserable and helpless. Memories of attacks by dive bombers entered his consciousness. Without being afraid, merely curious at first, the children had left their place of safety in a basement. When shots were fired, panic erupted, and farm animals broke lose and were wounded.

I picked out "injury" and "loss" as important themes, intentionally emphasizing at first his successful life-long effort to overcome the loss of all his belongings. This confirmation of his successful reacquisition of property would alleviate the trauma when he reexperienced it and would facilitate his efforts to cope with it.

The patient then described scenes in which he had felt fear, fear of the Russians and fear for his mother. He established a relationship to his later conflict in the triangle formed by his mother, his wife, and himself.

P: I can't make a decision in favor of my wife the way she wants. I can't swear at my mother; there simply is the fact that we belong together.

He told me that his wife's mother had died while his wife was a small child. Maybe that was the reason she expected him to belong entirely to her. He then complained about how he missed his father.

P: Why was he the one who had to die; if he had still been alive we would have had more security.

His grandfather graciously stepped in, and his values were a major factor that contributed to forming the patient's superego.

At my initiative we then considered what functions his father, who could have made the connection with the outer world easier, had for him. I stayed at the general significance of the loss and attempted to make his self-representation in the dream more accessible to him by describing the fact that "the crane towered over the region" as standing for his wish to compensate for the numerous deprivations he had had to endure while fleeing to the West together with his mother and brothers and sisters. These experiences of suffering were the subject of the rest of his associations. "We were treated like the plague." He traced his feeling of inferiority and his striving to make something of himself back to these humiliating experiences as a refugee.

The impression I had from his further associations strengthened my assumption that the defects in his body image had to be seen as derivatives of his castration complex.

I then made a summarizing interpretation, intentially employing a *dreamlike language of images* to revive his physical sensations.

A: You would like to hold your head up higher and move the crane and its boom around, high above everything else. But then along comes this despairing feeling of insecurity; all kinds of things are missing. It's not just the symptom as such that's obstructing you. You cannot show what you actually are. In such moments you recall all kinds of losses. What is visible are your injuries and the effects of injuries. And today you recalled threats and being shot at. When you stick your head out, then somebody lets you have it.

The patient then complained once more about his lack of security and that he always took two steps backwards after he had taken one forwards. He said that if he is attacked or simply even challenged in a discussion and doesn't react optimally, then he simply thinks he is a "loser."

The patient's reaction made it clear once again that the reference to traumatic events can only be a preliminary step to coping with them, which is the way to rediscover security.

From today's point of view I can note self-critically that in my enthusiasm for the psychodynamic connections I overlooked the situative damage caused by the overly talkative neighbor (the analyst) and in doing so possibly missed an opportunity to make transference interpretations starting from the here and now.

I prepared the following psychodynamic summary in order to demonstrate the reader the theoretical background that apparently somehow, has more or less consciously, influenced me. The patient's wishes to stick his head far out and be big and strong are defeated by his unconsciously precipitated anxiety of only being able to show himself as someone who is defect. His neurotic defects, such as the idea that his penis was too small, his chin too short, and his nose unsightly, were reinforced by his neurologic symptom of wryneck. A real defect was there for everyone to see. This was a vicious circle in which traumas from his distant past became linked with the way other people looked at him as a "cripple" and made him feel ashamed. The defect he had previously only imagined had become reality, first because a physical illness occurred, and second because the disturbance of his body image appeared realistic within the group of events described above.

I connected his castration complex with a deficit and a defective self-representation. This statement contains numerous intermediate inferences. There was no description of a human torso lacking a phallus, just of a crane without a boom. A metaphor was used that was based on the primacy of anthropomorphic perception and thought. Man-made machines were extensions of the patient's own body and were guided by him in his dreams as in animistic thought. The crane is a means serving the patient's self-representation, which we arrived at via the interpretative step of identification. Numerous questions had to be solved in this way. Why did the patient not portray himself as a human torso without a phallus? And when he used the crane, why did he not append an enormous boom to it instead of desparately searching for a missing part? At least at this point an omnipotent phallus wish did not manifest itself distinctly. He described a deficit and sought a substitute. In the dream the trauma seems to have really occurred; he sought help. I needed the hypothesis that the pain of separation from a vital and pleasurable body part was so excessive that the dreamer resorted to an indirect portrayal, one which was compatible with the possibility that he himself may still be "whole." In this way the patient gained some room to maneuvor so that he might still overcome and make good the feared trauma which had already appeared as an impressive defect. There was thus an analogy between dream representation and dysmorphophobia. I emphasize once more that the etiology of his wryneck is at a different level.

From this description we can deduce how it is possible to interrupt the circle of events therapeutically and thus to keep the situative precipitating factors (e.g., being stared at) from attaining any significance for the manifestation of such a disturbance of movement that is primarily neurologic in origin. The point is to transform the clinically well founded theory of situative precipitation and the connections described above into therapeutic steps.

5.2.3 Dream About Automobile Repairs

In the accompanying commentary I have included thoughts that ground my interpretations. My considerations are based on the feelings precipitated in me by the topics that were discussed.

The first part of the 153rd session was concerned with a fight the patient had had with his wife. He concluded this part of the session by deciding to find a constructive solution.

P: I tried to talk to her. "Tell me what's wrong. Let's talk about it." I can tell when she can talk about it in a way that makes her aggressions go away. I have to become more resolute toward myself and try not to always feel attacked, but try to see what she wants to shift off onto me because she thinks that I'm responsible for the fact that she has become the way she is.

The fact that he had become better able to respond to his wife was one positive result of his therapy.

After a pause the patient talked about a dream he found peculiar.

P: Last night I had another dream that was very peculiar. I was in a garage again because I was having problems with the car exhaust. It was broken. They were having difficulties because new ones didn't fit right. Then they started to make a new exhaust. The problem was the muffler, and more and more people got involved in making the muffler. At the end everybody at the garage was busy working on the exhaust. And suddenly it was finished. My car was ready, and I could hardly believe that so many people had been involved in helping me. Then I was supposed to pay for it, and I said of course I would.

Consideration. This dream made me assume that there was an anal source for his hypochondric disturbance of his body image.

The patient commented about the many helping hands.

P: While praying this morning I thought about it. I suddenly had the idea that it was my brethren who had given me so much when I couldn't find any help anywhere else. They still accepted me. And you were one of them too. The last time I wanted to say that the more I am freed of my troubles, the more devout I become, and find so much . . . so much security.

A: Yes, in the dream things are recreated; things that were broken become whole again.

Consideration. At first I was irritated by being included among the group of bigotted brethren with whom he was linked in a sect. Then I felt that the patient apparently needed this harmony and had to include me to reinforce his feeling of security. I was enthusiastic about his dream and its anal symbolism. It was the first dream on such a topic in the entire analysis. I thought about the fact that some extrapyramidal disturbances are accompanied by coprolalia. Such patients have the compulsion to say obscene words, especially those related to feces.

I referred to his self-representation in the dream and to the latent anal significance that I assumed the dream to have, and specifically mentioned anal references – letting air, fizzling, having fun, giving gas, and stinking. I also mentioned the words "fart" and "shit," and used the word "pot" literally. I assumed that he would reject this anal aspect and that his longing to be loved, even as a stinker, was large.

P: Funny, but I just had the thought that there was also a single woman in the garage. I was a bachelor and was immediately fascinated by her. This doesn't go together at all with the exhaust.

Consideration. This addition was presumably triggered by my interpretation of his longing to be loved anyway. The woman did not fit into the anal world of men and boys.

The patient made longer statements about sexual games he had played in childhood, which provided some new details.

A: You feel secure when you pray together with your brethren. Then you're not a bad guy or a stinker or a fart.

P: I have a different attitude toward sexual things, but my wife still condemns me when I massage her, pet her on her buttocks, her breasts, and her genitals.

A: What I said about exhaust, bowel movement, and stinking seems to be foreign to you; I have the impression that you weren't convinced.

P: Not entirely.

Consideration. My forced attempts to make interpretations went too far. The patient did not respond to them. I therefore attempted to build a bridge for him by returning to it again and doubting my own assertiveness. Although I was sure of my assumption about the unconscious meaning, I had doubts about the timing of my intensive allusions. I therefore attempted to remind the patient of observations he had made at home on the farm. The patient responded by remembering many details.

P: And there was a village bull, and the cows were led to him to be covered. And now I recall something, an experience, while I was an apprentice. A journeyman asked me to undress and to play around with my genitals on his behind.

I was surprised that this forgotten experience, which was very explicit thematically, became conscious again. The patient did not clarify how far the seduction went, and I did not want to be intrusive. The patient talked about this experience until the end of the session, and about his fears about getting caught and punished, about his subordinating himself to somebody else, about his fear that something might be damaged, and also about his pleasure and curiosity.

5.2.4 Dream About an Agent

Before relating the following dream in the 216th session, Erich Y said that it was "typical," meaning that it fit well into the framework of his problems.

P: They were looking for an agent, and I was their suspect. To avoid being discovered, I had to move around as if I were a cripple.

The patient continued and enriched this simple description of his dream. He was being followed by someone hot on his heals, followed wherever he went, whether on trips, at the train station, or to the toilette.

P: I had to use force on myself, because I couldn't stretch out or stand up straight in order not to be recognized and discovered.

It remained unclear why he was being followed in the dream and what he was accused of having done. He was simply being sought as an agent, and hiding was at the focus of his experiencing.

His vivid description of his hunched posture and the way he anxiously avoided stretching himself, because he would have been recognized and taken into custody, led me to allude to the way in which he choked off his gestures. I pointed out that many of his actions were linked with feelings of guilt. As an agent, he did things secretly and in a concealed manner.

By referring to the ambiguity he attributed to my role, I cautiously prepared the way for a transference interpretation: For his conscious experiencing I was the one who offered him help; unconsciously, however, he was afraid of what might be discovered and come to light.

A: That is something that always worries you. How can you keep your aggressive fantasies and fantasies about being an agent a secret? How can you hide them? You're not supposed to get mad or let anyone know who you really are.

P: That's right. There are a lot of things I have to keep in mind just so that I don't give them a reason to suspect me.

A: So you stay hunched over where it's not at all necessary, like here with me.

Commentary. Since the patient knew that the analyst was neither a policeman, secret agent, nor state's attorney, readers may be amazed that the analyst acted so cautiously. It was nevertheless clarifying to refer to discordant ambiguities by name. Many analysts do not bother to do so because they assume that such simple clarifications of what the patient very well knows are superfluous or can be made when the situation demands. We believe that the reference to the double function in this specific transference interpretation is reassuring, but that in precisely this way it is possible to unravel the entire extent of the unconscious secret actions.

I concluded my interpretation by suggesting that the patient put himself into his favorite roles when watching movies about detectives and agents, in order to learn more about himself.

The patient then looked for the reasons that he "increasingly adopted the bent over and hunched posture to keep from being recognized." He accused himself of being a coward, and out of the blue he suddenly said: "Becoming a father isn't hard, being one is." We were both surprised by this sudden thought, and without beating around the bush I referred to the patient's association in an interpretation: "You can become a father fast if you don't hide your tail between your legs. You alway had to hide your tail so that nothing would happen."

The patient responded to the metaphoric nature of this colloquial manner of speaking and mentioned numerous examples. He was still afraid I would throw him out if he succumbed to his aggressive fantasies. He described himself as a captive bird that would like to escape or, having learned to fly, left the nest only to immediately succumb to his anxieties about being punished and causing damage. "Yes, they took my wings away from me."

I now made an interpretation offering several possible reasons for this behavior, which the patient had previously helplessly sought. To indicate the spectrum of reasons and open the perspective as wide as possible, I spoke in general about his desire to be active. I described hands - agent's hands - that were not permitted to reach here and there. The dialogue also contained the direct statement: "You are an agent. You see a lot more, even here in my office, when you look around. But even then you think you're doing something illicit."

Encouraged by my direct allusion, the patient then made the helpful discovery that he himself bound his wings, although he had previously always assumed that others had imposed this restriction on him.

Consideration. This discovery cannot change the fact that - in accordance with Freud's theory of anxiety - Erich Y had been exposed to real dangers and had not escaped them unscathed. Yet what remained was the therapeutically important question as to why the patient still behaved like a coward and ducked his head.

P: I keep myself in this position. I tie my wings.

A: Your fear of punishment is revived over and over; you're afraid that even more will be clipped off if you don't tie yourself down.

P: Hum.

A: How was it in the other dream when you underwent an operation?

P: Yes, hum, on my head; my brain was cut open.

A: You protect yourself in the dream to keep even more from happening, to avoid even more injuries.

P: Yes, the peculiar thing is that I let my body and everything available to me, that I let myself be pushed so far that I walk around crooked and like a cripple, that I don't fight against it. Why?

The subject at the end of the session was the relationship between persecutor and persecuted. The patient turned to these ideas by listing what it would be like if he were to turn the tables and pay back all the humiliation and shame he had suffered. This reversal appeared in drastic form in the following dream about an amputation.

5.2.5 *Dream About an Amputation*

In the last third of the 223rd session Erich Y happened to mention a very drastic dream. In a certain context the word "foot" had reminded him of having had a very gruesome dream.

The dream was preceded by a subject that was on the patient's mind a lot and that was active as a day residue. He was worried about the future willingness of his insurance company to pay for his treatment, and he therefore wanted to reduce the frequency of the sessions. The patient paid a small portion of the expenses himself, about DM10 per session. Since he was a voluntary member of a public insurance fund, he was treated as a private patient. This precipitating factor, i. e., his concern, has to be mentioned at the beginning because the patient was strongly affected by it, showing again that minor causes can have large effects. Unconsciously he experienced this fee to be a significant loss of bodily substance.

At first we discussed the matters of financing treatment, saving, and stinginess. He and his wife had differences because of their differing attitudes to money. Erich Y was extremely upset by minor debts he had after buying a house. After considering the rational and irrational sides of this issue for a long time the word "foot" happened to be mentioned and it reminded him of a dream.

P: I want to be free, on my own feet again. The word "foot" reminds me of a gruesome dream I had last night. I was here, with you and you were limping. After you had sat down, I asked "What's wrong?" "It's my other foot, they've amputated my other leg." "What do you mean, your other foot?" "Well, one of my legs is already made of wood, and now I've lost the other one, too." I just couldn't believe it at all. I hadn't even noticed that you already had a wooden leg, and now the other one. You were pretty composed. I just couldn't get over it. It's very peculiar which mental combinations take place and appear in a dream.

A: Yes, you would like me to stay in one piece and not get injured, and be sure that nothing happens to me. That means that you have to pay attention here and be careful not to offend me. Well, in the last session we talked about persecution and being a victim, injure versus attack.

The associations and interpretations proceeded from the day residue. The patient had viewed my request that he personally contribute to the fee as a threat to his bodily existence. He was amazed and even shocked by the highly emotional consequences that my expectation provoked.

I focussed my interpretations on the fact that the patient attempted to secure his peace and harmony through subordination and that he at the same time felt he was the victim. By stingily holding on to and keeping what he owned, he had established a balance and overcome the damages he had suffered.

A: My request is an intrusion on your substance. Eye for an eye, tooth for a tooth. As you do to me, so I do to you.

P: I can really imagine that if I had to pay all the expenses for these sessions here, then so much pressure would develop that I could progress as much as possible and as quickly as possible in order to get out of here again and to get some relief.

Commentary. The patient's unconscious wishes and expectations would have found some other plausible linkage to a realistic perception if the question of the patient contributing to the fee - a slight increase in the total fee from about DM 80 to DM 90 per session, which was of course also a welcome increase to the analyst - had not arisen. Asking the patient to contribute was not a means the analyst had intentionally introduced to guide transference in a particular direction. It is not necessary to artificially create plausible and realistic perceptions that can turn out to be offensive. The utility of the small private fee in this case is demonstrated by the patient's further thoughts.

A: Yes, you'll be under so much pressure and it would be easier for you to be angry, because I would be the one who's reaching deep into your wallet and taking the leg your're standing on. If you had to pay everything yourself, that would really be a tremendous burden. And you feel it when it's only 10 marks. Of course, you can always minimize its significance, that it isn't so bad after all even though you experience it to be very bad now. The dream shows it, too. My request is an attack on you. An eye for an eye, tooth for a tooth. It's fortunate that you remembered it and that you were able to dream about it at all, and that you told me about it. You suddenly thought about the dream.

P: Hum, yes, I thought of the dream a couple of times over the weekend. And I asked myself, "Why?"

Commentary. As a matter of principle, and not only because of the disturbing strength of the unconscious dynamics, it is advisable to focus interpretations on the issue of security and to begin from the longing for wholeness, the reaction formations, and the efforts to overcome deficits. The analyst followed this rule in this treatment. He proceeded from the assumption that the patient would like him to remain uninjured and had the wish that nothing should happen to the analyst and that any injuries be overcome. Otherwise he himself, a cripple, would not have a chance either.

This transference dream provides an insight into the genesis of defects in body image because in it the injury was translated back into the context of its interactional genesis.

This topic was continued in the decapitation dream described below.

5.2.6 Decapitation Dream

Erich Y opened the 230th session by mentioning the worsening of his symptoms in connection with a family quarrel. According to my impression, the patient occasionally reacted to his wife's pedantic behavior by trying to do everything right - which was of course beyond his ability. In view of these marital problems I was also helpless because his wife's behavior influenced his psychic life by reinforcing his superego. Yet she had refused to attend counseling herself, although she also accused the patient of being the only one who had the opportunity of speaking his mind and finding some relief.

After a short pause the mood changed and the patient, now dismayed, told me about the "gruesome dream" he had had last night.

P: We were in a small company that I wasn't familiar with. Two men were quarreling, but then it got serious and turned into a fight. One man tore the other's head off and threw it around, and the man whose head was torn off was suddenly gone. Although I had been there, I asked where he had gone. He was gone, they had gotten rid of him, without a trace, just like with a girl who had also been missing for some time. She disappeared just the same way. Not that she had lost her head, but she was simply gone. [Short pause] Peculiar, such a gruesome dream.

A: Yes, it's a sequel to your dream about my missing leg. The intensity of the fight, the fighting, the struggling to have your way is clearer now.

Consideration. This was meant to emphasize the continuity of the castration theme in transference.

P: In the dream I helped to destroy all the signs of the fight, to make an investigation impossible. There was an oven and what do I know what else, and the contents were destroyed and removed, so that nobody would could find anything, even though I had only been an onlooker of what happened. [Long pause]

A: You always had to appease people or conceal and hide things, hide yourself, and not be aggressive or competitive or fight a duel to the bitter end. Partly because you were afraid. Then you were the loser, the little boy, the refugee, who had to hide his tail, who watched two men fighting for their lives. Although you were just an onlooker in the dream, you participated actively in covering things up.

Consideration. I viewed the fatal and gruesome duel both as a symbol of transference and as multiple self-representations of the patient, who - as a result of working through the consequences of earlier duels at the unconscious level - thought that he was the one walking around with a deformed head. Yet he had also distanced himself, or split himself off, if you will, so that he was only an innocent bystander. The defensive aspect of the dream was most important to me at first.

P: But it was so gruesome.

A: It was no coincidence that a head was involved. A head is involved in a lot of things. Your idea of being small is partly a result of thinking that something is missing there, although it's obvious that nothing was ever missing. But at the level of images, fantasies, and the unconscious, wishes are transformed into actions, for example when people say that someone is risking their neck.

P: Hum.

A: Hum. You also asked yourself why you pictured me as being injured.

Consideration. I established a connection to the dream in which the patient had visualized me as having an amputated leg, and drew his attention to the fact that there had been a change. At the dream level he was now also a culprit, no longer just a victim. This change from passive suffering to active participation is important not only for general therapeutic reasons. I repeatedly had the idea that action potentials could assert themselves in the automatized sequnce of movements in the way Lorenz described vacuum activities (Lorenz and Leyhausen 1968).

P: Hum.

A: For a long time you portrayed yourself as being the one who was injured, as the victim.

P: Hum.

A: Because you are very afraid of yourself, you were the victim, not the culprit. And otherwise you also try to cover up all your tracks, so that nobody notices anything and nobody knows that are involved in this and that. Just like everyone else, you are a person who competes, who is involved in violent disputes and rivalries, even in murder and manslaughter, no, not in reality, you have such impulses at the fantasy level.

By making the generalization that the patient is human just like everyone else, I attempted to weaken his anxiety about fatal aggressive actions so far that he could give more room to these unconscious aspects. For the same reason, I emphasized the fantasy level, after I had gone a little too far by using the words "murder" and "manslaughter," which had shocked the patient. While reading the transcript I thought about how the patient had had reservations that I could somehow use his thoughts, possibly not in his best interest.

P: This sensitivity, that's it. Yesterday at work. Right now there's a man in the office who's supposed to make a carreer for himself in a subsidiary. He's collecting information from us and being trained, and he came to me and asked me about this and that. I gave him the information, documentation, and a copy of the monthly report so that he knows what to report to the management. Afterwards a colleague said that he's being supplied and armed with the best materials. He meant that we shouldn't help the new man to get off to such a good start.

Consideration. There was another, insincere side to the patient's extreme willingness to help. Rivalry and competition entered into it at the level of the day residue, as competition between ideas. As the following associations demonstrated, the patient had had a good idea that someone else had snatched away. The issue is that something that originated in his head was taken away from him.

The patient had had a very good idea to significantly improve the routine at work. In embittered silence he had accepted the fact that his department head had taken credit for it and acted as if it had been his idea.

P: It hurt me very much, but I accepted it.

A: See, he took what was in your head. He took your head away, in the language of the dream. There is a little rivalry in the situation. You hid your tail, well . . . .

My interpretation corresponded to my theoretical reflections. The day residue is a minor cause with a large effect.

P: Hum.

A: You can see that the others are fairly envious or don't try to control their envy.

P: But when I put myself in the limelight [the patient sighed], I feel as if I'm showing off.

A: Yes.

P: It still hurts. I actually ought to be satisfied that I had the idea and that it was successful. Yes, alright, there would be advantages if the boss at the top knew that everything was my idea or somebody else's.

A: You see how much rivalry is involved. You have your duels. When you touch your head, then apparently the duel you are fighting in your head becomes one between your head and your hand.

In this interpretation I attempted to focus on the internalization of a duel. Erich Y was always dismayed at how he used his hand to struggle against the involuntary twisting of his neck. The angrier he got and the more force his hand applied, the stronger the counterforces twisting his head to the right. His observations were noteworthy. In addition to the duel described above, other types of contact such as shaving or touching his cheek caused his head to turn. My interpretation was based on the assumption that at, the unconscious level of this symptom there was an internal duel, and in my interpretations I attempted to shift the conflict back to the level of interpersonal relationship, including the *transference*.

A: Your hand is your own. It belongs to you just like your head, but when you touch yourself, touch your head, then your hand apparently turns into a foreign object . . . .

P: Hum, hum.

A: . . . into something attacking you.

P: Hum. [Long pause]

A: When I ask for money, even if it's a small sum, it seems like a substantial amount. As if it cost a piece of yourself. It unconsciously touches on an immense feeling of losing something, triggering rage, which in turn leads you to chop off my leg.

It was important for me to refer to this conflict in transference at a level that was concrete for the patient. That is where the affects reside.

P: That this feeling, this tension as it's expressed in the dream, is so immense, in other words, right to the end, like in the dream, head off....

A: Yes, yes. [Long pause]

P: ... as if there weren't any alternatives.

A: Hum. Yes, it's not for nothing that there are headhunters.

P: Hum.

A: Besides, a head is something magical. Having a head means having strength. Just like cutting off genitals and drawing strength from them; it's at the same level. [Long pause] Cannibals consume human flesh to incorporate their foe's strength in themselves.

In these interpretations I attempted to revive the magical components at different levels, in order to make the patient more receptive for his own unconscious motives. I immediately had the feeling that I had gone too far, and therefore in my next comments returned to the level of symptoms and the associated envy for the healthy heads of the people around him.

P: Hum.

A: A lot of things are precipitated by your complaints. "If I could only have another head, if I could only have his head." And now personally, "You could have my head." Remember, I copied the circuitry in your head, stealing your ideas just like your supervisor did.

Consideration. I recalled one of the patient's earlier dreams, which I referred to now to make it even clearer to him why he attempted in his dream language to get my head, too, and to appropriate the substance of my ideas.

P: Yeh, yeh, yes, yeh, yeh. But those are ideas - stone age, that's how far back they go.

The patient had become extremely animated. While showing his confirmation by repeating the yeses, his voice was full of enthusiasm, which was followed by the slight restriction about the primitiveness of his thoughts.

A: Yes, they are in each of us.

P: Of course everyone carries them around in their unconscious, like in a backpack, but that I can't control them, and when I control them, then there are these repressions. But this desire to possess and this force, that can't come to the surface, it can't be done. If everyone were to act according to this principle, then there would only be murder and manslaughter. [Long pause] Now I'm thinking about human relations and about complaints. Sometimes you notice how the customer tries to find out what's really happened. The way I see it, he doesn't have control of himself, overshoots his goals, and things are no longer in proper perspective. People who act this way, even in daily life, are repulsive.

Consideration. It was logical that the patient tried to direct the intensity of the competition and rivalry into reasonably acceptable forms, as all the other day residues indicate. It was important to me to further clarify the transference components, specifically in connection with his personal contribution of DM10 to my fee, which he experienced to be a loss of substance.

P: There are definitely capabilities, possibilities, and thoughts that can be awakened without becoming brutal. Yes, what good is it for me when I tell my colleague, "Do you think it was right to take my idea like that?" What good is it for me now? He knows that it wasn't right. I ought to have enough control of myself that I don't have to give him a piece of my mind to be satisfied. Hum. Yes, naturally, I would also like to do good compared to the others.

The rest of the session was concerned with this topic and competition.

P: Naturally it's an important point, feeling hurt, the feeling you've been passed by. As you say, something is taken away from me, and it means I get shorter, am constrained, yet to me that's a petty way of thinking.

A: Yes, I think it only looks that way. It's not petty, because of the immense consequences we experience. It's really almost the opposite of petty, something important, because the consequences that we experience are immense and because it conceals how much it affects you. Yet you experience it as something petty because consciously it really isn't so terrible.

P: Hum.

A: On the one hand it's a ridiculous event, yet on the other it's an enormous experience.

P: Yes, emotionally.

A: When I take DM10 from you, then I'm attacking your substance, to be or not to be.

P: Yes.

A: Or when I have your circuits in my head, then you want to have my head and wear it prominently, not hunched over like the agent. You would like to get into my head, yes, to have everything that's inside, what do I know. Then you would have everything yourself. It's human. Then you would be free and . . . .

P: Hum.

A: . . . and would be strong and potent and whatever else you attribute to my head. As if I had a superbrain or were a bigshot.

P: Hum.

A: The bigshots are the ones who have lots, lots of money, who are rich, and have the power, the powerful fathers, like the one you especially longed for after losing your own so early and being on the run and abandoning house and home.[Pause]

P: Maybe I'm deceiving myself when I think that the other person, the big shot who has everything under control, can immediately tell that I want to use it.

A: Hum. But covering up isn't the best solution either, is it? We have to stop now.

The patient said good-bye, also wishing me a nice weekend, and I did the same.

Commentary. The way in which sessions are ended and which words are used to announce the end is more than incidental. Both participants are subject to time, even if in different ways. The "we" form emphasizes the shared element, which analysts should not routinely suggest because the patient is only entitled to 45 or 50 minutes. It is the analyst who must end the session if he is to adhere to his schedule. To remind the patient of this, we recommend that the analyst use the "I" form in announcing the end, switching to the "we" form when the mood makes it seem advisable.

5.3 Dream About the Symptom

It is not unusual for symptoms to appear in dreams. According to wish theory, it should even be a frequent occurrence that individuals overcome their symptoms in their dreams and portray themselves as being healthy. In the following dream, described in the 268th session, Erich Y suffered from wryneck. This fact would not deserve special comment except for the context that the patient and I gave the event. The patient's associations and my interpretations show that the twisting of his head in his dream represented searching movements that could be analogous to those of an infant at its mother's breast.

Erich Y said that in the dream he was wandering around aimlessly and anxiously. The company he worked for was spread over a large grounds. The canteen was separate, with the plant set back in the countryside.

P: I had the feeling I was small and lost. Then I met a secretary and an assistant, who were talking. It seemed to me that I was standing off to the side. Then we walked some distance and my head turned to the side. I couldn't get it under control; no matter how much force I used, I couldn't do anything. My head twisted to one side just the moment it was important to be in the middle.

Consideration. The patient's feeling in the dream of being lost and his great insecurity made me think of childhood situations in which helplessness and lack of motor coordination are especially conspicuous.

A: Yes, and what can you recall about your mood in the dream? Could it be that you portrayed something in the dream? Out in the big wide world you're very exposed. The patient expressly denied that he felt observed, and then continued:

P: I wasn't feeling well. I was standing all by myself and didn't have contact to anyone. The company directors were discussing something. I felt left out. For me it was like being in a different world, something .... [Long pause] It has something to do with "child," but I can't really say, it's so far away.

A: In a large room, at their mercy and exposed to everyone, without support and without a hand to hold on to.

P: Yes, I was superfluous, maybe because I walked along without saying a word, or that I didn't have contact because of my appearance or reserved behavior. Maybe I wanted to go along and take part, but that wasn't at all possible because of my attitude and behavior. People can somehow tell that I cannot let others get close to me, even though I would sometimes like them to. It's very funny that I have to think of a woman's breast now.

A: How? Think of it right now?

P: In my thoughts, like a child looking for its mother's breast, to gain strength – not at all ironically.

A: Yes, yes. You were worried that I would react *ironically.*

P: But I didn't have any sexual feelings.

Consideration. The idea of deducing the patient's searching and rediscovery of the primary object from sexual desire in a narrow sense was so distant to me that I could not take the patient's concern personally that his pregenital sensuality might provoke ironic ridicule from me. For a long time I had been aware of not blurring the qualitative differences of pleasure within the libido theory.

A: Yes, as if I would only think that you are following sexual desire, and not another one. Even children turn their heads.

P: At the moment I can't get it out of my mind.

A: Yes, but why should you get it out of your mind or turn away from it? That's what you mean, isn't it?

P: Hum.

A: Just while you're in the process of looking for it in the dream, in the large room.

P: It's the anxiety again about turning to the breast and taking something from it, because someone else might misinterpret it, think that I am doing something wrong, always when I'm expressing my feelings – the inhibitions – the others. [Pause] In my imagination it's always the same, just like in this dream. The secretary and the assistant seemed so large to me because I magnify them.

A: Yes, but, just like the breast also somehow probably seems very large, in comparison to a mouth. The mouth grasping for it, or the eye when it's close to the breast, then the breast is very large. If only a part is visible, then it seems very large.

P: And then I have the feeling as if I have many more sensations toward my mother than I want to believe and than I show, and that I was always looking for love and affection even as a child, but that even as a child I was very reserved and didn't say anything about my feelings. And then at times I act a little like a child to my wife when we snuggle, when I embrace her, hold her, and touch her, she says, "Hey, what's going on. This isn't normal, you're exaggerating so." And there's a parallel to now; it's always been this way. I sought it in love too. Love, love, affection.

Erich Y was referring in this passage to a comprehensive sense of love, and mentally protected himself against his wife, who misinterpreted his gentle sensuous feelings because their ultimate goal was sexual in nature and complained even after "harmless" contacts. In this way she extinguished his independent searching for nearness and tenderness from the very beginning. The relationship between tenderness and sexuality in the each of the sexes frequently leads to serious misunderstandings in relationships between men and women. Thus it is no coincidence that Freud developed two theories of tenderness, which Balint (1935) in particular studied extensively.

5.4 Thoughts About Psychogenesis

The restrictions on Erich Y's self-feeling that resulted from his imagined physical defects were at the focus of therapy from the very beginning. As early as in the fifth session the patient had described a dream in which he had been injured in a traffic accident. In the 35th session, in the context of controlling movements and actions, he discussed the puppet theme for the first time, and later it appeared in numerous variations. Defects were a frequent part of the patient's self-representations, both in the dialogue between him and the psychoanalyst as well as in his dreams. The dreams we have selected mark points at which themes come to a climax that exhibit a tendency of a shift in the objects chosen for his self-representation, from inanimate objects to persons. This shift was no simple linear progression. The questions as to which modifications can be demonstrated by studying a series of dreams and which diagnostic and prognostic conclusions can be drawn from the initial dream have been discussed in earlier publications by close associates (Geist and Kächele 1979; Schultz 1973). Here we employ a dream series to demonstrate problems that have been worked through since we consider the treatment process to be an ongoing form of focal therapy with a changing focus (see Vol.1, Chap. 9). We have tried to center attention on self-defects in dreams and consequently have neglected the other dimensions of the therapeutic process that are relevant for a synopsis.

We believe that consideration of this dream series contributed substantially to clarifying the genesis of the dysmorphophobia. This symptom is at the same level as the dream if we assume that the compromises are similar in structure. According to the psychoanalytic psychopathology of the conflict, the symptom and the dream are linked together by the idea of compromises between the repressing and repressed forces and ideas (Freud 1896b, p. 170). We apply the idea of compromise to the genesis of symptoms just as much as to dream interpretation and the entirety of items produced by the unconscious. Freud emphasized

> that neurotic symptoms are the outcome of a conflict.... The two forces which have fallen out meet once again in the symptom and are reconciled, as it were, by the compromise of the symptom that has been constructed. It is for that reason, too, that the symptom is so resistant: it is supported from both sides. (Freud 1916/17, pp. 358-359)

Yet what is the case with Erich Y's *wryneck*? According to the distinctions made in the initial diagnosis, it was a neurologic illness that was precipitated by psychic conflicts and whose course was codetermined by them. In the therapeutic interviews the differences between the purely *neurotic* symptoms of dysmorphophobia and the *physiological nature* of neck twisting were occasionally blurred. The neurologic disturbance of movement was placed in the context of expressive and emotional movement in the dream about the agent and in the patient's image of the movement as the search for the mother's breast. One consequence of the fact that human experiencing is *holistic* is that patients often do not distinguish between whether the source of their physical limitations is psychic or physical. An analyst's task in this regard is complex, including examining the reasons for a patient's ideas about his illness. A patient's explanations for his physical ailments, which he often experiences, for example, to be a form of punishment, are an important aspect. Even a scientifically incorrect subjective theory of the genesis of an illness is a part of how an individual copes with his illness. A patient's observations and conjectures about his illness often constitute an access to psychic factors that may have been involved in its genesis and course. The analyst has the task of making diagnostic distinctions and clarifying the respective roles that the physical and psychic components played in the origin and development of the illness. On the other hand, it is important for the analyst to take the patient's personal theory of his illness seriously because the two parties otherwise talk at different wavelengths.

Erich Y's condition was strongly dependent on whether he could stand up straight or whether, because of his social and superego anxieties, he had to sneak around like a cowering coward to keep from being recognized or - as in the dream about the agent - being caught. The conspicuous twisting movement of his neck, which was beyond his conscious control, increased his feeling of insecurity, creating a typical vicious circle in which the physical ailment reinforces the psychic disturbance and vice versa. Erich Y's neurotic ideas about his disfigured head and other constrictions that Reich might have referred to as character armor (see Chap. 4) had for decades even made him incapable of moving around freely and without inhibitions. Conflict had characterized much of his marriage and was one reason that his self-security was very weak. Important in this connection is the existential significance of upright posture and standing straight for an individual's self-feeling and self-confidence, because the ability to stand up and stay erect belongs to man's fundamental experiences and has been the source of a wealth of metaphors. In the last few decades systematic studies of the development of infants' ability to walk upright (Mahler et al. 1975; Amsterdam and Levitt 1980) have supplemented earlier phenomenological and psychoanalytic studies (Freud 1930a; Erikson 1950; Straus 1952). It seems obvious that a physical disturbance that appears to the subject to be an incapacity to control or coordinate movements revives latent insecurities rooted deep in his past. In this particular case a very large role was played by the conditions under which the patient's loss of autonomy was accompanied by a feeling of shame and his self-confidence was transformed into bashfulness, and by the way in which this change could be reversed. Neurotic symptoms of this kind are conducive to change.

Erich Y experienced his physical symptom (his wryneck) to be related to guilt, anxiety, and shame. The analyst pursued the patient's personal theories in order to eliminate secondary neurotizations. It was plausible to assume that freeing the patient from his neurotic suffering could also have an affect on his physical symptom because it would reduce his anxious expectations and the accompanying increases in both general and specific excitatory potential.

Since we have discussed the general principles of examining hypotheses in therapy research in Chap. 1, we will limit ourselves here to considering the analogy between the searching movement for the maternal breast and the (pathological) twisting of the patient's head. We recall that one of Erich Y's associations to one of his dreams was about a woman's breast, which turned into that of a nursing mother. In transference the patient feared being rejected, and consequently tried to find reassurance by emphasizing that he had not sought anything sexual. The momentary cause for his anxiety that the analyst too might misunderstand his longing for nearness and tenderness was the fact that his wife had frequently rejected him. This scene was definitely very important therapeutically. Yet what does this mean for the suggested analogy between the searching movement and the pathological twisting? Is it possible that the torticollis, i. e., the twisting of his head, was an expression of an unconscious reflex of searching for the oral object?

These issues are related to the question as to the degree that psychogenic factors were involved in the development of this patient's illness. Knowledge of the course of this treatment supports the view we presented in the introduction, namely that psychic factors contribute to the manifestation and exacerbation of a symptom. Of interest here is whether the observations made in this individual case throw some light on how the psychic precipitants and psychogenic conditions functioned as contributory causes as Freud suggested with his term "complemental series."

To help readers keep their orientation, we will reveal the outcome of the following discussion by weighting the various factors in the complemental series according to the theory that we adhere to, namely the nonspecific nature of the pathogenesis of psychosomatic illnesses. Physical disposition in the most general sense of the term determines which illness occurs. The individual symptoms thus follow biologically given patterns that are rooted in the patient's physical constitution, as described by Freud's notion of complemental series, and that are referred to as "organ vulnerability" in Alexander's schema (see Sect. 9.7). Incidental items that can be found in the different psychological dimensions are factors contributing to the modification of physical reactions. With regard to the speculations raised below, right at the outset we can pose the critical question of why an early disturbance presumed to constitute the psychic prerequisite of an illness does not become manifest until so late in life.

Melitta Mitscherlich (1983) applied this general assumption of an early disturbance to the genesis of wryneck. In earlier studies she had described, in spite of the problems that had become manifest during Abraham's (1921) and Ferenczi's (1921) discussion of tics, torticollis as being (preoedipal) conversion hysteria, and in her 1983 study she argued that torticollis represents a *preverbal symbol*. According to her, such patients regress so deeply that they become incapable of using linguistic symbols to express their affects. In such a condition of deep regression such patients resort back to motor forms of expression whose counterparts are in the infant's pre-ego stage, because no other means of expression are available. The motor patterns used in such cases correspond, according to her, to rooting, the infant's schema for controlling sucking and touching movements that Spitz described. Starting from Ferenczi's (1913) omnipotence of gestures, M. Mitscherlich spoke of the magic belief of the torticollis patient in the "omnipotence of movement." Motor activity itself contains the profound ambivalence of turning toward, as by a hungry infant, and of turning away, as by an infant whose hunger has been satisfied.

An infant's rooting and the analogous searching movements in a regressive state are one thing, and the extrapyramidal head movement in wryneck is another. We have to emphasize that the twisting in torticollis must be considered in light of the results of neurophysiological studies, and cannot be considered to parallel any natural schema of infantile motor movement. The muscle activities or hyperkinesia demonstrated on an electromyogram can be interpreted neurologically as disintegration taking place within the extrapyramidal programs of motion schema, which leads to a false activation of the relevant muscles by the central nervous system. The coinnervation of the antagonistic muscles that are already tensed in the relaxed state which occurs in voluntary turning of the head is, according to Fasshauer (1983, p. 538), "another argument, in addition to already very substantial complexity of this movement anomaly, against a psychogenic cause of spasmodic torticollis." In other words, the anomolous movement in torticollis is not an isolated psychogenic symptom in the sense of a regressively deformed searching movement. In order to prove such a theory it would be necessary to test and verify many hypotheses, for example which cognitive affective processes in the adult precipitate infantile searching movements and, more importantly, how these searching movements can be transformed into the motion in torticollis through regression. The concept "presymbol" is no more a substitute for plausible hypotheses and their examination than the assumption of a preoedipal conversion. The concept "presymbol" contains, just like all other speculation about the alleged early genesis of physical ailments, highly speculative assumptions about splitting processes. In order not to be misunderstood, we would like to expressly emphasize that Freud and Breuer's discovery of the consequences of inhibited affects and the significance of abreactions and catharsis in therapy belong to the fundamentals of clinical psychoanalysis. Yet if this twisting movement were based on a splitting off of circumscribed instinctual or affective oral object relations, then it would have to be possible to discover them in the cathartic primal scream or in some physical therapy, and no such discovery has been made. It also cannot be expected that an abreaction can be therapeutically effective in cases of torticollis or of similar physical ailments because these symptoms do not originate from a split off quantity of affect.

Although these critical comments about the psychogenesis of somatic illnesses and of torticollis in particular limit the range of psychoanalytic therapy, they also give it a solid scientific foundation. Proceeding from those factors that maintain a set of symptoms, one encounters the typical basic anxieties that are precipitated and reinforced by the illness and occur in a form corresponding to the patient's personal psychodynamics. The result is a group of special targets for the therapeutic technique. In accordance with the Ulm process model outlined in Vol.1 (Sect. 9.4), we have described several issues from the psychoanalysis of Erich Y as thematic foci. In the theory of the genesis of psychosomatic illnesses that we have adhered to for many years, these foci are in a nonspecific relationship with the torticollis. We thus share Bräutigam and Christian's view "that in most psychosomatic illnesses *the formative elements, i. e., those that are specific to the illness* are already present in the *physical disposition*" (1986, p. 21). Our experience also indicates that the manifestation and course of the illness depend on both psychic and social factors.

The variety and diversity of psychic problems mean that it is in principle improbable that specific correlations of wryneck – or of other somatic illnesses – with specific conflicts can be found. Nonetheless, the impression of many doctors that, for example, patients with wryneck somehow differ from others is probably not only based on an uncritical generalization of individual observations. The observed or presumed similarities result from the fact that the same illness provokes similar psychosocial problems, which in turn influence the further course of the illness and reactivate typical anxieties and feelings of insecurity. This is also the basis of the approach that psychoanalysis can follow to favorably influence the course of the illness as well as to reduce subjective suffering. Thus it would be a mistake to conclude from the nonspecificity of the pathogenesis that psychic factors play a minor role in the manifestation and course of the illness. If the analyst makes his psychodynamic diagnosis from the perspective of therapy, i. e., by determining thematic foci, then he and the patient will proceed in a manner that makes it possible to achieve changes. Conducting a group comparison is something else. The question of the typology to which an individual case is assigned depends on the perspective of the person conducting the examination. Because of the lack of prospective studies and of knowledge about the consequences of the illness on the patient's subjective condition, it is impossible to generalize from the results we have collected. The fact, which is beyond all doubt, that a *secondary neurotization* frequently or regularly takes place must be considered especially important and, in our opinion, sufficient for a psychoanalytic therapy to be indicated.

It is especially burdensome for patients who are already neurotic to experience their helplessness toward a socially conspicuous chronic illness. Existing social and superego anxieties frequently reinforce each other when there are conspicuous physical symptoms, leading patients into isolation in order to avoid being exposed to the humiliating glances of others. The resulting insecurity leads to increased self-observation. The patient's own eyes, in addition to those of others, are now directed at himself, creating the millipede phenomenon, i. e., causing him to stumble over his own feet because of his increasing self-consciousness. The therapeutic liberation from self-observation takes place hand in hand with the liberation from being the object of observation by others, enabling the patient to have exemplary experiences in his relationship to the analyst.

From this perspective it is simple to explain the dependence of the symptoms' manifestations on the situation, mood, and the spatial situation (described by Bräutigam 1956), such as the automatic reinforcement of symptoms that results from the individual worrying about being seen. Christian (1986) followed a similar approach in explaining writer's cramp, which he considered a result of the excessive burden of simultaneously processing affective and cognitive demands. Fluent actions are disturbed because the simultaneous processing of conflicting affective and cognitive demands exceeds a patient's capacity to coordinate them. Agonists and antagonists literally work against each other instead of cooperating harmoniously. Writer's cramp is purposive behavior and obviously has an instrumental side, while the pathological twisting in wryneck has none. Writer's cramp is precipitated by touching a writing implement or by the act of writing itself. The critical glances of others frequently function as factors reinforcing the symptoms. Often writer's cramp occurs only in specific situations or after specific actions, such as writing one's signature for a bank teller. This makes it clear that writer's cramp, just like other cramps and unsuccessful actions - e.g., while playing a musical instrument - and other tics, must be viewed *primarily* in a context of unconscious meaning; this context is missing for torticollis.

In light of the results of research on affects we believe that these processes are subliminal for long stretches, i.e., they are not conscious. Since, for example, the cognition of danger is simultaneously accompanied by anxiety and the latter triggers the motoric disposition to move (away from the object), it is quite likely in subliminal anxious tension of unconscious origin for muscles to be innervated and hyperkinetic activity to be precipitated by the automatic elaboration of possible movement by the extrapyramidal motor system. This state of affairs might apply to all habitual "tensions" that are manifest as personal dispositions to react. Psychoanalytic therapy proceeds from them and from their relationship to neurotic or somatic symptoms.

6 From the Initial Interview to Therapy

Introduction

This chapter focuses on the all-important step from the initial interview to therapy, complementing the corresponding chapter in Vol.1. This step can be demonstrated particularly clearly with regard to those patients who are often considered unsuited for psychoanalysis or analytic therapy. Experience shows that social class, delinquency, and adolescence are factors posing special problems, at least in the initial phase (see Sect. 6.2). The manner in which the analyst deals with the patient's family is another of the factors that can influence therapy one way or another (see Sect. 6.3). In this chapter we extend the detailed description of the problems associated with third-party payment, given in Vol.1, by referring to a concrete example (Sect. 6.4). We also devote a separate section (Sect. 6.5) to the consequences that peer reports within the German health insurance system can have on transference.

6.1 An Initial Interview

The initial interview was preceded by a brief telephone conversation. A psychiatrist, after having conducted numerous diagnostic examinations, had recommended that Ludwig Y undergo analytic therapy and given him the addresses of several psychotherapists in private practice. In the following months Ludwig Y had not succeeded in arranging an appointment with any of these therapists. I had several reasons for offering him an initial interview at short notice. The polite and modest way in which he posed his question, which seemed to be completely devoid of emotional involvement, led me to ask myself if this might have contributed to the fact that he had been turned down or referred to other therapists. During our telephone conversation I began to assume that he needed help much more urgently than he was able to express.

Ludwig Y arrived right on time. He was about 30 years old, tall, very slender, and looked miserable. For months he had been vainly undergoing examinations because of his diverse psychosomatic symptoms, which affected especially his cardiovascular system and digestive tract. Despite his bad condition he had not stayed home from work, but rather demonstrated that he was a very conscientious employee.

At the very beginning of the initial interview I noticed the contradiction between his tenacious and untiring search for a psychotherapist and a certain incapacity to convey the fact that it was urgent. This impression, which I had also had when he called to make the appointment, became the focus of my thoughts that he was in bad condition and just managing to keep his head above water. My first intervention was to refer to his ability to keep going, which he had retained despite his worries and helplessness. He was pleased when I told him that he had taken the advice to undergo psychotherapy seriously and not ceased to call and try to make arrangements for therapy. He confirmed this in his somewhat reserved manner, saying that persistence was one of his strengths. Then he turned to me and explicitly repeated the word "persistence."

I could hear how proud Ludwig Y was of this word and how it touched him. His rapid reaction to my reference to his surprising persistence had reinacted something between us. He and his father had often held their conversations in a refined language that was a level above ordinary life, and had felt close when this enabled them to forget the very simple circumstances in which they lived. Later another aspect of Ludwig Y's relationship to his father became clear and made his persistence in looking for a psychoanalyst comprehensible. This was that his father had pedantically followed recommendations handed down from above and that he considered his father a model of how to assert oneself in a friendly way.

A: What makes you so persistent?

P: My second marriage is in danger of breaking apart! One fight after another. And we exchange terrible words.

A: Words that go back and forth between you and your wife?

P: [Silent for a while] For me, arguing is almost out of the question. And I can't get mad, either. I learned from the psychiatrist that the reason for everything is that I don't have a personality. He gave me a kind of homework. I was supposed to think about what I really like, but I don't like anything; there's nothing at all that I could say I like. For example, when I look at someone else's record collection, then I can say, "Yes, he loves classical music!" But my collection is complete chaos; jazz and classic are all mixed up. And something else, when someone tells me that he is overwhelmed by a Mozart mass or that a Beethoven sonata brings tears to his eyes - no, that's entirely foreign to me.

A: You've just taken a look around here.

He was encouraged by my comment, and glanced again, this time openly, from one corner to the other. I referred to his curiosity by saying, "Now you're starting from the beginning!" and we both laughed.

P: Yes, I can see flowers. And there are flowers in the picture, too. I have to tell you that I am surrounded by a layer that prevents everything from pentrating deep into me. And if nothing can penetrate inside, then there isn't anything that can stay inside either.

A: And so you think that if there's nothing that can stay inside, then there's nothing that can stir. You cannot get angry. As a result, you are at peace with other people.

P: Yes. But *now* I'm foundering. My wife criticizes me for often being innerly uninvolved and not having any initiative. It makes her furious, and then she makes a fuss and tries to provoke me by using ugly words.

He mentioned several examples of how his wife complained about how she had to do almost everything by herself because he didn't make any suggestions or take responsibility. Then he changed the subject.

P: I've observed myself a lot recently. I didn't have a girl when I was younger. I couldn't ask anyone because I was always afraid I would be left standing there alone. So I just didn't bother. Until one came and asked me, and I married her because *she* wanted to. It was destined to fail. We had terrible scenes before getting divorced. I let her have everything, made debts, and fled home to my parents. I was depressive then. I had to have psychiatric treatment. They examined me for some mental illness, which I didn't have. Then they gave me tablets.

Ludwig Y summarized his thoughts in conspicuously short sentences. He had apparantly already thought about it for a long time. Now and then his eyes turned moist, but he quickly suppressed his feelings as if he thought it might bother me. He also excused himself when he thought that he had interrupted me or that I had wanted to say something. I briefly summarized this observation, which gave me an explanation for my first impression that he let himself be bossed around.

A: I have the impression that you're making an effort to give concise and objective descriptions of what concerns you, and that you're being careful to let me go first and to refer to what I say because something in you wants to give me the impression that your're a particularly pleasant person.

P: [Laughs a little, as if he knew it] But if the results are different, they turn out to be all the worse.

The patient returned to the fact that he was very worried that it was impossible for him to hold on to anything. He said this had even made him once think that there was something wrong with him, i. e., that he might be mentally ill.

Consideration. I had not told the patient anything new when I commented about the polite and modest way in which he adapted himself to a situation. But feeling himself understood, he began to describe the *new items he* had discovered in himself with greater urgency and emotional involvement. I again noticed his capacity to make precise perceptions and statements, which confirmed how much he was able to absorb and retain.

A: There's an apparent discrepency between your thinking that you can't keep anything and your subtle descriptions, in which you note everything that's necessary to get an idea of your difficulties.

P: Yes, I'm proud of my ability to express myself.

Immediately after this positive statement I ended this first interview by referring to the fact that our fifty minutes had elapsed. We agreed on an appointment two days later to continue our discussion.

Ludwig Y brought his referral from his family physician along to the next meeting. He was wearing - as became apparent at the end of the session - a watch with an alarm tone set to go off after 50 minutes. He drew my attention to a mistake in the personal data contained in the referral, but did not say anything about the fact that "psychosis" had been entered as the presumed diagnosis. I thought I could tell that Ludwig Y wanted to tell me something important.

P: Something has been on my mind. Sometimes I'm a rebel and go on the attack. But all of that comes from my head. That's where things are stirred up, while inside I feel empty. It's all very confused.

A: It's associated with your anxiety that what you say might be very confused.

The patient did not react to this comment and continued to speak about the emptiness inside him.

A: I think that you use the emptiness you're talking about as a kind of fantasy object. If it's empty inside you, then there isn't anything else left to make you feel dangerous in the role of rebel and attacker.

P: [Beamed at me] So, I have a fantasy object that I use to protect myself? Yes, if I have to go that far to protect myself, then it would really look bad inside me. I wonder what's going to come out.

A: People have such thoughts when they're considering whether to undergo psychoanalysis.

P: So I'm in good company, with a lot of others.

A: Yes, and some of them don't dare to have any therapy, because of this anxiety.

P: I'm sure that I can't continue living like I am.

Consideration. At the beginning of the session the patient had provided bits of information that belonged in the context of his adaptive behavior in the first hour. I waited for further material to find out more about his anxiety and defense in the brief framework of the initial interviews. I had probably referred to his anxiety too early. Yet the patient had not completely disregarded my comment, but simply continued talking about his *feeling of emptiness.* On his own he took the step from my interpretation that his feeling of emptiness was a fantasy object to using the word "protection," while still remaining relaxed. I also used the situation to further the process of making a decision about psychoanalysis. I wanted to inquire about other data for the insurance application. The fact that the patient did not mention that psychosis had been entered as the presumed diagnosis might have indicated that he was worried that his feeling of emptiness might be an indication of something worse.

After a pause Ludwig Y asked, completely out of the blue:

P: Is my *instability* a part of it?

I pushed the referral, which was still on the table, in his direction.

A:Have you read the diagnosis, and is it what you're referring to?

P: Read it, yes, but I don't know what it means.

A: Psychosis means mentally ill, something we mentioned in our previous talk.

P: So? No, I don't have it.

A: And you've never been in a psychiatric hospital?

P: No. [He added quickly] And neither has anyone from my family.

A: In your opinion, which diagnosis applies to you?

P: I don't know enough to say.

The patient listened to my explanation of the difference between psychosis and neurosis, without showing any interest. He apparently wanted to continue talking about his instability.

A: Perhaps we should go back to what you referred to as instability. I think you wanted to say something else about it before I changed the subject.

P: When somebody leads the way, I always go along [laughed a little]. Well, I was once magically attracted by slot machines. I'm ashamed of it now. I got into bad company, a bunch of drunks! [The patient laughed at me out loud and nodded.] Everybody was bragging. That was at the time I separated from my first wife.

A: Alcohol helped what was going on inside you, and otherwise stays inside, come to the surface.

P: Drinkers and children tell the truth. Well, then it looks bad in me. It makes me feel afraid.

Consideration. I did not believe that he was one of those who made big claims when he had been drinking, and assumed that he participated - in his fantasy - in the actions of the others when some of their inhibitions were washed away. This led to my next intervention.

A: Primarily you *observed* and attempted to find out more about yourself by observing the others.

P: I love doing that. [He described, very vividly, how he watched people, for example, at the train station and later told his wife long stories about what he had seen.] Naturally all of this is my own story. I know that.

Toward the end of the session he asked a question that was directed to each of us:

P: Will I manage to achieve anything?

A: The way in which you picked up what I said today, and further elaborated on what I showed you, specifically what goes on in you to enable you to avoid anxiety - you used the word "protection" to refer to it - shows that it will be possible to continue.

The alarm on his watch rang, announcing the end of the session. Both of us, of course, had to laugh. Such moments as this, when we both laughed, played an important role later in the therapy.

Consideration. During our discussion of his referral, my attempts to get more information out of him and to give him information went, at the level of his consciousness, against the grain. I somewhat excused myself by saying that I had changed the subject, and returned to discussing the subject of instability. But in the following material, the patient returned to his anxiety about becoming crazy, although he did not use the word. In replying to his question about whether I believed that he could achieve something by working with me, I did not refer back to the subjects of mental illness or being crazy, but summarized the points about which we had been able to reach an understanding in our two diagnostic interviews. Specifically, he had feared that he would be considered an alcoholic because he had participated, rather passively, in drinking bouts; he used the term "instability" to diagnose his own overall condition; and he felt understood as a result of my comment that he had gone there in the attempt to find himself by observing others.

Ludwig Y did not wear his alarm watch to the third interview.

P: I left my watch at my father's yesterday. But first I have to tell you something. There has been a change. This morning while I was waking up I noticed what was happening outside through the slits between the shutters. I heard the birds. I had the thought that something in me had opened since our last talk, just like the slits between the shutters. I can perceive a little of what is inside me; I understood something. I see that my lack of inner sensations is connected with my fears. What am I afraid of?

A: Yes, that is the direction to go.

P: I've already taken a big step forward.

He talked a little about the relief he felt from having more confidence in himself. We spent the rest of the time gathering some more information for the application for insurance coverage.

In his first few sentences the patient wanted to express his regained hope. One cause of concern for him was the amount of time he would need and the tempo of change. Since he made frequent reference to his anxieties, it was apparent that Ludwig Y was concered about how quickly he would be exposed to deeper anxieties and how he could master them with my help. As is frequently the case in initial interviews, he tested how the tempo is set. His question about how much confidence he could have in himself also implied the question of whether he can trust me - a subject that obviously was frequently raised later on.

Summary. There was a direct transition from these three interviews to analysis. It was possible to recognize significant conflicts and to take the first steps toward problem solving. The substantial inner pressure on him declined significantly following my interpretations of his defenses against his anxieties. He described his insights and his hopes, and began to reorder old observations and new perceptions. His anxiety about becoming crazy came to include many different kinds of contents, whose equivalents were expressed in psychosomatic symptoms and partially resulted via regression in a depressive reaction. From experience it is known this anxiety about becoming crazy declines if it is possible to link the *psychotophobic* ideas with individual contents that have accumulated. In the three interviews there were first indications of this. A primary goal was to clarify these anxieties in order to establish a more relaxed level for the therapeutic relationship. In our first meeting there were signs of how he resolved his conflict with his father. This theme was easy to follow in the reenactment in transference. His thoughtful manner and his accurate expressions pleased me, and he laughed together with me at himself and the world just like he had with his father.

6.2 Specific Problems

There is good reason for us to give ample room to the discussion of the specific problems encountered during the transition from the initial or diagnostic interviews to therapy. An analyst does not need to display any special skill in beginning an analysis with an educated patient from the upper middle class whose suffering makes him highly motivated for psychoanalysis. We have given several examples of a smooth transition from the initial interview to therapy in Sect. 2.1. The initial interview summarized in the previous section (Sect. 6.1) also did not place any special demands on the analyst to apply the psychoanalytic method in a flexible manner. The anaylst's ability to employ indications in an *adaptive* manner is put to a test, however, by the task of motivating patients to undertake analysis who are less accessible for various reasons. Disregarding psychotics, addicts, and borderline patients, who frequently first require inpatient treatment, there are primarily three groups that pose special problems. The groups are identified by categories of social class (Sect. 6.2.1), delinquency (Sect. 6.2.2), and adolescence (Sect. 6.2.3); they are associated with specific difficulties, at least in the initial phases, i. e., during the transition from interview to therapy, regardless of the differences between these groups or between individual cases. Our concern is to test the application of an *adaptive* indication on patients who would not fulfill the criteria of a *selective* indication and would therefore be turned away as unsuited for the standard technique of psychoanalysis. Yet if the analyst adapts himself to the expectations of the individual patient, the group of inaccessible patients is reduced to special problem cases. Thus an adaptive indication saves many patients the depressing fate of being shoved around from one office to the next. There can be no doubt that it is often very difficult to convince an unmotivated individual that psychotherapy is advisable. As a consequence, patients who do not consider it likely that there is any connection between their experiencing and their numerous symptoms are unpopular with psychotherapists whatever their color. Such patients are frequently even rejected on the telephone. Of course, it is a favorable sign that a patient does not let himself be discouraged and makes an effort to find treatment. In this regard the patients we can report on-because they found their way into our offices - are in a special category.

6.2.1 Social Class

Although in this section we discuss case material that is primarily associated with patients from the lower social class, we have given this section a more inclusive title. The reason for this is that we want, in agreement with the study by Cremerius et al. (1979), to emphasize that social class in itself constitutes a factor that can pose characteristic technical problems. It is no coincidence that approximately two-thirds of the patients who have received analytic or psychodynamic treatment in the FRG since the public health insurance companies agreed to accept such claims are white collar workers and that only one-third are skilled and unskilled laborers, the group of the populace insured by the original - and least selective - public health scheme (the *Allgemeine Ortskrankenkasse*). On the other hand, the rich and the powerful also make their way to an analyst relatively infrequently, as can be seen in Cremerius et al.'s study.

We will restrict our discussion to technical problems that occur at the beginning of therapies with patients from the lower class. We follow the definition of class based on the widely used criteria established by Hollingshead and Redlich (1958) and described by Menne and Schröter (1980). Occupation and education served as their criteria for social class.

Lower class patients are blue-collar workers (including skilled laborers), employees who perform primarily manual labor, and small farmers who have not graduated from a regular school or from a vocational or commercial school and whose father's education and occupation - and possibly also those of the mother--were similar. The occupation and education of the spouses of married women also had to fall into these categories since the social status and socioeconomic situation of a family is largely determined by the husband's occupational status and income. (Menne and Schröter 1980, p. 16)

Thus with lower class patients the following points should be paid special attention, at least during the initial phase of psychoanalytic therapy. The analyst should provide these patients with an especially large amount of explanatory information. The autonomy that these patients experience their physical symptoms to possess should be taken even more seriously than usual since these patients as a rule do not make the discovery that symptoms play a role until later. Psychodynamic interpretations that are made too early provoke mistrust and reinforce the distance separating analyst and patient. If the analyst cannot put himself into the position of those from other social classes, which includes the conditions under which they live and work, then he lacks the prerequisites for empathic understanding. In the initial phase, abstinent behavior by an analyst who believes he is not permitted to answer any questions repels such patients, for whom this effect is much more pronounced than for better educated and situated patients. Yet if the analyst follows the rules of everyday communication, as Freud spontaneously did in his informal consultation with Katharina, then it is possible to establish a psychoanalytic dialogue step by step. Otherwise reactions such as those described by Schröter (1979) occur. The lower class patient, for example, experiences the dialogue (and the analyst) as "unnormal," is disturbed, and rejects what must seem foreign and incomprehensible to him. Schröter described the formal aspects of the psychoanalytic dialogue as if it were a sin to adhere to everyday forms of communication in the beginning. Yet if interpretations are embedded in a dialogue that by and large corresponds to the needs and expectations of the patient and if their contents are adapted to his experiencing, then in our experience the reactions commonly attributed to lower class patients do not occur. The observation that lower class patients frequently take interpretations to be criticism, insults, and derogatory statements is thus a result of the unempathic application of the psychoanalytic method.

Some of the experiences gained from a comparative study of analytic group therapies (Heising et al. 1982) can be applied to individual therapy. For various reasons lower class patients prefer to maintain some distance. Because the patient is looking for a better world and the talk with the analyst constitutes a new and unusual experience for him, he finds certain positive and negative transference interpretations incomprehensible. It is more usual for conflicts to be carried out with substitute figures, and it not possible to bridge the underlying division into good and evil and to work on it in transference until later. Such secondary transference can be productive for the analytic process. A certain idealizing transference is formed in this distance, and it is tinged by unconscious envy and class hatred. It is necessary to modify the interpretive procedure in which the analyst offers himself as a transference object. Heising et al. (1982) referred to the fact that analysts feel offended when working with lower class patients because the specific satisfaction analysts experience as the object of transference, especially if it can be interpreted, is restricted with this group of patients. The authors raised the question of whether this fact might be related to the failures described in the literature of analytic work with lower class patients or to the view that such patients cannot be treated analytically.

A longer period of preparation is recommended when working with lower class patients, who require explanatory information about the purpose of the treatment. Initiating a comprehensive learning process in group therapy has been shown to be effective (Junker 1972; Reiter 1973). For reasons similar to those in treating somatically ill, it is essential that the analyst first respond to questions very concretely and answer them realistically. If the analyst observes these simple rules, which seem obvious to common sense, many of the alleged features - such as limited fantasy, rigid superego, and fear of authority - attributed to lower class patients (and psychosomatic ones, see Sect. 9.9) and specified as the causes of their being inaccessible to analysis vanish. The inability to view inner conflicts as meaningful and the opposite tendency of holding external sources responsible for an illness are frequent artifacts originating from the impatient expectation that the patient should already have gained insight into his inner conflicts.

According to this incorrect specification of typical features, lower class patients exhibit considerable similarities with many of the wealthy private patients who are unsuccessfully treated for years for a "psychosomatic structure" (see Sect. 9.9). Every indication is that both diagnostic classifications are artifacts. If the analyst gains a feeling for the world of a laborer and makes an effort to employ indications in an adaptive manner, then the initial difficulties recede to the background and the analyst's interest in the life of a patient whose educational level differs from his own if often richly rewarded.

Leodolter (1975) and Wodak-Leodolter (1979) have shown that it is impossible to adequately describe the communication between a patient from the lower class and a middle class doctor by using Bernstein's (1975) code theory. On the basis of his code theory, Bernstein rejected the possibility of a successful psychoanalytic interview between a lower class patient and a physician typically from the middle class. Since in his opinion the patient lacks the necessary capacity to verbalize, it is impossible for the physician to find a means of access to the patient's world. Bernstein, just like Schröter, apparently proceeded from the fixed rules of the standard technique, which in fact do not permit a dialogue that satisfies common sense expectations. If the analyst frees himself from such restrictions, many observations turn out to be the products of an restricted application of the psychoanalytic method. In any case, one prerequisite for examining verbal and nonverbal exchange is to acknowledge that the range of problems is much more complex than described by Bernstein. For example, Wodak-Leodolter (1979, p. 187) raised the following questions:

1. Does the lower class patient really lack the capacity for verbalization? 2. What are the differences between lower class and middle class sozialization; what forms of distorted communication are present in each case; what is therefore the form of therapy suitable in each case? 3. What does cure mean to the lower class patient; it is at least necessary to discuss the criticism that psychotherapy means "adjustment" to middle class norms.

Moreover, in our opinion it is not sensible to consider "capacity for verbalization" to be a global feature; more appropriate is to distinguish between its various elements and thus be able to realistically consider the particular capacity for simple individuals to express themselves.

First Example

Susanne X, a nearly 40-year-old housewife, came from a rural area and was married to a laborer. The reason she gave coming to her initial appointment was that she frequently got into hopeless situations in which she ultimately became extremely agitated. In her frequent states of psychogenic semiconsciousness she could not remember what she had said or done. She ran away aimlessly. These states were preceded by violent arguments with her husband; the reasons were trivial, the shouting terrible. The tension would not resolve until the next day at the earliest, sometimes taking up to three days. Years of drug therapy did not produce any change. Her family doctor and a psychiatrist responded to her questions about psychoanalysis by telling her, in essence, that she lacked both the money and the intelligence for such treatment. Having grown up in poverty, she had had to work even as a child, and immediately after finishing elementary school she had left home to work.

The previous rejections of psychotherapy had confirmed her expectation that she was too poor and stupid, yet she did not let this stifle her desire to learn more. She had acquired a wide range of information about psychotherapy and psychoanalysis from the media (magazines, books, radio, and television), and then turned to another psychiatrist, who referred her to a (female) analyst in the expectation that she would talk her out of all of these unrealistic ideas. This was supposed to help her bury her wish for psychotherapy for good. In response to my questions, this psychiatrist told me that in his experience analysts frequently did not establish an indication for therapy for the lower class patients he referred.

Susanne X had tried to learn more on her own, out of a mixture of spite, anxiety, and mistrust. She had felt that she recognized herself in various book titles, and after reading Richter's (1976) book *Flüchten oder Standhalten* (Flee or Stand Firm) she made an effort to obtain psychotherapy. After about one hundred hours of treatment, she brought me ten of her favorite books. After even more time had elapsed she asked me why I did not tell her not to read them. The confidence I placed in her capacity for learning encouraged her.

Going through the protocols of the first ten hours of treatment from her analysis, which took place three times a week and lasted three years in all, I noticed that the patient had tried in almost every session to provoke me into stopping the therapy, as if she felt she could not be rejected often enough since she belonged to those from the bottom.

In the initial interviews she described the extreme poverty, the misery, and especially the corporal punishment she had experienced in her childhood and adolescence, and several times responded to my attentive and empathic behavior by saying quite unexpectedly, "Am I in the right place here with you?" She repeatedly gave me such "shoves." I showed her that she expected the beatings she had received from her father to be repeated in the analysis and that she actively worked toward restructuring it accordingly (via identification with the aggressor). She said her father had been course, would shout and hit her, and was only interested in money. She had married her husband because he was the exact opposite, i. e., good natured, but then it was precisely this quality that she complained about in their arguments; for her, he was just too lax with everything and everyone. She said that this put her in a state of helpless rage and anxiety. Her last sentence in the first interview was, "Whoever has experienced evil will always be tempted to be evil themselves."

I made an effort to provide the patient sufficient information in response to her questions about being at the right place. She had told me that she read a lot. I limited the information I provided to saying that I wanted to try to understand her, and that I wanted to get to know her and that she should get to know me before we made any further plans. Everything that was unexpected and new disturbed her, and she would have liked to pick an argument with me right away.

She started the second session by glancing at me provocatively and asking, "Is there any point to this?" My comment that I first wanted to listen to what she had to say to me led her to talk about two subjects in detail. First, she said she was listening to a radio program called "Talk and Let Talk." In telling me about the program she described in detail the features that had fascinated me during our first interview. Yet neither of us verbalized this fact; we simply agreed that this manner of conversing could be very positive. Then she switched to the second topic, describing a couple she knew. In person they acted very endearingly, but otherwise they gossiped and said bad things about her. Yet the patient claimed that she knew precisely what happened since she had grown with evil people.

The patient said the situation of her sister, whose husband had committed suicide, was similar. She went on, saying that if everything continued as it were, then she would not have any alternative to suicide either, and she had everything ready. I inquired about her preparations, and told her that she had the feeling that she wanted to end everything with an evil deed - by committing suicide - precisely when someone was friendly to her, the way she felt I acted toward her. Then she would willingly put away everything she had prepared, only to immediately think about another means of killing herself. What followed was a life-and-death struggle.

I met Susanne X in the hallway near the waiting room before the third session and said, "Be right there." When I opened the door to my office five minutes later, she was standing right next to the door. She had taken my comment literally and explained that she had stood there to hear what I was doing. She complained that since nobody had been in my office, she could have come in immediately. I was there after all! She dealt with this topic by referring to the couple she had mentioned before, who always acted nice but were really only interested in their own good; how mean they were to other people. Then she said that two people had hanged themselves, one just recently. In this session she said three times that "Now I'm going to settle with them; I'm going there on Saturday." She recalled that the man was like her uncle, who - like her father - was only able to shout, be violent, and chase after money. She thought that confronting a person and asking for an explanation did not lead anywhere but to an argument, and therefore she would have to settle things on her own. She claimed she had already learned something from me; yesterday her husband had made an idiot of himself again by working far too long because everyone wanted him to do something, and then had come home exhausted. This time she had just listened to him, nothing else, while she used to show him what an idiot he was.

Susanne X said I had been right that she would let loose with words because she felt at home in mouthing off. As a child she had not learned how to discuss things. She recalled that her mother had only known two sentences: "You're not supposed to steal" and "You're supposed to obey." In the fourth session she told me about having taken some pictures of trees the day before; she wanted to have pictures of them from each of the seasons. Until then trees had only meant leaves to her, leaves that had to be raked. She concluded that for her even trees represented evil. The patient demonstrated her own psychological talent, which I did not elaborate on, by recognizing her own potential for change and development. She cooperated, and she changed, such as listening to her husband. It was obvious that in acting this way she was imitating our interaction in analysis; if I had mentioned this transference aspect to her she would have had to reject it because she would have thought "What does that have to do with what a doctor does?" At first she refused to think that she had anything in common with people like me; she consciously rejected any such connection. She told me repeatedly that she belonged to those down below and I to those at the top. If I had established some connection between this theme and me, her reaction would have been to raise her defenses against anxiety. She would have started complaining that what she did didn't have anything to do with what I did, and would have referred to the flattery of her friends which she at this moment could have handled better. It was possible to therapeutically exploit the fact that the patient used largely the same adjectives to describe members of her own family and other people, and that it was thus easier to establish a direct connection than it is with fairly mistrustful patients. I was at first surprised that the patient used the same expressions to refer to her husband as to her father and uncle, namely avaricious, domineering, and inhuman.

The fact that the patient had adopted, via identification, her father's manner of complaining was a frequent cause of conflicts with her husband. She adopted insults her father had used, calling her husband a poor joker, a good-for-nothing, and complained that "You're nothing if you don't have any money." In the following sessions the oedipal seductive side with respect to her father became stronger. Unfortunately I very prematurely offered the interpretation that this was how she seduced her father. She looked at me aghast, rejected (as has often been described) any interpretation of her inner conflict as grotesk, and thought I was not credible and strange.

In my opinion the reasons that oedipal conflicts cannot be interpreted or at least not until much later still have not been clarified. Many people live in polarized circumstances or according to a law of all or nothing; for many members of the lower class this has specific connotations. Static descriptions about the presence of rigid superego or weak ego functions are completely inadequate to describe these complicated processes.

I then became more cautious, being careful not to precipitate any new defenses against anxiety. More quickly than might have been expected, Susanne X began to assure me that I should not send her away. "You have to pay attention that I don't go the wrong way!" She spoke more frequently about her mother. She came to the next session wearing a bright red jacket and, laughing, asked if I knew what it meant. She came as little red riding hood who had been sent away by her mother. She had felt sent away because I had not explicitly affirmed her wish for me to look out for her–I had avoided answering her request. From her point of view I should have said to her, "Yes, I will now take over your mother's functions!" She claimed it was my duty as a doctor. In the following period she quickly transformed such disappointments and disparaged the doctor's function. This theme reached its climax much later, in the *final phase* of treatment, when she acted through the deprivation of power at different levels.

After the difficulties related to her social standing had diminished in the initial phase, as described above, it was possible for me in the particularly helpful periods of the analysis to show the patient which items of unconscious oedipal and preoedipal envy she actually meant when she referred to her de facto lack of education. It also became clear that this deficit was reinforced in a vicious circle, both in her experiencing and in actual fact. Once the patient recognized which needs she was additionally trying to satisfy, she learned to distinguish between her different conscious and unconscious intentions and goals. Also instructive was how she restructured commandments and prohibitions, i. e., her superego, that she had internalized and initially felt to be foreign; she substituted her own words for the foreign dictates. This change led to a partial restructuring. About 18 months after the termination of analysis, Susanne X called me to say that she was feeling well. She said she was still struggling against the feeling that the separation from me was a rejection, but that her confidence in herself - in identifying with what she had gained for herself in the course of her analysis - helped her get over it. However, she still sometimes had doubts about whether she had profited less from analysis because of her past.

Second Example

The following example demonstrates that we can employ ego capabilities peculiar to a certain profession in order to balance social differences and the feelings of inferiority associated with them.

Victor Y was 37 years old when he came to me because of insomnia and somatic symptoms; he had suffered from them since his "defeat" - a test he had failed. He had worked as an electrician since he was 17. Because of his skills he had felt confident enough to take a test for a promotion, but the conflicts he had with persons in positions of authority ruined his opportunity.

A period of several weeks elapsed between his telephone call for an appointment and the beginning of his seven-month therapy. Referring to the fact that *he* had requested this delay, he explained his technique of coping with conflicts with authority by distancing himself. He realized, however, that this also had disadvantages for him. I replied that he had also given me the impression of apparently being disinterested. He confirmed this, but added that he definitely wanted therapy.

The patient then provided a precise description of the test whose outcome had been so disastrous for him. In even more detail he told me about how supervisors and ordinary staff acted toward one another and vividly described typical experiences; there were even some humorous moments.

Suddenly he looked at me and stopped, just as if he had wanted to ask me, "Did you start at the bottom too?" He wanted me to understand him. He had done everything to get a promotion - "And now!" He suddenly began crying and said that he was losing his friends now too. The only thing the others could talk about was cars. He claimed he wanted to get out of this situation. Friends and relatives would also poke fun at him, saying he was just taking the easy way with his job. He felt misunderstood and continued having difficulties falling asleep, but added that he had so much on his mind, yet was still against taking tablets. "But now, my parents," he suddenly said; "you'll have to excuse the sudden change in topic. They were just visiting. I noticed that I don't want to turn out to be like they are. My mother only knows how to consume and keep father under her thumb. Father had once been the authority; he had been a corporal, and everybody had had to obey him." He told me that he tended to exaggerate his symptoms, just like his mother did. As soon as he would feel any pain, he would tell anyone and everyone about it. He added that his wife could endure a headache or backache for days without mentioning it. The patient wanted me to understand him correctly; he said he did not start screaming, just acted grumpy, but that this might even be much worse. He also told me that one other thing he did passionately was to straighten up the house, such as in the kitchen, but without it being any help to his wife. And he always had to sit on *his* chair. He went on to describe several other compulsive and superstitous actions.

Victor Y was the parental advisor to the class one of his children was in. He described how, prior to a meeting of the parents, he would feel pressure on the chest, and pointed to his heart. Then he would let someone else talk first, gather some information, and then it was easier for him to speak. I said that he was afraid of being attacked if *he* went first. He agreed, saying he avoided it by always letting the others speak first. He now felt he had to change the subject again suddenly; he said his face would turn red when, for example, his supervisor came, and there was absolutely no reason, none at all. Before falling asleep he would prepare long speeches he wanted to hold the following day, but then he would improvise instead of saying what he had prepared. I answered that he did possess self-assurance if he could improvise like that. Rejecting my comment, he said he would let off a tirade, attacking others, and then could not stop feeling guilt. He thought it would be better if he did not say anything at all, adding that his neighbor acted the same way and quarreled with everyone.

In the next session he was quiet, expecting me to give the command, "Start talking!" He said that he was busy sorting out his thoughts for a while, and that he would say something when he was finished. He claimed he did not need the therapy, and then commented about how bad he felt. "So," he said, "do something about it!"

He then started to tell me everything imaginable, in a dialogue all his own, even referring to himself by his first name. By doing so he made it impossible for me to say anything, yet he apparently was also giving me a picture of how he talked with himself before going to sleep at night. While on night duty now something had happened to him. "It was just time to stop and the phone rang. It was Mr. Z, and was I ready for him! He asked why there was still snow in front of his workshop. Because it had snowed. Why hadn't it been cleared away. Because the people clearing the snow hadn't got there yet." *Then* he had felt well, saying that Mr. Z was the kind that blew up right away, and adding that he could argue with him because he asked such stupid questions. He blushed. It had not been until he was standing in the shower that he had known he should have done it differently, namely listen first, then say "yes," then that something had gone wrong and that it would be taken care of. If it had happened in the evening he would not have slept a wink all night. "He, he must pay attention to everything, he thinks it's his responsibility." The patient said he would like to have a job like that, too, because he could do it. He confirmed my comment that he picked the wrong time to say out loud how he felt inside and made himself guilty. He recalled a few examples of how others coped with their aggressions.

In the next few days he felt bad, walked around stiffly and awkwardly, and at work only did as much as was absolutely necessary.

This patient, who described several versions of his conflicts with authority in the first two sessions, had shown me in the very first quarter hour - by nearly asking if I had had any vocational training - that my development as a doctor had naturally been different from his and that *he*, not I, was competent with regard to his vocational situation. I listened attentively to his long explanations and knew that this was how he could draw pleasure from his competence. I was thus able to recognize the patient's ego capacities that he, because of the dominance of his superego and his compulsive traits, would otherwise not have been able to portray in such a natural, secure, and unanxious manner. He then described how he had to make competent and responsible decisions at work, and that when making these decisions he very rapidly felt he was being insulted. As I told him that he did not feel secure with the real authority he did possess, he suddenly started to describe the company doctor. The patient described him as someone who did not achieve enough for a qualified physician, despite everything he was responsible for. This doctor had prescribed him a cure at a spa that had been very nice but had not helped at all; the medication he had prescribed had not helped either. In the next three sentences the patient, who was not very articulate, described how *he* viewed the development of his difficulties. When his father had said something, it meant having to obey the earlier corporal, but when his mother said something, it meant he was under her thumb and lost all independence. He feared he was like his mother, adding that he did not want to be like her.

By means of the dialogue that he initiated with himself at important spots, the patient showed me, first, his symptom - his brooding that kept him from falling asleep - and, more importantly, how he avoided transference. Sometimes he quite consciously took control of the session. The dialogue and cooperation between us was able to continue because I did *not* offer the interpretation that he had to start a power struggle with me because of the omnipotence he feared I possessed.

After working through his unconscious (oedipal) aggressions he was freed of his neurotic inhibitions, yet certain intellectual inhibitions continued to obstruct his advancement. On the other hand, he no longer needed this advancement in order to come to terms with his rivalry with his father (and substitute persons).

In the last session of his therapy, Viktor Y used numerous technical terms to describe an event that had occurred during his night duty. My statement that I could not say anything about it because I did not know enough about the subject made him laugh triumphantly. Then he was pleased by my comment that he had made a decision in a difficult situation, responded flexibly, and did not postpone an inevitable repair. Yes, he agreed, he thought he had become more humane. He said he was no longer the eternal grouch that he had been known as, and people did not even recognize him any more. He made me laugh again by suddenly saying, "Just don't be afraid that I'm going to go screwy!" He summarized what had changed and came to speak once more about the test he had failed. Half laughing he said, "I'm beginning to accept the fact that I will remain an electrician instead of going straight on to an institute of science and technology." I then briefly summarized the difficulties he had complained about at the beginning and had now overcome, such as losing his temper, becoming furious at the wrong instant, and not finding the right word at the right moment. Agreeing, he said he had stopped playing this game. He added, after pausing to think, he would have to live through, experience, and also create the strength he might have, even though his nerves might not always be strong enough. I replied that this was a good conclusion. He stood up and said "Yes," and that he would inform his doctor, and in doing so mischievously avoided the usual good-byes.

6.2.2 Delinquency

By employing an adaptive indication, as we explained and grounded in Vol.1, it is possible to successfully use psychoanalysis to treat delinquents. Yet it quickly becomes apparent that this designation is misleading since it is by no means the case that only the families of delinquents and society at large suffer from such asocial and delinquent behavior. This is a very divergent group of persons, and many delinquents who have been written off and are apparently beyond hope do in fact suffer from their incapacity to control their own behavior. Approximately thirty years of experience, especially that gathered in Dutch institutions of forensic psychiatry, justify cautious optimism that such persons are accessible to psychotherapy (Goudsmit 1986, 1987). Given the appropriate modifications, the use of the psychoanalytic method is far less heroic than indicated by the Menninger Project. At the time the Menninger Project was conducted, it was a "heroic" undertaking – according to Wallerstein (1986), who referred back to Ticho – to continue using the standard technique even in cases that, as we know in hindsight, would have required greater flexibility in combining therapeutic techniques.

The modifications, whose effectiveness has in the meantime been demonstrated everywhere, are directed at establishing a therapeutic relationship. Many delinquents have not experienced reliable family ties in childhood and adolescence.

If an analyst has established a therapeutic relationship with a delinquent, it is important that he be particularly cautious because subliminally a disturbance might develop. Such individuals all too often know that they can take another person for a while before it comes to a surprising end, and from the perspective of the patient the end is almost always the other person's fault. As is well known, the favorite defense mechanism of these patients is projection to the outer world. The fear and anticipation of this expected end leads some patients to undertake the unconsciously guided attempt to bring about the termination themselves. In this case there is a tendency for patients to flee from inpatient treatment, or to pretend to achieve satisfactory cures in outpatient treatment. It is important for the analyst not to fall for such attempts at self-deception, which may be very tempting. If he does, the two parties may decide to terminate treatment as successful although each of them privately suspects that the patient will subsequently have a relapse. The continuity of the therapy can be assured by soberly evaluating which length of therapy is required. Thus it is also in the patient's interest for the analyst, despite his empathy for the patient's momentary situation, to maintain a friendly distance and not to let himself be used by the patient, such as to obtain short-term satisfaction.

It is often necessary for the analyst initially to accept the patient's notions about therapy, in order to gain his confidence, and not to attempt to impose rules that the patient will rebel against because for many patients rules have always been handed down from above. In the case described below, hypnosis was performed several times at the patient's request, and psychotherapy was subsequently combined with kinesitherapy. With many delinquents it is almost essential that a social worker participate in the course of the therapy.

Example

Initial Interview and Biographical Data

We will follow the detailed notes that the analyst made, summarizing them with the author's approval.

Simon Y's treatment began with a telephone call, followed by an initial interview the next day. He was 37 years old, had a police record, and came to the analyst in an emergency. The analyst offered "first aid"; decisive was that the analyst did not primarily view the patient's wish for hypnotherapy - that the patient tied to a threat to commit suicide - as a kind of extortion but rather as an indication of the severity of the emergency. Otherwise their contact would not have extended beyond the telephone conversation, which the patient would have taken to be another rejection. The analyst's willingness to adopt a comprehensive view of the repertoire of therapeutic techniques and to take Sandler's (1983) adage seriously that psychoanalysis is what psychoanalysts do was an essential factor is creating a basis of confidence. There must have been a fortunate coincidence of factors on both sides that enabled a supportive relationship to be established in the very first interview and that this even enabled the patient to wait three months for therapy to begin.

We presume that the patient managed to wait for such a long time because he viewed the analyst's offer as his last chance and because the initial interview had given him sufficient hope of being able to find support and security. The patient had expected a repetition of his earlier experiences, which he described in the following way: "I'm afraid there's no hope for me any more; that's what all the other doctors have said before turning me down." After sobbing for a while, he asked the analyst, "Why are you wasting your time with me? Nobody has ever spoken with me as long as you have." At this moment the analyst could truthfully assure the patient that he had decided to try to assist him in his struggle to change his life, yet without knowing whether hypnosis was the right method. However, if the patient believed it would help, he was willing to try it.

Several reasons that provided the subjective basis for the analyst's decision to attempt therapy can be gleaned from his thoughts and feelings, which he described in the following way: "It's a mixture of great pity and indignation at the manner he has been treated, and a feeling of impotence: What can I do to help in this case? Nonetheless in the course of the initial interview I gained the impression that I could work with the patient and that a genuine attempt to treat him has never been undertaken .... I feel I have to emphasize that I did not have the feeling that I was coerced into making the offer."

When the analyst made his offer of therapy he was not familiar with any of the details of the patient's case history or with the records from other institutions. With the patient's approval the analyst requested and studied these reports. The external data about the nature of his delinquency corresponded with the information the patient had provided; we now cite from the analyst's brief summary of this information in order to make the course of Simon Y's treatment more comprehensible.

This patient was borne out of wedlock, was unwanted, and has been pushed back and forth, i.e., away, for his entire life. From the fondling home after his birth he was sent to the prejudiced parents of his mother, who thanked God that his Dutch father - who had been a member of the resistance - had been arrested and killed in a concentration camp. In elementary school he was isolated and handicapped by his stuttering that became progressively worse. He had cried a lot as a child, which was a symptom that later so irritated professional helpers that they did not know how to handle him. The well-meant advice of a school doctor that the 11-year-old and weakly boy be sent to a reformatory in the western part of the country led to new and severe traumas. Because of his dialect he stayed an outsider among the local youths. He vividly recalled the separation from his mother at the train station as an example of evil betrayal because she did not heed - and as he later realized, probably could not have heeded - his begging and pleading to let him stay. He described the two years he spent in the home as terrible.

He was discouraged by his isolation and his incomplete education, and after returning to his home town he broke off two attempts to obtain training to be a mechanic after just a few days. After working irregularly as an unskilled laborer he passed the driving test. After being convicted of burglary he was sentenced to 6 months on probation. Then, during a longer period in jail awaiting trial he rejected the company of other prisoners and the work he was assigned to do. After being released he did odd jobs working as a truck driver. He was often off because of headaches and backaches. The usual referrals back and forth between the social and psychiatric services were intensified. He did not know how to use the help he was offered, and stopped two stays in a psychiatric hospital. At the age of 22 he was sent to a center for crisis intervention, where he became fully aware of his pedophiliac tendencies, which he had hardly practiced previously. He had lived with a younger (male) friend and had hoped to establish a stabler life with him. When his friend ended their relationship, he fell at first into desparate rage and then into depression and thought about committing suicide.

Simon Y fell through the cracks in the network of social psychiatric services and consiliary examinations that are the consequence of the divisions in responsibility and competence. On the basis of thorough psychological testing, his IQ was determined to be 104. His drawings were at the level of a 12 year old. His capacity for social adjustment was considered minimal, yet the result of an MMPI was surprisingly normal. Over the years he had been prescribed large amounts of psychopharmaceuticals, which he had stopped taking long before the initiation of psychotherapy. Finally, the result of further psychiatric examinations was that no help could be offered to him; it was at this time that he mentioned his pedophiliac tendencies for the first time and asked whether hypnosis could not free him from them. Reading about yoga had given him this idea. As a result, he was referred again to the department for social work with the instruction that other housing be found for him. Simon Y had lived for years in a dilapidated house, in isolation since the separation from his friend, his only companion being his dog.

Simon Y had thought a lot about the meaning of his life and his difficulties and sought solutions on the basis of his belief in reincarnation. He feared he would no longer be able to escape his isolation and was insecure as to whether he was truly pedophiliac or not. He had not been moved by his brief sexual relationships to women, but he was enthusiastic about being with teenage boys. "Maybe they give me the love that I was denied earlier." The fact that this thought might have been suggested to him in one of the many talks he had had does not alter the fact that Simon Y still accurately described his situation from his perspective.

The analyst who offered him treatment divided the therapy into phases according to external data and thematic focus. Below we give several passages verbatim and summarize others. After approximately 9 months of work the therapeutic relationship was sufficiently consolidated that it was possible to initiate analytic psychotherapy. For didactic reasons we are interested in this long phase of preparation and how the analyst structured it. We conclude this description when the shift to psychoanalysis took place.

First Phase of Treatment

Simon Y's personal and social situation did not deteriorate during the three month waiting period. He arrived punctually at the agreed time. Looking embarrassed and as if he had been crying, he only said "Here I am." Since a pause at this moment can be disastrous, I asked him once more how he had had the idea of undergoing hypnosis and what he expected from it. He told me about his earlier experiences with yoga. His yoga teacher had told him that an individual has a very deep unconscious life and that it was sometimes possible to look behind the mask by using hypnosis. I replied that this was true, but that looking behind the mask was in many cases insuffîcent for really working through what was hidden there. I also pointed out that it was quite possible that we might encounter very shocking things behind the mask. Furthermore, I mentioned that it was possible to record what happened during hypnosis, thus giving him the opportunity to hear for himself what he said during the hypnosis. He answered that he thought it was a little horrifying, but rejected my offer to leave out very troublesome topics, saying "If we do it, then everything" - he could take it.

To test his ability to enter a trance, we began with the relaxation exercises from autogenic training. This was a failure since the patient was unable to concentrate.

Commentary. The analyst's intention was to direct the memories about affectively strongly prominent, forgotten, or repressed experiences that the patient recalled during hypnoanalysis to a more intensive conscious study and therefore suggested that the dialogues conducted under hypnosis be recorded. In the process hypnosis would lose it secretive and magical character, becoming part of the analytic procedure and allowing the transference and countertransference processes taking place in it also to be worked through. In this regard the introduction of the tape recorder into the therapeutic situation made it possible to expand the range of adaptive indications. It thus became possible to carry out the transition from the preanalytic treatment provided during a flexible introductory phase of unspecified length to an analysis of transference and resistance in a methodologically correct manner. Thus, to supplement our comments on this topic in Sect. 7.9, an analyst can undertake such analyses precisely by means of using a tape recorder, instead of despite using one. Even patients whose mistrust of the analyst's secret means of influencing is so large that they bring their own recorder can also be given therapy according to an adaptive evaluation of indications.

The patient began the second interview a week later by commenting that there had been hardly any change. Then he had to laugh and said, "Funny, but you hope for some change although it's clear to me that it's not at all possible." He wanted to try the relaxation exercises once more, and this attempt was also a failure. The patient then asked whether it was possible for me to record the relaxation exercises on a tape he could take along to practice at home, which I agreed to do. With a small smile he concluded, "But I'm going to continue coming. You can depend on it."

As was to be expected, it was not possible for the patient to do the exercises at home with the tape recorder either. Since the Christmas break was approaching, we talked in detail about how to proceed. I made the patient the offer that he could call me at home if he had any serious difficulties. After the break he told me that he had had a very bad three weeks; he had felt terribly lonesome and had been repeatedly overwhelmed by the idea that his life was meaningless and that everything was useless. He was also plagued by frequent headaches, which forced him to lie down. The rest of the time he had taken care of his dog: "Without my dog and the prospect of coming here, I wouldn't have managed to survive these three weeks."

Simon Y did not have a clear idea of what he wanted or did not want in life, or of what he wanted more and what less. I therefore advised him to prepare a list of what he wanted and what he did not want at all or not much, which he brought to the next session. It was apparent from his list that what he did not want was associated with assignments he was given by third parties, especially by the authorities. The things he wanted were all connected with improvements in how he lived, with his ailments, and with his limited opportunities for having contact. The biggest item in our interview consisted of his insecurities in life. It became apparent that it was impossible for him to feel at ease in any area. The only area he did not have any problems was with his dog; he knew his dog understood him without him saying a word.

Commentary. The analyst took over the functions of an auxiliary ego by making clarifying suggestions. The patient managed to gain a better impression of his own goals, which were quite vague, by preparing a list. Identifying his goals in this way facilitated the course of the interviews because it was possible to refer back to something tangible.

Second Phase of Treatment

Simon Y talked in detail about his feelings of inferiority, which started back in kindergarten and were reinforced at school. His teacher stopped asking him questions because he was too dumb. He said it was like that everywhere. I expressed my conviction that he had many profound ideas. And furthermore, the psychological examination had clearly shown that he was not dumb. The problem was that all of these experiences had given him an inferiority complex, and it was our task to overcome it.

He talked about his being alone, his feeling of being alone, and pedophilia, in addition to about his inability to concentrate and his inferiority feelings. He said that he meant something to "the boys." Almost blushing, he added that he was not thinking about sex. Then he gave me a lecture explaining that pedophilia was caused by a predispositon and that it was impossible to do anything about it. Since I did not make a comment, he asked, "Or is it possible that all of this is somehow related to my own experiences as a boy?" I gave the simple answer, "I think so."

Consideration. The identificatory character of his love to the boys seemed clear to me, yet it was still too early to make any allusions to it.

In the next session Simon Y first talked about the feeling of insecurity he had in all of his relationships. He asked me again whether it might not be connected with his earlier experiences. Then I reminded him that we had wanted to make an attempt at hypnosis in this session. Relieved, he answered, "Yes, naturally I've thought about it but I didn't want to be the one to mention it because you might have thought that I want to have my way at all cost." Less clearly he then stammered, "And besides I wanted to see if you hadn't forgotten it."

To achieve a trance, I chose the fixation method since the patient had amply demonstrated how bad his concentration was. It took a rather long time for him to enter a slight trance. He was visibly dissatisfied with what he had achieved, as shown by his statement "I didn't notice anything." It was obvious that he had doubts about my skill. When I told him that it was often difficult at the beginning, he did not seem convinced.

I was not amazed that Simon Y came to the next session complaining. "A bad week, didn't do anything, didn't feel like doing anything, and lots of headaches." I did not tell him that this stemmed from his disappointments at the last session, but suggested that we continue with hypnosis. This time he entered a trance more quickly and it was much deeper. He recalled his departure from his mother, when he was sent to the home in the western part of the country. He immediately began to cry, telling me between his sobbing that he had felt terribly abandoned. He was completely lost in his pain and asked repeatedly, "How can a mother do such a thing to a child?" He also remembered that he had vomited on the train platform because he had felt so agitated and anxious, but his mother had been unrelenting. He was so agitated that I suggested that he would feel better and relaxed after he woke up. Simon Y was conspicously composed and calm after the hypnosis. He was silent for a while before saying that he could recall everything. After a pause he added, "I don't dare even think that I'm in treatment here and that it's going to continue."

Consideration. I did not tell him that he feared that I might send him away, just as his mother had done. Such an interpretation would have constituted too great a burden at this point.

Commentary. The patient's fundamental anxiety about being sent away and pushed around, i. e., his lack of security about having a fixed place in life, and his anxiety about being sent away again led the analyst to first strengthen the therapeutic relationship and not to interpret the anxiety. In our opinion the most important issue is to put the interpretation of anxiety about a renewed loss into a proper context. The rule that the analyst should interpret the anxiety at its point of urgency is frequently understood to mean that this is the deepest or strongest point at which the anxiety originated. If, in contrast, the analyst orients himself on which anxieties a patient is momentarily able to master, then the urgent points are different and the analyst can refer to a wide spectrum of affects. From this perspective there is no reason not to refer to the patient's anxiety by name and to assure him at the same time that as far as anyone can judge the continuity of the therapy is assured for quite a while.

The patient came to the next session in a fairly good mood, which was conspicuous. It had been a good week, at least for him. After he had made some introductory comments, I suggested that we continue with the hypnotic treatment. He could not concentrate and perspired, finally entering a trance and returning to kindergarten. Somewhere there were some other children, but he could not give more precise details. The teacher was nice. Simon Y saw himself in a sandbox, where he felt satisfied. He was not being teased.

After the hypnosis I asked him if he had not felt lonely playing in the sandbox while the other children were playing together. Simon Y gave me an amazed look and said, "Haven't you realized yet what a relief it was for me that the other children weren't bothering me? Being left alone was precisely what was nice. And the teacher wasn't bad either." He also told me that his mother had got rid of his little toy bears while he was in the home; "She didn't realize how important they were to me." I thought to myself that he had thus lost a transitional object.

At the end of the next session I gave him a small package containing a small toy bear and said, "It's not the same as you used to have, but maybe you will like it anyway." Simon Y beamed from one ear to the other when I gave him the package. He did not open it and silently left for home.

This week went very well for him, and his headache went away after a half a day of quiet. He told me how much he had enjoyed getting the little toy bear. "What a wonderful gesture that was." Then we returned to hypnosis, and this time he entered a fairly deep trance very quickly, a present for me. At first he was silent for a while, but then he became increasingly tense, swallowed several times, looked around anxiously, and said that he had previously not known that he had been sent to Amsterdam. He was just told, "It will be good for you to be together with other children." He now said that his mother and a social worker from the foundation supporting war victims had accompanied him to Amsterdam. Then he cried again for a long time. "How could my mother do this to me? She didn't know better, but as my mother she should have understood me." He added that every inmate in a jail was better off than he had been because the inmate knows what he has done. Simon Y had not known why his mother had sent him away. At the home he had learned to be disobedient.

During the hypnosis there was a catharsis, and afterward I asked him if he had later ever spoken with his mother about this terrible time. His decisive answer was, "No. That was completely impossible. Mother would have been mad if I had wanted to talk about it." Since then he had given up the idea of talking about it with her.

At the end of this session Simon Y asked me if I agreed that we could now proceed without hypnosis. He said that not very much new material was appearing, and he had now learned to overcome his shyness and talk with me frankly. I agreed, adding that we could still try hypnosis again if he wished.

Consideration. Giving the patient the little bear was an unusual intervention. I had of course thought for a long time about whether I should do it and whether I was buying the patient's affection. I finally did it because I thought that it was a good idea for the patient to have a visible and clear sign of my presence and my involvement, especially since the treatment could only take place once a week. The further course of the treatment showed that my assumption was correct. The therapeutic relationship was strengthened considerably, which in turn had a clear influence on the therapeutic process.

Third Phase of Treatment

Simon Y was feeling much better. He raised the question of whether his frequent outbursts of crying during hypnosis had been a revival of his earlier suffering or an abreaction. I answered that it was probably both.

After the Easter break he told me once more about his youth, this time in particular that he had not had a father, and also about all his feelings of powerless and humiliation. In the next session he spoke about his pedophiliac behavior, saying that he found adult men repulsive and did not know how to act toward women. He preferred 15- to 16-year-old boys because a relationship with them was not binding. It was impossible for him to establish a firm tie. Yet he also regretted the fact that the boys all grew older, ceased to be interesting to him, stopped exciting him, and usually went their own ways. It was a disappointment built into such relationships. He then raised the question again of the sense of life "on this lonely star." I let him tell me a lot about himself, not making any interpretations and only asking questions to keep him talking. The topic of the following session was his passivity. He said he was able to do nothing for days, got terribly bored, and became tired very quickly. At times he would get very angry with himself, but was unable to understand why. Nonetheless, in the meantime he had registered himself for an athletic project where he lived. He had done it in such a way, however, that nothing could come of it. I told him about the possibility of kinesitherapy and asked him what he thought of the idea that I register him for it. He reacted unexpectedly positively, saying that it appeared to him to be a good thing to do.

Just one week later he asked whether there was any news about the kinesitherapy. He said he had had the idea that he had to organize his life differently, that things could not continue as they had, and that nothing was free either. During one of our first sessions I had told the patient that it would be good if he got more exercise and that his dog was bound to enjoy it, too. It was easy to see that the patient was not in good condition. He told me that he had walked and cycled a lot in the last few days, leaving him suffering from muscle aches. He was so isolated from others that it was impossible for him to bear permanent company. And he was angry once again that his life was wasting away so senselessly. Then he mentioned a new factor. He had had a conflict with the municipal administration, having been given a reminder to pay his dog tax, which he found completely unfair. Simon Y complained bitterly about the bureaucrat's unfairness. But then a miracle happened. Completely by surprise, he had received a letter from the city informing him that because of the special situation he was being freed of the obligation to pay the dog tax. Simon Y was happy about his victory, but at the same time said that he was not really concerned with the tax, just with getting his way.

My assumption that winning this conflict would strengthen his self-esteem turned out to be an illusion. In each of the following two sessions Simon Y complained that he felt lonely, that his situation was hopeless, and that everything was senseless. He had received news that he could move into a small new apartment at the beginning of July, but he reacted ambivalently to it as well. "There's no purpose left." His attraction to the boys grew stronger and stronger. "Nothing works any more; there's just misery and frustration." Although I had just been informed that he could soon start the kinesitherapy, I did not say anything about it in this session.

Consideration. I had the impression that I would only have given him some superficial consolation by telling him about the kinesitherapy and would actually disturb his efforts to solve his conflict. In addition, the summer vacation period was approaching, and it seemed a good idea to me not to give him the good news until shortly before the summer break.

In the next session I told him that he could start the kinesitherapy after the summer break. Simon Y replied, "If you had told me that a year ago, I wouldn't have accepted. I wouldn't have believed it would happen. Today I intend to continue." Afterwards he told me about a dream in which he was in prison and felt sullen and completely indifferent. It was at this point that he told me for the first time in detail what had happened when he committed his crime.

Consideration. I thought that his dream reflected his real situation, being alone, especially prior to vacations, but I still thought it was too early to offer an interpretation, especially considering the approaching summer break.

Simon Y asked what I was doing during my vacation. He had imagined something like Nepal, a safari in a reserve in Africa, or at least one of the Caribbean islands. I told him that I would spend my vacation in an ordinary mountain village in south Tirol, and gave him my address. Simon Y did not have any plans himself. How should he have any? Just some hazy idea about driving far away into the Sahara desert, together with his dog, in his old delivery van. At the end of the session he told me, "Don't worry about me, I'll get over the long gap in good shape."

Fourth Phase of Treatment

Simon Y was lethargic when he came to the first session after the summer break. He was not at all inclined to move into a new apartment. After remaining silent for a while he told me that he had met a 14-year-old boy about four weeks ago. The boy attended a school for children who were emotionally disturbed and had learning difficulties; Simon Y described him as being very sensitive and attached. The boy often spent the entire day with him, but they had not had any sexual contact yet, although the boy was seductive. We had a long talk about the pros and cons of such a sexual relationship with a minor. Simon Y was convinced that "If a boy wants this kind of thing, then it's a sign that he needs it, and then it couldn't be harmful." He himself referred to the legal difficulties; "If the boy were one year older, then the police would be more likely to look the other way." After Simon Y had raised the issue, I asked him whether he wasn't deterred by the risks associated with such a relationship. He answered spontaneously that he did think about them but that a person had to take some risks in life, and that in addition the boy had already had several experiences and would not say anything. Important for him was less the sexual contact than the tender feelings he felt toward the boy. He added, "But if he clearly leads me into having sexual contact, then I don't know if I can resist him."

Consideration. It was clear to me after this session that the therapeutic relationship was now secure enough for him to tell me about these things without being in the least afraid. At the same time I asked myself the question I had not asked the patient, namely if the fact that he had established ties to this boy was not a consequence of the summer break.

Several hours later Simon Y came into my office very excited. He had been threatened in his house by a group of older boys and managed to escape through the back door. In response to my questions he admitted that he had had sexual contacts to one of the boys several years ago, but that this boy now had a girl friend and was filled with hate toward Simon Y. We talked in detail about this being one of the risks of sexual contacts with younger boys, and I summarized: "The boys want adventure and sex, while you desire a relationship you cannot have with people your own age. The result is that you have diametrically different interests, and therefore such a relationship cannot offer you what you expect. And besides, it can only last a very short time." Simon Y said that this last point was especially important to him and that he shyed away from a longer-lasting relationship. Moreover, he said he could not act differently since pedophilia was inherited. I replied that we would continue talking about this topic later and that things were not as simple as he imagined. During the next two years we talked about this topic over and over again in different contexts.

I had the impression that the preliminary phase was completed after nine months of therapy and that the therapeutic relationship had been consolidated, permitting us to slowly enter the phase of analytic psychotherapy. It is usually impossible to clearly distinguish between the two phases, and this was true of this patient as well. The main result was that a fairly stable therapeutic relationship had been established and that the patient was ready to cooperate and was motivated. It was also important that the transition to analytic therapy took place as continously as possible and that nothing abrupt happened in treatment that came completely unexpected for the patient. It hardly deserves emphasizing that interpretations are always directed at the patient's experiencing and at his momentary understanding and insights.

The goal of the subsequent therapy had been defined, namely to give the patient the opportunity to find meaning in his life, which he had experienced to be senseless. The question that was always in the background was the degree to which he was "predisposed" to pedophilia. This case confirms our experience that an effective treatment of pronounced and fixed psychosexual disturbances is only possible within the framework of a comprehensive psychoanalytic therapy. Motivation, of course, plays a very special role in the therapy.

Summary of the Treatment

It is necessary to distinguish two periods in Simon Y's treatment. The first covered the period from August until October, the second from the end of February the following year until the conclusion of the period reported here in February a year later. Let me add that the treatment is still continuing.

Shortly after the beginning of the first phase the patient brought me a notebook containing his personal comments and asked me if I would be willing to read them during the next week. The primary topic of his comments was the story of the euthanasia of his dog, which had been incurably ill. To keep it from suffering, Simon Y had fed his dog the sleeping tablets he had saved "for an emergency." His notes revealed his intense emotions, his normal intellectual ability, and his state of neglect.

A topic that dominated the first period was his frequent crying. He began crying during the interviews after he had had a crying fit in one of his sessions of kinesitherapy. He viewed his crying as a sign of his inability, yet also felt a strong aggressive force within him, which he was afraid of. He requested hypnosis once again, in the course of which he had a crying fit, worse than anything he had experienced since the initial sessions. Conspicuous was the fact that the patient hardly cried any more after we had discussed the fit in the context of his most recent experiences. Other themes that frequently recurred were his loneliness and his inability to make social contacts. After this he made his first small and hesitating steps to make contacts; for example, he helped at a traffic accident and volunteered to help at an animal home. At the animal home he was turned down; he was very surprised, however, that he had accepted this rejection as something normal, not letting it affect his entire life. In this phase pedophilia was a secondary topic; occasionally Simon Y asked why it was that he found precisely these boys so interesting. Yet the time was not ripe to discuss this topic.

It came as a complete surprise to me when he announced in October that he wanted to end the therapy. He felt independent and strong enough to try to continue without therapy. He also mentioned that he had contacts to a commune that was ready to let him join. He was very impressed that there were people outside of therapy who accepted him for what he was; he could even bring his dog. He also asked whether he should get into contact again sometime, and I answered that I would be pleased to hear from him.

A few months later he called me, and it was more than a coincidence that he called at exactly the time he would have had a session. He told me that an acquaintance of his had committed suicide in an extremely dramatic way. He came the next day and gave me the impression of being calm and unexpectedly self-secure. He was very saddened by the suicide, yet was easily able to imagine what had happened since he himself used to have such thoughts for many years. He also made it clear that he no longer had such thoughts. Then he told me about the commune. Once in a while he had conflicts, but he was always able to talk about them. I had the impression that the head of the commune was rather authoritarian. Simon Y also mentioned the name of a girl who lived there, and after our conversation he seemed satisfied and returned to the group he lived with.

It was clear to me that the treatment had not been concluded; my impression was reinforced by the fact that the group he lived with seemed to exert more influence in the direction of dependence than of independence. After a few months Simon Y returned again. At first he was depressed by the fact that he had left the commune. He viewed this as a failure, and it was only after several weeks that he realized that it was a gain, not a loss. He had not given in to the pressure to submit to the others. This strengthened his self-confidence, even in some otherwise bleak sessions. At this point, therapy focussed entirely on his pedophilia. It was then time to offer the interpretation that he was looking for himself in the boys, that it was a matter of identificatory love, and that he admired them because they were - at least externally - the way he had previously wanted to be, namely independent, free, not tied down, and free of anxiety. He could see that his younger friends were psychosocially disturbed; he recognized that their behavior was almost exclusively subordinate to obtaining direct oedipal satisfaction, that they viewed others only as objects of gratification, and that they were not or not yet able to establish a permanent personal relationship.

Analyst's Concluding Commentary. At the time of this report, two questions are at the center of the interviews. First, why is it so difficult for Simon Y to free himself internally of these younger friends? And second, why does he have so much anxiety toward women? He rejects homosexual contacts. Finally it should also be mentioned that he has not had any sexual relationships to his earlier friends for a long time.

A lot has happened during Simon Y's therapy. In many regards he has changed in obvious ways, a fact that his acquaintances confirm with admiration. We both know that his therapy has not yet been completed. Its length depends on the specific goal we pursue in therapy.

6.2.3 *Adolescence*

The crises that occur in adolescence are signs of *new combinations* and *adjustments* (Freud 1905d, p. 208) that we today view, following Erikson, from the perspective of identity formation and the search for identity. Blos (1962, 1970) described other aspects as separation and individuation processes, while Laufer (1984) focused on the integration of sexuality. The adolescent has qualitatively new kinds of experiences with himself, his body, his parents, and last but not least in his search for people outside his family. These aspects are still being given too little consideration within the psychoanalytic theory of adolescence. The adolescent not only attempts to actively influence his enviorment, but in handling his conflicts also tests new strategies (see Seiffge-Krenke 1985; Olbrich-Todt 1984). It is in this context that Lerner (1984) referred to adolescents as the producers of their own development. These results of developmental psychology are important for the conceptualization of the treatment of adolescents because the technique and goal of therapy have to be formulated in correspondence with the dynamics of development.

In diagnosing neurotic disturbances in adolescence it is necessary to remember that the adjustments expected of adolescents can be avoided, blocked, distorted, or delayed for numerous reasons. The disappearance of traditional initiation rites in modern civilization isolates adolescents or leads to a new kind of group formation. As a result the familiar ambivalences, shifts in mood, and polarizations are manifested in particularly strong forms. The adult world loses its sense of being ideal, and the adolescent searches for new role models. Rebellion and admiration quickly trade places, and the therapist is usually viewed very critically as being an agent of parental and social norms. Frequently there are excessively strong desires for autonomy, which make it more difficult for an adolescent to accept the advice and help of an adult.

Problems of therapeutic technique even begin with a patient's increased inclination for self-observation, which, in the form of a disposition to reflect, is actually a desirable precondition for therapeutic work. Is it not inevitable that the adolescent who both observes himself more and yet also isolates himself would resist our offer to examine together the world of his thoughts and emotions - regardless of the nature of the disturbance? The analyst is thus not justified in automatically interpreting in a traditional manner the skepticism the adolescent brings to therapy, especially since the pubertal insecurity previously linked with sexual maturation is today given a different meaning and is expressed in various ways.

The other aspect of an adolescent's concern with himself is his craving to gain experience. The purpose of this craving is, admittedly, not primarily to turn away from thoughts and emotions. This is another of the traps awaiting therapy, for the analyst should not discredit this craving for experience as acting out. The adolescent's primary goal is to act and gather experiences to expand his still incomplete self-esteem. Self-observation and the craving for experience thus form the two poles of an adolescent's all-encompassing wish to experience himself and the world. Erikson (1968) has especially described the significance of *experiencing* for the resolution of developmental crises in adolescence.

The cardinal question is whether and how the relationship between the adolescent and analyst can be employed as a "means to a end" in order to facilitate changes without getting too entangled in the complications posed by repeated transferences. Blos (1983) considered transference in adolescence the vehicle of a blocked development, calling transference in the therapy of adolescents two-sided. By reviving infantile positions and transferring aspects of self and object representations to the analyst, the old versions are actively remodelled via transference, creating a new revised version. The question is how the transference should be interpreted when adolescents use regressions for neurotic reasons to block the processes of development and separation. The reverse is also true. The transference wishes directed toward the therapist contain the danger of reviving traumatic experiences and are therefore warded off. This is the reason that it is important for the analyst here - in contrast to analyses of adults - *not* to put himself at the center of the transference at the beginning and sometimes even not for a longer period of time. By offering rigorous interpretations of the regressive components of transference, the analyst would take the place of the real parental figures and actually impede the separation. One of the paradoxes of the therapeutic situation is the occasionally very rapid manifestation of intense emotional reactions, which usually reflect some justified intense anxiety about the revival of infantile positions of dependence. It is therefore very important to induce a we-bond, as first described by Sterba (1929), as was attempted, for instance, by Aichhorn (1925) and Zulliger (1957).

The adolescent requires more than just insight into defense mechanisms in order for the blocked process of development to resume. His desire for the analyst to be a person to help him out of his deadend has to be understood to be an expression of phase-specific endeavors, for he would otherwise remain anchored in unconscious infantile expectations. The analyst's task is to differentiate between past and present, inner and outer worlds, and transference and real relationship in the analytic situation. The patient's utterances are properly freed of infantile residues if the analyst's examination of them allows for phase-specific desires as well as repressed infantile wishes (Bürgin 1980).

The issue from the very beginning is to structure the analytic situation so that the adolescent can use it as a sphere for making discoveries. The goal is to achieve a balance between *discovery* and *disclosure.* It is more than an anxiety about passivity and regression that prompts adolescents to want to transform the analytic situation into a *real* one. One meaning of their wanting advice from the analyst, desiring to know what the analyst is thinking or feels, and their attempts to provoke him into making emotional reactions is that they are attempting to attribute the analyst a human existence and thus to prevent him from becoming an omnipotent and anonymous figure. The adolescent does not primarily want to identify with the analyst to become similar to him, but wishes to distinguish himself and thus experience his own identity.

The preconditions for the course of analysis are created in the initial phase of therapy, when it is essential that the patient gain insight into the particular nature of the analytic situation as a place where discoveries can be made. Much depends on the therapist's ability from the beginning both to develop an understanding of the fears that his adolescent patient really has and to keep an eye on the fact that he has come to receive help. The younger the patient, the more important the real relationship at the beginning; transference can develop out of it gradually, depending on how the analyst acts toward his patient. It could be said that the adolescent first has to determine how and for which purposes the analyst can be of help to him.

Example

The parents of Otto Y, who was 18 years old, had scheduled an appointment for their son because he had been collecting old shoes for about three years. At his parent's urging he had taken part in a group therapy 18 months before, and as a result of this therapy, which had only lasted six months for reasons beyond his control, he had become more outgoing and felt less dejected. Yet there had been no change with regard to his "shoe problem." Since I had this information before the initial interview, Otto Y was justified in assuming that I knew the reason he was coming. He was a tall young man who was very friendly but somewhat embarrassed when we met; he even bowed. To keep his embarrassment from becoming too great, I said to him that he probably knew that I had been told about his shoe problem and asked him to tell me what he himself thought about it. He responded by putting his problem out into the open: "I'm in love with shoes." This opening remark baffled me, yet I also thought it was very clever. He had cleverly managed to overcome the embarrassment of the situation and at the same time put me to a test. He wanted to know whether I, just like his parents, wanted to take the shoes away from him and to normalize him. I said, "I can imagine that it isn't always easy to be in love with shoes."

He then began to tell me the story of his shoes. He said he had collected shoes since he was a boy, but only shoes without shoestrings. He said he objected when his mother wanted to throw shoes away. His collecting had intensified about three years ago, and he also looked for shoes that people had discarded. At this point he did not mention the fact that shoe collecting also had a sexual signifance for him. He told me that he sometimes thought he was homosexual, because he did not have any feelings for girls. It became clear, in contrast, that shoes exerted a very decisive influence on his inner and his external worlds. While he did his home work he often had to think of shoes and lost his concentration. Yet there were also areas in which he functioned well; for example, he liked to paint in his free time.

The longer I listened to him, the more I noticed how well-behaved and willingly he related his anamnesis. Although it was possible for me to surmise something of his own unrest, the rather fluent manner in which he presented his report made me keep my distance. I therefore told him that he had told me a lot about himself, but that I still had the impression that there was something else that disturbed him more than the problems he had mentioned. He was silent a moment before telling me a little about his earlier therapy. In hindsight, he said that this therapy surely had helped him because he was less depressed, but there had been no change in his shoe problem. I then managed to show him that he was afraid of talking about his shoes with me as long as he had the impression that he was only coming to please his mother. I then referred to his parent's expectations; when they scheduled the appointment I had learned that they wanted at all cost to come to speak to me. I assumed that he knew about this, and therefore told him that he probably wanted to be present at this talk because he would like to know whether I let myself be influenced by their expectations. He would surely want to use the talk to find out what my attitude was to his shoe problem. We did not schedule a date for the beginning of therapy to let him make a decision about further talks.

Commentary. Whether it is necessary to talk with the parents of adolescents at the beginning of psychoanalytic treatment must be decided on a case by case basis. Contact to the parents is generally problematic if the adolescent seeks therapy himself because the consequence might be a breach of confidence. A discussion with the parents is also not necessary in the case of older adolescents if the latter have achieved a satisfactory degree of outward independence. If the analyst has decided to see the parents, then he should hold this talk in the presence of the adolescent patient. We recommend in such cases that the analyst not offer any interpretations about the dynamics of the family ties that they mention, but to restrict himself to learning something about the family's past and present situation.

During the family appointment Otto Y was a passive but attentive observer of what happened. In contrast to his mother, who had tears in her eyes when she talked about the shoe problem, his father did not seem particularly irritated. I was able to follow the roots of the still close ties between mother and son back to his childhood. In the period until Otto Y started school, Mr. Y was very busy in his carreer. I also obtained valuable information about the beginning of the shoe collecting. At the time Mrs. Y had been very worried about her older daughter, who had a serious illness that made a life-threatening operation necessary. She probably had felt very alone with her needs. It was likely that, in consolation, her son meant something special to her. This had obviously impeded Otto Y's separation from the family during adolescence. The occasionally fierce exchanges between mother and son were not only an indication of the separation difficulties, but they seemed to provide a disguised incestuous gratification, with which Otto Y secretly triumphed over his father and his world. At the end of our conversation I pointed out that Otto Y had used the shoes to build up a world of his own that was out of bounds to his parents. Something similar also applied to therapy. I added that if Otto Y decided to start therapy, then it would not be easy for them as his parents to accept the fact that they could not participate in it.

At his next appointment Otto Y acted as if the family conversation had never happened. In doing so he showed me that he knew how to cleverly avoid disagreeable situations by constructing two worlds for himself, a world of external events and his inner world that he attempted to make inaccessible for others. He was thus able to avoid conflicts in himself and in his contact with his role models. It also became clear that he had already decided in favor of therapy, yet he remained reserved and cautious. It was still his goal to find out whether I would interfere in his own personal affairs after all. He chose a topic that was particularly well suited for this, namely telling me that he wanted to be a conscientous objector but that he had not yet made up his mind entirely. And glancing at me, he said he would turn to somebody who should be able to help him for advice. There was a trace of his anxiety that it might turn out that he was really homosexual. It was easy to recognize his intention. He wanted to know how I would react to the topic "homosexuality," and mentioned further details intended to provoke me into showing my interest in homosexual experiences by asking follow-up questions. Two years earlier he had met a student in a recreational camp, which had stirred him very much. He had admitted his shoe problem for the first time to this student and later taken his advice to attend the group therapy.

It was impossible to overlook his anxiety about homosexual transference wishes. This anxiety had two aspects. On the one hand, it disturbed him that I left the opportunity open for him to find out if he wanted to be homosexual; on the other hand, he was anxious that I would try to "normalize" him in accordance with his parent's expectations. In order to keep the psychoanalytic interview open as a place for him to make his own discoveries, I told him that he wanted to know whether he could talk about everything with me here, including about his homosexuality, to clarify who he was and how he wanted to develop in the future. In doing so I asked him to accept a frustration, in that it was obvious that he was looking for immediate help to make a decision both with regard to the question of being a conscientious objector and to the possibility that he was homosexual.

Moreover, he also showed me how insecure he still felt about making his own decisions. It seemed as if he wanted to check if I would really react differently to his anxieties than his father-Otto Y felt his father had let him down - and than his mother - who interfered too much.

Otto Y now began to tell me about his more "normal" conflicts. He was having problems at school; for instance, he had to be tutored in mathematics and he even had the feeling he was worse than the others in art class, his favorite subject. The world of shoes offered him refuge. While doing his school work he often thought about how he could get the next pair of shoes. At the same time he felt the anxiety that he might be discovered by someone else or that his parents might observe him sitting at his desk with a pair of old shoes. At this point it was important that I show him how he suffered from being different than other adolescents his age. I interpreted his longing to be able to live like other adolescents who did not need any therapy, and linked his ties to the shoes with his ties to his parents, especially to his mother. He was afraid that he might offend his mother by openly admitting his passion for shoes instead of keeping it a secret. I therefore told him that he hoped that I would see both apsects, the one in him that was attached to his shoes and his mother, as well as the one that was seeking a way to separate himself and to go his own way.

At first this interpretation intensified the emotional tension in him. The more he opened himself to therapy, the more difficult it became for him to speak with me. His anxiety about feeling ashamed moved to the forefront, while he became franker toward his parents, even daring to mention for the first time that he went looking for discarded shoes. And he admitted to me that he liked to take the old shoes to bed, which made his parents feel disgusted. At the same time he denied that his passion for shoes had any sexual significance and pretended to be ignorant. For example, he claimed to have heard the word "masturbation" recently for the first time and not known what it meant. This was a sign to me not to attempt quickly to make the sexual quality of his shoe fetishism a theme.

It was not until much later that I learned that he had attempted for a while to masturbate with his old shoes, but had given up because he did not have an orgasm because of delayed ejaculation.

The fact that the periods of silence became longer stimulated the tendency in me to force my way into him by asking insistent questions. He apparently developed very intensive ideas about me, accompanied by corresponding resistance. My curiosity to inquire about the details of his fetishism made me realize that he both wanted to provoke me into overreacting and seemed to expect that I would free him of the burden of the hard work on this theme. For the patient, I was the expert who, in contrast to his parents, did not get disgusted and was able to listen to everything. My growing curiosity made it clear to me that I was supposed to assume the role of a clandestine fetishist. By making allusions and hesitating, he was attempting to make me eager to know more about his world of shoes, and he was apparently able to better control his excitement and the situation. It would nonetheless have been premature for me to refer to this regressive transference dynamic. It was much more appropriate to interpret his ambivalence toward me because it offered him protection against regression. I therefore picked up the idea that I was the expert for whom the patient was merely an unusual case, and told him that this idea represented his attempt to protect his private world of shoes from me and to keep me at a distance.

This interpretation seemed to be criticism, resulting from a disappointment I had experienced and was unable to recognize until later. Although I knew how sensitive precisely this patient must be to such ideas of adults, however well meant they were, I was still offended that he responded to my transference interpretations by saying "Oh, my oh my." Whenever I attempted to show him how he experienced the therapeutic situation, he felt forced into a corner "by these allusions to the situation," as he referred to them. "I don't have the vaguest notion what I should say." Gradually a little game developed. He said he was anxious that I might tear him to pieces if he told me more about himself – just to respond to my next interpretations by saying, in an offended and accusing tone, "oh, my oh my" again.

I came to understand this "oh, my oh my" as an expression of his anxiety that I would use the transference interpretations to talk him into accepting my view of things, thus undermining his independence, which was instable as it was. To have to recognize how insecure and uncertain he was would have been even more shameful than for other adolescents. After I was able to show him how he was putting me to the test by saying "oh, my oh my," to determine whether I would react by being offended or whether I would take it as an offer with which he indicated how difficult it was for him to face his inner contradictions, he began to speak more and more about how critically he acted toward himself.

His own values led him to condemn his passion for shoes, which he was only able to maintain by splitting it off from his everyday life. He therefore resisted my interpretations relating what he tried to keep apart.

Otto Y feared that the therapy might destroy his freedom to have alternatives. There were a number of examples of his anxiety about making up his mind. For instance, at the beginning of treatment he had expected me to advise him in deciding for or against military duty because he was actually innerly incapable of making up his mind. The same was true of his decision as to painting with oil or water colors; I had told him that "There are two sides. You desire to be clear and decisive, but are at the same time anxious. There is something grand in keeping alternatives and not having to make up your mind. This is the reason you're resisting me, because you fear that I'll take something away from you by forcing you to make up your mind." He agreed, but added the objection that he really wanted my advice and felt left alone when I did not give any. The goal of his desire for advice was to prevent a conflict with his inner world and to keep his anxiety about being ashamed in check, which was becoming stronger and stronger. He turned red when I told him, after a fairly long period of silence, that he apparently now felt that I was demanding that he unveil the thoughts he was ashamed of. He said he was afraid because he had no idea where the therapy might lead. I discovered that there was a concrete reason for this statement, learning that the sessions aroused him to such a degree that he would walk the streets and look at shoes. He had recently seen shoes that had fascinated him very much.

I thought this was an indirect reference to my shoes, and felt that he would have to feel ashamed and resist my discovering this connection instead of leaving it up to him to make this discovery himself. My request to reschedule one session created just such an occasion; in the following I give excerpts of the protocols of two sessions, which I wrote from memory immediately after the sessions. The rescheduled session began with ten minutes of silence, which was unusually long for this patient.

P: At home I've misplaced a list of adverbs and searched everywhere for it.

A: Perhaps it's not a coincidence that you mention this list just now because here you often try desparately to find the right word.

P: Oh, my oh my, overinterpreted once again. That just fits the cliché of the psychoanalyst. I mean something entirely superficial, and you immediately assume something at a deeper level.

A: You are convinced that I constantly want to learn more about your passion for shoes and don't even realize that right now we are talking about rescheduling a session, something that might make you angry you because you have to do as I request.

P: Yes, I was a little angry and had the feeling that you are deciding for me. But now everything has been decided.

A: So that we shouldn't concern ourselves with your anger at all.

P: At home I'm sometimes pretty angry at my parents. Often it's just some feeling inside, but sometimes I'm desparate and cry, for example when my mother criticizes me because I've misplaced something. It happens quite often, and then she complains that I'm unreliable.

A: And you often feel as if you have to cry here when you feel I'm pressuring you.

P: Yes, sometimes I do. The point is that you are not supposed to be just my psychoanalyst, but an average person, so that I can maintain my dignity.

I had to think about the word *Verlegen*, used in German both for *rescheduling* the session and for misplacing the list of adverbs. I wondered about how he used "oh, my oh my" to resist becoming dependent on me in the same way as on his mother. He thus also had to protest against transference interpretations that mobilized his regressive desires and conflicted with his desire to be separate. He offered me the following figure for a relationship: He was looking for a list of adverbs that he had misplaced, his mother demanded that he be neat and complained to him because by misplacing it he eluded her control. With regard to transference this meant that he feared I could adopt the role of a demanding mother figure who expected to be told about everything and whose interpretations destroyed his freedom to choose, undermining his own initiative. On the other hand, by putting me in this role he was able to avoid the conflicts with himself, his affects, and his fantasies by insisting that everything be taken concretely. Yet then there was the danger that we would get caught up in a vicious circle of accusations and counteraccusations. Thus it was necessary for me to make his part in transference clear to him. By returning to the idea that I was supposed to be just an average person, he referred to the fact that he felt embarrassed in my presence. He was embarrassed, in part, because he always felt insecure about how much he could reveal about himself without putting himself at the mercy of his own regressive desires. It was therefore also important for him to be able to determine the time at which he would open himself to me. Consequently, at the end of the session I referred to the fact that rescheduling the session had apparently reinforced his anxiety that he could lose his control of himself and of me. He replied that this made him feel very embarrassed, so that he was no longer sure whether he still wanted me to grasp what was going on in him. He saw me as a psychoanalyst who overinterpreted everything.

Otto Y arrived for his next session exactly one hour too early. Since he never waited in the waiting room, but always knocked on my door at precisely the right time, it was impossible for him to have noticed his confusion. After he had remained silent for a while, I opened the session by asking him whether he had noticed that he had come too early. At first he was certain that he had not confused anything, before becoming hesitant.

P: Oh, my oh my, then I must have really confused it with Friday's session.

A: "Oh, my oh my," you otherwise only say it when I tell you something that you resist.

P: Yes. [Longer pause]

A: Before you go any further, we first have to find out what ideas you have about what I should do so that you will come to feel secure enough again.

P: [Intensely] Well, everything I say disappears in the back of your head, and I have no idea what you do with it. Second, we don't have a goal here, not even a preliminary one, and third, I'm afraid that I'll lose the last rest of my dignity and self-respect when I'm here although I would like you to help me maintain my self-respect. But we talked about this in the last session too.

A: In the last session you apparently had the feeling that you might lose your self-respect.

P: [Confused] What actually happened? Just now I can't recall. So much has happened in the meantime, I was at a birthday party, there was a music festival, and yes, now you're certain to begin wondering why I can't remember it any more.

A: It's becoming clear to me how difficult it is for you to switch from the one world to the other each time. Here's everyday life, and here's therapy, where we talk about your shoes. [The patient interrupted me before I could continue.]

P: And here I'm always reminded of your shoes. [He smiled while he said this.]

A: Precisely, and then you have the desire to possess them.

P: In end effect, yes, when you stop wearing them some time. [Long pause]

A: At any rate it's clear that you're struggling against always being reminded of it.

P: Because I'm afraid that I'll let down and won't achieve as much. And there are two things I haven't told you yet. Since I was small I've had the problem that the thought that animals are killed to get leather is repulsive. And I think this is the reason I can't throw shoes away. And besides, it's extremely difficult for me to talk with a person wearing shoes that I like. A physical attraction develops. But if the shoes don't suit my taste at all, then it's even more difficult to start a conversation with the person wearing them. Your shoes have something that's very important – they don't have any shoe strings.

A: I think you're not only talking about shoes but about a longing linked to the shoes. Being very close to someone is the issue. And if I wear shoes that both of us like, then I come so close to you that for this very reason it's difficult for you to talk to me.

P: While you were just saying that, I had an unpleasant-pleasant feeling that went deep inside me. [While leaving, he added] At any rate I won't forget today's session.

This session marked an important step toward consolidating the working alliance. Otto Y had secretly included me in his world of shoes some time previously without being able to talk about it. My shoes had both excited him and frustrated him. Since he had become increasingly fascinated by them and them alone, he felt himself becoming increasingly dependent and was ashamed of it. He viewed the rescheduled session and the fact that he had come too early for the following session as embarrassing indications of how reliant he had become on me. To have admitted all of this to me would apparently have meant to him that there would not be any borders between us any more and that I would have complete control of him. By raising the question that we would first have to find out what I could do to help make him feel secure again, I gave him the opportunity to attack me and distinguish himself from me. And by stating that everything disappeared into the back of my head and that we did not have a goal that would distract him from shoes, he referred again to his anxiety that he might be completely dependent on me, making him lose all self-respect. He showed me how he lived at two levels and had already begun to exclude me from his world of shoes. He drew a boundary between his two worlds, and switched from one to the other; although this isolated him, in this way he was able to continue enjoying the satifactions offered by his shoe world. By asking him how disturbing it was to switch back and forth between these two worlds, of his shoes and of everyday life, I gave him the opportunity to let me take part directly in his world of shoes, opening it for a moment and thus integrating a little of his split off world. He both admitted something he had previously kept for himself and also partially identified with me. By making it clear to him that I wore this pair of shoes because *I* liked them, it became possible for him in this session to confront the conflict between his longing for physical closeness (the reason he wanted to possess my shoes) and his desire for separateness (the reason I should not give him my shoes but resist his desires). He began to let himself have insights into his unconscious conflicts, which was closely connected to the experience he had with himself and with me in this session. In this sense, this session can be considered a turning point in this therapy. Otto Y began to recognize that the issue was not his shoes in a concrete sense, but what they meant, for example his desire for closeness and his anxiety that this closeness would amount to self-sacrafice. In the further course of this therapy, the patient began saying "hum" instead of "oh, my oh my" in response to interpretations he felt touched by. The "hum" left him the alternative of either telling me why he saw something differently, or beginning to work with. He stopped experiencing my interpretations to be interference, and instead took them to be tools with which he himself could work.

Commentary. To determine the conditions under which Otto Y's fixation for this fetish developed, it is necessary for his fascination with the world of shoes to be retransformed into the story of the conflicts related to the unconscious fantasies and pleasureable desires that he originally had toward a role model and that he tried to express indirectly in the fetish. It is also necessary to start from the biographical fact that this patient had lived in two worlds since before he turned 3 years old. He lived in and with his fascinating fetish, which was a symbol that indirectly expressed all of his fantasies, imaginary thoughts, and illusions and which probably originated out of various transitional objects. Nonanimate objects, which do not have any disturbing activity of their own, are very well suited because there are practically no limits on someone using them as the object onto which all imaginable conscious and unconscious fantasies are projected. Separated from an individual's personal development and from interpersonal relationships, a fetish finally also becomes a sexual object in the narrow sense of the word. The fascination that certain shoes can exert demonstrates the immensity of man's imagination. Yet even it cannot ignore the fact that shoes can be beautiful, ugly, attractive, or repugnant. It is noteworthy that the patient suffered from knowing that his love was directed at an object that was only available to him because an animal had been killed. The leather was an unconscious reminder to him of the killing of a living being, i.e., of aggression and destruction. It is instructive that the patient was only fascinated by shoes that were closed while all shoes with holes for shoe strings belonged in a negative group and even exerted a disturbing sensation. It is possible that the patient unconsciously took the holes to be a mar that, according to the displacement of perception onto the smallest detail, reminded him of every kind of injury and destruction. Closed shoes reestablished an unblemished world, yet one that was burdened with guilt, i.e., with the killing of animals.

It must furthermore be noted, regarding the psychodynamics in this case, that the patient's fear of possibly becoming homosexual - precipitated by his close friendship with a university student in whom he had confided - was another sign of his tie to the fetish, which inhibited his development. This tie apparently completely restricted his freedom for heterosexual contact and led to an absence of pubertal changes, disturbing both to him and to others.

This description of the psychodynamics, intentionally kept very general, integrates many important points of the psychoanalytic theory of fetishism and yet does not preclude any possibilities about what might occur in the course of therapy. The symptom formation was able to ward off conflicts from both the oedipal and the preoedipal phases of development (Freud 1927e, 1940a, p. 203; Greenacre 1953; Stoller 1985).

If we attempt to identify the common denominator of the views of different authors on the psychodynamics of fetishism, we discover that these views are focused, on the one hand, around pregenital and androgynous desire, and on the other, around the themes of controlling and exerting power. The fetish that is later sexualized frequently originates from a transitional object; the intensive satisfaction and security provided by the fetish is associated with this transitional object. As a result, therapy first leads to a disturbance because the patient's anxiety that the analyst will take away the object with which his entire happiness and feeling of security is associated. Although the analyst in this case was aware of this problem and made an effort not to appear as an agent of the patient's parents whose goal was to normalize him and take away his fetish, he still got into a dilemma that was closely linked with the development of transference. Especially with symptoms as in this case, there is an intense feeling of shame tied to the revelation of perverse practices. The patient was able to open himself step by step despite serious inner difficulties. In some instances, however, we can see that the analyst's interpretation of the patient's strategy to separate himself contained elements of criticism although his intentions were just the opposite. Thus the patient must have taken it to be unspoken criticism when the analyst offered the interpretation that he, the patient, wanted to keep all his options open instead of making up his mind and that he struggled against the analyst because the latter might take something away from him. This type of interpretation can be found very frequently, being made by well-meaning analysts who assumed that the patients would understand on their own that it was obvious that nothing would be taken away from them and that any anxiety that this might happen was unfounded. We recommend that the analyst, instead of suggesting that the patient realize that his resistance to transference is unfounded and give it up, examine the momentary genesis of the resistance together with the patient, i. e., that they look for the causes of the resistance in the here and now. In doing so, they must assume that the patient has good reasons for being disturbed. A good example can be seen in the passage of this patient's therapy in which he overcame his confusion. After the analyst had asked the patient for his opinion about what should happen so that he would again feel secure enough, the patient mentioned three points that have to be realized step by step in every analysis in order for it to reach a positive conclusion, i. e., achieve therapeutic change. Every patient is dependent on what the analyst thinks about him and where analysis is going, and the patient's self-respect is regulated by his relationship to the analyst. The comments that this analyst made about how difficult it was for the patient to switch from one world to the other sufficed to stimulate the patient to describe his transference fantasies about the analyst's shoes. In this unforgettable session the fetish became manifest in the transference neurosis. The analyst provided sufficient support in the process so that the working alliance was consolidated. Of course, this merely established some common ground, i. e., a similarity in taste regarding shoes. The task then became to work with the patient to develop positions at other levels that could lead out of the fetish. Such a tight "shoe" can only be overcome if the individual already has one foot somewhere else.

6.3 The Patient's Family

As we explained in Vol.1 (Sect. 6.5), it is necessary for the analyst to act toward the patient's family in a manner in accordance with medical ethics, which includes maintaining discretion. This sounds less rigorous if we say, along the same lines, that the analyst is bound to serve the patient's best interests. It is the goal of every psychoanalytic therapy to promote the patient's autonomy. Since it thus automatically impinges upon ties the patient has already established, the consequences of psychoanalysis have always been significant for spouses and the couple (Freud

1912e). Under exceptional circumstances, e. g., if there is a psychotic illness or a serious danger of suicide, it is both legally unproblematic and medically necessary for the analyst to keep in contact with the patient's family and for a decision to be reached that is acceptable to all the parties. Yet there are also indirect ways in which the patient and analyst can involve or exclude absent third parties.

Before we turn to a few typical problems, we would like to describe treatments that transpire to everyone's satisfaction. There are several reasons for choosing this point of departure, one very important one being that in recent decades there has been too little awareness of the fact that the improvement or cure of a patient with a neurotic or psychosomatic illness is a process that, taken as a whole, provides the participants and everyone else concerned far more pleasurable moments than disturbing ones. Just to consider our experience in this regard since an earlier publication some 20 years ago (Thomä and Thomä 1968), we can see that one characteristic of therapies that are largely free of complications for the families is the fact that the changes the patient undergoes extend and enrich the *scope of family life.* An important precondition is that the relationship possess a viable basis that has been strained primarily by the neurotic symptoms of one of the partners. In a different situation, for example if the partnership originally developed on the basis of neurotic ties or has been sustained by them, changes in the neurotic equilibrium lead to substantial complications. The partner not in therapy naturally responds negatively, suffering, for example, from the fact that the partner who previously was dependent has become more autonomous and freed himself of his neurotic dependence.

Let us consider treatments that are free of complications more closely, starting from the one position that we believe is appropriate, namely a three-person psychology as elaborated by Balint. In the actual psychoanalytic situation this triad is abridged to a dyad, which we would like to refer to as a "triad minus one." The fact that the third person is absent, present only in the participants' thoughts and not in reality, has far-reaching consequences. The resolution of the dyadic and triadic conflicts that develop depends on all three parties. Keeping one's eye on the patient's own best interests may well permit the analyst to lend an ear to the patient's spouse, to allude to the apt title of an article by Neumann (1987). These metaphors are not intended to distract analysts from the responsibilities that follow from their clearly defined therapeutic task. To lend a ear to the patient's spouse means to us above all applying our psychoanalytic knowledge about triadic (oedipal) and dyadic (mother-child) conflicts in such a way that the individual patient attains autonomy compatible with a happy relationship. The goal of achieving a postoedipal heterosexual relationship is a guiding utopian fantasy, probably reflecting a deep-seated human longing that is apparently represented by the psychoanalytic pair. It is the object of envy and jealosy from without. On the other hand, the analyst, precisely during the development of transference, must also be aware of the voices of those outside therapy, even though he generally only hears these voices through the patient's mouth. This is the reason that members of the patient's family frequently assume that it is impossible for the analyst to obtain an accurate picture of what the patient is like in reality and how he really acts. This results in tensions, which however can be alleviated or defused. Each of the three participants can contribute to this, and the typology of complications depends on the attitude and behavior of each of party and on their interaction. Since we have described the typical constellations in Vol.1 (Sect. 6.5), we will now provide an example of how a spouse can be involved.

Our frankness about the consequences that analysis may have for a spouse has led us to pay special attention to whether, for example, patients use their spouses for negative transference. If the analyst pays attention to the types of transference, analyses are freer of complications and fewer family members express the wish to speak to the analyst. For therapeutic reasons we prefer the patient himself to provide his spouse sufficient information that the latter does not insist on satisfying a wish to speak to the analyst. It is a cause for concern if a patient completely excludes his spouse from his analytic experiencing. We therefore discourage analysts from recommending, as part of the basic rule, that the patient not speak with others about the analysis. Such a recommendation, which many analysts even used to give in the form of a commandment, only leads to unnecessary stress and is never completely obeyed anyway. It is all the more important for analysts to pay attention to what patients tell others regarding either what they have experienced in analysis or the analyst's comments. The masochistic component of many neurotic disturbances, including the tendency for patients to inflict an unconsciously motivated injury on themselves, is another reason it is essential to pay attention to the manner in which patients let their spouses participate, or keep them from participating.

A Case of Possible Suicide

In the analysis of Martin Y, who suffered from compulsive symptoms, there was a manifest danger of suicide that was situational in nature, in this case being resticted to marital conflicts that hardly ever rose to the surface. The result of the equilibrium that had developed in his marriage was that each party avoided emotional involvement with the other. In a typical expression of turning aggression against himself, the patient thought more frequently about suicide, which he kept a secret from his wife. In analyzing transference I was not able to interrupt this development. Patterns of interaction that the patient had acquired since childhood were repeated in his five-year-old marriage. His wife had partially taken the place of his mother, and the patient retreated into spiteful passivity, as he had done before his marriage; she did not have any idea that his symptoms were actually reinforced by her behavior, which was soothing and avoided insisting on clarifying differences. The approaching summer break caused me some concern because I feared that without therapy the unspoken tensions between the couple would grow, as would in parallel the risk of suicide. In this situation I made the recommendation that the three of us have a meeting. The patient was relieved. It turned out that his wife had already wanted to turn to me because of her husband's isolation, but believed that she was not supposed to disturb the analysis.

In order to make the marital conflicts that reinforced the patient's symptoms and the three-person consultation presented below more comprehensible, I will first describe several particularly grave features of the patient's personality that were the determining factors behind his symptoms and behavior in private and in public. Martin Y had tried since his school days to function as unemotionally as possible, and thought he therefore seemed cold, arrogant, and funny. He led a constricted and withdrawn life, as if he were in a cage. He recalled that as a boy he had often said, "This is no way to live." Another noteworthy feature was that something in him only became alive after others became excited. This usually concerned situations in which a life was in danger. Most of all he would have liked to break out, run away, take his backpack, and emigrate to a foreign country to risk his own life. By referring to repulsive examples, his wife managed to make him give up his plans. But then he would think about other ways of breaking out. At work, where he was a model of orderliness and conscientiousness, he intentionally made gross mistakes, risking his job. He said he wanted to be fired.

During the first few months of his therapy, Martin Y caused an automobile accident, missed sessions, and came late. If he felt that I was worried, he livened up. He described how he had grown up in an environment void of emotion. His parents had led a withdrawn life after the death of his younger sister, and for many years he had felt accused of having caused her death. There had not been a chance for him to clarify anything by talking with his parents, which strengthened his idea that he was guilty - after all, he had once overturned his sister's buggy. He later discovered that she had died of a congenital disorder. And because on the day of the funeral he had run with delight toward an uncle who had come from far away and whom he had loved, his father had spanked him, which led Martin Y to have to stutter for some time.

Martin Y cried and felt liberated by being able to recall these memories from his childhood and talk about them. The proximity to his repressed aggression was made clear by sentences such as, "I only want to inhale because I'm afraid that something evil might come out when I exhale." He became able to mention one of his most frightening ideas, which had kept him from having intercourse with his wife for a long time, namely that he was afraid that he might fatally injure her in doing so. His wife's consolation helped him get over many things. He described her infinite patience that everything would take a turn for the good one day.

The patient had fewer compulsive ideas, anxieties, and impulses. I attributed this improvement to the fact that he had begun clarifying the background of his unconscious guilt feelings. Aggressive impulses had been repressed after the birth and death of his severely handicapped sister. Both verbalized and fantasized feelings of guilt, isolated from his experience with his sister, had led him to expect punishment. This expectation manifested itself over and over again throughout his life, tormenting him yet remaining imcomprehensible to him. It was the consequence of his unconscious guilt feelings, such as Freud (1916d) described for several character types.

One Sunday, just prior to a longer vacation break, Martin Y stayed in bed all day. He said his wife was not at home and he had dozed. Gradually he admitted that he had been making plans for committing suicide. Yet he had always come to a dead end because he was not able to decide whether he should get divorced first and then take his life, or whether he should act first. His wife was shocked when she returned that evening, but was apparently able to quickly regain her composure and distract and raise his spirits. Somehow they managed to patch everything up again, yet even after these tormentous hours there was no clarification.

It was after this event that the three of us met as agreed. Martin Y's wife said that her husband had become quieter and quieter. Often she did not know what to do. When she asked him a question, he would not answer; he would just let her hang. It was completely incomprehensible to her that he wanted to give up at work and still managed to appear happy. She said he was actually very conscientious, just as she was.

I said the point was now for us to clarify the situations that were incomprehensible to each of them, and to examine why he alternated between giving up or wanting to be fired, on the one hand, and, on the other, felt that he had to do everything to complete perfection. Martin Y, who had been silent until now, suddenly came live, saying it was indeed necessary to find a new solution. He claimed that everything would clear up after he gave up his profession to do something else. His wife immediately tried to talk him out this hopeful idea that gave him relief. She reminded him of friends who had flipped out and of the catastrophies that had happened, and demanded that he finally talk with them to find out for himself. Yet she was full of despair, she said, because he refused to do it; he would never talk. Then she began crying.

The patient sat sunken over his chair with his face, emotionless, turned away. After a while he said it was rediculous for her to talk this way and to dictate what he should do. She would say what to do, she would say what he should say and do. And somethimes she would kick him under the table to liven him up even more.

The cool manner in which he raised these accusations probably added to his wife's despair, prompting her to mention other complaints. She said that this was exactly the way things went at his parent's house. He did not say anything there either; he would, especially, simply not respond to his mother's questions. Then *she* answered for him because she felt sorry for his mother. He was outraged again, saying that when she started in this way, then it was impossible for him to do anything. It would be just the same when they went on an excursion and she would constantly say, "Look there, can't you see . . . there . . . and over there . . . how beautiful!" He had eyes of his own, after all. Then both of them had to laugh.

In this more relaxed moment I summarized that our conversation had followed the same course. *She* spoke, she answered, she was the first to show emotions, and she had to cry. It looked as if *she* had to speak, answer, feel, and cry for *him*. The wife interrupted me rather abruptly, saying that no, this was not the way she acted, but with time she had gotten to know him so well, she did not want to be this way, and it was impossible for her to be this way because she sometimes had no idea what was going on inside him. This was true, she said, especially when her husband blurted out terrible words. I remarked that this must make her anxious, particularly when he talked, as he had recently, about wanting to commit suicide. It was understandable that she then reacted so quickly and used all her strength to calm him down and distract him. Well, she responded, she often preferred that he talk like this instead of not saying anything. Of course it was better for him to say more about what he thought. She added that he had recently really pleased her. He had woke her in the morning, saying "Come on, get up! We can't arrive too late." He had been so decisive and had for once taken the initiative, making it really nice. She said she did not want to always be the lead dog, to make his decisions for him, and to have to tell him everything including which clothes he should put on. The patient became excited and interrupted her, telling us that he knew which clothes he should put on. Then *she* interrupted him, claiming he was like his mother; if someone told her "Put on your new dress, you look so good in it," she would start finding reasons not to - this, that, and everything would be wrong and she should have bought an entirely different dress, it was too warm and too expensive. Her husband would not say anything about how nice she looked in the dress. Nothing would be decided. Meals were the same. Although each of them knew exactly what he would like to eat, they could go on for ever. Neither of them would ever say what they wanted to eat. This made the patient angry. He said it was typical. His wife was fast to make a decision in everything. He said the point was now not to disregard others but to take their indecisiveness into consideration. He asked if it were not possible for her to try to understand what his reasons were. We went on to discuss this theme with regard to other everyday examples.

It was the first time that the couple had been able to talk openly with one another and think about their disappointments for a long time. Each of them promised to make an effort during their vacation to break this vicious circle of being silent, letting the other one play their role, and withdraw feeling enraged and not understood.

After the vacation break the patient said that our conversation had enabled them to become more willing to face conflicts. Another result was that the patient had experienced my behavior as taking his wife's side, because I had shown too much understanding for her anxieties instead of helping him clarify *his* anxieties. In transference I had protected his handicapped sister, and his negative mother transference now began to play a role in therapy. How often had his mother and sister taken sides against him! The patient became able to express his outrage and feel his aggression. Subsequently the patient felt less isolated and the risk of suicide decreased. It was possible to partially free the couple's relationship from the patient's acting out.

6.4 Third-Party Payment

Under the same heading in Vol.1 (Sect. 6.6) we described the general implications of third-party payment and, specifically, the principles according to which German compulsory health insurance programs cover expenses from analytic psychotherapy. In the meantime similar guidelines have been adopted in Germany by the private health insurance organizations and by the state in its subsidies of the health expenses of government employees. Thus it is now necessary for analysts in Germany to submit applications for payment for practically all of their patients to the appropriate health insurance body or government agency; these applications are then reviewed by peers with regard to the indications for psychodynamic or analytic psychotherapy. The guidelines of the compulsory health insurance programs (latest version from May 1990) differ, however, from the government subsidy policy with regard to the length of treatment. There are also differences between the various private insurance organizations. Internationally, the third-party payment is also gaining increased attention (Krueger 1986).

German psychoanalysts now have to file applications justifying their therapeutic approach according to the principles of the etiological theory of psychoanalysis. In these applications the therapist must make it plausbile to the reviewing analyst that the recommended treatment can lead to a alleviation, improvement, or cure of the patient's neurotic or psychosomatic illness or that it promotes the patient's rehabilitation. He must estimate the chances for change, i.e, make a prognosis. The purposes of these applications, which are submitted to reviewing psychoanalysts who then decide whether to *recommend* approval or continuation of analytic psychotherapy to the health insurance organization, are similar to those of diagnostic case conferences. It has to be demonstrated that the psychodynamic explanations are in agreement with the steps in therapy. Another purpose is to show how the patient reacts to the therapy, i. e., to describe changes in symptoms within the context of transference and resistance. The guidelines explicitly state that regression must be evaluated according to its therapeutic utility; the appropriate passage in the guidelines currently in force reads:

> Analytic psychotherapy refers to those forms of therapy that treat the material in the neurotic conflicts and the patient's underlying neurotic structure, together with the neurotic symptoms, and in the process initiate and promote the therapeutic activity with the help of the analysis of transference, countertransference, and resistance and of regressive processes.

This passage makes it apparent that the guidelines are oriented on a theory of therapy based on ego psychology. Applications for continued payment encounter no problems as far as "regression in the service of the ego" is necessary to master psychic conflicts in a manner that alters symptoms. Yet many analysts find it difficult to justify applications for continuance in the manner that Freud demanded for especially deep analyses. This is particularly true in those cases where therapy exceeds the customary length of time; Freud then linked etiological and therapeutic considerations and justified the different lengths of treatment by referring to the fact that although some problems and symptoms occur late in an individual's development, they can only be resolved therapeutically when their causes in the deepest layers of psychic development have been found. It is in this sense that the guidelines for the payment of analytic psychotherapy require a causal explanation. Regression for its own sake agrees with neither Freud's etiological principles nor his therapeutic ones. In this regard Baranger et al. (1983, p. 6) spoke of a widespread prejudice, arguing that retrospective attribution, one of the most important factors in Freud's theory, has been one of its victims (see Sect. 3.3). The fact that a "cause" does not acquire its causal force until much later and under the impact of subsequent events casts doubt on those theories that view the cause of later psychic and psychosomatic symptoms as lying in the earliest phase of development. Baranger et al. directed this criticism especially at M. Klein's theory. Such neglect of the causal significance of subsequent events is linked with a widespread tendency to consider "regression ... *in itself* the essential therapeutic factor." An analyst adhering to this understanding of therapy attempts to arrive at deeper and deeper levels of regression and encourages the patient to reexperience early, ideally his first, traumatic experiences. Baranger et al. referred to the illusion, which has been repeatedly contradicted by experience, that reaching archaic situations - whether as a result of drugs or of systematically favoring analytic regression - suffices to achieve progress. The examples of such experience that they mentioned are "the reappearance of the initial symbiosis with the mother, the birth trauma, the primitive relationship with the father, the paranoid-schizoid and depressive positions of suckling, [and] the outcroppings of 'psychotic nuclei.'" They explicitly emphasized "that re-living a trauma is useless if not complemented by working-through, if the trauma is not reintegrated into the course of a history, if initial traumatic situations of the subject's life are not differentiated from the historic myth of his origins" (p. 6).

Medical and scientific responsibility dictates that regression during analysis, i. e., charged by resistance and transference, be considered from the perspective of the *mastering* of conflicts. In our opinion, the concept of working through must also be subordinated to it, because otherwise illusory hopes are created and, under certain conditions, forms of dependence extending to malignant regression are created iatrogenically. Based on our experience as reviewers, a frequent indication of such a course is the disturbing statement in applications for continuation beyond 160 or 240 sessions that there is a danger of a relapse or even suicide if therapy were discontinued. Without wanting to dispute that such situations can arise even in an analysis that is properly conducted, we would like to summarize the essence of our experience both as practicing analysts and reviewers. It is therapeutically decisive that *malignant* regressions be prevented. In our opinion, the ego-psychological understanding of regression means that the best conditions are created in the analytic interview for helping the patient become able to master his conflicts. This includes coming to a realistic evaluation of one's life. To limit malignant regressions, we recommend that the analyst not lose sight of economic facts - an important element of the contact to reality-in the analysis of transference and resistance. In this sense the limitations on performance that the patient is familiar with can contribute to preventing malignant regressions. On the other hand, in some severely ill patients the limitations exert such pressure that neurotic anxieties increase. In our work it has always been possible for us to satisfactorily solve the problems that have resulted. As reviewers, we therefore frequently have the impression that there is a discrepancy between the disturbing statement of what might happen if therapy were discontinued within the periods set out in the guidelines, and the psychodynamic explanation of this condition according to logically comprehensible causal and prognostic criteria.

Application Procedure

We have chosen the following example for a number of reasons. The "report" that the physician conducting the analysis submitted to the reviewer for confirmation that the therapy conformed to the guidelines for insurance coverage, as well as his applications for continued payment were prepared before we decided to write this textbook or to include a description of a model case of an application for payment beyond the customary length of time. Thus the applications have not been fabricated extra for this purpose, and their size is, incidentally, not representative of such texts. This application for continued support is so comprehensive because the analyst filing the application had referred back to notes from a seminar on analytic technique. We profit from its unusual length, however, because it enables the reader to orient himself in detail about the course of the analysis.

In this case it was possible for the analyst to explain why treatment beyond the usual limitations on payment was justified etiologically and with regard to utility, economy, and necessity. Finally, it also lets us demonstrate particularly clearly what consequences the reviewing process has on the analytic process, i. e., on transference and resistance, which we cover in a separate section (Sect. 6.5). The choice of this example lets us, furthermore, save space and avoid repetition, because the coded case history, which is presented in detail under point 4 of the application form, is given in Sect. 8.2.1. Here we can avoid answering the question as to the information the patient provided spontaneously because several examples of the symptoms Arthur Y complained about can be located at other points in this text by referring to the index of patients. Moreover, it is especially important to provide as literal a reproduction of the patient's spontaneous comments as possible because the patient's complaints enable the reviewer to estimate his suffering and to relate them to the other points, particularly to the psychodynamic explanation of the illness.

The modalities of third-party payment are described in detail in Vol.1. To summarize them briefly, the patient who is a member of one of the compulsory health insurance organizations does not pay the fee directly and does not receive a bill. The fee per session is regulated, and furthermore, physicians and patients are not permitted to make separate financial arrangements. The situation is different with the relatively small group of patients who are voluntarily insured in one of these health schemes and who express the wish to be treated as a private patient. It is then permissable for the patient and analyst to negotiate the size of the fee, and it is the patient's task to turn to his insurance company for reimbursement of his expenses. Thus, here the analyst is not a contractual partner, via the physicians' association, of the health insurance organization. Yet even in this case it is necessary for the analyst to file an application for payment, in which he demonstrates that the indications and the severity of the illness conform to the guidelines, i.e., that an "illness" as defined by the insurance system does exist. An analysis for personal problems, for instance, is not covered by health insurance.

Arthur Y was a voluntary member in a public health insurance scheme and had taken out a supplementary policy to cover any additional fees. He was considered a private patient and the fee was agreed upon. Initially the fee was DM 138 per session, which was paid in full by the two insurance companies, who financed the treatment until it was no longer possible to reliably determine the severity of the illness' symptoms. After the public health insurance company ceased payment, Arthur Y paid for another 120 sessions by himself, now at a rate of DM 90 per session. At this point the analysis primarily served to help him develop his personality and enrich his personal life. Although there is no clear-cut transition from an individual's difficulties in coping with life in general to the symptoms of a severe illness, it is still possible to make distinctions. Yet even from the perspective of psychoanalysis, most important is that a patient learn to recognize the part he plays in living his life and the influence he has on his symptoms.

As mentioned before, the public insurance company paid for more than the regular 300 sessions in Arthur Y's analysis. It is therefore possible for us to refer to this case in order to familiarize the readers with the arguments for which we provided a general grounding in Vol.1 (Sect. 6.6). Moreover, it is our good fortune that Arthur Y belonged to the small group of patients who desire to read the analyst's report. In Vol.1 (Sect. 6.6.2) we recommended that applications be prepared in such a manner that patients can read and understand them. Although it is permissible to deny a psychiatric patient access to his case history and reports under certain circumstances (Tölle 1983; Pribilla 1980), refusing patients in analysis access to reports might lead to very exceptional burdens. These reports are legally not considered to belong to the analyst's personal records that, with regard to countertransference, are private in nature. Yet, whatever the case, we reiterate our recommendation once more, and give the following example. The analyst complied with Arthur Y's request to read (made somewhat later) the application for the second continuation of therapy. Incidentally, at the point in time at which his analyst had prepared the report, he had not reckoned with such a thing happening, either in general or in this specific case. It is surprising that so few patients express the wish to see the reports about them. Arthur Y read the application in the waiting room a considerable period of time after the continuation had been approved. He wanted to find out whether his analyst had reached some agreement with the reviewer behind his back. The therapeutic relationship was strengthened by the fact that the patient found the application contained his descriptions of his feelings. He also found that the psychodynamic reasons for the continuation corresponded to what he and his analyst had discussed and were reasonable. It was especially soothing to the patient that his analyst had agreed to continue the therapy after the discontinuation of insurance payments, and at a fee he felt *reasonable.*

The analyst's report to a reviewer is based on a preprepared form (PT 3a/E); point 6 of this form is particularly significant because it requests a description of the *psychodynamics of the neurotic illness.* This description is the basis on which the diagnosis, treatment plan, and prognosis of the analytic therapy, entered under points 7, 8, and 9 of the form, are grounded. The significance of point 6 is brought to the attention of the analyst filing the report by the statement: "The reveiwer cannot process this application if this question is not answered in sufficient detail!" What are the major points to be taken into consideration? What is expected of the analyst filing the application? He is supposed to describe the causal factors that led to the development of the neurotic or psychosomatic symptoms or that serve as precipitating factors maintaining the symptoms. At the core of this is a description of the psychic conflicts, especially with regard to their unconscious component and the subsequent development of neurotic compromises and symptoms. Furthermore, the analyst must describe both the point at which the symptoms became manifest and the precipitating factors in the context of the original psychogenesis.

We will limit ourselves largely to this aspect in citing from the description of the course of treatment that the analyst provided in the application. To make this more comprehensible we first cite from his description of the patient's psychic state (point 5a):

Arthur Y came during my office hours reserved for emergency cases, was driven by anxiety, and was seeking emotional support. A positive transference developed, which I deliberately promoted in order to help him get over the Christmas holidays. I prescribed a benzodiazepine preparation.

Commentary. By providing the prescription the analyst made the patient feel he could trust him. It is even probable that the patient would not have undertaken an analysis without the prescription. We discuss the general questions that are associated with this in Sect. 9.10.

To avoid becoming dependent on the medication, the patient only took about four tablets during the four weeks that have elapsed prior to this application. The patient's desparate mood of dispair must be seen as a reaction to his compulsive symptoms. Certain changes in his symptoms during the last ten years can be understood in the context of his situation, and because of the nature of their course it is certain that they cannot be traced back to a phasic depression.

The following summary of the patient's psychodynamic state was given in the initial application:

The patient correctly considers the fact that his brother had cancer to be the situation that precipitated the worsening of the compulsive and anxiety symptoms that he had had for many years. Subsequent to this fatal illness in his family, old ambivalent feelings were activated; he had been unaware of the intensity of these repressed ambivalent feelings although they had manifested themselves in numerous symptoms. The patient is losing his capacity for integration and fears he may become insane, just like his mother. He is considering suicide, to protect both himself and others from worse things that might happen.

The patient is suffering from a disturbance in which he must ward off strong passive feminine tendencies. The patient's character is generally marked by an extreme ambivalence toward his father. Several anal fixations and conflicts are obvious. It is too early to judge whether his mother's depressive structure is of significance. The patient was denied the phallic narcissistic confirmation he had required during his oedipal phase, as a result of the exaggerated demands his parents had made on him. The consequence was a severe narcissistic illness. The induction of his father into the armed services initially offered oedipal wish fulfillment. The patient's conflict consists primarily in the fact that he adopted the demanding ego-ideal from his father and therefore has to strongly resist his passive desires for emotional support. I assume that his conscious anxiety about some sinister "perversion" is rather a sign of his resistance to his own passive tendencies. For instance, when he strokes his son's head – i. e., when he is tender and, via identification, the one being stroked – both turn into devils. Stroking becomes killing. Omnipotent pleasure is contained in the numerous manifestations of his compulsive anxieties: "If I were free of my anxieties, I would be terrribly arrogant."

The initial application contained the following on *prognosis* (point 9):

Despite the long history, the prognosis is favorable, at least regarding the worsening. A significant improvement can be expected, enabling him to retain his capacity to work. The insight I have already gained into the psychogenesis, and particularly into the course of previous psychotherapies, leads me to assume that a fundamental improvement or even cure is possible because the patient is flexible and not a dried-up compulsive neurotic, and because the narcissistic delusions of grandeur and the negative transference were apparently neglected in his previous analytic therapies, which let them retain their strength to cause symptoms to develop.

Application for Continuation for Sessions 80–160

Questions 4 to 8 in the form are particularly important in applications for the continuation of therapy, and may be answered as a unit. The analyst must provide information about what he has learned about the psychodynamics of the neurotic illness (question 4) and make any subsequent addition to the prognosis (question 5). Of particular importance are the summary of the previous course of therapy and the evaluation of the prognosis, including about the patient's capacity for regression, the degree of fixation, the flexibility, and the potential for development. The following summary is taken from the first application for continuation:

The biographical and psychogenetic connections and predecessors of the compulsive neurosis are: sadomasochistic experiences in childhood - being severely punished and cleaned in the large basement where the wash was done and where animals were still butchered, because he would shit in his pants (now: compulsive neurotic anxiety about the color red and blood, together with defense rituals). The first manifestation of an obsessive thought at his boarding school: a brutal teacher on the one hand, a homosexual seducer on the other. As a young boy he coped with his ideas of grandeur by identifying with Hitler; his impotence and feeling of being excluded resulted in identification with the "dirty Jews." (He felt himself to be a Jewish boy because he did not meet the ideals of his parents and those around him.) The fact that his father had not returned from the war and was later declared dead without them reaching a reconciliation left the patient's ambivalence and idealization unmastered. His relationship to his depressive mother molded his entire life. When he would like to sit down and feel satisfied, he becomes just the way his mother had been, depressive and lacking the will or energy to do anything. His feelings of guilt because of his unconscious hatred of his helpless mother reinforced his identification with her. He is not able to enjoy his success. Just recently he recalled a positive side of his mother; she had had a small corner store, where she was happy and successful, but it did not fit in line with the prestige thinking of his father's family.

The *transference* and *working alliance* developed as follows:

It soon became clear that he followed the basic rule slavishly, but avoided anything I was actually or presumably sensitive to. He had a single recollection from his first consultation more that 15 years ago: "Come to the academic hospital," I am supposed to have said with a Czechish accent. The professor and acting director of the Heidelberg Psychosomatic Hospital, a refugee! Scorn and admiration at the same time. His anxiety about being hurt or offended, in particular by the discovery of what he was really sensitive to or by the observation of his personal peculiarities, is much larger than his anxiety about his fantasies of omnipotence or impotence, which have developed over decades as a result of his retreat.

I am proceeding from the assumption that the increase in his positive self-esteem can become such a threat - in his identification with Hitler - that he shifts everything to the outside, i. e., experiences them as split off from himself and foreign - foreign in the description of the compulsive neurotic perception of "whooshing" noises. He links whooshing noises with the whooshing of a knife being drawn from its sheath, with which a sheep was butchered in the "precipitating situation." Afterwards the whooshing noises were linked with the drawing of a knife and ultimately with murder and fantasies about killing. The patient reacted positively to my statement about the projection of his omnipotence and impotence onto whooshing noises and the sacrifice of the lamb, and emphasized that these ideas actually made it possible for him, first, to overcome the foreignness of his thoughts and second to learn, even if reluctantly, to see them as a part of his self.

Arthur Y, returning to an allusion he had made, asked if the old oak [the analyst] could take all the poison he could inject in the form of doubts. Adding to this vivid image, he said he naturally did not want to saw off the branch he was sitting on. We then talked about his idea that I might turn ill, die, and not be able to continue treating him to the end. For him this would mean being left alone again. My response that he was not completely *dependent* (i. e., that he was not like a day-old babe sitting on a branch who could fall down) was new to him. He was accordingly surprised when I pointed out to him that he had already acquired some autonomy and thus had enough muscles to hold on to another branch. It came as a surprise to him that I phrased the question of how far he accused himself of overburdening me when he was alone as a problem. I drew a parallel to his sister's illness and especially to his mother's chronic illness, which had made it difficult for him to be frank and express criticism. He made himself responsible for his mother's suicide, as if the determination he had shown one day had driven her into taking her life.

Arthur Y had hoped to be well after 20–30 sessions. Yet he noticed how much work still had to be done. He said he had stopped several compulsive actions, but would not have any alternative to committing suicide if he did not become healthy this time. Implicit was that I considered him "guilty" of the delay. I therefore referred to my earlier statements about therapy and emphasized my *sympathy* and *coresponsibility*. I interpreted his idea that I remained *untouched*, like a doctor in an intensive care ward who cannot let himself be affected, as an expression of his wish for me to be an object that was both timeless and immortal. I added that the idea that he was considered guilty must make him feel enraged inside.

Sadomasochistic ideas are often symptomatically tied with the crucifix and the sacrificing of Isaac by Abraham. The fact that he warded of his longing for love and his anxiety about homosexuality with these religious images has also become clear in the transference. We were able to work out that one issue is his longing for his father, which he wards off because of his ambivalence.

Application for Continuation for Sessions 160–240

Since I have already provided a detailed description of the case history, I will limit myself in this application for continuation to a description of the course of the analysis, summarizing several important points.

Therapeutically it has proven to be very advantageous that, especially because of the patient's previous experiences, I have directed my entire attention to the analysis of the psychodynamics of the here and now. The analytic consideration of the changes in his symptoms in connection with the transference processes is instructive, and these changes must be considered negative therapeutic reactions. Their purpose is always self-punishment, especially each time the patient frees or wants to free himself a little from subjugation and masochism. Then there is a reversal to sadism and rebellion, although each success and action is unconsciously tied for Arthur Y to a strong anxiety about aggression and its consequences. This problem goes back to his relationship to his depressive mother, which limited his expansiveness. He identified himself primarily with the rigid superego of his mother and grandmother. It came as a great surprise to me and the patient to note that he felt admiration and fright while listening to my interpretations, which contained words such as "lust" and "gratification." At the same time an identification with the pleasure I provided verbally, in the sense of Strachey's mutative interpretation, developed step by step. Of course the patient's anxieties about closeness and sexuality, including homosexuality such as he had encountered in his traumatic experience with a teacher, became visible at this occasion. These two figures, the sadistic and homosexual teachers, were indeed the central figures in this case; much can be done with reference to them and they also appear in the transference. In this transference constellation, of course, the variables in the setting are especially well suited to serve as issues for handling other items. With his increasing liberation, we also come to discuss sexual problems he has with his wife because of his anal regression and his mixing of pleasure with dirt. In his earlier therapies he took all interpretations referring to sexual topics to be demeaning. Apparently in them such interpretations were so much the focus of attention that the aspect of self-punishment was not given adequate attention.

Another important area is the patient's effort to capture some of what he had missed, by spoiling his children and identification. These processes have led him to feel unusually constricted, and limited his own scope for action. For instance, he has a bad conscience even if he only arrives home slightly later than usual.

The favorable course of the therapy can also been seen in substantial improvements in his symptoms, and not just in the good elaboration of the ones mentioned above. It must be emphasized that Arthur Y has been able to overcome his dependence on the consumption of a quite considerable amount of alcohol every evening without this being worked through specifically. He has reduced his weight by 30 pounds and has become fairly athletic. He had been dependent on alcohol for years, even decades, because he felt it was the only means for him to be able to bear the rest of the day and the following ones. It was impossible for him to sit down without drinking. This dependence made him feel very dejected. One cause psychogenetically was that sitting quietly reminded him of his mother's depression; for many years she had been passive, occasionally even falling into stupor. His greater freedom is also indicated by the fact that no separation problems worth mentioning have occurred during interruptions of treatment during this entire period and that the patient has taken hardly any sedatives during my absence.

Supplementary Application for Sessions 240–300

The patient read this application after it had been completed. He was surprised he was able to understand the text. It was soothing for him that the application described the continuation of therapy as we had agreed.

The frequency of therapy was increased from three to four hours a week at the patient's request because of the intensity of the therapeutic process and to provide him the opportunity to work through the unconscious factors behind his symptoms. The increase has had a positive therapeutic effect, for we are now able to immediately handle changes in his symptoms that occur ad hoc and are related to transference.

The end of a positive development was marked by my informing him of the dates of my summer vacation and by the approaching interruption. During my summer vacation the compulsive symptoms reappeared, taking various forms (fear of harming his son or another member of the family, of seeing his son as the devil, and of having to listen compulsively to the whooshing noises of his own language and suffering from it). It was unfortunately impossible to recognize, and therefore work through, the entire psychodynamic context until later. Whenever the patient felt aggressive impulses, he experienced himself unconsciously to be a devil, whom he got rid of in the person of his son by developing his symptoms. In the transference these became key words, with regard to which the thematic work can be demonstrated. The very fact that the patient felt I was inconsiderate because of the vacation interruption is a sign of his own inconsiderateness. The patient became increasingly aware that inconsiderateness and arbitrariness were his own form of fantasies about power and omnipotence, and his symptoms receded to the same degree. Naturally the earlier compulsive neurotic acts of control, with which he was able to establish a certain balance, are part of this. By means of the expression "devilish tricks," which the patient enjoyed using in our conversations, he became aware of his unconscious tricks, his anal underhandedness, and the pleasure he gained from intrigues. He saw them through a magnifiying glass, and his punishment and self-punishment took on correspondingly strict form. The stronger his lust for life, the stronger his masochism momentarily became. It became clear that there used to be only *one* period of time during which he felt happy, namely during his vacation, but only if it turned out to be successful after intensive preparations. Vacation was about the only time in which he might have pleasure "because of his health." Thus it was all the more serious when he once said that he would not be able to go on vacation because his wife had overdrawn their account for some allegedly thoughtless reason. I, in contrast, became the well-to-do, even uncommonly rich "king" who can do whatever he wishes. In this passage the patient had made himself small, exaggerated the thoughtlessness of his wife, and not taken his secret financial reserves into consideration. Miserliness and envy entered into the analysis. Particularly impressive is the immediate improvement that occurs in the patient's symptoms after he experiences an insight in a very strongly affective manner. He himself draws hope from this, and although he has apparently been completely broken by the remanifestation of his symptoms, the spiral of progress he is making is obvious.

The *prognosis* is favorable despite the severity of the symptoms because the patient is able to work through his problems step by step and to free himself.

Supplementary Application for Sessions 300–360

This application for additional sessions, which went beyond what is foreseen by the guidelines, gave the reviewer the opportunity to make a positive recommendation. One of the reviewer's duties is to interpret the guidelines in a manner that the rules can be applied to special cases. The analyst wrote in this application:

The exception can be seen in the fact, first, that this is a very severe set of symptoms, which, second, it has been possible to influence positively in the previous therapy, and which, third, can be expected to undergo a further improvement, or even reach a cure, if the analysis is continued. This optimism is justified because the psychodynamic explanation given below not only provides an adequte explanation of the still existing symptoms but also clearly indicates that the patient is making an intensive effort to overcome his resistances. He is cooperating very well in integrating previously split off components of his personality. My prognosis is based on an agreement with the patient that after discontinuation of payment by the health insurance organization he is willing to finance a continuation of therapy out of his own resources and that I will substantially reduce my fee. We have already reached agreement on this. I believe that a further continuation of payment is justified on social grounds, because the patient will surely need a longer period of time to succeed in integrating the unconscious components of his ego, which still manifest themselves in symptoms because they are split off.

I will now refer to the central aspect that has been worked out in the previous period of treatment.

At the beginning of the therapy the patient had emphasized that sexuality was the only area where he did not have any problems. Now he has had an important insight that will certainly lead to further substantial changes. Let me add that although I never shared the patient's opinion, I have been very restrained in referring to it. My assumption was that because of the linkage of anality with sexuality every active step in this direction would have made the patient feel humiliated and would only have been a repetition of what he already knew, namely that his nose had been rubbed in his own feces. Sexuality consequently became associated with punishment and humiliation. After he had secured himself sufficient self-esteem in our numerous transference struggles, he risked an attempt to break through his self-punishment and the circle of executionists with whom he had previously identified in combatting his lust for life and any pleasure from life. He discovered that by subordinating himself to a sadistic figure in his childhood he had attempted, in his anxiety and compulsive symptoms, to destroy every pleasure and all sensuality. The result was murder and destruction in subjugating himself to an omnipotent god and its representatives on earth (Hitler, priests, SS thugs, etc.), to whom he offered himself as a love object.

The deep dimensions of this identification can even be seen in harmless anxieties and symptoms that disappeared after he had identified with me in the form of a friendly father figure.

It hardly needs to be mentioned that the patient also has deep anxieties because of the aggression in him that is directed against symbols of power. Restructuring has enabled the patient to face all of his libidinous and aggressive impulses with much more tolerance. One symptom is particularly obstinate, namely his extreme sensitivity to whooshing noises whenever the general level of his anxiety is increased because of unconscious processes.

On the basis of this psychodynamic explanation I request that an exception be made and 60 additional sessions be approved in this case.

The therapy was continued with a reduction in fee and frequency after discontinuation of third-party payment. The patient and analyst were in agreement that the primary goal of the analysis was now to overcome general problems he encountered in his life and whose status as an illness was becoming increasingly dubious. The relatively infrequent and successful continuation of the analysis, which Arthur Y payed on his own at a rate of DM 90 per session, served to stabilize his self-esteem. The judgment that the analysis was successful was based on several criteria. Decisive in our opinion is that the curing of the symptoms can be related to a psychoanalytic process which permits one to infer that a deep-reaching structural modification had taken place. We recommend that the reader follow this process by examining the excerpts of Arthur Y's analysis given in this book (see the patient index).

6.5 Reviewing and Transference

All of the analyst's actions must be examined with regard to their consequences on the relationship and transference. The question of whether the analyst provides a prescription or not, or prepares a certificate or not - everything has an influence on the relationship between the patient and the analyst.

The manner in which the analyst handled a certificate in the context of a substantial worsening of Arthur Y's symptoms became the focal point for working through negative transference. This was a theme that covered several sessions; similar situations occurred several times in the course of the analysis.

Arthur Y was a voluntary member of a public health insurance scheme and was treated as a private patient. Years before he had taken out a supplementary policy to ensure complete coverage. This latter insurance firm had notified him that outpatient therapy was not covered by his policy, but offered to consider some coverage if an illness were present and if the physician providing treatment would prepare a detailed statement supporting psychoanalytic therapy, specifically about its necessity, economy, and utility.

We now give excerpts of two sessions on this theme.

P: Yes, you always return to the business with the insurance and the certificate that I need from you. I had the feeling you thought that I shouldn't leave everything up to you and take account of realities.
A: No, I wasn't thinking about any given realities, but about disappointments. You have already been waiting about a week for the attest.
P: I just have the feeling that you are intentionally holding it back because I haven't said enough about it yet.
A: No, but you see that this is apparently a very important point.
P: I'm amazed that you think this business with the health insurance company is more important than I do even though it affects me directly. I think it's outrageous for the insurance company to deny me something I'm entitled to.
A: And now you've had the idea that I am also denying you something in order to make you angry.
P: Yes and no.
A: Hum.
P: To move me to say more about it.
A: But you have the feeling that you yourself can't do any more, and I referred to the longing about how nice it is if someone can organize everything well.
P: One person.
A: If possible, someone who is strong. It would be funny if this longing weren't there.
P: Yes.
A: Whether you have this longing now?
P: Naturally.
A: Such longing can lead one to not fully utilize his own ability. I've made you aware of this, and perhaps you've drawn the conclusion that I have delayed giving you the certificate, or perhaps you had the idea that I would not do as much for you. Longing, disappointment, or rejection?
P: Yes, if you're in the shape I'm in, then you have the immense desire for somebody to come and straighten everything out.
A: Yes, yes, not just this business with the insurance, but also the anxieties and everything, of course.
P: That there is some danger of not developing one's own powers, that's clear to me.
A: This is probably linked with the fact that you are cautious and don't say, "What a nasty thing for him to make me wait so long before giving me the certificate."
P: Yes, I actually had the feeling that you would not give it to me until I got pushy in some way.
A: Thus, on the one hand you have experienced this as a rejection, but didn't get nasty with me or the insurance company. You didn't get nastier, just your anxieties and thoughts.
P: Sure, when I think about it in this way, it's logical to ask if the certificate is finished, if I can take it with me now. Perfectly clear.

The patient ended a longer period of silence by saying that his thoughts had now slipped away, moving on to his conflict with his boss.

My hesitation to give him the attest immediately had led the patient to change the subject. Yet later he returned to the subject.

P: You still haven't answered my question.

A: Yes, I've just wondered what I could say now, but I haven't thought of anything else. But the matter isn't closed. You would like to hear if you're going to get the certificate now.

P: Yes, precisely.

A: And you've also had another idea, but it isn't closed either.

P: You still haven't answered my question of whether I'm going to get the certificate. Now, yes, so what, then I'll ask again.

A: But then it would have to have been typed already or being typed right now, that is, already have been dictated.

P: Then I'll take it with me the next time.

I raised the question of whether the patient was wondering if he would not get it at all, which he denied. Then the subliminal feeling that I might deny him the certificate developed after all.

P: Now we're getting somewhere. You might say that I haven't developed my own strength and as long as I haven't done that . . . but then I can wait a hundred years if you say that, that I have not yet developed my strength. My impulse now to say, "Damn certificate, there!"

The patient recalled that the receipt of the insurance company's rejection after returning from vacation (just like the delay in receiving the certificate) had led to a worsening of his symptoms, and that everything had been less stable since then.

At the end of the session I summarized what had happened. Since he had the impression that he was being harassed, his rage had mounted. The effect via displacement was a worsening of symptoms.

Commentary. The analyst had required several days to draft the text that was ready at this point in his secretary's office. The patient's uncertainty and anger had increased, largely unnoticed, and expressed themselves in his symptoms, through a return of repressed affects. In order to reconstruct this sequence of events, the analyst intentionally kept the patient in suspense in this session. Although leaving the matter open at first was productive in this case, this procedure is not free of danger because it is risky to follow the adage that the end justifies the means.

The analyst gave the patient a certificate he had not yet signed in which he drew attention to the fact that the open questions had already been clarified by the decision of the public health insurance company to provide payment. A detailed report, if still required, would only be prepared for a physician competent to judge psychoanalytic issues.

In the following session it became clear that Arthur Y had thought intensively about the certificate.

P: If I had been in your place, I would have bowed to the wishes of the insurance company more than you did . . . . I would have tried a subservant approach. Maybe I would have come to the same result. If the insurance had then paid the rest, then my thesis would have been confirmed – you reach your goal if you are subservient. Your attitude is different, and I'm not yet completely sure how I should formulate my own letter, whether I should express a request or insist on my rights. I believe I am entitled to compensation.

The patient offered further alternative formulations for the text that he himself had to write to the insurance company. He was impressed by my clear and brief statement and found it to be a model of a courageous attitude toward an institution.

A: Hum. Those are two entirely different worlds, and there is the fear that the insurance company might react with spite if you demand something.

P: If I use the subservient expression, they may have sympathy with me and say, "What a poor soul. And it's the poor soul's turn again. We, the big, powerful insurance company can help the poor soul for once. It's just a couple of marks. Throw it out to him, let him chew on them." Yes, this affair is awfully difficult.

A: You know that I haven't signed the certificate yet.

P: Yes, I want the certificate as you have drafted it.

A: You can send it in together with you own letter.

P: I want it as you drafted it; I think it's right, perfectly ok.

With a view to the entire application procedure, I then made a few comments to the patient about the terms "necessity," "economy," and "utility," and also about the concept of illness that the insurance companies employ when determining their responsibility to pay and that peer reviewers employ in their evaluations for the insurance companies. I also explained the meaning of medical confidentiality and mentioned the fact that the applications are handled in an anonymous manner. The patient then ended this theme:

P: I still haven't decided about how I will express myself. Perhaps I can use both forms. Well, somehow I'll think of something. I'm just amazed that such things can have such a strong impact on my mood that I almost feel destroyed. What would it be like then if I got into a real crisis, was out of work, lost my job, had difficulties with my wife?

A: It's sometimes easier to survive struggles with a real and actual opponent than to fight an opponent who is so hard to grasp and where you have to be on your guard.

P: Today you're always referring back to yourself. Well, if I experience you emotionally just like I did that teacher, if that's the case, what consequences can I draw from knowing this? I still don't know, and it makes me feel insecure.

Arthur Y focused on the theme of dependence and considered his efforts to retain my favor.

He mentioned the tape recorder.

P: I still haven't really come to terms with that thing. I have the feeling I am helpless, defenseless, violated. [See Sect. 7.5] Maybe it's because I fear certain parallels. I would probably be a good piece further if I could completely admit to myself that this experience back then was really bad for me instead of always wiping it away. As if it hadn't happened, as if I only wanted to make myself important. [He was referring to his experience with a homosexual teacher at boarding school.]

A: It's terrible to have such an unfulfilled longing and to experience how it is misused without being able to defend oneself and simply being helpless.

P: And it's really comprehensible that you get terribly angry.

A: And it's also comprehensible that you prefer to minimize it.

P: And now I would like to ask you whether you believe that these experiences with the teacher were a substantial factor in the anxieties I developed later.

A: Yes.

P: The answer is a big help to me – a clear answer .... The whole muddy business. I just thought of it. I just thought of a comparison. Somewhere I am running in mud up to my waist, keep on sinking down, and then somewhere always manage to get my feet on solid ground, but it's still more or less a coincidence. I don't know

> whether the next step will be in a vacuum again .... But now I at least have some orientation to continue in a certain direction despite the mud .... Everything is very difficult. In the words "devotion" and "trust" I see the danger of being mawkish.

The session ended on the theme of the patient's longing for his father, which occurred after he had mentioned the first manifestation of his neurotic anxiety symptoms in prepuberty.

7 Rules

Introduction

Psychoanalytic rules have multiple functions, a fact that is a consequence of the tasks and goals of the psychoanalytic dialogue, as we have explained in Vol.1 (Sect. 7.1). This is the reason that the corresponding chapter in Vol.1 is focused on the thesis that the efficacy of each rule has to be proven for each and every patient. The rules are put to a test when the analyst pursues the question of whether the system of rules provides a given patient the best possible conditions for therapeutic change. The issue of the utility of rules is a good starting point for using them in a flexible manner, i. e., one in which they are applied in a manner appropriate to the individual patient, and for guiding the dialogue toward therapeutic goals. Since the rules are subordinate to the dialogue, we assign the latter a prime place in this chapter (Sect. 7.1).

Since the other chapters contain many examples of free association (Sect. 7.2), we restrict ourselves here to excerpts from the initial phases of therapy. The same is true of evenly suspended attention (Sect. 7.3); we describe its fluctuations retrospectively.

A flexible application of the counterquestion rule is possible within the system of rules if the analyst responds to the questions the patient inevitably asks instead of following the rule stereotypically. We criticized this stereotypical application in Vol.1, and in Sect. 7.4 we give examples of a flexible application of this rule.

The study of metaphors and the changes they undergo in the psychoanalytic process is especially fertile. Since their significance in the language used in therapy can hardly be exaggerated, we cover the psychoanalytic aspects of metaphors in a separate section (Sect. 7.5.1). The linguistic examination of a psychoanalytic dialogue in Sect. 7.5.2 gives special consideration to metaphors and impressively demonstrates that scientists who come from other fields and study analytic texts independently are able to extend our knowledge significantly. They provide insights into the style of the language that are generally inaccessible to the treating analyst.

The two sections on value-free attitude and neutrality (Sect. 7.6) and on anonymity and naturalness (Sect. 7.7) deal with interrelated problems that were not given adequate consideration in Vol.1. Examples from case histories demonstrate that the resolution of these problems is of great therapeutic relevance.

Many of our examples are based on transcripts of tape-recorded analyses. We have included a larger number of examples in this chapter that demonstrate the influence of tape recording on transference and resistance. Following the general discussion of this topic in Sect. 1.4, we have good reason to include these instructive examples in precisely this chapter on rules. Our purpose is to demonstrate that the psychoanalytic situation is influenced in numerous ways. The introduction of a technical aid must be examined particularly critically, just as are the consequences that rules have on the dialogue; in Sect. 7.8 we give thorough consideration to this topic, including the counterarguments that have been raised.

This volume would not have been written without this innovation. The especially instructive experience we have had has convinced us that the influence this technical aid exerts on the patient-analyst relationship can be considered just as critically - i. e., analyzed - as that of any other variable. The manner in which analysts describe a phenoneon as having been analyzed refers to a genuine quality of the psychoanalytic method, namely that both the influence of the analyst and the setting are made the object of joint considerations.

7.1 Dialogue

The psychoanalytic interview is often compared to classical dialogues. It is therefore natural for us to reconsider the origin of the word "dialogue." Its roots, just like those of the word "dialectic," go back to the Greek *dialegesthai*: to dissect, consider, and consult, or in its transitive use, to discuss something with others. Originally, "dialectic" characterized dialogue as consultation. *Dialegesthai* meant to come together and consult. According to Plato, the dialectician was the one who knew how to ask questions and to answer them. Where, furthermore, the consultation in the dialogue is subject to rules, the word "dialectic" is employed "to refer to the use of such rules or to an institutionalized dialogical practice" (Mittelstrass 1984, p. 14). It is not unusual for the style of the Socratic dialogues, whose goal is summarized by the famous sentence "I know that I know nothing," to be viewed as an ideal. Socrates' students suffered from the superiority of their ironic teacher; Alcibiades is said, for example, to have called out: "What else do I have to endure from this person! He wants to show me his superiority everywhere." Socrates referred to his method as *maieutic*. His comparison with the art of midwifery, his mother's profession, is taken up by some psychotherapists who compare their work with the Socratic maieutic. The metaphor of midwifery is occasionally used for psychotherapy to emphasize the new beginning that self-knowledge leading to change is an important element of. The use of metaphors, however, must take into account any dissimilarities, which motivates us to emphasize the autonomy of the psychoanalytic method.

The style of dialogue handed down from Plato shows Socrates to be a midwife who knew precisely where he had to apply the forceps and who always anticipated which ideas he was really helping to attain life: his questions inevitably determined his students' answers. Socrates produced his own philosophical child. He did not shy from incorporating Sophist devices into his dialectics. If a psychoanalyst were to pose questions the way Socrates did and direct the patient's answers by means of his style of dialogue, then he would be accused of manipulation. In the psychoanalytic maieutic the patient sets the pace of the events. He has the initiative and both the first and last word, however important the psychoanalyst's contribution to the search for liberating solutions to problems may be. An issue in therapy from the beginning to the end is the creation of the best possible conditions for helping the patient achieve change.

It is doubtful, for example, whether Alcibiades, if he had been a patient, would have rapidly regained his composure after admitting his complete ignorance and having his self-security destroyed. Every act of subjugation provokes much aggression, and it in turn can lead to acts of depressive self-humiliation if it is directed against the individual himself. In *psychoanalytic* dialogues the issue is to create the best possible conditions for the patient's spontaneity, and to enable him to act on a trial basis in a manner that itself is indicative of the change he desires. The analyst must subordinate his role to this goal.

To arrive at (self) awareness and reasoned actions is the ideal of the psychoanalytic dialogue, which is rooted deep in the intellectual history of the West. Thus it is no exaggeration to view Plato's idea of anamnesis, or recollection, as a predecessor of Freud's emphasis on remembering as a part of psychoanalytic insight. Freud described psychoanalytic treatment as a special form of dialogical practice:

> Nothing takes place in a psycho-analytic treatment but an interchange of words between the patient and the analyst. The patient talks, tells of his past experiences and present impressions, complains, confesses to his wishes and his emotional impulses. The doctor listens, tries to direct the patient's processes of thought, exhorts, forces his attention in certain directions, gives him explanations and observes the reactions of understanding or rejection which he in this way provokes in him. The uninstructed relatives of our patients, who are only impressed by visible and tangible things - preferably by actions of the sort that are to be witnessed at the cinema - never fail to express their doubts whether "anything can be done about the illness by mere talking." That, of course, is both a short-sighted and an inconsistent line of thought. These are the same people who are so certain that patients are "simply imagining" their symptoms. Words were originally magic and to this day words have retained much of their ancient magical power. By words one person can make another blissfully happy or drive him to despair, by words the teacher conveys his knowledge to his pupils, by words the orator carries his audience with him and determines their judgements and decisions. Words provoke affects and are in general the means of mutual influence among men. Thus we shall not depreciate the use of words in psychotherapy and we shall be pleased if we can listen to the words that pass between the analyst and his patient ....
>
> The information required by analysis will be given by him only on condition of his having a special emotional attachment to the doctor; he would become silent as soon as he observed a single witness to whom he felt indifferent. For this information concerns what is most intimate in his mental life, everything that, as a socially dependent person, he must conceal from other people, and, beyond that, everything that, as a homogeneous personality, he will not admit to himself.
>
> Thus you cannot be present as an audience at a psycho-analytic treatment. You can only be told about it; and, in the strictest sense of the word, it is only by hearsay that you will get to know psycho-analysis. (Freud 1916/17, pp. 17-18)

Twenty years later Freud (1926e, p. 187), responding to the question of a fictive "impartial person" as to what psychoanalysis does to the patient, gave a very similar answer: "Nothing takes place between them except that they talk to each other. The analyst makes use of no instruments - not even for examining the patient - nor does he prescribe any medicines .... The analyst agrees upon a fixed regular hour with the patient, gets him to talk, listens to him, talks to him in his turn and gets him to listen." Freud even interpreted the impartial person's presumed skeptical attitude, saying "It is as though he were thinking: 'Nothing more than that? Words, words, words, as Prince Hamlet says.'" Such reactions can still be frequently heard in discussions about psychoanalysis, and can also be expected from patients until they have convinced themselves of the power of their thoughts and the effects of their words.

Although Freud swore by the power of words and referred to both emotional impulses and affects, the sentence that *nothing else happens but a verbal exchange* in psychoanalytic treatment has unnecessarily restricted the therapeutic range and the diagnostic understanding of psychoanalysis. For Freud, in fact, "words" were not the beginning, and in his theory of development the ego had its origin in the body ego. It was the *physical* symptoms of hysterical patients that were accessible to the "talking cure." The ideas these patients had about the origin and significance of their physical symptoms did not fit into the sensory motor disturbances that neurologists were familiar with. By paying attention to body language and to what the physical symptoms had to say and by letting himself be guided by what is today referred to as the patient's personal theory of his illness, Freud transformed himself from a neurologist into the first psychoanalyst. We mention this origin in order to weaken the assertion that nothing else happens in analytic treatment but an exchange of words.

Many things that take place in the relationship between patient and analyst at the unconscious level of feelings and affects cannot be completely referred to by name, distinguished, and consolidated in experiencing (see Bucci 1985). Intentions that are prelinguistic and that consciousness cannot recognize can only be imprecisely verbalized. Thus in fact much more happens between the patient and analyst than just an exchange of words. Freud's "nothing else" must be understood as a challenge for the patient to reveal his thoughts and feelings as thoroughly as possible. The analyst is called upon to intervene in the dialogue by making interpretations, i. e., with linguistic means. Of course, it makes a big difference if the analyst conducts a dialogue, which always refers to a two-sided relationship, or if he makes interpretations that expose the latent meanings in a patient's quasimonological free associations. Spitz (1976) has also referred to the nonverbal interaction that precedes language acquisition as a dialogue (see Vol.1, Sect. 7.4.3). The child learns to communicate through actions before it begins speaking. At a surprisingly early moment it enters into complex social interactions with its mother (see Vol.1, Sect. 1.8). A wealth of forms of preverbal communication are present in the body ego and in the preconscious and unconscious dimensions of the psychoanalytic dialogue; their relationship to the experiencing ego is very obscure, yet they do codertermine the quality of the patient-therapist relationship. In Chap. 5 and in Sect. 9.10 we discuss the importance of the analyst taking both the patient's ideas about his body image and medical knowledge seriously in psychoanalytic treatment and of not diluting the difference between them.

Research on the dialogue between mother and child has provided a wealth of new results about the role that affectivity plays in the child's acquisition of language (see Klann 1979). These results will have far-reaching consequences on analytic technique. The studies by Stern (1977, 1985) were, among others, important in providing a foundation in developmental psychology for Buber's philosophical ideas about the *dialogical principle* and the interhuman. Buber's ideas can be used to better understand the psychoanalytic dialogue, as demonstrated by Ticho's pioneering study:

If the [therapeutic] relationship is seen exlusively in terms of transference and countertransference and its dynamic understanding, then there is a danger that the analytic situation will become a monologue. If a dialogue is maintained, a careful observation of transference and countertransference manifestations enables us to reconstruct the environmental past. The multiplicity of infantile environmental factors may make this very difficult sometimes. But analysts at times want to avoid the painful involvement with a patient that interferes with their need to stay "independent" of their patients. In such a situation, the analyst is carrying on a monologue, and the dependence-independence conflict will likely be repeated in the analytic situation. (1974, p. 252)

Ticho's original comparison of Winnicott's and Buber's theories can be profitably applied to therapeutic technique in many ways. In the psychoanalytic exchange, the dialogical principle approaches the Socratic form of dialogue if the latter is understood as a dialogue in which the discussants are led by insight to submit to reason.

Most analysts have some image of an ideal type of dialogue. Yet since the rules that psychoanalysts apply in analysis have to prove themselves anew in every case, it is alarming for any kind of rules to impose a rigid style on an interview. In the present stage of development of the psychoanalytic technique it is more important to compile precise protocols and conduct empirical studies, including interdisciplinary ones, about how and what analysts discuss with patients than to establish the pure form in which the psychoanalytic discourse is supposed to be led. Although it has become customary to emphasize the difference between the therapeutic interview and everyday conversation (Leavy 1980), we feel compelled to warn against an overly naive differentiation since everyday dialogues often are:

characterized by only apparent understanding, by only apparent cooperation, by apparent symmetry in the dialogue and in the strategies pursued in the conversation, and that in reality intersubjectivity often remains an assertion that does not necessarily lead to significant changes, to dramatic conflicts, or to a consciousness of a "pseudo-understanding" .... In everyday dialogues something is acted out and silently negotiated that in therapeutic dialogues is verbalized in a systematic manner. (Klann 1979, p. 128)

It is impossible to establish an overall relationship between similarity and difference in the patient-analyst dialogue. It is disadvantageous from a therapeutic perspective to proceed from the differences and view the dialogue as an extremely asymmetric structure. Empirical studies confirm what seems obvious to common sense, namely that a helping alliance is especially likely to form when a correspondence develops between the views of the analyst and those of the patient that both parties acknowledge. The correspondence may be in apparently very banal items that the patient does not have to be consciously aware of. A workable relationship is more likely to develop if similar views exist on some things and if the patient can somehow sense them. Although the proverb "birds of a feather flock together" has its counterpart in the idea that opposites attract each other, that which is different or completely foreign is more likely to be sinister for most people, and this is especially true for anxious patients. It is therefore reasonable to proceed from the familiar to the unfamiliar in structuring therapeutic interviews. While common sense can be deceiving, it is still advisable not to simply disregard the judgements that result from it.

The analyst and patient live, after all, in the same sociocultural reality even though they may have different attitudes toward it, a fact the patient cannot help noticing. Most importantly, each is subject to the same biological laws governing the life cycle from birth to death. Every patient senses from the very beginning that his analyst is not above the rhythms of nature and that he is thus familiar with the vital needs which provide the patient pleasure or cause him pain. These features that they have in common are given, and the fact that these features are commonplace has deeper implications because the manner in which the patient learns that the analyst is not spared the consequences of aging or illness itself has significant consequences.

The analyst's role in developing a helping alliance is always in part mediated by something general in nature, i. e., that goes beyond his specific professional role as prescribed by his therapeutic tasks. The resulting relationship is characterized by numerous forms of interdependence and by an abundance of discordance; the manner in which it is structured determines in large measure the success or failure of the therapy. Although it may seem banal, the fact that the interdependent nature of the relationship between role and person and between intervention and relationship has been verifed by empirical research into psychotherapy, such as that summarized by Garfield and Bergin (1986) in the third edition of their handbook, is not unimportant. This leads us, to go beyond our discussion in Vol.1 (Chap. 2), to the question of whether the psychoanalytic therapeutic alliance, which is related to a specific definition of roles, also contains those items that in Luborsky's opinion constitute a helping alliance, i. e., a therapeutically effective relationship. Even the therapeutic relationship is based in large measure on the formation of a "community of feeling" and the emotional ties created "by means of identification," two phenomena Freud (1933b, p. 212) identified in his correspondence with Einstein as being at the basis of human society.

Dialogues demonstrate that significant processes take place in the medium of conversation. This understanding is threatened by one-sidedness if we assume that it is sufficient to describe psychoanalysis as conversation (Flader et al. 1982). Speaking and remaining silent are dialectical elements of conversation that link acts - silence as the act of not speaking and an independent factor - with the verbal acts that, as a rule, negate other acts. This alteration of positions is the means by which the exchange process that is decisive for both parties takes place.

In Vol.1 (see Sect. 8.5), we have already described several features that characterize the occasionally extreme polarizations of the style of interview specific to psychoanalysis. The following example features the significance of speaking and of remaining silent in the analytic process, events that are frequently observed and clinically very familiar.

Example

Arthur Y told me that he felt very well and that he was on the right path. He added that he was not sure where he should start, and mentioned business problems and conflicts with competitors. The patient was unusually silent in this session. Most of all he would have liked to fall asleep.

A: You used to feel the pressure from thinking about the fact that being silent was a waste of money - so and so much per minute.

Arthur Y was pleased by his increased calmness.

P: Yes, I have much better control of myself today; the basis has become much wider. Still, I don't have as many debts as I used to.

A: You used to always overlook the credit side when you thought about financial matters.

P: Yes, the calmness I have today that the world is not going to collapse when I let myself go a little, well I'm very pleased about it. That I can do it without immediately becoming anxious that everything will get confused, as implied by the questions "What's going to happen to me if I blow the hour here?" and "Does my financial existence depend on it?"

Commentary. In our opinion this is an example of productive silence because the patient was able to allow himself the experience of being calm and thus of displaying some passivity without experiencing feelings of guilt. He displayed increased self-security, and he passed his test. In other words, he managed to deal with his time in a generous way and to overcome his anxieties associated with impoverization and the reaction formation of miserliness.

7.2 Free Association

At the beginning of treatment it is important for the analyst to familiarize the patient with the fundamental rule. He must decide in each individual case which information he should provide about the multiple functions of the rules (see Vol.1, Sect. 7.2). Since elements of psychoanalytic theory and technique have become part of general knowledge, although frequently in caricatured form, numerous patients now come to psychoanalysis with more or less accurate expectations.

First Example

Franziska X told me in the first session about the information she had received from her health insurance company. She also asked me about the report I was supposed to write. After I explained what this was, she asked how long the therapy would last and expressed her concern. Her brother, who claimed to know something about it, had told her that she would need at least a year. After reflecting briefly, I said that it was impossible to make any precise predictions and that it depended on what kind of progress we made.

I then informed Franziska X about the formalities of treatment, saying it was advantageous for her to lie on the couch and that I would sit behind her. She was supposed to try to tell me everything she happened to think about. After I had inquired whether she had any more questions, to which she said no, I suggested that we begin immediately.

P: Can I now tell you what I'm thinking about?

A: Hum.

P: I have to think right now of the lullaby about the seven angels around me [laughed in embarrassment], because you are sitting behind me, at the head of the couch. Last night I even dreamed about it; I wanted to come here, but I couldn't find you or the right room. I'm bound to tell you about a lot of dreams. I dream almost every night. When I wake up, I can usually still remember them. Yesterday I got terribly angry. I spent the weekend in the town of X, where I attended the university. I liked it so awfully much, and I always get mad when I have to come back to Ulm. Everything is so ugly in Ulm, no pretty girls.

A: Are they important to you?

P: I'm just not interested in men. In Ulm it's as if the clouds always have it covered up.

Commentary. It is not difficult to see that this is a well behaved patient who promptly followed the analyst's instructions. Her first association about the situation - she on the couch, the analyst behind her - was about a childhood scene in which she calls angels for help, to protect her during the night. This precipitated an anxiety that the patient related to being left alone in childhood, which was ameliorated by her embarrassed laughter. The next (second) association continued the subject of insecurity. In a dream Franziska X looked for the analyst's office, but found neither it nor the analyst. Her third association loosened the tension; she assured the analyst that she was ready to cooperate and added that he might even find her dreams interesting. Her fourth thought was indirectly related to a substantial anxiety symptom, which began when she started working in Ulm. She longed to return to her student days.

The patient expressed further associations about her student days and about visits to bars in the evenings, where she would sit around with friends until late. This had made her husband mad, even before their marriage; he would get tired and go home alone.

The patient then accused herself on not being able to say no, and changed the subject. She asked about the results of the psychological test. She said she was definitely inadequate in intellectual matters, yet she still wanted to get her Ph.D., as she had realized in the last few days. The brother she had asked for advice about treatment had just finished his dissertation.

After a moment of silence Franziska X wondered whether everything would not just get worse if she thought about it too much. She said her parents would not have wasted a thought on it, and that it would be completely pointless to talk with them about it. There was another pause in which I did not say anything. She continued that she was afraid of making debts; she always needed a cushion at the bank, and this was her sole concern in analysis.

In the pause that then followed I noticed that the patient was examining the room and her eyes had stopped on the old-fashioned oven.

P: Psychotherapy is in bad shape in Ulm [laughing].

A: Because of the old oven?

P: Not just that; the other house, too, the one I had my first interview in with Dr. A is almost falling down. When I visited him I was afraid that he would turn me down because my stories were so trivial.

A: Just like you couldn't find the room in your dream.

P: But my stories are trivial. This is bound to be an adventure. I'm curious to see what comes of it.

Commentary. The patient's associations have to be viewed as statements she made to the analyst. They do not create a simple story in which the plot is easy to follow, but a collage whose individual pieces are part of a more general motif that is often difficult to recognize.

The thought that "everything is ugly" was also directed at the office and the analyst, who related the comment about there not being any pretty girls here to the patient's negative self-feeling, yet without assuming that this allusion referred to an intention that had already become conscious.

The remarks the analyst makes while the patient is learning to freely associate have a significant function because they give the patient to understand that there is a counterpiece to how he is supposed to act, namely an answer to the jumps in his thoughts. Interventions inevitably direct the further course of events because they interrupt the process that tends to destabilize the patient. On the other hand, silence is frequently a comment after all, especially since the patient not yet familiar with the analytic situation will expect the interview to follow the rules of everyday communication (see Vol.1, Sect. 7.2).

Second Example

Linguistic studies on cases recorded in the Ulm Textbank document that in one sense patients enjoy a privilege at the beginning of therapy. According to them, patients can start by more or less holding monologues and in this way follow the fundamental rule. The analyst's role as a listener is then judged quite positively. This is demonstrated by the following short example from an initial session of a patient named Amalie X.

P: I feel something positive, that there really is a person to whom I can tell everything or who has to listen for better or worse and who can't complain when I say something stupid.

At the same time the patient developed her own ideas about the (listening) analyst, who usually participated in the conversation in a manner that did not meet the patient's expectations.

P: I have gradually realized that you more or less don't give answers; at the most you make something more precise. And I wonder why you act this way. Because this won't really become a conversation. I simply want to know what the reasons are. I really wonder about it, and it's an entirely different kind of conversation than I'm used to. [From the second session]

In the eleventh session the patient repeated her observation about the different nature of the situation and complained in more detail that there was too little response.

P: Well, I think it's an entirely different kind of conversation than what I'm used to. What bothers me the most at the moment are the gaps between what is said, because I don't know whether you're waiting for me to say something, or I'm waiting for you to speak. Always the pauses between what I say and what you say. It's pretty uncomfortable. And when I say something, then maybe it reaches you via some pneumatic dispatch. But then I'm not here anymore and I can't know and can't experience what you think the moment I tell you something. I don't even get an answer to my dispatch.

This excerpt demonstrates the stress that the fundamental rule can cause. The problems of technique that are encountered at the beginning are centered around the question of how we can facilitate the patient's transition to the specific kind of discourse that characterizes psychoanalysis without being able to eliminate every burden, but also without causing any unnecessary iatrongenic damage that we would have to expend great effort to overcome bit by bit. In this chapter in Vol.1, we argue in favor of flexibility on behalf of the analyst, in order to create the proper conditions in accordance with the patient's own circumstances.

At the end of the analysis the patient referred once again to her initial difficulties:

P: Moreover, in hindsight it sometimes seems strange to me that . . . well, I'll just say it in one short sentence. I sometimes thought, "Why didn't he say right away what he wants [laughed a little], and give me a set of instructions." I can remeber it precisely. I asked in horror, "Do I have to lie on the couch?" and I thought it was terrible. Then I said, "What do I have to do now?" and you said something like, "Tend more to say what you happen to think of." It was words like these. It may have been formulated differently, but the word "more" was there in any case.
A: More than in sitting.
P: Yes, you said it, and that was everything. That was the entire rule, the instructions, whatever it's called, and then I thought, "Boy, he's overestimated you; why doesn't he say any more, and then I wouldn't have to struggle so much myself." I often had that thought. He's looking at an entirely different person. He doesn't know me. He's just trying out how it works. He's starting from preconditions that are not very applicable to me, that are his own, and that only gradually became my own. It took me a good half year to get used to the couch. Even if it's theoretically clear, it doesn't help for a long time; everything you read about it doesn't help at all. Yet I wouldn't have dared to take a good look at you if I had been sitting. I don't think I would ever have managed to have that pleasure.

Commentary. Some years had elapsed since the beginning of this analysis. From our present perspective, we recommend that analysts provide more explanatory and interpreting answers in the initial phase, for example, in order to diminish the traumatic effect of pauses and enable the patient to use and master them more productively. The establishment of a helping alliance should be at the focus, and flexibility adapted to the requirements of the individual patient is necessary to achieve it. We have given several examples of the beginning of treatment that are of more recent origin in Sects. 2.1.1 and 2.1.2.

Amalie X made a significant contribution to the revision of our technique by drawing our attention to the significance of letting the patient be a party to the background and the context of the analyst's thoughts and actions (see also Sect. 2.4.2). We are convinced that this participation is neglected by many analysts, the consequences of which might be antitherapeutic. It is important for the analyst to structure the interaction in a dialogical manner and to reduce the asymmetry, especially in the initial phase.

Third Example

In the initial phase of therapy patients often pose the question as to what they should do if they cannot think of anything to say. The following example from the treament of Christian Y demonstrates one possible way of handling this difficult question; this procedure promotes the working alliance and is an indication of the first steps of interpretation.

P: What should I do in case I can't think of anything to say, if there's nothing of any significance on my mind.
A: Well, at first there was something on your mind. You said "nothing of any significance."
P: Yes.
A: Then just say what is on your mind, even if it doesn't seem siginificant to you.
P: You mean even a statement like "You have a lot of English literature here"?
A: Yes, precisely, that's a thought after all.
P: Or the noise from outside? I don't see that there's any connection to the treatment.
A: Well, we don't know. At any rate, it crossed your mind.
P: Yes?
A: Hum.
P: Am I making a mistake about what's important?
A: Right now, yes, inasfar as you assume and say that it doesn't belong here, for example the English literature you see here, that you've noticed, and that belongs here, and the saws outside that you can hear, and you notice it and it belongs here too.
P: I would have thought it was a digression.
A: Well, perhaps you went from the English literature to the saws because you might have thought that the idea with the literature was too personal, and therefore you quickly switched to the saws. That would be a wandering of your thoughts from the books in this room, which belong to me, to the outside, i. e., away from here. Insofar it could be a digression.
P: I just wonder, "Why?"
A: Maybe because a red light - to speak figuratively - lit up that told you not to think about the room or English literature any more.
P: Hum, yes. [Pause]
A: Do you have any other thoughts?
P: No, I've just thought a little about how good you are at remembering so many things, like a couple of words or a particular subject. Your concentration, how do you manage it. [Pause]
A: Yes, and then there is - the English literature, the masses of books - the question of knowledge. What does he know, does he know a lot, is his concentration good, and does he have a good memory, and maybe you feel envy?
P: Hum, not just envy, but interest too because I would like to know how you manage it. I'm not your only patient. You can't just concentrate on me because there are others you have to help in the same way, don't you?

Commentary. Digressions, which of course constitute an important part of association, can be used to clearly demonstrate a momentary resistance to association. In this case the analyst used the image of a red light to refer to it. The patient's digression seems to have started when he tried to find out whether and how the analyst maintained his concentration. Also involved was the acquisition of knowledge and the related comparisons, in which the patient did not fare well because his capacity to work and concentrate was severely disturbed. Every patient is interested in knowing how analysts manage to store so many data about a large number of people and their life histories in their memories and usually have it functional. By using suitable comparisons, an analyst can let patients participate in aspects of this mental achievement. The deidealization associated with it can also help the patient establish an access to his own cognitive processes.

It would certainly be wrong to belittle the analyst's trained ability to recall even apparently secondary details and dates. They are remembered by their thematic correspondence to categories or contexts and can be easily evoked by situative precipitants. Kohut, in particular, recognized the degree to which idealizations contribute to the maintenance of life. Of course, the more a patient falls behind his ideal and the more the latter becomes unattainable, the greater is the patient's envy, together with all of its destructive consequences.

It was wrong for the analyst to interpret the envy instead of continuing to focus on the interest the patient showed for the analyst and his collection of English literature. The patient's envious impulses toward the analyst's possessions, his knowledge, his abilities, his potency etc., which were disguised by the idealization, had a destructive effect on his imagination and paralyzed his thinking and acting. Many therapeutic steps are necessary to reduce the self-destructive consequence of such envy, and the first is for the unconscious envy to be thematized. Although this patient did not reject the interpretation, in the initial phase it was too early to mention envy. It would have been better to extend the theme of identificatory interest - How does he do it, and how can I do it - in order to establish a helping alliance.

7.3 Evenly Suspended Attention

Freud's recommendation that the analyst surrender himself in his evenly suspended attention to "his own unconscious mental acts" describes in more precise terms the nature of the participative observation that facilitates the perception of unconscious processes of emotional and cognitive exchange. The variety of the associations the analyst can have in the state of evenly suspended attention was clearly demonstrated by a thorough study of retrospective comments about analytic sessions that we conducted together with Meyer (1981). The analyst's associations can be classified according to their source and goal (Meyer 1988). They occur at various layers, some of which presumably became clear to the analyst during the session, while others appear to be independent continuations of affective and cognitive processes and were only recognized in hindsight.

Thinking Out Loud

The therapy of Ignaz Y was recorded as part of a research project on the origin and goal of interventions. As part of this project, the analyst dictated his afterthoughts immediately after the session, partly in response to predetermined questions (Kächele 1985).

P: That's really a funny microphone; it's got three parts. [Pause] This morning I'm so tired because I drank two big glasses of wine last night. [Long pause]

A: Any other ideas about the funny microphone?

P: I'm a little startled; I thought of a bug.

The patient concerned himself with where the tape recordings go; for a long time he had thought that I was not really recording "his shit," and now he was concerned about what might happen to his career if it got into the wrong hands.

P: It's gradually getting eerie, I mean everything I say here .... Maybe it's my need to run away from my own trash .... I don't think I've ever mentioned my dumb slogans; I've always felt so terribly ashamed about them .... Maybe you'll understand .... A thought just came to me, but I'm afflicted with new words just coming to me and that I completely ruin names and terms.

The patient described how he twists names around, even the names of his children and his friends, and that these words were filled with a special meaning for him, representing a kind of secret language. In puberty he had invented entire sequences of syllables and amused himself with the idea that he was the king of this empire. He noticed that he only twisted the names of people to whom he felt a positive tie.

A: It might be that this junk is only junk for others but that it is something valuable for you personally.

P: Yes, that's true, even though it's awfully childish, but I have the time of my life with these sounds, as if they were toys .... I turn the others into my toys a little .... That's how I reduce my fear, even with my children, when I'm sometimes afraid that they'll devour me.

In the further course of this session it became clear that the first name he had twisted was that of the most important role model in his childhood, namely that of a half-sister who was 7 years older than he was and whom he gave the name Laila. With this endearing nickname he was able to find consolation and to fill his empty early years. After he admitted how he distorted my own name toward the end of the session, he was also able to express his concern that he experienced the analysis as a threatening vacuum cleaner that sucked his inner world out of him and captured it.

The analyst's summary of the session, which was dictated immediately afterwards, contained the following unstructured report, which we have only slightly edited:

A terrific session; I'm really surprised at what came out. Even before the session began I had hoped that he would continue to talk about the tape recordings because this was the only way I felt that I could reexamine if I could still abide by the agreement we made about the recordings; it would make me feel less disturbed and worried. What was good was that the idea of shit was developed further, that the patient spoke about his relationships, that anxieties developed, that he was punished for them, and also that he constructed a world of transitional objects, which he had not mentioned before.

I had already had the feeling that the thematization of shit also expressed the magical animistic stage. It was only in response to his question whether the analysis was supervised [it was not] at the beginning of the session that I had not known what to say; I thought that he had to have the idea that I was also supervised and that it might be connected with the mastery of anxiety, since he was very anxious about an indiscretion occurring .... Of further importance from the session is that the theme "Laila," the important person from his childhood, has now reappeared after it had been dominant for the entire year .... I even felt his comment that he used these playful neologisms to be a great present; I recalled a patient with a skin disease who had just recently told me about such games, very private things that are both much more intimite and shameful than all possible object-related acts, this jabber, this stammering, the onomatopeia, and therefore the idea suddenly seemed very sound and fitting that in the small boy's perception his mother only consisted of a Laila, a dear Laila, and that this neologism had remained so vivid. And I never understood where the name Laila came, nor do I really know now who Laila actually is; is she a stepsister, is she another illegitimate child of his mother? I don't know anything about it; she is simply both hidden and present, the one who replaced his mother. That was actually the image, that Laila was actually only a figment of the patient's imagination, and yet a unimaginably important figment. I have always compared the Laila with a film from Agnes Varda about happiness [the reference is to the film "Le Bonheur"], the bright colors, the overpainted and apparently completely unaffected world of happiness. The magical creation of the name led me, via thoughts about Carlos Casteneda and Schreber's protolanguage, to the idea that he had created a world of his own that offered him autonomy.

I also liked his reference to a "private sound shift," and I had the idea that he was able to avoid depressive moods. He had obviously felt understood when he had read A.Miller's book on depressive constellations. He had been able to get over his depressive moods by inventing a children's zoo with the help of a fairy.

I have the impression that he departed rather quickly; his sorrow is genuine.

My interpretation that the neologisms represented creative achievements took a great burden off him, and also calmed him by removing his constantly returning anxiety of being schizophrenic. At the end he will probably have told me several specific distortions of my name and of that of his second boss in his home dialect. I hardly expected it any more; he transformed it into his own Swiss dialect.

The subject of his return to Switzerland and his comments about this idea stimulated a number of thoughts. Was he looking for the language of his father and mother? Why did he distort my name? He distorts names when the relationship is dear and tender. He did not have to distort the name of his stupid administrative boss because such disappointments did not go so deep; the frustration of tender, merging impulses, in contrast, apparently made him feel the need to make the fairy come alive. I believe the patient took a large step forward here because he was able to view his clowning and silly behavior from this perspective without my having to do much about it; I even have the feeling that my reports about the sessions are not yet very freely associated, but maybe it is also a matter of time before one can let oneself have more space.

Commentary. The task of associating about a just ended session cannot simply be conceived as an uninterrupted continuation of the analyst's "unconscious mental activity" during the session. One important result of this study was the impact the separation from the patient had on the analyst's hindsight. The transition from the therapeutic situation, in which a dyadic and a monologic (partly verbalized, partly nonverbalized) level exist in parallel and which both promote and inhibit each other, into an externally monologic position, in which the analyst's task is to associate by reflecting on the dyadic situation that is only present in his memory, led to a rapid reorganization of the analyst's psychic situation. The retrospective report demonstrates this.

The analyst expressed his pleasure very directly, even grasping the comments that had disturbed him as presents. The analyst's style of language makes one sense an identification with the patient's game, and enabled him to reconstruct what advances the patient had made. The unmentioned idea the analyst had about the film by A. Varda was from the realm of his own personal experience, in which he felt the hypomanic defensive character of the patient's self-invented happiness was convincingly demonstrated. The reference to the motive of the proto-language emphasized the character of this language game, which was not only based on a childhood world but that expressed a defensive formation in the patient's present. In the further course of his fantasies, the analyst again achieved some distance and reflected on the outcome of the session. He then said goodbye to his imaginary listener (who stands for a real person who does research) with an act of distancing that was less justified by the factual content of his comments than by the emotional content of the session. Such an assumption seems logical since the analyst immediately thought of this session - which had taken place many years before - in response to a question as to the choice of a suitable example of evenly suspended attention.

7.4 Questions and Answers

We have discussed this subject in detail in the context of the *counterquestion rule* in Vol.1 (Sect. 7.4). Today most analysts reject the method of directing questions back to the patient in a stereotypic manner - such as with the phrases "What are you thinking of in connection with your question?" or "What thoughts enter your mind when you think about why you wanted to ask me this question?" - because it frequently has antitherapeutic consequences, and not just in severely ill patients.

Example

Arthur Y, my patient, and several of his relatives were involved in a conflict over an inheritance. Apparently uncertain about what to do, Arthur Y asked me: "Now I'm asking you for your private opinion, not your analytic one." The patient emphasized the urgency of the matter by referring to his increasing uneasiness and a worsening of his symptoms. My thoughts about the difference between private and professional opinions was initially linked with an embarassed feeling of insecurity.

A: Since my private opinion is probably the common sense one, our opinions on this issue are probably pretty similar, but it is my professional task to help you solve the matter in your own best interest. I'm asking myself why you want me to reinforce you in something you already know.

Consideration. Although doubts about common sense are sometimes quite justified, an issue we discussed later, I made the remark about probably having similar views after considering the matter carefully and not out of embarassment. It was clear that the way the patient behaved would either aggravate or moderate the conflict between the members of the family entitled to an inheritance. Such simple reactions are a part of common sense. Yet the patient was uncertain as to which direction he should go and wanted to have my advice, which I was unable to give him. Yet I did reinforce his anticipatory knowledge of the consequences that this or that act would presumably have.

P: It's a very normal human trait for your opinion to be important to me.

A: Certainly.

P: With my earlier analysts I always had the feeling "Don't get too close to me." Especially Dr. X gave me the impression that by asking such questions I was transgressing a limit, as if to develop a relationship among pals. Maybe that's the reason I formulate everything so awkwardly or in such an involved manner.

We spoke about the fact that is satisfying to reach agreement and share an opinion, i. e., to become pals. Then one aspect of being pals became clear that had bothered the patient in a previous therapy. We spoke about the various possibilities to defuse or resolve the family conflict. It became clear to the patient that the consequence of one particular action - correcting something and thus acting correctly - had to be to continue the war in the family. By acting in this way he would really draw people's attention to the feud in the family.

P: I've just thought of a phrase from Schiller, that I can mold to fit you: From a safe refuge it's easy to give advice.

A: Yes.

P: Yet if I want to have my peace and quiet, I cannot continue to shoot. But I can't let myself get shot either.

A: But you haven't been shot and killed.

P: My feelings have been hurt, I've been insulted.

A: You've been gravely insulted because you experience yourself to be so powerless.

P: Yes, sure. My brother-in-law took it differently. He didn't get excited at all. My self-esteem sinks to zero. Then I don't have any ground to stand on any more. There's no limit to how far I could fall.

A: And that's why it was so important to you that I reinforce your common sense, because otherwise you wouldn't have thought about asking for my private opinion, which you somehow already know.

P: Yes, I do know it already.

A: Well, you cannot always assume that the other person has common sense.

Apparently encouraged by my comment, the patient then mentioned sectarian thinking in psychoanalysis, but immediately became anxious that this might have offended me: "I hope that I haven't attacked anyone here who means so much to me or made him my enemy."

Consideration. In this session there was a turn toward an intensification of transference, which my comment had made easier for the patient. All too often in his life he had submitted to others and appeared to adopt their opinions, but inside he had retained his doubts, which increased with time. By asking for my private opinion, the patient was seeking a means of access to his own unvarnished needs, which gained in strength during the conflict over the inheritance and which he was afraid of.

The Request for a Book

Erna X was interested in books on psychoanalysis. A friend of hers had drawn her attention to the book *Les mots pour le dire* by Marie Cardinal (1975). She had been surprised and astonished when her friend asked her whether she would dare ask her analyst for the book. The closer the session came, the uneasier she became. Erna X immediately raised the question, which contained two aspects. I could take her question about whether I possess the book, which according to her friend was out of print, and would lend it to her to be presumptuous. After examining the intensity of the potential presumptuousness in detail, I answered her question realistically, also emphasizing that in view of all the books in the room, which however did not include the one she desired, I thought it was logical for her to ask and that I did not take it to be presumputous at all. Then the patient turned to the second aspect. Would I lend her a book, and would I expect her to read it thoroughly? Erna X feared that in this case she would be put to a test and queried about what she had learned.

P: I expect to be checked.

A: So you would have to read it so thoroughly that you would be ready for every possible question.

P: Yes, I don't know whether I really want to read it that thoroughly.

I emphasized to her that I did not have this expectation and that it was up to her to read what she wanted.

Commentary. The patient's thoughts show which inhibiting responsibilities would have resulted if the analyst had actually been able to lend her the book. Of course, these consequences could have been worked through by interpretations. The consequences that rejection and cooperation have on the relationship and on how they are to be interpreted differ from case to case.

There are various means to meet a patient's interest in obtaining publications on psychoanalysis. We consider it to be wrong to discourage or forbid patients from gaining information about psychoanalysis from books. As impressive as it is, for therapeutic and scientific reasons, for an analyst to encounter a completely naive person who retains his naivete in treatment, it would be just as antitherapeutic to stifle this emerging interest. The problems of rationalization and intellectualism that are occasionally associated with it certainly do cause problems, but these cannot be compared with the consequences of forbidding a patient to read. Initially Freud seems to have discouraged patients from reading publications about psychoanalysis; later, however, he expected patients, at least analysts in training and educated patients, to inform themselves by reading (Doolittle 1956).

Erna X described the typical feature of her story:

P: It was clear to me that I would ask you until I sat down in the waiting room. Then I had one doubt after another. It's the same way with other things. I get the doubt that this or that might get disagreeable. It's the same way, too, with my career. Then I let everything go.

A: It's the subject of being presumptuous again, about your taking something for yourself when you want to advance, when you intrude into my library, or when you want to learn something about my thoughts during the analysis.

P: So deep inside I knew that you aren't mad at me for asking for the book. Where does my anxiety about being presumptuous come from?

A: Probably a lot of curiosity has accumulated because of the restrictions you experienced when you were small. Your interest is so intense that you fear your desires might be excessive. The desire for a book then becomes an example of a presumptuous and illicit desire.

P: Yes, that's right. My desire for the book might be considered too personal. I wouldn't have had any inhibitions about asking a friend to lend me a book. But you're the doctor, somebody special, somebody I look up to. I can't let myself do this or that.

A: That would create something you have in common. You would take part in what belongs to me.

P: By no means do I want to be obtrusive. You would have to look for it; it might be bothersome. But there isn't any way out if you think like this. If I hadn't asked, I would have left feeling very dissatisfied.

Erna X then spoke about the things that currently were a burden on her, in particular about her mother's illness.

P: I have more responsibilities. I need more time to take care of my family. I need someone more often for my children. My husband suggested that I cut back on therapy, and I had a dream about it. I was at home, and you drove over to visit me. You excused yourself, saying you had to interrupt the treatment because you were overworked. I felt honored that you visited me and accepted your suggestion. I accompanied you to your car and saw two young and attractive students sitting inside. It puzzles me that in my dream I accepted my husband's suggestion and that *you* interrupted the treatment.

A: It's a reversal. To return to the subject, it is probably an expression of your concern about being presumptuous when you want more and I reject your desires. Your dream indicates that other things are more important to me than you are. Maybe it's the two pretty students who are more important?

P: Yes, presumably that's true. At the end I was in a ridiculous situation, rejected, alone, sad. I'm thinking about something else. The rejection. You were friendly, by no means cold and rejecting, not brusque like my husband - "Just leave me alone" - but just like you always are. You explained something to me. I understood it and accepted it although I didn't like it.

A: But you didn't object. You felt I had paid attention to you by driving extra to see you and to turn you down.

P: Dreams are really often surprisingly amazing. It's unbelievable, everything that took place in this dream. You forget a lot. Did I really want to go with you? You left so abruptly.

A: You wanted to come along, and in a particular sense you did come along, only indirectly, in the form of the students. The fact that you lost out and were turned down was terrible for you, but indirectly you were there. The rejection probably had something to do with the pretty girls who take part in what happens here at the university. That's the reason you were so astonished. It would be presumptuous for you to want to have a book.

P: Yes, that's what I thought. I asked myself if it would be presumpuous if I studied psychology and went to hear your lectures. I'm sad that I've missed my chance. I get angry when I think back about how I chose the simple and safe way.

A: Yes, you've missed some chances, but there are others, for example in your profession.

Commentary. It should be emphasized that the analyst referred to the positive opportunities at the end of the session, stimulating hopes that also have a transference component. It was realistic for the analyst to help the patient perceive her future opportunities in the profession she had learned.

7.5 Metaphors

7.5.1 Psychoanalytic Aspects

In Vol.1 we considered the meaning of metaphors in connection with the controversy about Strachey's translation of Freud's works and discussed the role that metaphors play in the language of theory (Sect. 1.4). In accordance with Arlow's (1979) reference to the fact that metaphoric thought predominates in transference, we have assigned the clarification of similarities and dissimilarities a prime role during transference interpretations (Sect. 8.4).

Similes, metaphors, and allegories play an important part in Freud's style, as can also be seen from the size of the corresponding section in the index to the *Standard Edition.* It contains a list of the shorter quotations or peculiar uses of language that are directly related to psychoanalytic concepts. As this special index demonstrates, Freud frequently used similes to illustrate psychoanalytic theory.

Metaphors are a figure of speech that originated in rhetoric and that have finally become the object of an independent *metaphorology* (Blumenberg 1960). Original metaphors make a special contribution to helping new ideas acquire vivid substance (Lewin 1971). Metaphors have played an oustanding role in all the sciences, especially with regard to discoveries, because they link that which is known and familiar with that which is still strange and unfamiliar. They are well suited for achieving the balance that is implicit in Kant's (1965 [1781], p.A51) aphorism that "Thoughts without content are empty, intuitions without concepts are blind."

The problem posed by metaphors has attracted many researchers since Richard's (1936) pioneering study. Various linguistic and multidisciplinary studies and symposia, such as those documented by Ortony (1979), Miall (1982), Sacks (1979), and Weinrich (1968, 1976), demonstrate that metaphors are obviously an object of great interest in many disciplines in the humanities. In the psychoanalytic literature, however, there is still an insufficient number of publications dealing explicitly with the significance of metaphors in the language used in theory and in practice, a fact which Rubinstein complained about in 1972. Psychoanalytic papers are almost completely lacking in multidisciplinary studies. In 1978, Rogers published the results of an interdisciplinary study group on psychoanalytic aspects of metaphors, but it attracted much criticism (Teller 1981) because it followed the tension-discharge model of cognitive processes. Göbel (1980, 1986) discussed the relationship between metaphor and symbol with reference to the distinction that Jones made, and took newer publications in philosophy and linguistics into consideration.

In order to gain a better understanding of the meaning of metaphors in the psychoanalytic dialogue, we should look at the origin of the term, which makes it logical that a psychoanalyst thinks of the process of displacement. The term, taken from the Greek, originally referred to a specific act, namely the carrying over of an object from one location to another. Aristotle referred to the metaphor as "the right carrying over" (*eu metapherein*), as the ability to recognize similarities. It was not until later that the word came to refer to a figure of speech. Such carrying over becomes a metaphor when it is taken *figuratively*, not *literally*. Metaphors represent an intermediate stage to the complete use of symbols. They are rooted in the anthropomorphic world of images and in man's bodily experience.

Characteristic for metaphors is their mixture. The concepts "image," "simile," "allegory," and "metaphor" are frequently used synonymously in works on literature (see Köller 1986). The distinction between these concepts is not complete even within linguistics. "Image" often serves as a generic concept for metaphor, simile, and allegory. A simile is a construction referring to an image that contains the words "as" or "like."

The tension between similarity and dissimilarity in the transference from the original object, or referent, to the new object is central for understanding metaphors. In contrast to simile and allegory, in which image and object can coexist, in all metaphors the image takes the place of the object. It is therefore logical to assume that a statement such as "I feel *like* a wilted primula" expresses a weaker identification in a dialogue than do the sentences "I *am* a wilted primula," "I *am* a jellyfish drying up on the sand," "I *am* a desert," "I *am* a porcupine," or "I *am* a heap of shit."

The fact that metaphors play an outstanding role in the psychoanalytic dialogue is due to this intermediate position; the clarification of similarities and dissimilarities is a constant issue in the dialogue (Carveth 1984). This was the reason that Richards, writing 50 years ago from a linguistic and philosophical perspective, classified the phenomena of transference as examples of metaphorology, a field his concepts greatly enriched. Black (1962) summarized these concepts in his "interaction theory of metaphor."

Considering that the carrying over was originally taken literally, it is also logical that many metaphors originated in analogy to the human body and lead back to it. From a therapeutic point of view it is therefore essential to rediscover the unconscious physical starting point in figurative language and to refer to it by name. Of course, we cannot expect it to be possible to trace all metaphors back to particular bodily experiences. Such a general reduction, which Sharpe (1940) defended and explained with reference to case histories, is not appropriate for the diversity of metaphoric language. We share Wurmser's (1977, p. 472) view that the metaphor is "a guide to unconscious meaning - not unlike dreams, parapraxes, or symptoms."

Since the analytic dialogues cited in this volume contain numerous metaphors and allegories and the following section contains a thorough linguistic study, we will only mention three examples here. The world of images exerts a great fascination. Metaphors are well suited to be used as flattering descriptions of concrete bodily needs and the feeling of shame associated with them, since theories and concepts are not the only instances in which rationalizations can serve resistance. This is also true for metaphors. After unfolding a figurative language related to emotions, it is therefore advisable to locate and call by name the bodily and sensual source of perceptions expressed in metaphors. The concern that this might destroy meaningful images or even the creative foundation of fantasizing is unfounded; our experience is just the contrary, namely that the world of images becomes even more vivid and original when it is linked to the starting point of the analogy. It is, of course, no coincidence that the intermediate position of metaphors makes them well suited for elaborating the struggle between iconophiles and iconoclasts. Grassi (1979) demonstrated that this involves recognizing the power of fantasy, which is the reason that analysts are always on the side of the iconophiles, i. e., those that revere images, and not on that of the iconoclasts, who destroy them. The function of metaphors in psychic life should be examined from psychoanalytic points of view. For example, negative metaphoric self-representations are frequently encountered in therapy, and the allegories invented by patients are therefore useful as indicators of altered self-esteem.

The Analyst as Irrigationist

At the beginning of his therapy, Gustav Y had described his world as a desert in which only meager and resistant plants could survive, and afterwards he compared the consequences of his therapy with the effects that an irrigation system has on barren desert soil, making it possible for rich vegetation to develop. Metaphors related to plants are especially well suited to represent the inconspicuous aspect of the development of psychic processes (Kächele 1982). Yet it is impossible to be satisfied with the fact that the desert lives, as pleasant as the changes are that produced the new metaphor. For this patient it was just as surprising as it was important that the analyst asked him why he structured his world in the form of a desert. In doing so the analyst assumed, contrary to the given facts, that this was not necessarily the case - an assumption that is always justified with neurotic patients because of the functional character of their inhibitions. It was also important that the analyst asked him why he had made him into an irrigationist. This attribution served the anxious defense of the patient's own pleasureable oedipal and preoedipal fantasies of fruition. As was shown in the further course of the therapy, the specific forms that his symptom and character took were a consequence of the repression of desires that stemmed from a variety of sources - a metaphor that Freud (1905d) used to represent his libido theory.

Commentary. Although specific urophilic and uropolemic memories themselves were not mentioned in the analysis, it would have been helpful in this case for the analyst to have been aware of Christoffel's (1944) theories. As with everything that is human, even the bodily experience linked with urination has been portrayed poetically. The figurative language of poetry has been used to express the unconscious fantasies, to use psychoanalytic terms, that Freud described with his theory of *psychosexuality*. The step from the poetic description to the scientific discovery introduces connections into human nature that are reminiscent of the laws of nature. For instance, in his famous novel Rabelais described the omnipotent and uropolemic fantasies of Gargantua, the main figure of his novel who was able to flood all of Paris by urinating. Christoffel integrated such urophilic fantasies into the theory of psychosexuality. For a patient to experience himself and his environment as being a dried up desert goes back in part to the repression of his impulses, which he then tries to find as an irrigationist in the person of the analyst.

The Source

Erna X used to withdraw quietly when she was disappointed and felt tense, to be alone and simply to cry out of desperation. She was now able to express her conflicts more openly, but she was still helpless as to what is to come next.

She finally came to speak of her reserves. I picked up this train of thought by comparing her reserves with a source she could tap. She turned it into a flowing fountain. The bubbling water became an allegory. Erna X laughed. "Now that's a picture," she said, "that makes it possible to have lots of ideas, in contrast to the picture of a pool of standing water. I think of myself more as the standing pool than a bubbling fountain. Bubbling is impossible for me - it was turned off." The session ended with the patient expressing her satisfaction that she was returning to the source, and that with analytic help she would make fewer mistakes in raising her children.

I was all the more surprised when Erna X began the following session by stating that she had not wanted to come. She felt she were in a void. She answered my question about whether the last session had been unproductive with a clear no, saying the business with the bubbling water had just carried her along. Such figurative comparisons exerted a strong appeal on her. While in the waiting room she had still thought about the bubbling. She described the vitality of her daughter, who really bubbled with high spirits. She said her daughter took great joy in life, her eyes sparkled with pleasure, she exuded a feeling of satisfaction, and she could also go wild. Bubbling was, according to the patient, a normal manifestation in childhood. Erna X reflected on her own childhood and the limitations that had been imposed on her.

I expressed the assumption that this was the reason that she-had not wanted to come or that she had wanted to stay away for good because she had been raised to have the idea that she had to come with a clear programmatic purpose and only if she were sure that she had something to offer. Her uneasiness increased when we discussed spontaneous statements. I reminded her that her wish to touch my hand had previously filled her with anxiety. To give her relief I mentioned that all ideas and fantasies are directed to the outside.

Commentary. We would like to draw particular attention to the analyst's helpful comment that gave a general meaning to the patient's transference. Such actions thin the transference, which can have negative consequences if the patient experiences the generalization as a rejection. In this case the result of the generalization was rather that this patient became much less shy about including her analyst in her fantasy world.

P: I may have started to bubble here but the big flood can still come, the full-fledged bubbling. It's like with a water tap that was turned off so firmly that it's extremely difficult to open it bit by bit. I couldn't think of anything else, although I've had the opposite experience.

I then gave the interpretation that her thoughts about stopping might be motivated by her concern that she might think of too *much*, not too *little*.

P: The tap was closed. It's just as simple as it is extremely difficult, because in opening it I'm also trying to turn it back bit by bit. I try to tell myself, "Be satisfied with what you have and get along with it." I don't see any alternative.

After a long pause Erna X posed a surprising question.

P: Have you ever sent a patient away and told the person that there wasn't any point in coming any more?

In the pause that followed I could sense that the patient was urgently waiting for an answer.

A: I'm thinking about it.

P: What prompted me to ask? I can tell you that. An acquaintance was in therapy that her analyst ended with the justification that there wasn't any point in continuing. Subliminally I'm probably also afraid that there isn't any point.

A: You're anxious that too much might bubble out of you, and fear being sent away, not because you have too little to offer, but rather too much.

P: If I don't bubble enough, then you send me away, and if I bubble too much at home, then my husband sends me away. I'm more spontaneous that I used to be, and rasher. I feel as if I were left in between.

I agreed with her that this was a genuine difficulty that would be gone if she did not come any more. The session then continued along the ususal lines. I explained that it was natural for both the patient and the analyst to occasionally raise the question about the sense of continuing.

P: If you're asking me whether I want to make more progress or not, I couldn't answer spontaneously with a clear yes or a no.

She described her ambivalence by referring to the example of her desire for children, on the one hand, and the rejection of a further pregnancy on the other.

P: If I made more progress, what then? It's awfully difficult.

A: What bubbling are you afraid of? What minor bubbling could turn into a full-fledged one?

P: That I can't continue to live under the momentary circumstances . . . . I made a mistake that I have to fix. At the same time, it's impossible to change it.

A: Do you think you have so little influence on your husband, or that he has so little scope for acting? Have you already tested the various possibilities you have for influencing your husband?

The patient answered in the negative.

A: You still haven't discussed a lot of things, and your husband doesn't give you any encouragement. A lot is still overcontrolled, so that what in reality is there somewhere – your desires and your fantasies, presumably of both of you – has disappeared.

P: I am reluctant to do everything myself. I would much prefer having a husband who is active.

A: It's a natural expectation to want more stimulation, but there is probably another side, namely that it is not proper for you to mention some things, e. g., sex.

P: Yes, sex is something that men are supposed to control. It's like a cliff – do I jump into the water or not? That's what I'm struggling with right now. I'm looking for a way out, to leave it alone. If I had had a little more time, then I would have read something. Then I would have come here better prepared. But even then I wouldn't have the session under complete control and somewhere the bubbling would start. If I'm the one to start, then I might reveal too much of myself. Waiting makes it possible for me to feel my way. My wishes and needs must have been completely strangled. And not just wishes and needs, abilities too. I would never dare to say that I'm capable of doing something. [Long pause] I can't get over that figurative comparison. I'm thinking about a pond, on a fountain that is flowing and bubbling. That's not how I want to be. I don't want to stand there and be seen, standing out there alone and in the open. I would stay down there in the water and cautiously look up, but prefer to stay down there, surrounded by warm water. That's more my style.

A: It's probably connected with the fact that in the figurative language of similes, talking about bubbling, showing, and flowing out expresses a strong relationship to an entire individual and to his body. This is the reason water streams out of the mouths of statues at fountains, and nymphs are there, and so is urination. A person is the source of a stream in urination. That's why there is that famous little statue in Brussels, the Mannikin piss, where the water comes out of his penis. That is what is suggested by these images.

P: [Laughed] I know it. Years ago, I might have been 10 or 12, my father was in Brussels and brought back some pictures, including one of the Mannikin piss. I looked at it without saying a word. I thought it wasn't important, but even then I probably had questions that were simply brushed aside.

Commentary. The analyst's idea might seem farfetched if the anthropomorphism contained in all metaphors were ignored. Metaphors and allegories start from bodily experiences, which are always present at an unconscious level. This is not the least important reason for the fascination that metaphors exert. Nonetheless the analyst made a considerable jump here. Was the jump very risky? No, because water and urination are closely associated in unconscious anthropomorphic thought.

The Metaphors "Porcupines" and "Barbed Flowers"

Clara X returned from a vacation in the mountains, which was hoped to have a positive effect on her daughter's chronic illness, in high spirits. While we greeted each other, she beamed at me, which led me to respond in a particularly friendly manner. At the beginning of the session Clara X uttered a sound that I took to be a grunt of satisfaction and involuntarily responded by making a similar grunt. This echo died away without having any effect.

After some silence I spoke about the two sounds. Her friendly greeting at the beginning and the onomatopoeia of the sounds created an intimite atmosphere in which closeness and warmth could be felt - or so I thought. I referred to Schopenhauer's allegory about the porcupines in order to discuss the subject of how distance is regulated. Clara X had frequently used, in various forms, the porcupine as a metaphor for herself.

An abbridged form of the allegory, which reappeared in in the patient's self-representation without her knowing its source, is:

> A group of porcupines gathered very close together on a cold winter day so that the warmth they emitted as a group would keep them from freezing. Yet they soon began to feel each other's barbs, which caused them to move apart again. Now when they felt the need for warmth and moved closer together, that second evil repeated itself, so that they were torn back and forth between the two sources of their suffering until they had found a moderate distance from one another, at which they were best able to stay.... Social needs drive... men together in the same way, but the numerous repulsive qualities und unbearable mistakes they have repel them from another.... Yet whoever has much inner warmth of his own prefers to avoid society, in order neither to give cause for complaints nor to receive any. (Schopenhauer 1974, p. 765)

Believing that Clara X had moved closer to me, I mentioned my assumption that the grunts symbolized the steps from a hedgehog to a pig. Clara X, however, had taken the grunts to be more the cry of a sow who was warning her piglets. She did not feel that the sound she had emitted expressed satisfaction, even though she did feel at ease. She said she was once again faced with the questions of whether to continue and which goals might still be achieved in therapy. She could not really imagine getting much further. For a long time she felt she had been running in place, not getting anywhere. While she did feel at harmony with herself, both she herself and her relations to others were still full of contradictions and rough edges. She felt she would just have to accept it as a fact, and asked me if I believed that she would manage to be able to change her behavior in any way.

At first I told the patient that I shared her doubts, emphasizing the difficulties that stood in the way of change. Once again she employed the image of a wild rose, which she had mentioned in an earlier session, asking what kept it from flowering. Long ago she had described how she had rejected a boy who had approached her - as in the German folk song "Sah ein Knab' ein Röslein stehn," based on a poem by Goethe - in a fantasy in which a seagull released a stream of excrements on the boy.

Commentary. Coming closer apparently precipitated significant defense processes. The seagull served to illustrate anal aggression.

Being more satisfied with herself as a woman and having an appearance that others find more appealing was linked for this patient with a mortal threat, which was expressed in her associations. She referred to a frank statement I had made emphasizing that I liked her more when she felt more comfortable as a woman and that this good feeling, stemming from inside, made itself felt in a change in her figure, i.e., in her appearance. I had thus also expressed the conviction that she would also like herself more and could then achieve greater harmony in her interpersonal relations. Referring to the autobiographical stories of anorectics, she expressed her doubt as to whether truely fundamental changes inside would ever really effect changes in external things and vice versa, so that an anorectic girl might be reconciled with her condition and even become a happy woman. She had simply, yet with disbelief, accepted the positive reports I had given earlier about anorectic patients. She said she would not overcome her doubts until she herself had met one of these cured individuals and might use her as a role model. Knowing that it would not be easy to fulfill such a wish, she would continue her search for a role model but without any prospects of success.

Clara X admitted that she occasionally had a feeling of complete happiness, but only for a few brief seconds. I responded that the issue was then to determine how the length, intensity, and frequency of these moments might be increased. She used exclusively oral topics to describe these moments, speaking about nursing a child.

The patient explained that she might like to have the feelings of confidence and security. It then came out that for the patient the word "please" (or "like") was linked with a mortal danger, i.e., with the word "fall," the two words having the same root in German. This was the reason that she was so irritated when I used this word. Clara X referred to a story to illustrate the danger she might get into; at first she referred to it as a joke: A man had attempted to convince a woman that she could jump off the tenth floor of a building without injuring herself. He had said he would catch her. In response to her disbelieving questions, he had assured the woman that he had just recently caught a woman who had dared to jump off the twentieth floor. Now the woman started having even more objections, asking about the injuries that the man must have suffered while catching her. He had only said that nothing had happened to him because he had let the woman bounce first.

The terrible end of the story was made ridiculous by her allusion to a bouncing ball, and the patient's ironic tone of voice was perfectly attuned to the story.

Each of us immediately realized the dangers that Clara X would be exposed to if she relied on me. Her story had expressed what could happen if she surrendered herself to her spontaneous needs, including that of wanting to please people.

Commentary. To turn to someone in confidence implies intimacy, and just the thought of it was repulsive to this patient. In such moments she might have the satisfying feeling of nursing, i. e., the fulfillment that posed such a danger to her. It was impossible for her to experience this satisfaction as happiness because every satiation was a withdrawal, and to avoid this feeling of withdrawal she had put herself into a state of autarchy, i. e., into a position of almost complete independence. That in the process her longing had become immense could be seen in the destructive force she attributed to her hunger in the widest and deepest sense of the word. If, namely, she did not restrain her lusting for life and her craving, the object - the world - would be destroyed. The patient's radical abstinence was her attempt to preserve the object and - as paradoxical as it might sound - herself as well. Fusion and union can be experienced unconsciously as destructive self-dissolution if aggressive instincts predominate. A fasting that is undertaken for primarily other reasons, which may frequently be superficial, e. g., a person's figure, can subsequently turn into a vicious circle. The frustration of the nurturing impulse, which requires great effort, leads not only to a loss of differentiation in orality if the impulses break through, but also to a continous stimulation of aggression. In every kind of surrendering, the patient experienced anxiety about the destruction of the object or herself instead of experiencing a pleasurable "oceanic feeling" and an unlimited union with the world. It is thus no wonder that Clara X and her analyst found it very difficult to modify the form of self-preservation she had established in her illness.

Some time later Clara X starting using the *echinoderms*, e. g., a starfish, as her symbol.

P: I have to maintain an external skeleton, because when the external skeleton is removed from an echinoderm then it flows apart, like a mollusc. Then there's nothing left. Everything dissolves.

A: Then it's logical that you've put on such a skeleton.

P: Yes, it's so dangerous if you don't have one that you can't . . . nothing . . . .

A: . . . then the fear that . . .

P: . . . that if the external skeleton is removed, that they sill simply collapse. Molluscs.

The analyst referred back to the hedgehog.

A: Oh, the *hedgehogs* have an internal skeleton.

P: But then I don't have one at all.

Commentary. We would like to draw attention to the smooth transition from one sentence to the next. The patient completed the analyst's thought and vice versa. The analyst took up the new metaphor, the *echinoderms*, for the old one, the *hedgehogs*.

The analyst continued by asking a question.

A: Where does the idea come from that you could dissolve if you stopped showing your external skeleton?

P: From real experience. I can start crying and, independent of the reason, get into a state of utter helplessness. Then it's impossible for me to say why I have lost control. Perhaps it's the wish to be understood and for my weaknesses to be accepted, and not have to be big and brave. It's my wish to let myself fall down and to say, "I can't do any more, you do it now." Besides, I don't want to be able to do any more. But then from others all that I encounter is displeasure, embarrassed concern, and awkward situations – "My God, what's wrong now?" It's terrible. It's bad enough in itself, but it's made even worse by the others. So I naturally think, "See, now you're being left alone, to punish you because you've been so childish." It was a feeling I often had when I was a child.

A: Then you have the feeling of dissolving, of being carried away by the immense stream from inside you.

P: Yes, precisely, that's how it is, dissolving into tears. Dissolving in tears. That's where it comes from. It's a part of oneself. Or losing the ground under one's feet. There is only one kind of reaction that makes it all bearable, namely if other people let me cry, and if something has been accepted, then I don't need it any more. Then I only cry as much as I need, and then it's over. But most people react differently – fussing, becoming disconcerted, being startled, and so forth, and then exactly what I don't want sets in. I cramp. Recently I even cried in front of my husband, and neither of us was moved. It was impossible for him to misunderstand it, which made it possible for me to cry in front of him without triggering his usual reactions. Sometimes I start crying in a way that I just can't stop. Right now I imagine that you can't understand me, partly because you're a man and crying is something that stopped when you were a 4-year-old boy.

A: Well I did contribute the expression "dissolving into tears."

P: Oh well, but that came through your head. My father also always stood outside the matter, or at any rate, yes, somehow above it.

A: But it isn't entirely negative for someone to be above the matter in such moments.

P: But I don't have the feeling I've been understood. In this point, not at all, not at home.

Consideration. Since I had been very involved with this patient, her criticism hit me very hard. Of course, it was also a kind of transferred disappointment, as shown by her reference to her father. I had a consoling thought, namely that it seems inevitable for there to be a certain distance between someone who is crying and the others around them. The tears of another person, even those of a significant other are not one's own tears; they are the tears of someone else. Empathy seems to approach a state in which two people feel as if they are one, yet without them forming *one* identity.

7.5.2 Linguistic Interpretations

In the current phase of the development of psychoanalytic technique it is important for precise protocols of analyses to be compiled and for empirical studies, including interdisciplinary ones, to be conducted about how analysts talk to patients and what they say. As early as 1941 Bernfeld entitled one section of an article that has remained relatively unknown "Conversation, the model of psychoanalytic technics" (p. 290). In a subsequent stage of development the dialogic orientation receded in importance. The Study Group for Linguistics at the New York Psychoanalytic Institute, under the leadership of Rosen (1969), concerned itself with language, especially from the perspective of ego functions. The study of dialogues entered another new stage when the step was taken to record and transcribe therapeutic interviews.

It is important particularly with regard to interdisciplinary cooperation that the participants remember what they have been trained to do; otherwise there is the danger that, for example, linguists who have some knowledge of psychoanalysis will not do a proper linguistic examination but will ask what psychoanalytic interviews would presumably be like if analysts followed the basic rule. It is a fact "that the character of psychoanalytic therapy as a special kind of verbal exchange (in the sense of a regulated performance of discursive activity) has hardly been discovered in the psychoanalytic literature as an object of specialized study, let alone researched in detail" (Flader 1982, p. 19). Mahony and Singh (1975, 1979) reached a similar conclusion in a critical discussion of Edelson's (1972, 1975) efforts to make Chomskian linguistics applicable for a revision of dream theory.

In linguistics there are various theoretical perspectives. There are theories that view metaphors as a unit of "langue," following the Swiss linguist F. de Saussure - who viewed language as a sign system - and others that see metaphors as the unit of the "parole," i. e., the actual, "spoken" structure of language. The starting point of langue theories is that metaphors are a feature of expressions or sentences within an abstract system of language. They follow Aristotle's definition of metaphor as a simile without the word "like" or "as."

Parole theories accept as given that metaphors originate in their actual use. One school of thought is interaction theory, which assumes that there is no actual expression for a metaphoric one. Weinrich assumed that the significance of a metaphor results from the interaction between the specific metaphor and its context. According to Kurz (1982, p. 18), "The metaphoric meaning is thus more an act than a result, i. e., the constructive creation of meaning that somehow takes place via a dominant meaning, a movement from ... to .... "

Keller-Bauer distinguished between two fundamental manners of understanding metaphors: "The metaphoric use of X, which can only be understood on the basis of the literal use of X," and the "metaphoric use of X, which can also be understood on the basis of previous metaphoric uses of X, via precedent cases" (1984, p. 90). These forms of understanding have a common basis. Although literal communication is dependent on conventional knowledge, nonliteral communication is based on nonconventional knowledge. Precisely the nonconventional thoughts are relevant in metaphoric understanding, and awareness of such "thoughts" is necessary to understand them. "We understand a metaphor via such associated implications" (Keller-Bauer 1984, p. 90).

These "associated implications" play a significant role in the mutual interpretation of the meaning of metaphors in the dialgoue between the analyst and the patient, and they can be seen in the symptoms that are formed.

Kurz (1982) saw only a difference of degree between a metaphor and a symbol. In his opinion, attention is directed at words in metaphors, i. e., at the semantic tolerance and intolerance. Linguistic awareness is stimulated. In symbols, in contrast, the literal meaning is retained, and the referent, the consciousness of the object, is stimulated. The question is how we proceed when we understand a text element symbolically. To clarify this process of symbolic understanding Kurz distinguished between pragmatic and symbolic understanding, considering pragmatic understanding the elementary form of understanding. In everyday language we ask, for example, what the reasons and motives are, i. e., what the relationship between the means and ends is and, thus, what the empirical facts are. In symbolic understanding the issue is to understand the meaning "beyond the given," i. e., to understand that a knife can also be a symbol of aggression. What is symbolized is not a pragmatic empirical element but always a "psychic and moral object of meaning in our own environment" (Kurz 1982, p. 75).

An allegory is a constructed simile. To refer to a dictionary definition, "While the simple simile links two individual thoughts to one another, the allegory extends the comparison to an independent connection, as is often characteristic of epic allegories, especially Homer's. In contrast to the metaphor, the simile does not put the image in the place of the object, but presents each as linked together by an explicit conjunction" (Brockhaus 1954, p. 699).

The Interpretation of Metaphors: Relating Different Images and Referents in the Psychoanalytic Dialogue

In this section we present a linguistic study of a psychoanalytic dialogue that demonstrates which linguistic acts can be determinative in the dialogue between the analyst and the patient. Our purpose is to describe linguistic acts; we will not make any conjectures about how, according to the rules, the psychoanalytic dialogue is supposed to take place or be interpreted. The text following the introduction by the analyst who provided the treatment is from the perspective of a linguist.

Introduction. This linguistic study made much clearer to me what actually took place in the dialogue. The spatial and temporal connections that were identified and that utilize metaphors based in an individual's subjective experiencing contain important curative factors of general importance. A patient acquires a new attitude to the present as a result of viewing himself from different perspectives and at different points in his biography.

Linguistic Study

Arthur Y spoke about the tension between confirmation and devaluation. In describing a problem, he first stated what it was, viz. the doubts that plagued him when he received confirmation.

P: When someone confirms something that is positive for me and that, although I also know it to be a fact, still somehow cannot believe, that in some corner of my inner self I feel is impossible . . . .

Then the patient described his self-doubts.

P: Somewhere there is still a lot left in me that tells me the entire time: Regardless of how you act and whatever you do, it doesn't matter. It won't change anything in the fact that ultimately for the others, your surroundings, for everyone who sees you, you are just a pile of shit, just lying there and stinking and smoking and for all I know steaming. You will never manage to hide this reality, this shit, this pile of shit, from others for long. You won't even manage by resorting to some tricks or by hiding behind some kind of endearing way of acting or behind professional success. In other words, you can do what you want.

The patient even let this "something" comment in direct speech. Furthermore, he spoke at first as though the identity with the pile of shit only existed for the other one, not for himself. Yet then the patient said that he was not only speaking from the perspective of the other one, but also from his own: "Sooner or later everyone who has any dealings with me will find out that I'm nothing but a pile of shit." Then he referred to the image of the jellyfish and that "it looks quite attractive in water, but if you take it out and throw it on the sand, then it just lies there like a pile of slime." With that the patient concluded his description of the problem and made a longer pause. He then got ready to start his next statement.

In everyday language it is normal for an individual to expect another person to raise some questions or make some comments after listening to such a description of a problem - such as "That's terrible!" or "That doesn't bother you, does it?" The analyst, instead, responded in an unusual manner by mentioning the following thoughts: "Yes, and this image makes me think of the following idea that your image refers to .... " Here the analyst used the concept "image" as a synonym for metaphor. As we mentioned above, the terms "image," "simile," "metaphor," and "allegory" are frequently used synonymously in literary studies. Firm distinctions are not even made in linguistics. Weinrich, for example, used the word "metaphor" to refer to all forms of linguistic images. And "image" is often used as a generic term referring to metaphor, simile, and allegory.

The analyst referred explicitly to the patient's *image*, to his jellyfish metaphor. He referred to the experiencing of the jellyfish and thus also to that of the patient, who identified himself with the jellyfish.

A: ... how the condition was as long as you were still swimming on a feeling of well-being, you had a feeling of well-being, namely in the feeling of well-being on the throne. And I can imagine that you still experience this much humiliation because you do *not* compare this state with what you are today and what you ....

P: That's the problem, yes.

A: ... have achieved, but with the state of admiration, with the jellyfish state, with the state of sitting on the throne.

The analyst emphasized the patient's feeling of well-being as long as he (as a jellyfish) was in water or sat on the throne. i. e., before he became a pile of shit. So while the patient only emphasized the aspect of external attractiveness, the analyst referred to the patient's inner experiencing. He thus expanded on the patient's use of the metaphor (an extension of the meaning and the frame of reference), and in the process changed the focus (a change in the focus of attention). At the same time he established a relationship to the patient's earlier experiences.

In making this interpretation the analyst performed several linguistic acts simultaniously. We would like to examine one of these acts in more detail, namely the act of using language to indicate something, which opened new realms for the patient's thoughts.

On the basis of studies by Bühler (1934) and Ehlich (1979), Flader and Grodzicki viewed the use of deictic (showing) expressions "in connection with certain spheres of reference, which a speaker opens each time in order to demonstrate something specific to the listener" (1982, p. 174). They distinguished three spheres of reference: the spheres of *perception and time spoken*, often referred to with deictic means such as "I," "you," "that there," and "now"; the sphere of *speech*, which is opened by something being shown within the temporal or local organization of the development of a speech or a text, with means such as "Before I explain how . . . " or " "Later I will develop . . . "; and finally the sphere of *imagination* (or Bühler's term "fantasma"), referred to with expressions such as "then," "afterwards," "there" (at an imagined location) (Flader and Grodzicki 1982, p. 174).

In the recorded session being considered here the analyst opened the sphere of perception and time spoken, using the personal pronouns "me" and "you" and the expressions "By means of this image" and "in this image." He referred to the sphere of speech by means of the expression "have the following ideas." He opened several spheres of imagination at the same time in order to link the experiencing of today with that of prior times.

Three spheres of imagination can be distinguished in this analytic dialogue: first, previously (before his sister was born); second, then (after his sister's birth); and third, today. The analyst established a connection between these three spheres of imagination and demonstrated the degree to which the patient's present experiencing is determined by "previously" and "then." This act of showing is performed in terms of language in part by the deictic expressions "as long as," "still," and "today."

In the framework of his interpretation the analyst returned to the meaphor of "throne," which had already played a role. For the analyst the jellyfish's feeling of well-being in water corresponded to the patient's sense of well-being as long as the latter was on the throne, i. e., as long as he gets the admiration of being the first born (renewed reference to the past world of experience; the first imagined world - the experiences of the first born, the time of admiration).

Afterward, i. e., after the birth of his sister and after the patient had lost his throne, he was only a pile of shit. Afterward came the disparagement following the embarrassing acts of shitting in his pants every day in kindergarten. The temporal deictic word "afterward" referred to another, a new imagined world (2). By referring to the meaning of the metaphor "pile of shit," the analyst emphasized one feature, i. e., the patient's experiencing of disparagement (change in focus).

The analyst created a reference to the patient's world of experience at the time of the therapy (third imagined world) in the statement: "And I can imagine that you still experience this much humiliation because you do not compare this state with what you are today and what you . . . . " This emphasized the experiencing of humiliation. Here, too, the analyst incorporated the level of experiencing into his interpretation of the metaphor "pile of shit."

The analyst pointed out to the patient that he was still experiencing the same humiliation as previously (linking the second and third worlds of imagination) because he compared current confirmation ("earned" admiration) with the admiration of the previous period (admiration paid to the first born, admiration for free), thus disparaging the confirmation that he was now given.

The therapist was able to speak in such a differentiated manner here about the patient's disparagement and humiliation because of his knowledge of the events. The patient had frequently talked about the conflicts in him that the birth of his sister had precipitated, as reflected in the symptom that he began to shit in his pants, to which his mother and grandmother reacted by scorning, disparaging, and humiliating him.

In summary, in the interpretation analyzed here, in which the interpretation of the metaphor was one act in the behavior pattern "interpretation," the following points should be emphasized. By referring to the patient's experiencing, the analyst carried out a change in focus in each of his interpretations of the metaphor. At the same time, he also established a connection between the different experiences "then" and "today." The analyst indicated the continuity between "at first," "earlier," and "today," which the patient experienced, and then interrupted the continuity by pointing to the difference between then and now. This passage also indicates the amount of work done by the therapist in putting all these images into a coherent relationship.

Clarifying Symbolic and Vivid Meanings in the Analyst-Patient Interaction

Arthur Y described his feeling from the day before, which he characterized as "stable, surprisingly so." This was just the opposite of his experiencing in the evening, when he noticed the pocket knives his son and daughter had. The patient described the unease and anxiety that the knives has precipitated in him that night.

P: And then yesterday evening I discovered this knife, and then it started all over again, the fear that I might go after someone in my own family - this fear is always strongest regarding my children.

His attempts to defend himself against this threat - to get it under control - became clear in the very orderly manner he described the situation and his behavior (then, at that time) and mentioned his subjective experiences (fear, frightened). He attempted to determine what significance the knife held for him, considering it at the pragmatic level of symbolic understanding.

It was conspicuous that the patient emphasized the normalcy of the situation and used a series of techniques indicating that he attempted to master his feelings. Both of these probably enabled the patient to maintain distance to his experiencing to keep him from getting lost in it (an indication of a borderline situation).

This distancing was strengthened by the allegory about the hamster, which Arthur Y explicitly referred to as such.

P: And then I remembered our hamster. When I, when we set him on the chair and put something in front of him, a spoon or something, then he would take it with his snout and mouth and throw it on the floor. It's funny to watch [sniffled]. Apparently it bothers him. This knife in there bothered me in the same way.

This night the patient's distancing was a success, as might be indicated by the fact that he subsequently only referred to "the thing," saying that he actually did not need to fear it at all.

In the following passage Arthur Y established a connection to a knot that had already been a topic in therapy. The knot probably really existed in some staircase. For the patient, it had something to do with his aggressions, which the analyst often referred to by name.

P: That I would have such difficulty realizing that I too have aggressions.

He said when he reached this point, then his feelings of both anxiety and real opportunities became all entangled. The patient then developed this metaphor of a tangle, which led to the association with "disentangle," into an allegory or a simile.

P: I can't find a better comparison, and if I had the beginning of the string or the other end, then I could try to disentangle the mess, but somewhere I would have to, I mean, of course I have the beginning, I would have to try with the help of the beginning to get somewhere.

The patient not only explicitly described this allegory about the tangled mess, which clearly indicates the patient's inner confusion, as a comparison, but also described its quality - "I can't find a better comparison." This kind of explicit description of a comparison or allegory might, in turn, be an indication of the distance between the patient and his inner experiencing.

That the patient experienced his feelings of anxiety and being threatened as coming from outside himself might be indicated by his impersonal statements: "And then it started all over again, and the reason that this thing made me feel so anxious receded into the background once again."

After having discussed another topic, Arthur Y returned to the knife. He said that he had actually wanted to examine this problem in the session under study. He expressed doubt as to whether he had benefited from the session, expressed criticism, and retracted the criticism immediately. He did not say explicitly, "The session was a waste of time." but expressed himself in the following manner: "And now, although I don't have the feeling - when I think about it - that the session was a waste of time, really I don't, although I almost said just as much, and now nothing has come of it."

The patient used various techniques to retract his criticism: (a) the conjunction "although," (b) the negated feeling "don't have the feeling," (c) the reiteration "really I don't," and (d) a fictive double backdating, expressing an incompleted act, "although I almost said just as much."

A ten second pause followed, before the analyst picked up the topic the patient had started on, not by thematizing his criticism but by directly referring to the topics of "pet" and "knife." He referred to the allegorical meaning of the story about the hamster who used his snout to push everything that bothered him onto the floor.

A: You thought about the hamster, so, whatever bothers him, well, push it out of the way . . . .
P: Yes.
A: . . . push it out of the way . . . .
P: Yes.
A: . . . whatever bothers it.
P: It looks so funny.
A: Hmm.

The patient applied the story about the hamster directly to his own personal situation, until it became complete nonsense. His interpretation of the hamster's symbolic meaning was entirely at the level of pragmatic understanding.

P: Well, yes, I could take the knife and destroy it, but that's silly. That's no solution. In reality it's not the knife at all, I think, and if I throw it away, then there are more in the kitchen, then I could throw them away, too. [laughing] And when my wife starts looking for them and says, "Damn it, where are all the knives?" then I can say that I've thrown them out, and she would reply, "Your're crazy." All I could say then is simply, "Yes."

In the following passage the analyst was concerned with the symbolic meaning of the hamster.

A: Yes, yes, the hamster gets hit and is killed . . . .
P: Yes.

The hamster and especially the butchering of domesticated animals, e. g., pigs and rabbits, had already been mentioned several times in therapy. These animals represented for the patient enslaved and powerless beings that get hit and are killed. Thus the analyst established a relationship from this session to earlier descriptions (linking different spheres of imagination). The patient agreed with the analyst, but relativized the analyst's reference to the association about the hamster, saying it was a coincidence.

By saying "It's a coincidence," Arthur Y rejected the connection that the analyst had established. At first the analyst agreed that the association was coincidental, but then relativized his agreement by saying "perhaps" and then reiterated that the hamster had a symbolic meaning and that the association had probably not been a coincidence, saying "but I'll classify it as such."

A: That's a coincidence, yes, yes, perhaps a coincidence. Yes, definitely, but I'll classify it as one.

Here it is clear that from the analyst's perspective the patient had not entirely understood something he himself had said. By referring to the fact that the hamster had frequently played a role, the therapist left the interaction at their common level to move to the "analytic" level, in order to make something that was incomprehensible (nonintegrated) to the patient comprehensible (to integrate it). By means of his rejection, the patient attempted to reestablish the cooperation at the first level, which the analyst did not accept, insisting instead on his perspective.

The patient's rejection of the analyst's interpretation led the analyst to begin a discussion of a series of further aspects of the symbolic meaning of the hamster, the rabbit, and the knife, which the patient accepted in the course of their interaction, i. e., the patient accepted the analytic level of interpretation.

A: Namely, inasmuch as knives disturb you because they pose a threat, and the hitting, then a person can't do enough to avoid getting hit if he's, so to speak, a guinea pig . . . .
P: Yes.
A: . . . a hamster that's equated with these objects . . . .
P: Oh, yes.
A: Let me anthropomorphize this for now.
P: Yes.
A: . . . Gets hit and stretches out, then he can't do enough to get out of the way. But if the issue is different, if he's not the hamster, but the one who has power and therefore, in order to defend himself, needs . . .
P: Hum.
A: . . . a knife, then he naturally doesn't want to get rid of them, but . . .
P: Then he can't have enough of them.
A: Yes, then he can't have enough of them.

Here the analyst interpreted the hamster as a symbol in a general manner and without making an explicit reference to the patient, using the indefinite third person. The hamster symbolized the patient's powerlessness, yet according to the analyst the powerless patient had also maintained unconscious fantasies in which he was the one who had power, namely the knives to protect himself. The patient was thus not only the one threatened by the knives but also the one who needed the knives to defend himself. The analyst attempted to make it clear to the patient that the knives both symbolize the external threat and represent the patient's own possibility to defend himself, i. e., repesent his own aggression (which can injure others).

By making the short comment, "Then he can't have enough of them," which the analyst picked up and repeated, saying it almost simultaneously, the patient confirmed the analyst's interpretation. The patient recalled that he had thought that he was not afraid, telling himself "You know that you would never hurt a fly. So why are so afraid of this thing?"

The analyst picked up this line of thought and related it to the patient's son. He then relativized the patient's statement to the effect that it was not the patient's intention to hurt anyone but that it was an "inevitable side effect."

A: Somewhere you know that you didn't want to hurt anyone, but hurting someone was a kind of inevitable side effect, but . . .
P: How do you mean that?
A: I mean that you are not the one who is enslaved; I mean that you, when you tell X to go to hell . . . .
P: Yes.

The analyst thus made it clear that the patient's current identification with the hamster was not logical, because in current reality he was not the one who was enslaved, but the one who told X to go to hell and who then thought about "rationalizing away" the job of his less successful colleague.

In the following interpretation the therapist attempted to convey to the patient that he was the one who has power and who has the ability and desire to hurt others:

A: The point is that you are no longer the one who is oppressed and beaten, but that you have power and thus can turn the tables. Then the other person gets hurt, not you. In turning the tables, you also want to hurt the other person.
P: Yes, that's precisely it, now we've reached the knot.
A: Hum.
P: Hurt someone, yes, hurt someone, take revenge.
A: Yes, yes, hum.
P: It would be nice if . . . .
A: But precisely the moment you take revenge, hurting someone is part of it, and then you immediately feel . . . [the patient sniffled] . . . the tables are turned around again. In other words, you know how it hurts to stand there and have your pants full.

In this interpretation the analyst established a relationship between the patient's experiencing in which he was the one who was enslaved (then) and (current) reality in which the patient was the one who was powerful and who can/will turn the tables (sphere of imagination 4). Yet precisely the moment the patient realized this, the tables were turned again (today) because he knew what it was like to stand there and have your pants full (then). In other words, he knew what it was like for someone to be despised and hurt. The analyst had thus put all the symbols and metaphors the patient had mentioned into a coherent whole.

After a long pause the patient returned to the knot (here as a block to thinking), which the analyst used in the following allegory:

A: Yes, where would you go further - maybe you don't have the confidence in yourself to go any further, now that you have reached some end.

This challenge was followed by a longer pause, following which the patient only concerned himself briefly with his own aggression. Until the end of this session the patient talked about the humiliation and aggression he had suffered and about his helplessness. The powerless hamster was again in the forefront.

The patient thus introduced certain empirical facts into the conversation (here: knife, hamster, knot) and attempted to understand the meaning they had for him (pragmatic level of understanding). The analyst referred to the other kinds of meanings that these empirical facts could also have for the patient. He interpreted their symbolic relations and extended them allegorically. At the same time, he indicated the limits of such symbolic meaning.

Summary

The linguistic analysis crystalized the following facts out of this text. This was a patient who frequently used images, allegories, and symbols in therapy. In contrast to everyday communication, the therapist and patient were not restricted to the manifest meaning of the images, but attempted to find their latent meanings. In other words, the therapist worked with the patient to discover the biographical significance of words - metaphors and images - that the patient was only familiar with at the level of their manifest meaning.

The therapist helped the patient understand his own comments, to put them into context, to go beyond their incidental nature, and created the biographical continuity between "earlier," "then," "today," and "tomorrow." He achieved this by means of linguistic acts such as extending the meaning and the connotation, changing the focus, opening spheres of reference and imagination, and linking different spheres of imagination.

This linguistic study demonstrated that in this dialogue the analyst examined all the patient's comments systematically for their latent meaning and that he created biographical continuity by linking various comments the patient made. This study is also a demonstration of how productive interdisciplinary cooperation can be.

7.6 Value Freedom and Neutrality

Values play an important role in psychoanalytic therapy, which is inevitable considering the fact that a large number of normative questions are at stake for patients. These questions concern, for example, the most favorable resolution of conflicts, the issue of happiness, and the justification of certain desires. This, however, does not in itself imply that a analyst introduces his own norms into his discourse with the patient.

Freud related the value free nature of psychoanalysis to scientific research, not to the therapeutic sphere:

> Moreover, it is quite unscientific to judge analysis by whether it is calculated to undermine religion, authority and morals; for, like all sciences, it is entirely non-tendentious and has only a single aim - namely to arrive at a consistent view of one portion of reality. (Freud 1923a, p. 252)

Freud's goal in this passage was to uphold the scientific nature of psychoanalysis, against critics both outside and inside psychoanalysis. Freud felt that the greatest threat to its scientific nature was posed by countertransference (see Vol.1, Sect. 3.1). In his warnings against countertransference reactions he used in 1914 for the first time the German word *Indifferenz*, which Strachey translated as "neutrality." In doing so, Freud adhered to an understanding of science that was characteristic of nineteenth century empiricism. He adhered to a "positivistic philosophy" (Cheshire and Thomä 1991). According to this view, the acquisition of knowledge must be kept free of subjective factors, to ensure that statements correspond with "external reality." One purpose of this neutrality (or *Indifferenz*) was thus to guarantee the objectivity of analysis. Yet it is just as impossible to uphold this claim as it is the demand that the analyst pursue the goal of objectivity by remaining neutral (*indifferent*). Kaplan (1982) has shown that Freud himself did not follow this ideal, frequently making normative statements.

Despite the fact that values are implicit in psychoanalytic therapy, the utopia of a value free science is commonly mentioned in the literature, especially when the issue is analytic neutrality. This is the result of deep-rooted conceptions about the nature of objectivity. Making value judgments is frequently identified with being subjective, which makes it impossible for them to be grounded rationally. Since there are no intersubjective rules for applying values that can be grounded, an individual's freedom to make his own value judgments is thus opposed to the open or manipulative coercion of the individual to adopt particular life styles. Yet if one aspect of psychoanalytic therapy is that values are implied somehow in "neutral" interpretations, is it then not true that psychoanalysis violates the idea that each individual should be happy according to his own wishes? Or can we justify our actions by claiming that psychoanalytic therapy does not impose any values, only helping people to achieve self-awareness? The argument is frequently raised that psychoanalysis does not promote norms, only the self-determination of individuals, and that it therefore, for example, regards symptoms only as posing a limitation on self-determination that can be overcome by means of self-knowledge. According to this conception, the ideal analyst limits himself to understanding the patient and communicating what he has understood.

In our opinion both alternative views of psychoanalysis as either a clandestine normative manipulation or as value free enlightenment are themselves incorrect. The therapeutic and explanatory functions of psychoanalysis can only be fulfilled if the *relativity* of values is acknowledged. We would therefore like to contrast the two opposite interpretations of psychoanalytic neutrality, i. e., of its alleged value freedom and its manipulative character.

According to the first thesis, therapy can only be grasped as a process of enlightenment. The most important therapeutic means are, consequently, interpretations, which are statements about unconscious determinants of behavior. Although these interpretations frequently refer to values, a distinction must be made between the description of the patient's judgments and the stance the analyst takes to these decisions. Incidentally, it was precisely this difference between empirical facts and an independent judgment of facts that interested Max Weber (1949 [1904]). According to the thesis of value freedom, analysts are not to make recommendations as to how conflicts should be solved, but should make patients aware of the implications and causes of their conflicts.

The opposite thesis maintains that the idea that therapy is a value free undertaking is a contradiction in itself, the reason being that therapy implies an initial constellation that is negatively valued, for example one characterized by symptoms. Moreover, therapy also has goals that are positive in nature, just as it has means of realizing these goals. According to this thesis, it is impossible to assert that psychoanalysis is value free and at the same time put forward the maxim that what is unconscious should be made conscious. This demand itself is said to contain the judgment that unconscious strategies of conflict resolution must be considered to be less favorable than conscious ones, for example because of the consequences in terms of symptoms. Equally justified is the reference to the fact that the autonomy of the individual is also a value that contradicts the ideal of value neutrality in psychoanalysis.

Even a proponent of the value free position would acknowledge that the attempt to assist a patient reach self-awareness is based on a value judgement. This position asserts that this is a precondition for therapy, whose justification lies in the unprejudiced conviction that symptoms are caused by unconscious processes. Furthermore, it claims that there is a categorical difference between the identification of specific goals and the formal matter of whether an individual is in a position to make a decision regarding goals. In this sense, autonomy is not a value like hedonism or asceticism because it concerns the manner in which individuals are able to determine their desires. For example, symptomatic behavior is not defined as mentally ill on the basis of the nature of the goals but on the basis of the fact that individuals do not have the choice to decide against the symptom. Tugendhat (1984) asserted that symptom-dependent behavior impairs the practical nature of wanting. Meissner (1983) has formulated a series of values that he believes belong to the essence of psychoanalysis: self-understanding, the authenticity of the self, truthfulness, and the willingness to remain committed to specific values. He referred to the fact that these values are located at a higher level of abstraction than concrete value-related decisions in daily life. The call for an unbiased attitude therefore has to be restricted to concrete decisions and must take into consideration the normative nature of values that are located at a higher level.

The ideal of overcoming normative prejudices is strained especially when the issue is the role that understanding and empathy play in psychoanalysis. Precisely with regard to this issue we believe, however, that it is impossible for the analyst to attain either unbiased behavior or unbiased understanding if a more inclusive notion of values is used. We do not have the option of behaving in a nonnormative manner in interpersonal relations. Even a decision to take the status of a pure observer with regard to another person would be the result of a value judgement to which there may be better or worse alternatives. To ask such an observer whether it is correct in a concrete situation to behave as a passive observer could well be a meaningful question. A relationship without value judgements would only be conceivable if the analyst could simply escape from a relationship to a patient; otherwise he cannot evade the question of whether his behavior was appropriate to the situation or not.

Consequently, the call for the analyst to remain neutral cannot be grounded in the ideal of value freedom, just as strict neutrality in psychoanalysis is no guarantee for value freedom. The insistence on neutrality must, on the contrary, be considered as the expression of a particular normative attitude toward therapeutic work, one which corresponds, for example, to the view that indoctrination of a patient is impossible. This normative attitude, probably just like other such attitudes, is specific to particular situations as well as to particular personalities. In psychoanalysis it is linked to the fact that the understanding of the unconscious conflict is given precedence to other interests. If the analyst and patient agree to assign preference to the pursuit of these tasks and the values attached to them, then other values and differences lose in significance. Naturally, this does not result in value freedom in a philosophical sense, but it does create something that can be referred to as an open space, which is characterized by a pluralism of concrete values. The establishment of such a space free of any pejorative connotations is of eminent significance for a relationship of trust between analyst and patient. It provides the patient the security to confront impulses and thoughts that he is ashamed of or for which he feels guilty.

If it is possible to make the patient's system of values and his criteria for making judgements just as much an object of analysis as his view of reality, then who provides the criteria on which values and reality can be measured? The purpose of the recourse to analytic neutrality is to refute the argument that analysis indoctrinates patients by declaring the analyst's criteria to be final. On the other hand, neutrality is supposed to prevent the analyst from adopting in an unreflected manner criteria that are dictated by the patient's environment or that soley represent id or superego aspects. Here A. Freud's recommendation that the analyst maintain an equal distance literally imposes itself:

> It is the task of the analyst to bring into consciousness that which is unconscious, no matter to which psychic institution it belongs. He directs his attention equally and objectively to the unconscious elements in all three institutions. To put it in another way, when he sets about the work of enlightenment he takes his stand at a point equidistant from the id, the ego and the super-ego. (1937, p. 30)

The analyst's objectivity is supposed to contribute to avoiding partiality in the choice of perspective, and insofar it makes sense to speak of technical neutrality.

There is a similar problem with regard to the understanding of transference. If the relationship between the analyst and the patient itself is examined from the perspective of two-person psychology and transference refers to more than the biographically explicable distortion of patterns of relationships, then there is no secure perspective from which the relationship can be considered because both of the parties involved in the interaction influence the "reality" of the relationship to varying degrees. Freud and later Hartmann still opted for the relatively simple route of uncritically adopting common sense reality as the criterion for what is normal and distorted. Since psychoanalysis has become aware of the relativity of our reality (Gould 1970; Wallerstein 1973), it has become impossible for reality to be considered independent of the particular social norms and conventions. In this context, analytic neutrality also became an important concept, which was supposed to prevent the analyst from taking his own theoretical and personal presuppositions as the basis for evaluating transference and from letting himself be taken captive in his efforts to acquire an empathic understanding of the patient's presuppositions (see Shapiro 1984).

Yet this is where the immunizing and consequently ideological function sets in that the concept of analytic neutrality has increasingly taken on. The reason is that the dilemma resulting from the fact that it is possible to evaluate psychic topics from different perspectives and thus to arrive at very different interpretations continues to exist. Although it is definitely commendable for the analyst, as A. Freud demanded, not to become blindly subservient to the demands of the id or thesuperego, it is still impossible to assert that maintaining an equidistance to all the instances itself guarantees that the perspective is correct and appropriate. In the case of conflicts, "truth" is not always in the middle, but can take on different appearances, according to the specific situation. For better or for worse, we have to acknowledge that the moment we adopt a specific perspective we no longer see other psychic mechanisms, including their unconscious implications, and that attempting to resolve the problem by avoiding taking a position leads us to even overlook quite decisive mechanisms. One-sidedness is an inevitable aspect of our work with the unconscious. Yet nonetheless many publications surprisingly create the impression that all forms of one-sidedness could be avoided if analysts would only demonstrate *even* more neutrality and would be *even* better analyzed. Such an unrestricted idealization of the psychoanalytic method corresponds to the hesitation to make judgments that currently characterizes clinical work. The underlying ideological tendency of this apologetic approach is evident even in the use of language. You only have to pay attention to how often sentences occur in psychoanalytic publications that specify what "the analyst" has to do or what psychoanalysis is, the result being that whoever rejects the alleged features (e. g., being neutral) is not really an analyst or that he is acting in a nonanalytic manner. In this way, the psychoanalytic method is kept free of any doubt. It is such definitions of psychoanalysis that obstruct the dialogue between psychoanalysts and representatives of other disciplines and that have given psychoanalysis the reputation of being an orthodox school of know-it-alls. They have also prevented the subjective influence that the analyst exerts on the therapeutic process, including his influence as a human being, from being sufficiently observed and empirically studied.

The process of finding an adequate position from which to make judgments in psychoanalysis or for an examination of reality can thus be slightly facilitated if the analyst takes a neutral attitude, but neither neutrality nor objectivity provide a definitive answer to the problem. Reality is determined for the specific situation by means of a consensus of those participating. Thus analyst and patient must be willing, despite resistance and all of the problems associated with countertransference, to let themselves be convinced by the other; this is a precondition for the creation of a consensus (see Vol.1, Sect. 8.4). The social contact of each of the participants, i. e., the confrontation of the patient with his environment and of the analyst with the opinions of his colleagues, provides the guarantee that this consensus does not develop into a folie à deux. The consensus that the participants in the process reach has to prove itself in this social environment even if it does not prove capable of changing possibly divergent opinions. If the patient in analysis retreats from social life or is no longer interested in a consensus with his social surroundings, there is an increased danger of a restricted view of reality. The same is true if the analyst stops facing the judgments of his colleagues or if the professional group he belongs to withdraws from the scientific discussion. In the latter case, a folie à deux is only replaced by an unjustified one-sidedness in which many participate. The great significance that case reports have had since the beginnings of psychoanalysis is based, in our opinion, on the necessity of overcoming a folie à deux by means of reaching an intersubjective consensus.

The fact that this problem has been mixed together with the rule of abstinence has had unfavorable consequences on therapeutic technique. The abstinence rule is based, as we explained in Vol.1 (Sect. 7.1), on the libido theory. It is supposed to prevent gratification via transference. As explained above, the purpose of the neutrality rule is to promote a properly understood autonomy on the part of the patient and to create a space free of value judgments. The word "neutrality" does not describe this attitude any better than Freud's original term, "indifference." We therefore suggest that the term "neutrality" be replaced by the concept of an "unbiased and balanced" attitude.

The unbiased quality is threatened in therapy from several sides. It cannot develop if the patient insists on being offensive and argumentative in asserting particular values against the analyst. This can be the case, for example, with religious patients or patients who are firmly bound in an ideology. In this case the patient must always experience any attempt to achieve an unbiased situation as a "no" to his own hierarchy of values. It is not unusual for a longer period of an exchange of ideas to be necessary before a common basis is created; in some cases therapy even founders on the lack of agreement. This is particularly the case if the analyst attempts to impose his own idiosyncratic values on the patient.

The limits of impartiality also become visible if the patient acts, either within or outside the therapeutic situation, in a manner that makes it impossible for the analyst to focus his concentration on the psychic conflicts. Neutrality can no longer be responsibly upheld if the patient becomes brutal or is grossly inconsiderate to himself or people in his social surroundings. It is then necessary for the therapist to set limits, until the patient himself is in a position to recognize that his system of values is distorted and to correct it. On this point Heigl and Heigl-Evers (1984) emphasized the importance of testing values in the analytic process and pointed to the limitations of neutrality.

If a correctly understood sense of impartiality is to be retained as an ideal of therapeutic technique, then it is necessary to specify the issues and the concrete goals under which the analyst can remain neutral or impartial. Exaggerated abstinence is just as incompatible with such an ideal of therapy as is insufficient distance to the patient's conflicts. As is frequently the case with ideals, there are no criteria that are simple to identify; neutrality refers to a particular position in a specific situation that is characterized by the integration of opposites. These poles can be described in more detail in several different dimensions.

1. Openness - Neither Prejudiced nor Uninformed

The analyst takes the first step away from the ideal of objectivity when he begins to create his own image of the patient. He inevitably classifies some information as important and discounts other information as being unimportant, and activates preconceived patterns of anticipation and experience. These patterns, first, stem from the analyst's practical experience in life, and second, correspond to psychoanalytic working models of a patient (see Vol.1, Sect. 9.3). If this model gains too much influence on the further processing of information, it can disturb the process and lead to prejudice, as Peterfreund (1983) has shown. It is thus quite sound for an analyst to leave his image of a patient incomplete and not to believe he already knows everything that the patient will say and experience at some later point.

If the goal of being unprejudiced becomes an ideology, the analyst ceases absorbing important information and does not draw important conclusions, in an effort not to be prejudiced. A spectacular example of this is the practice common in many places of strictly avoiding every kind of advance information before the initial interview. The reason given for this is to avoid any contamination. What is achieved is that the patient meets an analyst who in the patient's eyes is obviously uninformed regarding important information such as letters from referring practitioners. This creates distortions in communication and the patient takes such a refusal to provide information as disinterestedness on the part of the analyst. It also obstructs the analyst from obtaining a comprehensive image of the patient. Even if one follows Hoffer (1985) in acknowledging the priority of working through intrapsychic processes, there is a big difference between whether this priority is within the context of knowledge about the patient's social reality or whether it is simply linked to an ignorance of the patient's social frame of reference. A properly understood sense of neutrality is thus a balance between prejudice and being uninformed.

2. Cautiousness: Avoiding Domination and Aloofness

Caution toward feelings coincides to a large extent with the problem of handling countertransference (see Chap. 3). Here we will only explain the problem of drawing a line. The analyst is advised to display reservation in paying attention to or acknowledging countertransference because there is the danger that the analyst might seduce the patient or vice versa. On the other hand, an extremely souvereign and objective treatment of countertransference leads the patient to have the impression that the analyst can never be reached, injured, or offended. This experience might ultimately so discourage the patient that he gives up his efforts to please the analyst - out of resignation, not out of insight.

For the patient to achieve structural change it is necessary for the analyst to admit that he has human reactions and yet to retain his professional role and thus to resist being seduced or destroyed. In this regard it is also necessary for a balance to be recreated in each and every session in the therapeutic process.

3. Openness in Values - Neither Partial Nor Faceless

Freud's warnings apply to the danger that the analyst might impose values on the patient. This danger seems minimal if the analyst and patient share the same sociocultural values. We know, however, that the chances of success sink the greater the discrepency between the systems of values. The distance can only be overcome if the therapist is able, at least temporarily, to identify with the patient's system of values; othewise he sacrifices the opportunity of adequately understanding the patient and of helping him make progress within the framework of his understanding of the world. Depending on how flexible the analyst is, at some point a limit is reached at which this identification is no longer possible, which makes it necessary for the analyst to depart from his ideal of neutrality (Gedo 1983). The large scale on which some analysts reject patients because they "simply can't" work with them reflects, on the one hand, wise foresight; on the other hand, the spectrum of patients that are not excluded very clearly demonstrates how rigid or flexible the analyst is toward his own system of values.

An analyst's neutrality toward his own set of values quickly reaches its limits in the daily work of analysis. He inevitably provides at least some indication of his own attitude when he confronts the patient's values. The patient interprets every "hum" at an appropriate spot as a confirmation of his view of things, and comes to demand it as something he is entitled to. In contrast, the patient may interpret any omission of a "hum" where one might be expected on the basis of the style of the presentation to be a sign of skepticism and disguised rejection. Although the analyst can mention his doubts about such interpretations, it is very difficult to convince a patient that such a perception was wrong, especially since patients' perceptions are frequently intuitively correct. The more alive and natural the analyst is in dealing with his patient, the more indirect expressions of opinion are contained in the concrete interaction.

Greenson (1967) has described a vignette exemplifying how the analyst's political opinion can be made visible in paraverbal expressions, which can make the patient feel that he is under pressure. Lichtenberg (1983b) has also described a case in which the analyst's actions expressed specific values that were visible to the patient and that obviously exerted an influence on him.

An apparent way out of this dilemma is for the analyst as a matter of principle to restrict himself to a minimum in providing confirmation, making it more difficult for the patient to perceive where the analyst secretly approves and where he has doubt or is being critical. Although this enables the analyst to gain better control of the danger of indirectly expressing an opinion, it also makes him appear impersonal to the patient, making it impossible for him to fulfill his function as an object of identification (see Sect. 2.4). The amount of involvement that is necessary in an undisturbed course of therapy depends on the personalities of the analyst and the patient. Decisive is probably less the degree of the disturbance than the nature of the primary socialization of each participant.

4. Being Open to the Direction of Change

Especially complicated is the relationship between analytic neutrality and the analyst's goals in therapy. Therapeutic goals are necessarily linked with values, and it is with reference to such goals that it is easiest for the analyst to assert his values. That Freud had concrete goals of change in mind can be seen in the fact that he actually assigned the analyst the task of improving and educating the patient (1940a, p. 175). Yet in the same breath he warned analysts against misusing this function to create the patient in his own image. Clinical experience demonstrates that an analyst succumbs to this danger most easily when he knows that he is close to the patient and feels bound to him by strong sympathy. The situation in which the analyst indirectly influences the decision-making processes usually coincides with the patient's willingness to please the analyst; such behavior can therefore take on very sublime forms.

A questionable solution is for the analyst to forego the determination and pursuit of therapeutic goals or to phrase them so loosely that they become meaningless. It is in this guise that "nontendentious psychoanalysis" celebrates its revival: the only goal that remains is "to discover the traces and dents that growing up in our civilization leaves behind" (Parin and Parin-Matthèy 1983), if one then does not want to pursue the general goal of transforming terminable analysis into an interminable one, and in the process making the psychoanalytic process into a goal of its own (Blarer and Brogle 1983). Here, too, idealization and immunization are at play; in very few cases is it sensible to have only the patient's self-analysis in mind and leave its consequences entirely up to the patient - and even in these few cases, this can only be done in an especially satisfactory phase of analysis. Self-analysis is no sacrosanct value that is never misused and whose independence from the social context is guaranteed. We tacitly link the ideal of self-analysis with the idea that it proves to be worthwhile in each individual situation. The specific meaning of "proves to be worthwhile" depends on the criteria that both the analyst and the patient apply to their situations in life. As a rule, it is the patient's neurotic problems that cast doubt on the worthwhileness of the psychoanalytic process, and an analyst demonstrates a substantial amount of disinterestedness if he remains indifferent to the consequences of the analytic process, even if they violate the patient's own best interests.

Even Hoffer, whom we referred to above, succumbs to the danger of denying this empathy toward a fellow human being when he compares neutrality with a "compass [that] does not tell which way *to* go, but helps us to see which way we *are* going and where we *went*" (1985, p. 791). In this metaphor, neutrality denies the interest and influence the analyst has in and on the patient. The compass metaphor also recalls the metaphor of the analyst as a mountain guide, which Freud regarded highly. A substantial amount of knowledge is in fact required for the analyst to correctly estimate the dangers posed by different routes and the patient's capacity for solving problems, in order to avoid serious complications. The therapeutic ideal of impartiality cannot amount to providing rules of behavior that save the patient from making the experience of testing himself or to treating him like a child. Neutrality, however, cannot consist in leaving the patient alone with his self-analysis when it is proving to be a failure.

5. Cautiousness About Exerting Power

The influence that power exerts on the psychoanalytic process is rarely made an object of reflection, a fact that has often been the object of polemics by critics of psychoanalysis. These polemics correspond to a tendency of analysts to use a reference to the analytic technique as a means to avoid the real issues. Yet to argue that the analyst does not exert any power because he limits himself to making interpretations and to abstinent behavior is not an adequate response to these problems. Some elements of the analyst's behavior can play a role in struggles between the analyst and patient precisely because of the meaning the patient unconsciously attributes to them. It is well known that an analyst can employ interpretations to get the patient to accept certain conditions of the setting. The discrepency between the patient's power and the analyst's is further increased when the analyst makes deep interpretations utilizing privileged knowledge about unconscious truths.

The analyst can employ his silence as an instrument of power, just as the patient can experience it as being one. In a favorable case the patient can feel satisfied in a state of regression. The analyst should not ignore the fact that a lack of feedback during a long period of silence can have numerous consequences - the more silent an analyst is, the more powerful he becomes for the patient and the stronger is the reactivation of infantile patterns of experiencing (see Vol.1, Sect. 8.5). It may be a pleasant self-deception for silent analysts to believe that they behave particularly neutral because they never make statements of judgment. Yet in the process they deny the fact that a patient who has longed for some form of emotional response might gratefully accept the slightest statement or impulse. Even the fact that the analyst simply opens his mouth at certain places will direct the patient onto the analyst's unstated intentions. The analyst can in this way, of course, manipulate the patient's resistance, but not resolve it in an analytic sense. The analyst's inscrutability is a fiction concealing the misuse of power. Truly inscrutable for the patient would only be an unempathic analyst whose reactions are incalculable and inconsistent.

The misuse of power in deliberate silence or forced interpretations has been especially criticized by analytic self-psychology (see Wolf 1983). On the other hand, referring to the concept of empathy does not provide a guarantee against the misuse of power; even an empathic analyst has power and can misuse it. Therefore if neutrality is supposed to be realized as an ideal for therapeutic technique, then it cannot consist in abstinence, being silent, or making forced interpretations. The ideal position is in the middle, with the patient codetermining to an important degree the course of things yet without him having complete control of them. The danger of a misuse of power is substantially limited if the analyst makes his technical steps comprehensible to the patient and reflects together with the patient on the power contained in them. Reaching agreement on the delegation of power creates space in which the analytic situation can unfold.

Example

We would like to illustrate the different dimensions of neutrality by referring to an example taken from the analysis of a 30-year-old man. He sought help for anxieties related to his body, which were connected with problems in his relations to his partners.

At the beginning of approximately the 200th session Norbert Y expressed his concern at recent acts of terrorism. On the one hand, he was anxious about being affected by a terrorist act, yet he also thought wrathfully that it served people right for the terrorists to defend themselves. He said that inconsiderateness had become so widespread that life had become difficult to take. The limits of what people could be expected to tolerate had been long transgressed in the area of environmental pollution. In this phase I primarily listened to the patient, only asking questions or making comments to clarify what he said.

Next the patient described how he recalled a situation with an inconsiderate driver, who did not pay any attention to pedestrians. He had sometimes really enjoyed, when he had been out with a pushcart, pushing the cart so that he blocked traffic, making the drivers in back of him proceed at a slow pace. During this story I again mainly listened to the patient. He then described a fight he had had with his girlfriend, in which he tried energetically to resist her attempts to tell him what to do. The patient described a relatively harmless situation and his intense reaction to it. He had made a massive attack on her, calling her unattractive and an egocentric dragon and saying she did not have a trace of tact. It was possible to sense emotionally the patient's feeling of triumph at having so successfuly defended himself.

I was so moved by his report that I remained silent at this point although the patient was obviously waiting for me to make some approving comment. The patient then complained that I obviously did not support him in this point, but took his girlfriend's side. Becoming increasingly enraged, he then complained that I took his girlfriend's side more frequently than his although he had read that analysts are supposed to support their patient if they really want to provide help. He felt, however, that I had abandoned him in this matter, adding that maybe I was not an analyst who had the patient's interest at heart and I only gave therapy by following the instructions in some book.

I told the patient that he had apparently noticed that his report about his argument had irritated me, and that the fact that I had offered him so little support apparently hurt his feelings. I added that in that moment I was apparently interchangeable with his girlfriend, whom he had also picked to pieces. I had also become interchangeable with inconsiderate polluters and drivers.

Here the patient hesitated, saying after a pause, "First I thought that you were going to throw me out, and then I suddenly became afraid that you were really going to give me a grilling."

This comment in which grilling was the object of his anxieties attracted my attention, and I asked him about it. He had ideas such as that I first wanted to sound him out, only to then show him how confused, dumb, and clumsy his thoughts were. It was possible to relate these thoughts, which the patient himself experienced as being nonsensical and also embarrassing, to a part of his relationship to his mother. According to his recollection, she had spoiled him, but had also intentionally made him feel like a dumb and awkward boy, especially in the presence of relatives and friends. That he was so enraged in such situations that he began to cry just made the whole affair worse. I had already been aware of these individual items from his biography before the session, but it was only now that I was able to understand how immense his feelings of shame and helplessness had been, and how much greater was his need to act wildly, as it were, to liberate himself from his helplessness. His argument with his girlfriend had apparently reactivated this tendency to react uncontrollably as a preventive measure. When we had grasped this mechanism, the patient was able to reestablish a normal distance to me and to his girlfriend, whose opinionated manner continued to upset him but ceased to be a source of anger.

This example demonstrates that the analyst did not have to comment on the patient's political opinions and that this did not disturb him during his later critcal comments about me. In analysis, psychic problems take priority and political values become secondary. In the inital phase of this session the analyst was especially interested in the patient's affect, and it was not difficult to discover aggression in his comments, whose origin at this point was unclear.

The patient's story about the inconsiderate driver and how he had taken revenge on such people differed from his comments in the previous episode in that the patient in this case made his own behavior the object of discussion. His behavior contradicted the ideal of self-responsibility, since the patient interpreted the situation of a victim as justifying his own inconsiderate actions.

The patient's comments about his argument with his girlfriend was a kind of intensification of the previous episodes. The issue was once again a complaint about inconsiderate behavior and aggression, which led the patient to express massive criticism of his girlfriend. Here too the patient had obviously experienced himself primarily as a victim and expected the analyst to agree with him. The discrepency to the ideal of self-responsiblity was so large here that the analyst was moved and obviously was no longer able to follow the patient emotionally and denied him the sign of understanding that he expected, even if only in the form of a "hum." In doing so the analyst transgressed the limits of the kind of behavior that the patient expected. It is possible to argue that the analyst only refused to make an explicit value judgment or to take the side of either the patient or his girlfriend. For the patient, however, the analyst's explicit refusal to take sides was not an example of neutrality, particularly since the analyst had previously been understanding. Therefore the patient had to conclude that the analyst had secretly taken a critical stance toward his actions. It was therefore logical for the analyst to confirm the plausibility of his perceptions (Gill 1982).

This change in behavior made the analyst into an inconsiderate object for the patient, which he promptly attacked and whose value he denied. It was important at this point for the analyst to bear this criticism without being insulted or injured, but also without accepting a position of aloofness.

The purpose of the analyst's interventions at this point was to signal his interest in the patient's emotional reactions. The fact that the analyst's comments were *even* harmful remained secondary. Fortunately the patient responded to the offer; he did not rapidly retract all of his statements or intensify them defensively, but reported about a new emotion, namely his fear of the analyst. It was only at this level that the mutual interest in understanding each other took priority over the condemnation of actions and it became possible to understand the patient's anxiety and his overreaction as a kind of exaggerated preventive response that corresponded to his earlier traumatic experiences.

7.7 Anonymity and Naturalness

We contrast the behavior of an anonymous and impersonal analyst with his natural behavior because the latter definitely expresses a personal touch. We hope that the latter approach will help us resolve difficulties that arise within a relationship between two parties who have different interests. These differences do in fact exist, and even the legitimate criticism of the exaggerated stereotypical descriptions of these roles does not justify ignoring them. In the office the analyst's role is different than outside it, and the same is true of the patient. This topic therefore poses a challenge for us to locate the sensitive points at which they intersect. Meetings outside the office, which we will pay special attention to, must be considered in light of the analytic situation - and vice versa, i. e., the definitions of the different roles are interrelated. The problems that patients and analysts have when they meet outside the office add another perspective to the subject of naturalness in the office.

"If in doubt, act naturally" - this recommendation is only easy to make in a state of sociological naivete because the issue of being natural originates in man's *second* nature, i. e., from his socialization. For example, experience shows that it is difficult for analysts and patients to talk in an unconstrained manner when they happen to meet outside of the office. This is presumably related to the differences that exist between the psychoanalyst's office and other social situations. It would be inappropriate for the patient to let himself freely associate in public, and the analyst would behave conspicuously if he refused to talk about the weather or vacation plans and instead remained silent or interpreted the conversation. The contrast that each experiences is intensified by their inequality. The patient is insecure because he is anxious that the analyst will use what he knows from treatment; he feels embarressed. On the other hand, the analyst's spontaneity is restricted because he thinks of the consequences it might have on the analysis.

The intensity of the contrast between the therapeutic situation and outside it can be expressed in numerous forms, as can the topics, and numerous factors are involved in determining which forms are taken. This makes it impossible to provide a comprehensive description by compiling a list of examples. Acknowledging this situation is the decisive precondition for reaching an adequate solution to the problem it poses. By admitting that he is also affected by this contrast, the analyst makes it easier for the patient to find a suitable role and to be independent in it, which in turn makes it possible to fulfill the goals and tasks of the treatment. The analyst's functions in the therapeutic situation can be described in terms of role theory and then compared to other roles that the analyst has in other capacities, for instance as the head of a discussion group or as a politically active citizen.

The acknowledgment of this diversity of roles implies contrasts, and the patient and analyst classify the latter on the basis of comparisons with the experiences that they have had with each other in therapy. To take an example concerning naturalness, it was not until the end of her professional career that Heimann (1989 [1978]) discovered that it is necessary for the analyst to act naturally toward his patient. We refer to this as a discovery without a trace of irony because Heimann, who intuitively never had difficulties being natural as an analyst, was unable to admit until this late publication that acting naturally is therapeutically necessary and therefore justified despite her acceptance of neutrality and anonymity. It was hardly a coincidence that this publication had the involved title "On the Necessity for the Anaylst to Be Natural with His Patient." This text is relatively unknown, and has just recently (1989) been published in English.

Rules that exclude spontaneity and stipulate that the analyst must first reflect before reacting demand the impossible. If the analyst believes that spontaneity is incompatible with his professional role, he will feel particularly unfree when he is together with a patient in social situations. The patient, in turn, will be eager to make his analyst finally act or say something spontaneously in the analysis itself or to meet him on a person to person basis outside of analysis.

There are many factors that justify the assumption that the rule "if in doubt, act naturally" is easier to accept than to follow, whether in the analytic situation or outside it. We would like to mention several instructive examples. Many analysts avoid their patients if it is at all compatible with social norms. Candidates in training, who themselves avoid meeting their training analysts, are particularly affected. If a meeting does take place, any conversation that results is more likely to be inhibited than free. The unnaturalness is greatest in training analyses, which candidates assume to be a model of pure and untendentious analysis. The unfavorable consequences of a teacher-student relationship in which the master avoids even professional encounters, e. g., in seminars on technique, have been known for a long time. Fortunately there have always been some opportunities to make corrections. Each contrapuntal experience with a training analyst has a deidealizing function and is easily remembered. Although the question of whether all the stories that are later told can be believed is another matter, we must ask ourselves why a spontaneous comment by the analyst, which a third party might find completely banal, might retain a place of honor in a candidate's memory, and why many profound interpretations sink into oblivion. Everything exceptional occupies a special place in our memory. For example, the *one* and only direct confirmation that an analysand receives in analysis becomes something unique.

According to Klauber (1987), the analyst's spontaneity is necessary to enable the patient to moderate or balance the *traumas* originating in transference. Yet if the analyst's naturalness, which we equate with his spontaneity, has a compensatory function, then the strength of the traumas is something that depends in part on the analyst and his understanding of the rules. The problems that arise during encounters outside the office become greater to the degree that both participants avoid acting in a natural manner within therapy.

Acknowledging the diversity of roles that the patient and analyst play in public and private life can increase the tolerance for differences. It is therefore essential that in their training candidates develop an uncomplicated relationship to the various roles they will play in and outside their professional lives. The degree of natural behavior by their analysts that candidates experience both in and ouside psychoanalysis is an instructive measure for such tolerance toward the diversity of roles. We have investigated the changes in the system of psychoanalytic training from this point of view and reached a disturbing conclusion. Even into the 1940s it was frequently the case that analyst and analysand alternated roles and played different roles. The story of Freud's best known patient, the Wolf Man, was full of complications and entanglements that Freud and many of his students were involved in, as Mahoney (1984) described in his comprehensive report. The mingling of roles that M. Klein practiced was no less varied, as can be learned from Grosskurth's (1986) biography. This diversity of roles seems to have played a large role into the 1940s, particularly in the formation of different schools. Many of the analysts in training at that time were embedded in a frightful entanglement of personal, professional, and institutional interests. In hindsight it is easy to understand that reaction formations occurred, which after the experience of such "human, all too human" behavior swung to the opposite extreme. We gave too little consideration to this side of the development of the psychoanalytic technique in the relevant passages of Vol.1 (Chap. 7 and Sects. 1.6, 8.9.2). The painful experiences of many analysts have contributed to the sudden change from a diversity of roles to stereotype ones. Once schools have begun to form, then the adherents are always less tolerant of deviance than the master. By reactively adhering to written prescriptions, it is extremely easy for such idealizations to be combined with the interests of each group in professional politics.

Naturalness was lost in the stereotype role of the impersonal analyst. Although this apporach made it possible for much confusion to be avoided, the idea of finally being able to arrive at an analysis of a pure transference free of all outside influences proved utopian. *Traumas* resulting from *stereotype roles* took the place of the burdens resulting from a *mingling* of roles.

This dichotomy cries for a third option, which we have described at many places in Vol.1, in particular in discussing the extension of the theory of transference. Viewed from the perspective of role theory, the analyst's tasks imply certain definitions of his role that have practical consequences in therapy and with which the patient becomes familiar. The patient unveils his own world in the analyst's office, including the roles he plays and the ones that come naturally to him, where he is genuine and where he is phony, and how he can find his way to his true self. The fascination exerted by self-realization and even more by the search for one's true self is connected with the fact that precisely the latter lies in the sphere of unlimited opportunities or seems to lie in the still unconscious preliminary forms of one's own prospects in life. The dreamer's script contains foreign, supplementary, and desired self-representations. It is precisely the still unborn and the unconscious anticipations that are brought to life in the analyst's office. The patient knows from his own experience that the analyst also feels at home in many roles and is in a position to respond to certain roles that the patient offers and to react emotionally to them. The patient may pull all stops to test the analyst's capacity for empathy. If there were no natural reactions, transferences would be nipped in the bud and die off. This unique stage permits the analysand to perform trial actions free of all danger, the precondition being that the analyst provides confirmation and offers him roles that correspond to the patient's unconscious offers (see Sandler 1976). The professional restrictions on the relationship between patient and analyst become a symbol of *borders* that as such also provide *security*. The limited space in the analyst's office becomes a simile for protected naturalness.

The rediscovery of spontaneity and naturalness means that the patient may learn more from and about his analyst that he already knows about the latter's feelings and thoughts from the interpretations. It is precisely via interpretations that the patient gets to know himself from the analyst's point of view, and for this reason we believe it is extremely important for the patient to become aware of the larger context in which the analyst's comments, statements, and interpretations are part. *It is therapeutically essential for the analyst to let the patient share in the context and to reveal and ground the background of interpretations.* This must be distinguished from letting the patient share in the analyst's countertransference. The less the patient knows about the context, the more curious he will be to learn more about the analyst as an individual. It was unfortunately quite late when patients made us aware of these very neglected and yet easily resolvable problems of psychoanalytic technique (see also Sect. 2.4). From this position there is a rather simple answer to the question as to what the patient may learn in the office about the analyst as an individual, namely everything that promotes his knowledge about himself and does not obstruct it. Via the analyst's naturalness, the patient learns corresponding facts about himself. Even a deficit can be the starting point for discoveries because it would be a contradiction in itself to fulfill some conventional expectations or to equate them with natural reactions. Obviously, the analyst's spontaneous and natural behavior can stay within the code of socially accepted behavior or transgress it. The latter seems to be the case particularly when a specific countertransference is precipitated. The recommendation "if in doubt, behave naturally" is oriented on the rules of accepted social behavior, which meet in common sense.

Thus the analyst will behave naturally in his office and at coincidental encounters outside it if he structures the expectations associated with his various roles in a personal manner. This still leaves much room for spontaneity in connection with a patient's particular circumstances. A rich source of psychoanalytic knowledge would dry up if analysts adopted an anonymous stereotype role.

We would like to explain our comments by referring to two examples. First we describe how a female patient gave a bouquet of flowers to her analyst. Although we by no means categorically reject the rule of never accepting presents, on the basis of our experience we are convinced that rejecting presents often prevents analysts from recognizing their true meaning. Rejections and condemnations can have consequences that are very difficult to correct (see Van Dam 1987; Hohage 1986). Accepting flowers naturally has consequences on the analytic process, but more important is the question as to which form of behavior has the more favorable consequences in a particular situation and which criteria the analyst should use to make a decision.

In the second example we describe an encounter in the office building but outside the analyst's office. It would be easy to mention many more examples. In large cities many analysands belong to the same social strata and professional groups as the analyst, and encounters between the patient and analyst at cultural events can therefore be frequent even in large cities. In our opinion it is only natural for a feeling of insecurity to arise during such encounters.

First Example: Flowers

Amalie X held a bouquet of flowers in her hand as she greeted me.

P: It may not be very original, but it was my idea!

I accepted the flowers, noted that they needed water, and put them in a vase. Of course, there was the rustling of paper, action, brief comments, the sort of thing that happens until the paper has been removed and a suitable vase has been found.

P: They're bound to fit; I bound them extra tight.

A: The flowers are lovely.

The patient explained that she had had the idea the night before, and that just before the session she had received flowers herself, which made her think of it again.

P: I asked myself if it would be better for me to have them sent to you at home.

Yet then she added that this thought had probably been just an excuse.

A: There were other, more important reasons.

P: I thought that I wouldn't have to run amok as much here. [She laughed and corrected herself.] No, how do say, run the gauntlet [laughed again], yes, not amok or run the gauntlet if I have them sent to you at home, it would simply be more discreet and, uh, I don't know, maybe I didn't want to be that discreet . . . .

She herself discovered that the flowers "are simply a combination of things that happened on the weekend, so I don't know quite rightly what they mean either." She talked about the connections to the flowers she herself had received just prior to the session. And she mentioned the visit of an acquaintance who was a student and knew me.

P: And he talked about you from the perspective of a student, and somehow it bothered me terribly, because I suddenly knew things about you, not much but still . . . despite my great curiosity I have never heard much about you. You've never left your place, and somehow the flowers may be something like, well, I can't really say . . . .

Consideration. Amalie X forgot what she had wanted to say, and I could tell that the tension was gone. I assumed that she had encountered resistance, presumably because something critical had been said about me.

I pointed out to her that she had only given a very brief summary of what the student had said. It turned out that the young man had asked if she got along with me; he had said he did not because my manners were not direct enough, too involved.

P: And then I had the feeling, today with the flowers, it's a kind of compensation, but the word bothers me because it's not compensation. When my acquaintance said it, it didn't bother me, because I've often had the same feeling. Sometimes your sentences just never end. Just two sessions ago we talked about it, but I've sometimes asked myself, "Why does he intentionally want to teach me I can't think," and in a way this was just a compensation for these years . . . . For a long time I thought that you were trying to prove to me how complexly and multifacitedly you can think and leave it up to me to follow you or not. And the moment the student said that he looked at it the same way and when he even dared to call it "involved," it was naturally a relief for me, hum, and at the same time I thought that somebody should stop the nasty boy from talking that way [laughed while talking].

The patient then spoke about her experiences with difference acquaintances she had made via newspaper ads, and how confused it all made her.

P: Okay, somehow everything I do seems to work, and probably to keep it all and to guarantee it by linking it to you, I bought the flowers [laughed briefly]. Somehow that seems to come into it. Yes, I believe in such a superstitious talisman. You see everything you're good for, even right now.

A: As you said a moment ago, the flowers are supposed to end the confusion.

The patient then told me about another episode that confused her, in which she was supposed to give another man flowers.

P: I naturally wanted to give S. the flowers, but there was too much distance, in every sense, and then you had to stand in. It's not very nice. [Brief pause] Are you hurt? [Brief pause] Oh, yes, of course I won't get an answer.

A: And how could it hurt me if the distance is too large or that I have to be a stand-in?

P: The latter might hurt *you*. *I* am hurt that S. isn't close enough. [longer pause]

A: And the flowers here reduce the distance to me.

P: You sometimes have a way of taking things right out of my mouth and neutralizing them at the same time. Oh, it triggers different things, actually always two kinds of feelings. On the one hand I hold it against you, but it also fascinates me.

A: Yes, because you've used the flowers to neutralize it yourself. [Short pause]

P: Who or what?

A: Amok. [Patient laughs]

Commentary. This comment triggered a surprising turn in the conversation. The patient was in a state of inner tension before she gave the analyst the flowers, which caused her to make a slip of the tongue. Her anxiety about being criticized was expressed in her thoughts about running a gauntlet, but she fought against this subjugation and ended up with amok. There was thus a lot bound up with the flowers, even long before this session. If the analyst had not accepted them in a friendly manner, then this instructive dialogue would never have taken place.

P: I have to laugh because I believe I've hardly ever made a slip of the tongue. I believe that I've rarely done you the favor, don't even need two hands to count the number of times, but that's not much over a period of 4 years . . . . That it's not very easy with the flowers is probably clear, but it's okay. In the waiting room I said to myself that I would give them to the secretary. I had the feeling that you are mad, which was the reason I had to say that the idea was not very original, to excuse me as it were . . . . I had the feeling I would have been indiscreet, uh, showed something, I should have had them brought to your house, with a card and glove. [Laughed and sighed at the same time]

A: Why did you think that it isn't original?

P: Well, I have to say something. Most of all I would have liked to have simply beamed at you [laughed]. Now I've at least said it.

A: With your flowers, to show me your shining directness, namely that you've made the decision to answer the ads in the paper.

P: Yes, it stands for that, because the things I have experienced, especially in the last few days, but also in the last few years, the things I was terribly afraid of doing, that if I did do them then it has always helped me get a step further . . . . and without being here I really wouldn't have done a lot of things.

A: Yes, I'm very happy for you and thank you that you have mentioned it and that I was able to help you a little to do the things that you want to do.

Commentary. At the end of the session the analyst thanked the patient, in a context that offered encouragement and confirmation. This was the preliminary end of this interpretative work.

Second Example: Encounter Outside the Office

When patient and analyst meet outside the office it is not easy for either one to behave in a natural manner that is fitting to the situation or to talk in an unforced manner. The dialogue in the office is too intensive and too different in nature for them to be able to easily find their way into different social roles. We recommend that these difficulties be acknowledged, and in our experience this can have a liberating effect on both the patient and the analyst.

Erna X was walking past me into the building; I was standing together with a group of men. At first she thought it was the janitor, because my suit was blue. This thought startled her, and her insecurity about how she might get passed this group of men became unbearable. The following is a summary of her most important associations.

She said that Mr. Z, the janitor, is friendly, in contrast to many of the people she encounters in the building. It is unusual for anyone to say hello. Maybe the staff believes they're not permitted to look at the patients. The ladies and gentlemen whose rooms are up here would walk past you and would be unfriendly, dreamy, absent-minded, carrying books. The janitor's friendly manner was in clear contrast to their behavior. "Maybe that's I why I associate you with the janitor, because he's the only friendly person in the building."

The next theme was her double role as woman and as patient and being greeted as such. As a patient she should greet the doctor, but as a woman she should be greeted. My interpretation referred to her insecurity in these roles. "Are you the patient who greets humbly, or the woman who expects to be greeted and is pleased when people pay attention to her? Attention expressed in everyday life by the fact that women are greeted by men." The patient recalled memories of her childhood, and that as a child she had had to greet people. "It was very important to my grandmother that people thought I was a friendly child." I interpeted her anger at her having been so obsequious, which in turn increased her insecurity. I also mentioned the possibility that she might greet so rapidly in order to avoid situations in which she was greeted first. Thus she did not give male doctors the chance to pay attention to her and to fulfill her wish. She admitted that she avoided such embarassing situations; she put her coat on by herself and did not let anyone help her to avoid becoming embarassed.

She then recalled memories of her puberty. She was embarassed when her father or uncle helped her into her coat. "You feel you're being watched. He holds the coat, and I don't get in. If you held the coat for me, I would be excited and surely make a mess of everything. It's a form of attention that is irritating." She preferred to leave her coat in the car, to avoid the problem of putting it on and taking it off again. And on this day she would have gone a different way if she had known that she would have to walk past me. I related the previous role conflict with the momentary one in the following interpretation.

A: It wasn't right for people to view you as a growing young woman. Then you would have had wishes, wishes that in a broad sense have to do with getting dressed and undressing, with being seen and paid attention, with being admired.

P: I still feel like a small girl.

The subject of dressing and undressing had already been a topic the previous week. The patient recalled that she had thought for several nights about the following scene during the period we talked about someone helping her into her coat. Her aunt and uncle had often come to visit, and she went to bed early. Twice it happened that her uncle entered her room without knocking. She had been undressed, almost naked. To relieve the patient I first referred to her uncle's role.

A: Perhaps he was curious. It wasn't a pure coincidence, was it?

P: It was terribly nasty of him. He had had something to drink. It was all very disturbing. And I couldn't say anything because I was the little girl who wasn't supposed to be bothered by such things.

A: If you had complained, then you would have made it known that you no longer experienced yourself as a little girl, but as a young woman who was aware of her erotic attraction. You would have made this plain if you had complained.

P: He would have said, "What do you want?" And my parents would have said, "What are you thinking of? What dirty ideas do you have?" This uncle was always telling jokes, and I wasn't supposed to laugh. If I laughed, then I was asked "Why are you laughing? You don't understand any of it." I stopped wanting to laugh. I still haven't got over these two experiences.

She had come up with all sorts of tricks to prevent her uncle from entering her room.

Prior to a later session there was a comparable scene outside my office. I had seen the patient coming through the main door and was ahead of her on the stairs. To avoid having to walk up several flights of stairs together, I went into the office of a colleague, with whom I had wanted to discuss something anyway. My reaction was both reflexlike and intentional, and I had the preconscious intention of avoiding the complications that frequently occur from walking together. I had forgotten the earlier scene.

The patient thought that I had quickly gone into my colleague's room for her sake and to save her an embarassing situation. At some point I mentioned that I did not have any recollection of the janitor scene, which was long ago. I told her I had in fact had something to discuss with a colleague, yet added that it was not easy for me either to handle the problems that occur during encounters outside the office. I said I also felt a little embarassed and the situation would be awkward because making small talk would be very different from the analytic dialogue, but not to say anything would also be very unusual.

This comment made the patient feel very relieved. It was objectively, as she expressed it, not easy - even for me, the analyst - to solve this problem. Walking along silently would contradict accepted social behavior. It was, instead, rather customary to exchange a few words after greeting. I added, "That's also how I feel about it, but there is no reason we have to act that way. Why shouldn't we just walk together without saying anything."

7.8 Audio Tape Recordings

Instead of constructing an ideal of the psychoanalytic process, such as Eissler (1953) did, only to have theoretical arguments about which compromises are more or less acceptable, we believe it is more meaningful to investigate the influence exerted by various factors. One of these conditions that we have examined in detail is the subject of audio tape recordings (Ruberg 1981; Kächele et al. 1988). Our results indicate that the specific impact of this variable can be recognized and worked through in a therapeutically productive manner. Some problems are even encountered more rapidly, showing that projection onto the tape recording can be a starting point for a productive dialogue.

In our experience both parties become accustomed to the idea that third parties might listen to their dialogue. The tape recording then becomes a part of the silent background that, like all the external factors in the psychoanalytic situation, can have a dynamic effect at any point. The simple presence of both the silent recorder and the inconspicuously placed microphone remind the participants that they are not alone in the world. The procedures used to make the analysand anonymous and to code the tape can also become a topic for joint thought, even though confidentiality and the removal of names are two preconditions for the introduction of this aid. Of course, this protection only applies to the patient. The removal of the name of the analyst in question does not prevent colleagues from finding out who the treating analyst was. They can easily recognize in the published dialogues the analyst's manner of speaking and the way in which he thinks and acts analytically.

In our opinion there are many reasons it can be useful for analysts to inform patients about the purpose of the recordings of therapy. The most important is that the analyst is willing to consult his colleagues. However, the style of discussion that still predominates among analysts makes it comprehensible that the majority of analysts still hesitate to use this tool, although it is better suited than any other means to improve therapeutic skills by stimulating critical reflection of the transcribed dialogue.

The analyst has, of course, not only a right to personal privacy but also to organizing his professional sphere according to his own best convenience within the profession's system of values. A specific mixture of various character features, which have to be paired with scientific curiosity and a belief in progress, probably make it easier to commit such an act of largely unprotected self-exposure to the profession. At any rate, we have tried to make a virtue of necessity and ascribe a curative function to the introduction of audio tape recordings in several regards: for the individual analyst, whose narcissism is put to a hard test; to the profession, which no longer has to rely solely on recollection in scientific discussions, but can refer to authentic dialogues; and to the patient, who can indirectly profit from it. It is a sign of the times that some patients even bring their own tape recorders. It is advisable to reckon with such surprises. Since it can certainly be useful for a patient to reconsider dialogues, the analyst should take this interest seriously, even if such an action should be motivated by the unconscious intention of being well prepared for a malpractice suit. Shocking was a dialgoue that Sartre (1969) commented upon, to which a patient had coerced his analyst and which he had recorded. In that interview it had come to an reversal of roles; the patient tormented his analyst with precisely the castration interpretations that the analyst had allegedly given him for years.

For the psychoanalytic profession it can at any rate hardly be harmful if original recordings or transcripts are used to enable researchers to examine closely what psychoanalysts say and do in therapy and to identify which theories they follow. It might have a positive effect on the narcissism of individual analysts for them to be confronted with their own therapeutic behavior. To allude to a well-known expression of Nietzsche's, in the struggle between pride, deeds, and memory, the voices on the tape recording revive memories that make it difficult for pride to remain relentless and triumph over memory.

7.8.1 Examples

The community of psychoanalysts is apparently more disturbed by the introduction of audio tape recordings than are the patients. In attempting to locate the common denominator of their concerns we encounter once again Eissler's (1953) basic model technique and the "parameters" that belong to it, which we have discussed in detail in Vol.1 (Sect. 8.3.3). This model has created more problems than it has solved.

We have not yet experienced the situation that the resistances precipitated or reinforced by the presence of a tape recorder have not been accessible to interpretation. In the following we illustrate this with reference to our experience in using tape recordings, placing special emphasis on the interpretative response to the patient's reactions.

A Supercensor

Amalie X talked in the 38th session of her therapy about her experience with a therapy while she was at college. Her therapist at that time had not returned her diary to her, which had made her feel disheartened. I suggested that the fact that the analyst kept her diary corresponded to the tape recorder keeping her thoughts. The patient said that she knew nothing about the use of the recordings, adding "I also have to say that I'm not very concerned about it." In the following hour the talk also focused on *giving and taking*, and I again mentioned the idea that the tape recorder took her thoughts.
P: That probably bothers me less; it's such a distant medium.
This answer made it clear that this patient managed in the initial phase of the therapy, after working through a disturbing experience from an earlier therapy, to arrive at a clear statement of how she viewed the situation.

Specific desires for discretion sometimes lead to the request that the tape recorder be temporarily turned off. This patient, for example, talked about a colleague who was also in therapy; she did not want to mention the name of the latter's therapist until the tape recorder had been turned off (85th session). The analyst can accept such a wish or can emphasize the aspect of resistance or explore ideas such as whether the patient believes the colleague might be negatively affected. The phenomenon that the analysand wishes to protect others by being discreet and therefore suspend the basic rule regarding a specific item of information also occurs, incidentally, in every analysis, including those without tape recordings.

Analysts can repeatedly observe the fact that thinking about the tape recorder can stimulate a thought to suddenly come to the fore in the patient's free flow of associations, as shown in the following example.

In the 101th session Amalie X spoke with great decisiveness about her sexual difficulties and managed to disclose a relatively substantial amount of information; in the middle of the session she became increasingly horrified by the intensity of her longing. I interpreted her anxiety "that she views herself and her fantasies as an addiction or as being perverse after all, and somehow I do too, and I only act as if I wouldn't find it perverse or addicting." The patient herself arrived at a differentiated opinion; "When I think about it, I know that this is not what you think." Yet she herself saw herself in such terms and was afraid that others would say something like, "Yes, the old X." In this moment she asked herself, "Is the tape recorder still running?" The thought was linked with the idea that an older secretary might type the transcripts, and other associations led to the father confessor etc.

In her 202nd session Amalie X took a statement I had made to be an explanation of my therapeutic technique. She found it "unusually positive" and mentioned the inaccurate assumption that the tape recorder had been turned off and that I was thus able to act more freely and was less inhibited. The patient imagined that the presence of the tape recorder had the same inhibiting effect, as a supercensor, on me that the presence of her supervisor at work had on her. "If I don't see the black wire here some time, then you will feel freer and for once can say what you're thinking."

In the 242nd session the patient noted that the microphone wire was not on the wall. She speculated that the presumed disappearance of the tape recorder (or microphone) signalled the end of her therapy. She said she was afraid of the separation, and that her earlier idea that my colleagues would listen to the recordings and laugh at them had disappeared.

By the way, for this patient we can report that, based on the empirical research we mentioned at the beginning of this section, examination of a sample of one-fifth of all the sessions (113 sessions) of Amalie X's therapy showed that the tape recorder was a topic in 2.7% of them (Ruberg 1981).

A Fake

Franziska X had a positive attitude toward tape recording from the very beginning because her brother, who was a sociologist, had recommended that she use a tape recorder as a means of self help. The patient quickly developed transference love and exhibited the corresponding difficulties (see Sect. 2.2). In the third session she stated that most of all she would like to bracket out all the expectations, fantasies, and desires, simply everything that constituted the emotional involvement with the therapist.

P: Yes, if that would be possible, then it would probably be much easier for me to be uninhibited in describing things, if you weren't buzzing in my head, if I could turn you off completely, if I would just be lying alone in the room and talking to the tape recorder.

Here the tape recorder serves as an artificial psychoanalyst, not precipitating any anxiety about a loss of distance.

In the following session Franziska X asked if the tape recorder was turned on or not, since the cover was closed. She then told me that she had drunk a lot (several glasses) of wine the night before. I linked the two statements by asking whether she felt the desire for the recorder to be off. The patient responded in the negative, emphasizing, "No, I don't think so, it's never bothered me . . . [almost a little ironically] Perhaps I'm worried that my valuable comments won't be recorded . . . and perhaps it's running after all." Her ironic tone reflected her anxiety about her worthlessness, as was shown in the further course of the therapy.

The patient's reactions to the tape recorder changed in accordance with dynamic changes that occurred. In the 87th session she reflected on the pleasure and unpleasure she had in the therapy.

P: Sometimes I think about what we have already achieved in the analysis, and then I'm always overcome by the feeling that I would like to take all the tapes and throw them into the fire and start all over. I've talked the tapes full with bla bla. I imagine that in an session there might be one good sentence, and for this one sentence you have to sit and listen 50 minutes, hoping that one comes. Sometimes there aren't any. And that's why I believe that you then become dissatisfied and mad at me again.

A: That I use so much, use so many of the tapes, and get so little in exchange.

P: Yes, I feel as if I'm taking private lessons. I would like to be a good pupil, so that you might be happy with me.

In the following session Franziska X at first did not have many associations, but then explained that when she had the feeling she liked somebody, then she would "talk a lot, sometimes even too much . . . but if I have merely the feeling that they're cold, then it just doesn't work right." I related this to her associations about the tape recorder; "In the last session you had the feeling that you only reveal invaluable stuff; at least a good worm has to be in it for me." Franziska X confirmed again that she had the feeling that she always had to offer something special to gain confirmation.

Auditorium

Kurt Y, a scientist, was in analysis because of impotence and an incapacity to work. In the fourth session he glanced at the microphone as he entered the office, laid down, and after a short pause began to speak. He referred back to his experiences as a child, which had also been a topic in the preceding session. In general he had been a quiet, good boy; it had only been in his soccer club that he had been able to let out his pent up energy. He added, however, that he had always played poorly when spectators had been present.

A: As if you were afraid of the attention.

P: Yes, everything was over as soon as I felt the expectation that I would have to demonstrate my skills.

A: While you were coming in, you glanced at the microphone. Is there perhaps an expectation associated with it?

P: No, today I don't have to think about it much, but yesterday I noticed it. I had the strong feeling I had to fill the tape, that there couldn't be any gaps, that something had to go onto it.

A: These expectations, the ones you identify with the tape recorder, represent in your opinion the expectations I place on you.

Kurt Y began the 54th session with a comment about the tape recorder. He had the feeling he had to hold a speech, as if he were in an auditorium, and this was linked with the idea that what he had to say was not really finished and needed further elaboration. It was like in his workbook, where he recorded his notes about his experiments; he would not make it accessible to anyone prematurely. Kurt X talked for a long time about the tape recorder, leading me after a while to assume there was a resistance, and I told him that it seemed to be easier for him today to speak about the tape recorder than about other things. He then began to speak, albeit with many qualifications, about the sexual experiences he had had the past weekend with his fiancee.

At the beginning of the following session Kurt Y again referred to the tape recorder. He said it was much friendlier today, as if it were a third person in the room, someone he could imagine to be a young physician. He could bear it after all for someone to listen, adding that the recordings were presumably used for teaching.

The threatening, fascinating idea of the large auditorium had become milder, more realistic, and also easier to bear. This was accompanied by his resumption of his description of his sexual intercourse with his fiancee, which he told with visible enthusiasm. For some time intercourse had not been possible because of an illness she had had, and this had given him the feeling that the wall he had to scale was not so high after all. Yet as the weekend with his fiancee had approached he had registered how his anxious anticipation had constantly increased. And he had promptly been unable to do "it" that evening; in his helplessness he had not achieved an erection.

I offered the interpretation that he presumably had been unable to let himself fall, just like he here was unable to let go. I added that I assumed that he felt he was being watched and that he compared himself with other men, a fact he had not included in his description but I added.

He said that he had then slept "black," without dreaming, and tried to explain the color "black" from his dream, which seemed unusual to me. In the morning he had had a slight erection, and he had taken advantage of the situation to scale the wall.

I thought to myself that this had probably been a major barrier for him, just as talking about his sexual life was a major barrier that he scaled in this session. I told him so, and he was very surprised. Yet he agreed that it was true that he had never talked about it here although he had often felt the need to.

It was clear to me that the work on the meaning of the tape recorder, and especially the interpretations of transference that were associated with it, had reached him, and that he had therefore been able to scale the wall of intimacy in therapy.

In the 57th session I told Kurt Y about my vacation plans, including about a long absence that was partly for professional reasons. While thinking about the professional reasons that might lead me to make this trip, he had the idea that it might be to hold lectures. In this connection he mentioned the tape recorder again. This time it was an indication of scientific work, laboratory experiments, and that he himself was a guinea pig, all expressions of the therapist's coldness. The patient's mood changed, though, in the further course of talking about these feelings.

P: The tape recorder does have something positive to it. At the very least the tapes will stay here and thus something of our relationship will stay here as a kind of pledge.

I interpreted the connections between vacation, distance, and his reactions to them as a kind of fundamental question about what he was worth to me and how regularly I would be there for him.

Controls

In the case of Heinrich Y, my efforts to motivate him to undertake therapy were quite difficult, which let me envisage the problems that his general mistrust toward analysts would also mobilize against tape recording.

In the 16th session the patient surprised me by bringing a cassette recorder along, which he prepared for recording while he asked me whether he could use it. I pointed out the simultaneous timing of the two actions - the request for my approval and his actions as if I had already given my approval - and added that the recording of our talk had to be very important to him. Since I had previously obtained his informed consent for recording the sessions, I said it was only appropriate that I permit him to do the same. The patient laughed at this, obviously relieved. At this point I did not ask any more questions about the purpose of his actions.

Heinrich Y then began to complain intensely that, as is frequently the case at such an early stage of therapy, nothing was happening, that the therapy had shown little sign of success, and that his depressive states had begun to preoccupy him more again. On the previous weekend, he said, he had been at a conference on Zen Bhuddism, where he hoped to be able to obtain additional advice for helping him cope with his life.

A: Additional advice? That also means that our sessions don't provide enough.

P: Precisely, the sessions are over so quickly, and afterwards I can never remember exactly what happened.

A: But then tape recordings must be a desirable means to listen to everything in peace and quiet.

P: Yes, I hope to be able to work through everything in detail, to get more out of the sessions. I play them to my girlfriend Rita - who has had some experience with psychotherapy - and she can tell me whether everything is alright here.

A: Yes, in this initial period it seems natural to ask somebody for advice, especially since you were very reluctant in agreeing to undergo therapy. Your severe depression was precipitated, after all, by Rita believing herself to be pregnant. Might it be possible that the tape recorder permits you to exert some control on what you are able to speak about with me?

P: Rita should just find out how bad off I am and what part she's played in it.

A: So that this is an indirect means of telling Rita something that you cannot or don't want to tell her directly.
P: Well, things I say here, I can point out that it's part of the therapy.
A: That I'm responsible for it and you can't be held accountable for it.
At this point the patient laughed mischievously and emphasized that I traced his most secret thoughts. He added that it might be better after all for him to turn off his recorder and tell Rita that it simply had not worked correctly.
A: At any rate the space we share here would be protected from somebody's censorship. This would also provide some freedom.
This form of working through, however, did not deal with the other aspect of the conservation of sessions that the patient sought. I therefore emphasized once again that this observation was very important and that we together had to look for the ways and means as to how he could organize his review of the sessions productively.

Turning Off the Recorder

In one session Arthur Y requested that I turn off the tape recorder before talking about the subject he did not want to be taped. The subject was a conflict precipitated by the unanswered question as to which profession his daughter should choose. She had had doubts about whether she should continue her education at a vocational college or switch to a regular university. She wanted to first have a trial period at the university before making a final decision to leave the college, but universities required applicants to confirm that they are not enrolled at other schools before permitting registration. Arthur Y was afraid that the schools would check on this information. I interpreted his exaggerated concern in the context of his old anxieties about inflicting harm, similar to the way in which harm had been inflicted on him. In other words, the topic was once more the relationship between subject and object and confusing sadomasochistic identifications. By having the tape recorder turned off, the patient not only wanted to avert the practically nonexistent danger that something might become public; the real issue was once again apotropaic magic, namely the reversal of a potential harm by means of the magical power of his thoughts. The rest of the session was dedicated to this topic, and the tape recorder was not turned on again.

This was the first time that the patient had mentioned the tape recorder in a long time. Before turning it off, I had reminded him that in one session long before he had even requested that the recording of one session be kept at all cost. He said he always wanted to have a means of gaining access to his idea that he himself had felt like a brutal SS officer for a moment. This was linked for him with his insight into his punishment anxieties and the reversion from delusions of grandeur to delusions of nothingness and from sadism to masochism. The patient had also once had the desire to read the transcript of one session; we agreed that he could read one in the waiting room prior to his next session. He had made the arrangements to have the time, but the text had not told him anything new. The only important result had been that he had been satisfied with the coding.

A Disgrace

Following a clear improvement in his severe symptoms and a substantial increase in the pleasure he found in life, Rudolf Y wondered at the beginning of one session when he might be able to discontinue the therapy. He talked enthusiastically about his friendships and his growing capacity to make contacts. The dialogue then moved to the topic of the relative contributions each of us had made to the therapeutic progress.

P: Yes, that's it, that I don't let you have the pleasure of gaining knowledge at my expense, don't give you confirmation of how good you are and of how much you know about me.

A: So it isn't a pleasure related to you that you in turn might profit from.

P: Yes, I'm a means to an end. [Very long pause] The tape, it's in vain; there's nothing on it. [laughed]

A: So I, the one who would like to demonstrate something, to show myself, how good I am, can't demonstrate anything.

P: Yes, that's it.

A: I could show the collected moments of silence. [Both roared with laughter] It documents my powerlessness.

P: Yes, the silence.

A: So a balance has been created. Today's long silence on the tape is the compensation for the submissiveness with which you agreed that I may know so much about you. Today I'm the one who's been disgraced, shown to be powerless, and made the butt of laughter. You were pleased by the idea that my colleagues would laugh at me.

P: Yes, I still switch between these extremes of either complete submission to superiors or of thinking they're sons of bitches.

Commentary. The tape recording is a factor in the patient's alternation between these extremes and in the polarization into power and impotence. The laughter accompanied an insight into this distribution, which the patient's attribution had the effect of increasing and maintaining. Tape recordings provide a good occasion for considering the topic of transference, an example of which is given in the following section. Rudolf Y obviously realized that his silence might be a disgrace for his analyst. Old scores are settled in transference as well as in catharsis.

7.8.2 Counterarguments

We take counterarguments very seriously precisely because we place a high value on the use of complete original texts in clinical discussions and scientific studies. Frick (1985), for example, tried to support the assertion that tape recordings distort the therapeutic process. She reported that the associations of one patient, despite his having given his approval for the recordings, indicated that he felt latently exploited and seduced. It was only after the therapist had taken the initiative to give up the tape recording that the patient showed positive changes in several areas of his life.

Frick took this to be a confirmation of her opinion that Langs' idea of an ideal therapeutic framework had to be retained in order to protect the "sanctity" of the therapeutic relationship. Allegedly no interpretation was able to "detoxify" the negative and destructive consequences of the tape recording.

If this assertion were accurate for a larger group of patients, and not just in an individual case, then it would be necessary once again to submit the advantages and disadvantages of this tool to a thorough comparison. In fact, however, something seems to have gone wrong in this *one* case, which Frick blamed on the tape recording. The patient was treated in an outpatient clinic by two residents in supervision. The first therapist withdrew after four weeks, entering private practice, while the second therapy was limited to nine months, meeting twice a week. In the last quarter of the initial interview the therapist informed the patient about the basic rule and asked for his approval for tape recording all the sessions. The fact that the resident was being supervised was implicit, but was not discussed with the patient.

We assume that Frick functioned as the supervisor; at any rate, she has provided instructive commentaries to passages from the transcript. Completely open is, however, whether any interpretations were given, and if so which ones, in order to help clarify and solve any problems that the tape recording might have posed to the patient. If a larger numer of interpretations are not reproduced in context, it is impossible to clarify the influence the tape recording exerted or to assert that the process was distorted. In *one* interpretation an analogy was made between a situation with a girlfriend and the transference, specifically with regard to giving and taking, being exploited and being used, etc. In our opinion the most that such analogies can achieve is to direct the patient's attention to a possible connection without in itself providing a clarification. Without a deeper explanation, such allusions have rather a toxic effect than a "detoxifying" one; they even increase the paranoid meaning attributed to the tape recording.

This example in no way supports the author's negative conclusions and is at most suited to demonstrate once more that verbatim protocols can put the clinical discussion on a solid footing (see Gill 1985).

At the present state of our knowledge evaluation of the overall influence of tape recordings on the psychoanalytic situation is positive. Obviously, both participants are affected by the fact that third parties are involved.

What kind of a person would it take, we might ask in conclusion, who would not let himself be affected or let his spontaneity and freedom be restricted by knowing that unknown third parties studied his thoughts once they had been put into an anonymous form? This question is not far from another problem, namely at which stage of the psychoanalytic process do the analyst's thoughts about him become less unimportant to the patient? At some point the "interesting points" pale, to use the phrase Nietzsche employed in *Dawn*:

Why do I keep having this thought... that we *presume* that man's well-being depends on *insight into the origin of things.* That we now, in contrast, the further we go back to the origin, are less involved as interesting points; yes, that everything we treasure and the "interesting points" that we have put into things begin to lose their sense the more we return with our knowledge and arrive at the things themselves. With our insight into the origin, the meaninglessness of the origin increases, while the nearest objects, which are around us and in us, gradually begin to show their color and beauty and puzzles and riches and meaning.... (Nietzsche 1973, p. 1044)

8 Means, Ways, and Goals

Introduction

We discuss the important issues of scheduling, remembering and retaining and of anniversary reactions from the perspective of time and place in Sect. 8.1. Due to the importance of the reconstruction of the historical and political factors that exert an influence on an individual's life history, we dedicate an entire section to this issue (Sect. 8.2). This is followed by an study of interpretations, a subject which has been a focus of our interest for a long time; here we refer to a treatment that took place many years ago (Sect. 8.3).

A discussion of acting out (in Sect. 8.4) leads over to the topic of working through (Sect. 8.5). The first of the five examples of this issue that we discuss (Sects. 8.5.1-8.5.5) is a detailed description of a case in which traumatic experiences were repeated in transference and of how they were mastered.

Interruptions of treatment are accompanied by particular problems up until the final separation (Sect. 8.6; we discuss the significance of the latter issue in connection with termination in Chap. 9). It is impossible to restrict psychoanalytic heuristics to one section of text in this volume on the practice of psychoanalysis, in contrast to first volume on the principles of therapy (see Sect. 8.2 in Vol.1). Each chapter of this book illustrates the specific and nonspecific means the patient and analyst use to make their way.

8.1 Time and Place

8.1.1 Scheduling

The most convenient arrangement for the analyst is to schedule his appointments so that the majority of his patients regularly come and go at set times. Such inflexibility, of course, restricts an analyst to accepting those patients whose personal situation makes it possible for them to keep appointments several times a week and to pay for hours they miss. To avoid such a restriction, many analysts are willing today to plan free time into their schedules in order to accomodate rescheduling and to have time for emergencies (see Wurmser 1987).

Whatever solution is chosen has its own advantages and disadvantages, which can be different for each of the two parties. All other considerations become superfluous if the analyst cannot create the preconditions under which a patient can come to treatment frequently and over a sufficiently long period of time without being forced to accept substantial restrictions or deprivations in his private or professional sphere. We are therefore in favor of a certain degreee of flexibility, which of course is associated with problems all its own. For example, according to our experience it is primarily in the flexible part of the analyst's schedule that he is prone to make mistakes or overlook items, such as forgetting an appointment or scheduling two appointments for the same time.

Because of his limited amount of time and the need to be punctual, the psychoanalyst is under increased pressure; the consequence can be a form of countertransference that is specific to the profession and directed in particular at patients who are tardy. On the one hand, we must remember that the patient is free to dispose of the time he or his health insurance company is paying for; on the other hand, tardiness and missing sessions mean that valuable time is lost. Any financial compensation does not change the fact that in such a case the analyst can only think about the patient, not do anything for him. If the patient continues to disregard his appointments, the analyst has practically no chance to exert any influence. And having become powerless, all that remains is for the analyst to reflect about the absent patient's motives and about what he himself may have contributed to the situation.

The commitments that each of the two parties makes are supposed to *lead to* something by creating an atmosphere of freedom. If the patient and analyst do not lose sight of the goals of psychoanalysis, there is less danger that the discussion of appointments, missed sessions, or rescheduling appointments will degenerate into haggling.

The following example illustrates the issues of *punctuality* and *perfectionism.*

Arthur Y entered my office out of breath.

P: I'm late, I messed up.

A: A minute, isn't it?

P: Yes, but your clock is a minute fast.

A: Really?

P: I think so.

A: But then you're on time.

P: One minute late. But that puts us right back in the middle of our topic.

A: Yes, you can want to be emperor, not just king.

P: Yes, or the pope.

A: [Laughed] Yes, the one at the very top.

P: There's a nice fairy tale called "The Fisherman and his Wife." In essence it says that the fisherman caught a fish, and the fish said, "Let me go and I'll make a wish come true." The fisherman's wish was to have a normal house instead of his old hut, and when he came home and told his wife the story, she scolded him: "You could have wished a lot more." The next day he caught the same fish again, and well it happened over and over again. His wishes got bigger and bigger, until finally he was the pope. But then he wanted to be the Lord God himself, and then he was sitting in his old hut again.

A: Oh, yes.

P: Yes, I once wrote down the word "perfectionism," in order to think about it. When I'm in a race with time, like now, I get afraid and act irrationally. I drive much too fast, a lot faster than you're supposed to. And when I think about it, it's completely out of proportion to the minute or two here. [The patient's comments are only interrupted by an encouraging "hum" or "yes" by the analyst.] If I get caught in a radar trap, then it might get tricky.

A: And there's more and more inner tension, paralyzing you and blocking everything so that you can't think about anything else. The fairy tale gives a deeper meaning to perfectionism.

P: Yes?

A: Namely of being the best with regard to punctuality, but it's linked to your concern that the punishment will come some time. It's very pronounced in your case, the idea of being punished. The extreme was to want to be God, and if that is what you want to be, the biggest of all, then the arrogance preceding the ruin is complete.

Arthur Y then mentioned a problem with one of our next appointments. I made several suggestions, saying that I preferred 7:00 p.m. The patient agreed and added:

P: Then you'll have a long working day, although it's none of .... Yes, yes, I'm being impudent again.

A: Hum.

P: It's really none of my business.

A: But it's very much your business. Yes, for example, after a long day at work, "Can he still manage at 7 p.m.?"

P: Hum, yes, that's precisely what I was thinking.

A: Yes, it's very much your business.

P: Well, we were talking about the fairy tale "The Fisherman and his Wife." I love this fairy tale because it's so profound, it contains so much practical wisdom, about being satisfied with something. Perfectionism is something that professionally has always been on my mind. I enjoy it, I like being the biggest, and I am in one region. But I let my perfectionism maneuver me into a deadend .... I should be able to take it easy some time and say, "So what, then I'll be two minutes late." The worst thing that can happen to me is that the two minutes are gone. That makes three marks, and they're not going to break me. But that's not really the issue. I mean, you stand here, look at your watch, knit your brow, just like I might, and get more and more upset and angry, simply because it is 9:09 or 8:08, and there's no quibbling about it. Perfectionism, not liberal but stubborn.

Commentary. The patient's comment about the profundity and practical wisdom of the fairy tale was a reference to the different ways it could be interpreted. The topic of perfectionism was, in contrast, limited.

A: Perfectionism is the pearl. And why is it then so terrible ....

P: ... for the pearl to fall out of the crown.

A: A pearl so precious that your own esteem depends on it.

P: Yes, yes.

A: So it's not just stubbornness, and you even claim that I make it the most valuable item and raise my brow over it.

P: Yes, I transferred it to my own situation, and I think that if I'm this way, then the others are too.

A: I have to be this way, because if I weren't, it wouldn't matter to me if you came or not. If that were part of it, wouldn't it matter to me then?

P: I really don't think so. At least I wasn't thinking of it.

A: But why it is that way? Why does it become so awfully valuable?

P: Well, because it's the opposite of what caused me problems when I was a child. For example, if I'm on time, to the very minute, or if I double my turnover, or if the superiority of my company gives me power over the competition and it's really enough power to drive my competitors, the smaller businesses, to the verge of bankruptcy, then first of all I'm punctual, second the best, and third the most powerful. In other words, it's exactly the opposite of what I used to be.

A: It's wonderful that you can be exactly the opposite of what you used to be. And if you can get me to consider punctuality to be the most important value, then we have the proof that you're different than you used to be.

P: Yes, it's clear to me too from what I said that I have to be the exact opposite of what I used to be.

A: And that's why the fairy tale is so fascinating, because the old fisherman did change.

P: Yes, but then there was the other turn around, and I'm afraid that everything is going to break down and I'll end up in an institution or prison after all. [This was one of the numerous compulsive thoughts and anxieties that afflicted the patient.]

A: And if you come a minute too late, then I'm completely dissatisfied with you and lose all interest.

P: Yes, it's peculiar that this one minute is decisive for my esteem.

Commentary. The dialogue was focused on the struggle for survival and success, on the transformation from pope into devil, and vice versa, and on polarizations and antipodes, being the best in both good and bad. The analyst gave the patient support by referring to the unconscious aspects of his struggle for survival. If someone is the most powerful of all, then nothing can happen to him.

P: Yes, I understood what you meant. What I've achieved here - yes, just saying this causes me problems because the thought spontaneously crosses my mind that you might object to the word "I" when I say "what I've achieved." That you might reprimand me, "At the very least you should say 'we.'"

There was a momentary interruption of this line of thought.

P: I know that it's not true. Well, good, whatever the situation. Gone, shame, it's gone, what I wanted to say.

Arthur Y lost his train of thought.

A: Maybe you were blocked by the idea that you should at least say "we." But presumably you didn't like the fact that you deprecated your own importance.

P: Yes, maybe I can pick up my train of thought again. I started from the idea that I have achieved something here.

A: Then your train of thought was interrupted. When you say "I," then you get punished.

P: Hum.

A: Then the "I" is gone. And then you're small until you've recovered from the punishment.

Commentary. This "momentary forgetting," this interruption of the patient's train of thought and his rediscovery of it, deserves special attention. It belongs to a large group of phenomena that offer us insight into unconscious defense processes. If a parapraxis or a psychic or psychosomatic symptom appears during a session, it is often possible to clarify its immediate source. Very instructive is also what the analyst contributed to the weakening of the repression and the rediscovery of the line of thought, i.e., to the disappearance of the microsymptom. Luborsky (1967) discovered that momentary forgetting while associating can serve as a prototype for research to validate hypotheses.

P: Yes, yes, now I've got it. It's the independence, the freedom, I demonstrated today by not waiting in the waiting room until you came. But where's the limit? One minute, or two or five or even ten minutes? Maybe some day I'll say to myself, "Ha, I'm not going at all today!"

Arthur Y then related a story about how he had had his way. He made it clear that if someone were late for an appointment with him, he would choose a friendly but reproachful statement like "It's not so bad. The next time you're sure to be on time again."

P: And I felt so terribly liberal when I said it.

At another point Arthur Y asked anxiously whether he talked too much about himself, implying that it might become too much for me.

A: You would be getting too personal if you said that I had a long day. Why are you worried about it? Maybe one reason is the question of whether I can still offer you proper treatment after a long day, whether I still have something to offer.

P: One thing was primary for me, namely transgressing some border by making a personal comment.

Commentary. The patient's anxiety about committing some transgression was, as can be concluded from a more thorough knowledge of his psychodynamics and symptoms, motivated in part by unconscious anal sadistic impulses, which were contained in his masochism. At the same time the patient identified with the victim, i. e., the analyst who was exhausted in the evening. This was presumably also the mode of his empathy, which the analyst pointed out to him. Finally, the analyst drew the patient's attention to the fact that he had expressly said that the suggestion of a session in the evening was especially good. This made it all the more probable that the unconscious source of his concern was irrational.

8.1.2 Remembering and Retaining

We chose this heading to draw attention to a significant topic, namely the problem of establishing a connection to the preceding session and remembering what happened. Who remembers what the patient and analyst felt, thought, and said, and how and where is this knowledge retained? What about forgetting? In psychoanalytic theory the development of object constancy is tied to the continuity of a stable interpersonal relationship. Whose responsibility is it to ensure that this continuity is maintained despite the unavoidable interruptions in life and in therapy, and what can the patient and analyst do to ensure that it survives the inevitable crises and is strengthened? Such questions surface when the patient cannot recall his line of thought and wants the analyst to tell him what the contents of the preceding session were. Proceeding from the word "contents" we could have decided on a heading for this section that we intentionally did not chose, namely the word "container," a metaphor that Bion introduced to refer to the reproduction of a comprehensive theory of communication and interaction expressed in terms of specific variables and constants. This metaphor stands for a specific theory and, accordingly, has to struggle with its connotations and implications. Although it is obvious that Balint's two-person psychology does not exist in a realm free of theory, it is important to us to achieve as much frankness as possible toward the phenomena discussed below. This is the reason we have chosen a heading that is colloquial.

After remaining silent for several minutes, Clara X began with the words:

P: I've tried to think of what happened in the last session. I can't remember. Can you remember anything?

A: Yes, I can recall a few things, but I assume that a few points will still cross your mind.

P: I can only recall that I cried. Maybe you can give me a hint.

A: [After a longer period of silence] It's possible that you need a hint from me, yet I still hesitate because it's also possible that it would be better to wait until you yourself come up with something. You can surely remember something; it must be stored somewhere. But perhaps you can't remember anything because what's most important is whether I've bridged the gap to the last session and whether I've kept mind on you, so that you can forget it. If you or something of yours is safe with me, then you don't have to remember it.

P: Yes, that would be a wonderful feeling.

A: Yes, it would be terrible if I couldn't recall anything. As a matter of fact, this was even one of the topics in the last session. We talked about the session we missed. I had left it up to you to schedule an additional hour. The topic at the beginning of the last session was whether your reason for running away was your deep disappointment in me. I hadn't understood how important it was whether I thought about you or not or whether I missed you.

P: But I still don't know why I cried so much.

There followed a period of silence that lasted several minutes, which I interrupted:

A: Have I passed the test? No, I haven't said anything about your tears and why you cried. So I haven't passed the test yet, inasmuch as I can pass it at all.

Commentary. It is possible to feel how the analyst struggled to make the best of the patient's forgetting, but he was uncertain about what to do. He even doubted whether he could pass the test at all, yet it was not clear what the reasons might be. His admission of his helplessness took on a therapeutic function by relating the problem to their relationship.

P: Yes, I think that's an important point for me, I mean how it affects you, whether it repells you, whether you think it's impertinent, whether you're offended, whether you would like to ignore it or – as in behavior therapy – to erase it by disregarding it. Of course, it could also cause just the opposite to occur, all the more so. Or whether you would have liked to say, just like my earlier therapist, "Don't scream like that" and screaming referred to talking loudly or crying. Well, you've survived it, so it won't have been so terrible.

A: A number of things were terrible. There wasn't anything left. You've forgotten it. You gave it to me for safe keeping. You didn't think about the session or me.

P: I did think about you, but not in connection with the last session. If I can't get control of my eating binges, then I'll kill myself. I wanted to kill myself close to your office and leave my diary addressed to you. A pretty spiteful idea, to make you feel guilty, give you a bad conscience, for something that's not your doing. "Let him see how he handles the trash that's left over." Yet I can't relate this thought to the last session, only to my continued helplessness toward myself.

A: You experience this helplessness during the binges you have at night.

P: Yes, everything's part of a circle that I can't break out of. After eating I have such strong stomach cramps. It's the same thing every night. As far as my body is concerned, I couldn't get through the night without binging. It's a true compulsive act, a real parapraxis. It makes me sick.

A: Yes, at night it catches up with you. It's gotten to be a habit that you can't overcome, it's a nuisance and repulsive because you've got a full stomach, but you've transferred everything that wants to come out to your stomach, while you're dozing and without you're feeling ashamed. Then it comes out that you have needs you're dependent on. You can't suppress your longing any more. During the day you hardly experience it anymore, you've got yourself under such complete control. I think your feeling of shame has to do with this dependence. Your thoughts about committing suicide express the idea that I haven't helped you and you haven't been able to accept the fact that you are just as dependent as someone who can fast.

P: I would be glad if I were still someone who could fast. Good, that was my best time. But I'm on the verge of thinking that I could always eat a horse. I'm more afraid of binging than anorexia.

A: Yes, in anorexia you were independent. Had no reason to be ashamed. It's possible that you were excessive for a while, but that would took care of itself.

The patient mentioned her anxiety about becoming addicted.

P: I'm desparately looking for security, for an identity of my own. Otherwise I have the feeling I'm melting away or of adjusting and having to do everything just right so that I can survive. At the same time I have the feeling I'm nothing, an nonentity like a jellyfish that's spread out in the sand. Everybody can step on me and shape me the way they want. So it's still better, even if you don't like it, to be Death. That's me, I admit it. That's my feeling of identity.

Commentary. Just because two people may make the same statement does not necessarily mean that they mean the same thing. Although Clara X referred to herself as an anorexic and Death, as embodied by a skeleton (and contained in the German word *Knochenmann*), and thus disparaged herself by, in a certain sense, identifying with the aggressor, it made a difference if she referred to herself in this way, or if somebody else did, in which case the words had a very disparaging effect.

A: Excuse me for interrupting you at this spot. It seems clear to me that this is how you protect yourself. Otherwise I would walk all over you and you couldn't take the pressure any more. And what affects you from the outside is probably connected with it; it's your own activity and spontaneity that you attribute to people around you who influence you, who want to give you something. That's why you cling so tightly to your present identity; you use it to protect yourself against yourself.

P: I can't accept this in this form even if - to you - all of it seems clear and natural.

The patient complained about the gap between us.

P: An immense gap, a huge difference that makes my blood boil. [She became more enraged.] It's clear, obvious, natural, everything was clear and natural to my father too. He didn't have any emotional understanding.

Consideration. It's quite obvious that I let my countertransference maneuver me into a duel, so I made the issue into a mutual problem by admitting my helplessness.

A: Yes, I've exaggerated quite a bit, probably because your position is so strong. I took a position that was just as stubborn as yours, and you have good reason for criticizing me. There's no sign of compromising or listening to the other's needs even though this is your deepest wish. Something like this has happened here, with one rigid position confronting another.

The patient asked me which compromise I had to offer.

A: Yes, I'm also asking myself what I can do to make everything more appealing to you, instead of being so rigorous and reinforcing your position.

P: You could avoid the word "clear." When I mention something I've realized and you use the word "clear," then I can feel it. I feel like I'm a little sausage and the contrariness in me gets stronger.

I shared her opinion, and told her she was right.

The following session began with the patient telling me about her idea that she could lay down under the couch.

P: Once when my daughter was small I had the idea of crawling under her bed and not coming out any more.

A: And in the last session you talked about what I contribute to your hiding and not coming out any more. And that you don't have enough leeway. That I inhibited you by overusing the word "clear." My comments reinforced your opposition.

P: I think we just managed to straighten things out by the end of the session.

A: Yes, we were able to reach agreement. It ended on a good note after all, without an explosion. I really believe that you want me and your husband to see you in a different way. You don't want to be offended by being called an anorexic or Death.

Alluding to Rosetti's painting "The Annunciation" [as mentioned in Chaps.2 and 4], which Clara X had copied, I said:

A: I used all my powers of speech to describe the changes your body has undergone.

P: Yes, and I still prefer to be Death; it's my identity, externally to be a normal wife and innerly one making sacrifices.

A: The good wife who innerly makes sacrifices?

P: If I adhered to my husband's ideas about a woman's role, then I would have to sacrifice almost everything. Emotionally I would go to the dumps, even if I were completely normal. My husband wouldn't give me any encouragement to take a step toward being independent and having a life of my own. He sometimes accepts something, but sooner or later he rejects it and rides roughshod over me.

A: Yes, these are experiences you've had. Your husband doesn't make it easy for you to change the situation. You haven't tried much to see what would happen if you did do something differently here or there, if you were different. Perhaps you wouldn't still be living with your husband, perhaps you would have found a friend or your life would be different in some other way. Yes, I believe that most people see you just the way you described yourself - as Death. And although you've accepted it, comments about it still offend you and reinforce your attitude. In this way your environment and I contribute to maintaining your situation, for example when I say "It's clear, isn't it," when I trample you and strengthen the force that's already powerful in you, namely stubborness. Your special form of self-assertion, your special form of finding triumph in all the humiliation and insults that you have to bear. It must be horrible for you to sense that in several important points you don't please most people even though you have so much charm and a natural sense of humor.

P: What are the several important points?

A: Well, I'd like to leave it up to you to decide.

P: The question is really whether I still want to.

A: Nothing happens against your will, nothing, you can choose the dose. I can't do anything. Maybe you don't even know how powerful you are. Perhaps you feel threatened and disturbed by me and the therapy.

P: I feel inhibited and reprimanded. But I still haven't found out how I'm supposed to be different.
A: You sense serious danger when I try to make something appealing to you.
P: Why don't you ever say "It's good the way it is"?
A: Well, it is good the way it is. Yet I can imagine that it could be even better, that you could be more beautiful than you are, I can't hide it even though it is good the way it is. I can also imagine that you would feel better if you didn't have to hide yourself. You're hiding yourself regardless of whether you're on the couch or under it; you have a lot hidden in you, things that you still have to live out. In this regard I'd be sad if you left here, but it's good the way it is, relatively speaking. [Longer pause] You've reached the best possible solutions to a lot of the difficulties you used to have or have now. It isn't easy to find solutions that would offer you more pleasure and happiness. Once you asked me how I would feel if you stopped.
P: Yes, and?
A: I think you asked me if I would be sad or distressed.
P: Yes, and why do you mention it now?
A: Well, the core of the matter is satisfaction. Whether when you go away one day you'll go away feeling satisfied and leave me here feeling satisfied. To the question of whether I would miss you, I just had a peculiar thought. I would miss you more if you left with a big deficit, or in other words, if I had the feeling that there was a lot that was still unresolved where I could have provided you some help.

There was a pause that lasted several minutes, during which deep sighs could be heard - an eloquent silence. I added a "humm."

Commentary. The silence was a quiet continuation of this dialogue. How deep does the agreement and feeling of identity have to be to give the patient more security - that is the question that cannot be solved by contrasting verbal and nonverbal dialogue.

P: Just as I turned to one side I had the thought that we aren't getting beyond a certain point with words. This back and forth is like ruminating. Deep down inside there's something that looks an awfully lot like desperation. Death, pleasing or not pleasing, feeling well or not, it misses the point.
A: Yes, you despair about yourself and about me, and desperation has something to do with doubt about how you are and what you are. To avoid being torn back and forth, you cling to what you have, as the only certainty there is. [Renewed silence and sighs] Words aren't enough, nonetheless at the end I would like to ask whether there is anything you wanted to add.

The patient expressed the wish to shift the next session to the morning because she wanted to leave for the weekend. I was able to arrange it.

8.1.3 Anniversary Reactions

The doubts and criticism that depressive individuals have toward themselves are a sign of their being dominated by the past. Their lived time seems to stand still. The more the depressive person is overcome by the past and his feelings of guilt, the more the future is closed to him. The phenomenology and psychopathology of experiencing time, which we have discussed in Vol.1 (Sect. 8.1), makes it possible to determine the severity of depression. The more severe the affective disturbance, the grayer the future appears to the patient. The restrictions put on activity in psychotic depression takes the form of inhibitions of vital functions. From a psychoanalytic perspective the question is the extent to which the affective disturbance is caused by unconscious *psychic processes* that also manifest themselves in the symptom of a loss of a positive feeling for time. In depressive patients we can assume that the disturbed experiencing of time that was described by von Gebsattel (1954, p. 141) is a disturbance of vital fundamental activity that psychoanalytically can be explained by unconscious defense processes. There is no doubt that our experiencing of time is closely linked with the rhythym of instinctual gratifications. The lack of such gratifications therefore has to lead to a loss that takes the form of hopelessness and of there being no future. Thomä (1961) has described these problems for chronic anorexia nervosa patients.

In the interaction between analyst and patient the internalized time structure is transformed into the current, flowing, and experienced time (see Vol.1, Sect. 8.1). When Kafka (1977, p. 152) referred to the analyst as a "'condenser' and 'dilator' of time," he had the linkage between temporally very divergent statements and their possible meaningful connections in mind. The following example is intended to demonstrate how unconscious time markers can take the form of anniversary reactions.

Ursula X, who was approximately 40 years old, came to psychoanalysis because of a chronic depressive neurosis. The patient's depressive complaints had begun 12 years before, after her younger brother had committed suicide. He had been the first son in the family after three daughters and was admired and given preferential treatment by everyone in the family, but especially by their mother. By coincidence the first session of analysis happened to fall on the anniversary of the day he died, a fact the patient did not mention at first. In the course of therapy, however, it became apparent that the patient's depressive symptoms worsened on her brother's birthday and on the anniversary of his death, so that it was justified to speak of an anniversary reaction. The conflicts, which had remained unconscious, seemed to be labeled by a time marker, which made it possible for me to pay special consideration to the relations between the patient and her brother and between the patient and me in transference.

In the first year of analysis the close childhood relationship that had existed between the two of them - and that the patient had maintained - became clear. In her brother she sought the warmth and protection that she had not received from her mother. At the same time, she felt a special sense of responsibility for him and bound, as the oldest daughter, to fulfill their parent's will. The patient's inner conflict was shown particularly clearly on the thirteenth anniversary of her brother's death, i. e., after one year of analysis. In her severe depressive self-doubts and self-accusations she attempted to imagine what was going on in her brother before he was run over by the train. Her intensive desire to think herself into his situation and to understand him demonstrated her own struggle with her thoughts about death and her desires to die. For her, being dead meant being together with her brother and achieving her long-sought unity with him. The anniversary of her brother's death also marked the beginning of the second year of analysis, which the patient had undertaken in order to make a new beginning. The analysis documented that she wanted to live, and to the very day when she should have had to mourn her brother's death. Every step she took toward independence and out of her depressive withdrawal was associated with severe feelings of guilt about leaving her brother behind, dead.

In the second year of analysis an unconscious transference fantasy developed between the patient and me in which I assumed the role of her brother, which fit as far as our ages were concerned. As analyst, in the fantasized exclusiveness of our relationship I satisfied her longing for protection and warmth; at the same time she admired me. The manifestations of her feelings of envy became stronger.

In the last session before a vacation break (the 250th session) the patient was overcome by doubts about whether she should actually go on the trip she had booked with an airline. It would be the first trip she had gone on all by herself, and she said: "I've got pangs of conscience because I have to leave my daughter and parents behind, not to mention you." Then she made the serious suggestion that I should go on the trip instead. She had already gone through the conditions and told me everything she would do to make it possible for me to go. I said, "Okay, we can play through the idea of what it would mean if I were to take your place." Noticably disappointed, she told me how she had imagined that I could tell her about the trip upon my return. She knew that in a certain sense she was taking the easy way out. She would not have to leave her daughter, parents, or me and afterwards could still take part in my pleasure.

After a long period of silence she recalled that it was her brother's birthday. She had not thought of it until then. Her associations indicated that her brother had often gone on trips, taking her place and that of their mother, and was able to give vivid descriptions of what he had experienced. This was one reason she felt closely tied to him. She had the feeling of having gone on a trip with him, so that despite the external separation from him she still felt innerly united with him. After briefly thinking that she would therefore probably feel much worse for a few days, I offered the interpretation, "If I were to go on the trip for you, then mentally you would be linked to me although we were really separated. Yet if you were separated from me by the trip, then you wouldn't be sure if you would stay linked with me." She then recalled that she had always asked her brother to only tell only her about his trip upon his return. She felt ashamed about how she had kept him for herself. She also felt ashamed now about wanting to keep me for herself when I returned from the trip. I said, "Then I would go on the trip for you, you would be linked with me in your thoughts, but you would also bind me." Her response was to have stronger doubts about herself, but she had a better understanding that she wanted to avoid the separation from me in order to avoid having to assume responsibility and to retain her longing for unification. After a pause she had the association that a part of her inappropriate feelings of guilt for her brother's suicide might have resulted from her having sent him out into the world in her place. By doing so she did not have to give up her place next to her mother and was still able, by identifying with her brother, to hold on to him and to their mother. At the end of the session she sighed and was sad; "I would really have liked it if you were to fly in my place." Because of her ambivalence it was hard for her to enjoy her very own personal pleasures without the detour via altruistic transfer.

In the course of the analytic process the focus was on working through her separation traumas and their repetition in the analytic situation; one consequence was that the patient, during her fourth year of analysis, forgot her brother's birthday for the first time.

Commentary. Freud's original description (1895d, p. 162) of this phenomenon had been long forgotten when Hilgard (1960) and Hilgard et al. (1960) coined the term "anniversary reaction" to describe it and identified in empirical studies the psychic preconditions for its manifestation. They proved that anniversary reactions are significantly associated with traumatic losses in early childhood and that they lead to serious separation difficulties in later life. Mintz (1971) distinguished clinically between two types of anniversary reactions, depending on whether an event or specific date is conscious or unconscious. In the former, a date that the patient is aware of, such as a birthday or the first day of vacation, can provoke a current conflict that is associated with an earlier one and reinforced by it. The anniversary reaction occurs as a result of a specific response to this unresolved conflict. Characterictic is the annually recurring reaction to the conflict on a date that the patient consciously experiences. In the latter case, the time marker that is associated with a psychic conflict is unconscious. The date of a divorce and the birthday/deathday of a close member of the family are engrams that remain unconscious. They lead the person affected to suffer from puzzling emotional fluctuations or from a worsening of symptoms because on such days unresolved earlier conflicts regain importance without, however, reentering consciousness.

Mintz emphasized, similar to Pollock (1971), the connection between unconscious time markers and psychic conflicts related to death. Engel (1975) has reported numerous dream examples of this second type of anniversary reaction in his self-analysis; in them it is possible to recognize time markers that remained unconscious, for example, the anniversary of his twin brother's death.

Our example belongs rather to the first category. The precipitating factor is preconscious and easily accesible to the patient. The nature of her anniversary reaction - her stronger feeling of depression - illustrated her inner conflict. Her increased longing for union on the dates of her brother's birth and death led to a significant reinforcement of her own anxieties about death. The connection between the anniversary reaction and her pathological mourning, a feature that has recently been decribed by Charlier (1987), is impressive. Since the anniversary of her brother's death coincided with the "birthday" of analysis, unconscious feelings of guilt were activated. For the patient to have led a life of her own would have meant a complete separation from her brother. This conflict makes comprehensible the idea of a disturbance of one's experience of time.

The patient resolved her ambivalence toward her brother, whom she both loved and envied, with the aid of identification, which made it possible for her to maintain the relationship with the lost object and to control her strong feelings in connection with the separation. Thus anniversary phenomena are "manifestations and reactions that are related to time, age, and dates, and identifications and introjections that are complex and ambivlent" (Haesler 1985, p. 221).

We believe that this patient's anniverary reaction belonged to the context of ambivlent identifications. As long as she was able to act out the related conflicts with her husband, she was free of symptoms. It was only after her divorce that a reactive depression was precipitated because the patient did not feel permitted to feel free. Her partner fulfilled an important function as an object of displacement. The patient had unconsciously linked him with her brother. After the couple's separation this unconscious linkage revived old feelings of guilt, so that her reactive depression became chronic.

8.2 Life, Illness, and Time: Reconstructing Three Histories

This heading refers to the interconnections and complications that characterize these three topics. Our age is dominated by ideologies (Bracher 1982). Narcissism has become a collective metaphor (Lasch 1979). Considered from a psychoanalytic perspective, ideologies and narcissism have common roots. According to the definition given by Grunberger and Chasseguet-Smirgel (1979, p. 9), one inherent characteristic of ideologies is that they are all-encompassing systems of ideas and political movements whose goal is to make their illusions become reality. As we have explained in Vol. 1 (Sect. 4.4.2), man is susceptible to ideologies because of his capacity to utilize symbols, which is also linked to his capacity to be aggressive. Such ideologies can take on the character of delusions.

It must be emphasized that according to psychoanalytic criteria the contents a growing child attributes to his own fantasies are linked to the history of the time, particularly via the influence exerted by his family. The ideologically based, intolerant division of the world into good and bad individuals and the development of a system of values featuring mutually exclusive qualities are facilitated first by the family and later in school. Many people suffer psychic traumas but are able to liberate themselves from the unfortunate consequences, which sometimes seems to be a wonder. Others adopt the views that prevailed in their families, maintaining the unconsciously grounded prejudices of their parents. Others, finally, become ill from the incompatibility of opposing factors (Eckstaedt 1986; Eickhoff 1986). For example, such polarities are contained in the symptoms of compulsion neurosis, which is characterized by an alternation between extremes and the associated incapacity to be tolerant to one's self and to people with different opinions. The psychopathological *contents* of the compulsion change through history and from one civilization to another, yet the *forms* remain the same. This fact relativizes the causal role assigned to specific psychosocial factors in the origin of psychic and psychosomatic disorders.

Example

There was no doubt that the Nazi ideology exerted a significant influence on Arthur Y in his childhood and adolescence and on his entire life history and that of his illness. Yet it would be nonetheless misleading to overlook the decisive difference between the Jews who were the personal victims of the racist ideology, the individual who actively participated in the persecutions, and the compulsive neurotic. In this particular case, the patient's conscious and unconscious identifications with the Jewish victim and the SS officer who performed the execution paralyzed each other and protected the patient and those around him from the possibility that either tendency might manifest itself in reality. In this regard Arthur Y exhibited a structure similar to that of the Rat Man or the Wolf Man, Freud's paradigms for the unconscious mechanisms of compulsive neurosis. This phenomenon must be taken into consideration when discussing the question of how ideologies are handed down from one generation to the next. It is important to clarify which group the father or parents belonged to – the persecutors, the active adherents, the fellow travelers, the silent majority that adapts to the given political situation, or the victims.

The therapeutic work on several of the topics outlined in the following case study can be found under the appropriate patient code. The detailed presentation of this case history is intended to serve as a basis to help the reader understand the many vignettes of therapy.

This analysis concentrated on disentangling the extremely disastrous complications that consisted of personal, familial, and historical elements. As always, it is futile to ask whether the patient would have become ill if this or that had not happened, e.g., if he had not had numerous traumatic experiences before and after adolescence.

Arthur Y had suffered from the disorder for nearly 30 years when he decided to make a fourth attempt at therapy, which proved to be successful.

As the analyst providing treatment in this case, I was more than just a close contemporary of the patient. In this therapy I was able to reconstruct some of the history of the psychoanalytic technique, as it was reflected in this patient's experiences. To renounce the anonymity that I neither can nor wish to maintain in this case, in hindsight I can state that I rediscovered some of my own development in the therapeutic technique of well-known colleagues who were involved in the previous therapies.

More important was the fact that many of the stories the patient told me made me recall the experiences I had had when I was young. Many of my own experiences and events in my childhood were reanimated in this therapy. There are many faces to the relationship between agent and victim.

Familial Background

Many typical Nazi ideas were handed down in the patient's family just as they were in many others between 1933 and 1945. The racist division of people into Aryan and non-Aryan and into Germans and Jews was the foundation on which the idealizations and prejudices - which were linked with the drama of family life in a unique way, reaching down to the individual member of the family and into life in the small village - were erected.

Both of the patient's parents were enthusiastic supporters of Hitler, who was also the patient's ideal until late in his adolescence, i.e., until early in the 1950s. The patient's father was a prosperous mill owner and the second person, coming only after the major local landowner, in a small village in southern Germany that did not have any Jewish inhabitants. He served in the army from 1939 on until he was reported missing in action. He was declared dead many years later. The patient's mother, who bore four children for "the Führer and the volk," held particularly high expectations for her eldest son, the patient. After the war she was insecure and not up to the demanding work of running the mill. She was a chronic depressive, ultimately committing suicide. The patient had three siblings, a brother born in 1939 and two sisters, born in 1940 and 1942.

The familial background affected the formation of the patient's ego ideal, as a consequence of which the first-born son did not fulfill the expectations his parents had placed in him. According to the patient, it was rather inconceivable for his mother to have been proud of her oldest son. His memories did not take him far enough back for them to give him a feeling of happiness at having once been the object of admiration. His development did not at all correspond to the ideal for a German boy in the 1930s. Until far into the analysis the patient viewed himself and the world through his mother's eyes, as he described it. After the birth of his brother, his mother had treated him like a cry baby, and everyday in kindergarten he acted correspondingly - his reaction to his brother's birth was to dirty his pants every day. Since he was not allowed to stay home, walking to kindergarten and especially back home again became a source of torment and humiliation for him. He would be hosed off in the room where the wash was done and where butchering was also done. The totality of his traumatic experiences erased any positive feelings toward life that the patient might have had, since it is, after all, hard to believe that his mother's eye never shined when she looked at her oldest son, to use Kohut's metaphor.

The repeated traumatic experiences the patient had from dirtying his pants included the disparagement of being called a weakling and everything else other than being "tough as leather, hard as Krupp steel, and fast as a greyhound," to use a popular phrase of the time. He was not one of the boys who were big, strong, and good looking - the type he was afraid of in kindergarten as well as later on.

His annihiliation anxieties, which he retained throughout his life, were so extreme that it took a long time before the patient was even in a position to consider the possibility that he might have aggressions of his own and that he might project them onto others. He was free of anxiety, however, regarding the idea that a fast, painless death might rescue him from life.

The patient, who was raised an atheist, drew the religious contents of his compulsive thoughts from the years he spent in a boarding school. There his idea of God was also shaped by a sadistic teacher and a homosexual one; the latter looked after the sick children in particular. Although the patient did not submit to either of them, and was not used and abused "to the end," whatever that meant, his feeling of distress increased because of his longing for a father. The mixture of homosexuality and sadomasochism was so virulent that he had his first compulsive idea after reading a detective story, namely of committing the crime in the story himself - by killing the sadistic teacher with poison. In his panic he threw the book into the toilet. By getting rid of the corpus delicti that had given him the idea, the anxiety disappeared.

The patient's mother brought him home from the boarding school to become an apprentice in the family mill. An uncle had filled in as miller while the family waited for the missing father to return. The family did not believe that he was dead, and the mother and grandmother lived in the illusion and hope that they could keep the mill running until he returned, even though the mill did not produce a profit. The uncle, who had an affair with the patient's mother, and a business manager pocketed money from the mill, and after they left the patient attempted to keep it running, until he closed it down shortly before it would have gone bankrupt; this left him with substantial debts, which he was able to pay off by selling property. Since then Arthur Y worked in a related field as a salesman, where he worked his way up through hard work. Yet the success he had in his career increased his self-esteem just as little as the fact that he had established a family of his own and could have been proud of the fact that he had managed to find a - both attractive and intelligent - wife he had liked especially well ever since they had first met, and to have three teenage children who were developing well.

The Symptoms

Throughout his life the patient had tried desperately to overcome the irreconcilable contradictions inside him. Yet despite his strong anxieties of possibly committing a murder and defense rites that took the form of compulsive thoughts and acts, he was successful in his profession. He just managed to keep his dependence on alcohol under control; every day he lived for the soothing effect it had on him in the evening.

One far-reaching therapeutic insight must still be mentioned. He asked if fulfilling all the commands, in whichever form, that might come from an absolute ruler and whose common denominator for the patient was the fact that they were directed against pleasure and sexuality would lead to him being and staying the only and beloved son. These projections of power and impotence and his use of simultaneous and rapidly changing identifications to participate in them went far back, leading beyond the pathological resolution of oedipal conflicts.

It is known that such idealizations and prejudices can be linked with different meanings. Since masochistic self-denigration, e. g., "I am a pile of shit," are constantly linked with more or less unconscious anal-sadistic ideas of grandeur, diagnostically the one is implied by the other. Compulsive rites that lead to a temporary soothing of anxiety can take on numerous forms.

In object relations theories, i. e., from the perspective of the interdependence of inner and outer, the contents of value systems and the absolute division into good and evil are given the significance that Freud (1923b) attributed to the ego's object identifications:

If they [these identifications] obtain the upper hand and become too numerous, unduly powerful and incompatible with one another, a pathological outcome will not be far off. It may come to a disruption of the ego in consequence of the different identifications becoming cut off from one another by resistances; perhaps the secret of the cases of what is described as 'multiple personality' is that the different identifications seize hold of consciousness in turn. Even when things do not go so far as this, there remains the question of conflicts between the various identifications into which the ego comes apart.... (Freud 1923b, pp. 30-31).

Psychogenesis

The focus of the *reconstruction* of the different psychogenetic factors behind the patient's symptoms must be on the mutually incompatible identifications. They are related, to give an abbridged explanation, to attitudes of his parents that he internalized; yet viewing this issue in greater detail it is necessary, following Loewald (1980, p. 69), to assume that the contents and ideas of identifications mean that interactions are also internalized. For example, when the patient's mother believed - even before her illness, i. e., during the patient's childhood - that the mentally retarded should be killed - "wack off their heads" - then the object (the mentally retarded and his head) are internalized in this behavioral context. If the incompatibility of various identifications is taken as the common denominator, then it is not difficult to form a sequence that ranges from early ambivalences to the later splittings. Thus, the process that isolates individual identifications from each other may result in a self-reinforcing vicious circle existing throughout one's life. This patient, for example, suffered the misfortune that the manner in which he was raised underwent a radical change when he was 10 and after the death of his admired ideal (Adolf Hitler). Initially he was raised as an atheist, deifying the Führer and condemning the Jews; later he was submitted to an upbringing that confronted him with a punishing God, whose earthly representatives reinforced the patient's conflicts.

I will now reconstruct this process on the basis of knowlege gained during the psychoanalysis. In doing so I will follow the categories Freud set out in the passage quoted above. Involved is (a) a splitting of the ego into different identifications that alternate between grabbing power and isolating themselves from each other, so that (b) the later identifications refer back to the earliest ones. Especially important is the fact that Freud, in a footnote to the text referred to above, traced the origin of the ego ideal to the individual's "first and most important identification," that with his *parents*.

It is surprising that Arthur Y was able to hide his condition from those around him and that not even his closest relatives knew that he suffered from an abundance of anxieties and compulsive ideas. He feared that he might end the way his mother did and felt responsible for her suicide because he had no longer been able to take her complaining and had flown into a fit of rage the day before her death. He thought that by committing suicide he would keep much worse events from happening, such as being isolated in a prison or an insane asylum after a sex crime. Such compulsive ideas first surfaced when he was 20 years old, when he became optimistic that his later wife might return his affection. At that time Arthur Y secretly submitted to inpatient psychiatric treatment, which did not bring any improvement. Later, in the course of two long analytic psychotherapies, he gained some insights; these were then deepened during a classical psychoanalysis that lasted nearly 600 hours.

Although the patient suffered from strong fluctuations of the symptoms of his anxiety and compulsions, he was able to continue to work without therapy. His expertise in his field and his excellent ability to empathize with his customers enabled him to be fit and alert at the right moment even though he was rarely free of compulsive thoughts. Simply the sight of something red, a sishing noise, or the sound of certain vowels could precipitate severe anxieties and the compulsion to avoid them.

The fatal illness of his younger brother led to a worsening of his symptoms and to his decision to consult me. He had visited me once before, long ago. All that he could recall from the first consultation in the mid-1960s was my accent. At that time I had referred him to a colleague for the psychoanalysis mentioned above, since I had anticipated moving to another city. The patient, after completing his therapy, had happened to accept an offer for a good position in the same area I had moved to, so that it seemed logical for him to consult me again some 20 years later.

Arthur Y's professional success and the stability of his family did not diminish his feeling of negative self-esteem and submission toward the compulsion that overpowered him. It was only in abstract terms that he imagined he had retained some of his own will and skills. Yet when I asked him toward the beginning of the analysis what it would be like to be free of all anxiety, he promptly answered, "Then I would be intolerably arrogant." By means of his ego splitting he had retained more than just his unconscious arrogance. Existing side by side in him were incompatible identifications with victims and with henchmen. In the course of the years the contents of these identifications - the objects in Freud's "object identification" - grew and grew. As a victim he identified with the Jews who had been the object of scorn and destined for annihilation, and sadistically he identified unconsciously with heroes and their medals. Freud owed his discovery of the *omnipotence* of ideas to a compulsive neurotic patient. Arthur Y put the incredible into the sphere of *arbitrariness*. Establishing a connection between the victim and the henchman, or finding the connecting link, was almost like trying to square the circle. Fortunately, the patient precisely did *not* want to be both, yet in his later life he continued to experience repetitions of such thoughts whenever he was in the appropriate mood and it was possible to detect something horrible or incredible in something he heard or saw.

For theoretical and therapeutic reasons associated with Freud's alternative hypothesis on repetition compulsion, I viewed these repetitions as the patient's attempts to solve his problem that were destined to fail because the unconscious identifications were split off and juxtaposed. In explaining repetitive anxiety dreams, Freud considered their problem-solving function in the sense of retrospectively coping with or mastering traumatic situations. If the ego is assigned a "synthetic function" (Nunberg 1930), it is logical to view repetitions, including those outside anxiety dreams, from the perspective of attempted mastering and problem solving. In other words, it is reasonable to ask why the patient had not managed, even with the help of psychoanalysis, to free himself of the repetitions of his anxieties and compulsions.

It is obviously insufficient simply to ascertain that a patient has incompatible unconscious identifications and that they alternately dominate his thoughts to such an extent that his ego feeling is completely filled by a depressive affect from one minute to the next. The important question is how and why such splitting occurs. The reconstruction of the causes here was facilitated by considering the cumulative traumatic experiences that overtaxed the patient's capacity for integration in all phases of his life until late adolescence.

The consequences of the patient's experiences in adolescence were more far reaching than to simply determine the contents of his central anxieties and compulsive thoughts. Both the polarization of his inner self that had already been initiated and the splitting in accordance with the ideology instilled in him at home were reinforced at the boarding school by two teachers, who were the exponents of love and hate. These two teachers embodied homosexual and sadomasochistic expectations and fears in a manner that precluded any transformation in him. Just the opposite was the case; there was a stabilization of the existing structures at this time, although there is a high potential for transformation at this age (Freud 1905d).

The patient experienced - in the one teacher's attempts to gain his affections and in his observations of the punishments the other teacher inflicted - his own disturbing desires in the discord between pleasure and unpleasure. One scene from analysis is instructive in this context. It took a long time for the patient to feel comfortable on the couch and secure enough to use the blanket, without automatically becoming homosexual or having the feeling that the rumpled blanket, which he did not fold neatly at the end of sessions, disturbed my orderliness; he initially feared that I would therefore have enough of him and terminate the therapy. It is hardly necessary to mention that the idea of stopping was the patient's attempt to protect each of us from even worse events. Every time the patient reached a new balance, he attempted to assert his identity resistance, to use Erikson's terminology (see Sect. 4.6). Erikson has described identity resistance in the following way:

> Identity resistance is, in its milder and more usual forms, the patient's fear that the analyst, because of his particular personality, background, or philosophy, may carelessly or deliberately destroy the weak core of the patient's identity and impose instead his own. I would not hesitate to say that some the much-discussed unsolved transference neuroses in patients, as well as in candidates in training, is the direct result of the fact that the identity resistance often is, at best, analyzed only quite unsystematically. (Erikson 1968, p. 214)

The patient became more courageous, even though he continued to display the pleasure he found in his power by reverting to masochistic and self-destructive forms and by participating unconsciously in sadistic acts.

The constellation at the outbreak of his illness - at the moment he was loved and had achieved an unimagined success - belongs in a general sense to the typology of those who founder on success (Freud 1916d). Since then the patient's life had been marked by his unrelentless effort to attain narcissistic perfection, whether in business or family matters. His altruistic self-sacrificing behavior was the source of both his happiness and his enormous capacity for feeling offended, which continuously activated unconscious sadomasochistic identifications.

Although the patient had long freed himself of the Nazi ideology, the polarizing system of values that had been instilled in him continued to be decisive for his self-esteem. He had an almost unlimited willingness to be self-sacrificing for his family. When he was offended, he regularly turned his aggression against himself. In business matters he also achieved his successes more as a result of his empathy with the customer or, one might say, his identification with the victim he has to sell his goods.

In conclusion, we would like to emphasize a topic mentioned above, namely the problem of the origin of alternating object identifications and their splitting, to use Freud's language. In a more general sense the issue is the relationship between *contents* and their psychopathological *forms*. It is obvious that elements other than the influence exerted by the Nazi ideology affected this patient's identificatory processes and that they were largely incompatible. Yet it is just as clear that the primary identifications and the preoedipal and oedipal conflicts played an independent role. Multiple personalities and thoughts about a double and the alter ego were in existence long before this patient sought his ego-ideal in Hitler. We could easily describe the patient's desperate and vain attempts to overcome his psychic conflict between the representatives of his identifications in terms of Stevenson's story about Dr. Jekyll and Mr. Hyde (see Rothstein 1983, p. 45), yet this would underestimate the significance that the *summation* of effects of mutually incompatible contents of identifications have on a pathological outcome, i. e., on pathological forms. On the other hand, taking only the early defense processes such as projective and introjective identification into consideration would also underestimate their significance because this would disregard the role of the series of traumatic experiences a patient has had for years. This is the reason we pointed out above that the internalization (i. e., the formation of "inner objects") involves *identifications with interactive processes.*

The patient could not say as Faust did that "Two souls live, ach, in my breast," because the one soul - the identification with the aggressor - was deep in his unconscious, and the other one - the identification with the victim - filled him with panic-stricken anxieties. During the analysis Arthur Y managed to integrate the split aspects of his ego, which we have described in the context of the applications for payment by the health insurance organizations (see Sects. 6.4 and 6.5).

Whoever suffers from himself in this manner has empathy and sympathy for other people and is far from committing a crime.

8.3 Interpretations

The following treatment report contains selected interpretations (see Sect. 1.3) from the psychoanalysis of a patient with anxiety hysteria. It is taken from a therapy conducted long ago (Thomä 1967), and not based on verbatim transcripts of sessions. The purpose of such a selection, today as well as at that time, is didactic, namely to describe the resolution of hysterical symptoms in practical clinical terms.

During the therapy of Beatrice X anxieties about pregnancy and giving birth took the place of her previous symptoms of anxiety hysteria, which we describe in Sect. 9.2, where we report on the symptoms and the initial phase of therapy. The patient was unable to fulfill her own and her husband's wishes for children because of her nerotic anxieties of what might happen to her during pregnancy and birth, which compelled them to take rigorous birth control measures. The patient's progressive improvement revived both their wishes for a child and the older, oedipal reasons behind her anxiety.

Yet before we comment on this therapy conducted 25 years ago, we would first like to describe how our perspective has changed as a result of the *revision of the theory of female development.*

In Freud's opinion, the development of girls is complicated by the fact that they redirected their love from their mothers to their fathers. The significance of this change in object was substantially relativized in the 1930s through the work of women psychoanalysts. If we proceed from the assumption that a woman has a primary mother fixation and mother identification - which Freud (1931b, 1933a) incorporated in his theory of the development of the female sex - then all of the complications disappear that are incorrectly attributed to the object change that was initially assumed. If we take the significance that this identification has for a woman's life history seriously, then the unconscious and mimetic acceptance of women's manners of behavior is a means by which children prepare themselves for the mother role playfully, as it were. The normal woman, after all, finds her object relations by means of her identifications with her mother, according to Lampl-de Groot, who however did not publish these ideas until 1953.

Oedipal conflicts can take place without causing any significant insecurity, as a result of the formation of female self-esteem. Thus it is probable, for instance, that the triad of equivalent woman's anxieties described by H. Deutsch (1930), namely castration, rape, and birth, is only manifested in women whose underlying mother identification has been disturbed, as Thomä (1967) pointed out.

The revision of the theory of the development of a woman's identity and her sexual role is probably the most radical revision of the fundamental assumptions of psychoanalysis that has become necessary (Roiphe and Galenson 1981; Bergman 1987). The *psychosocial* source of sexual identity that is anchored deep in the core of an individual's personality in the form of the feeling "I am a woman" or "I am a man" begins immediately after birth. A mother and father indicate how they experience an infant's sex in how they take care of it - their gestures, words, and the manner in which they handle the baby. We would like to refer especially to the work of Stoller (1976), who introduced the concept of core gender identity and referred to primary femininity. Hand in hand with this radical revision in the significance attributed to a girl's primary identification with her mother, which has been documented in a wealth of publications, there has also been a change in the psychoanalytic understanding of female sexuality in a narrower sense (see Chasseguet-Smirgel 1974). A false understanding of the psychopathology of the female orgasm has for decades been the source of iatrogenic stress on women undergoing therapy. For example, Bertin (1982) has reported that Marie Bonaparte, an aristocratic analysand and later friend of Freud's, underwent plastic surgery of her clitoris to overcome her frigidity. Freud's inaccurate assumptions about the origin of frigidity, which he took to be a disturbance of the transition from clitoral to vaginal orgasm, and other mistaken ideas about the psychopathology of feminine sexuality have obstructed the therapy of frigid woman for many years.

The significance of primary identification for the origin of deviances, in the extreme even including transsexualism, should of course not lead to the incorrect conclusion that femininity or masculinity is fixed in the first year of life. Under favorable circumstances, much can still be made good by friendships made in kindergarten and school, especially during adolescence, and from meeting substitute mothers and teachers. After the oedipal phase has passed, there are still chances to establish new and supplementary identifications reaching deeper than imitations but taking the latter as their starting point. Seeking and finding role models promote the processes of self-cure.

The unconscious defense processes that Freud discovered are often stronger than an individual's innate vitality. Then, as in the case of Beatrice X, hysterical anxieties continue to exist as a result of oedipal conflicts. Regardless of the particular conditions in the life history of an individual patient that initiate the unconscious repressions and other defense mechanisms - indicated by neurotic anxieties about pregnancy and giving birth in the case described below - there are always oedipal conflicts in addition to the fundamental problems of identification.

In the part of therapy in which we discussed her oedipal conflicts in connection with her anxieties, Beatrice X was able to overcome these conflicts and to make up for emotional ties and identifications with women that she had not experienced earlier. Friendships became more intense, and Beatrice X, giving in to a deep longing, even visited her old nurse, with whom she had spent the long years of the evacuation during the war.

Beatrice X had many homoerotic dreams. In the 258th session she related a dream about my wife. She imagined she was her patient, and immediately reassured me that she was very satisfied with me. She continued to be very worried about losing her father's love in transference if she turned to her mother. It was natural for her to seek information from friends who were pregnant and from young mothers.

Commentary from Today's Point of View. Completely aside from the denial of her oedipal desires in transference, Beatrice X had good reason to be unhappy with her analyst and in her dream to turn to his wife. In a contradictory and conflicting back and forth, the analyst had reneged on his committment to give her the title of several books on sex education, which in this case did not result in any serious damage. If an analyst refuses to provide information because of the abstinence rule, he misses a chance to strengthen the helping alliance and - in mother transference - to make identifications possible. The rejection of a reasonable request that the expert provide some information prevents a patient from obtaining any indirect oedipal satisfaction, yet it also damages the identification. In this case, the analyst apparently let himself be guided by the idea that every indirect satisfaction would not be in the best interests of the analysis. Today we know that the frustration theory of therapy, which appeared to justify a rigorous application of the rule of abstinence, is misleading. It was poorly grounded from the beginning, and it is not surprising that Weiss and Sampson (1986) refuted it. Their study, just like clinical experience, proves the superiority of Freud's alternative hypothesis, which starts from the assumption that the patient attempts in psychoanalysis, by using the analyst's support, to overcome traumatic experiences and master conflicts that had appeared to defy resolution. In the present case the rejection of the patient's wish for the analyst to give her the names of sex education books complicated the transference and the helping alliance. It caused the patient to turn away from the analyst and look to women as more suitable role models for the information she desired. If the male analyst had acted differently and made possible a mother transference, in our opinion the patient would have been able to find opportunities to identify with him.

We will now reproduce the notes for several sessions that are instructive with regard to the patient's oedipal anxieties. These notes also provide an example of the protocol scheme mentioned in Sect. 1.3.

261st Session

Beatrice X said that she had looked forward to the session, but that once here she had become uneasy while waiting and had wanted to run away.

She said that she felt very good and was very happy with her husband, but that she was concerned about a planned party to celebrate the completion of a building's shell. She said she naturally wanted to be there, but that her attitude was split into both pleasure and anxiety. She emphasized that she was very happy for her husband, without being envious of his success as an architect.

Dream. She entered a room. A man was setting up spotlights and film equipment and did not have any time for her. She was disappointed.

After describing the dream, the patient repeated her feelings toward attending the building party.

Consideration. The session began five minutes late. I wanted to draw the patient's attention to her - presumed - disappointment and asked her a suggestive question: "The man did not have enough time for you?"

Reaction. The patient did not respond to it, but mentioned her desires instead, saying how nice it would be to be at the center of things at the party. Then she gave me precise details about her sex life. She said she did not use to have an orgasm because she had restrained herself and had not actively participated when she became more excited. Then somehow she had become anxious that she could be injured if she were very active.

She also said it was not right for her husband to have so little time for her. She added that it was her fault because she would do trivial things in the evening instead of enjoying a quiet evening talking to her husband.

Consideration. Unconsciously the patient wanted to exhibit herself, be at the center of attention, and have a particularly satisfying orgasm. She was anxious about injuring herself. To keep from exhibiting herself, in her dream she pictured the man as not having any time for her. Then it was the man who disappointed her, and she could complain about him. This enabled her to maintain her repression of her sexual desires.

Interpretation. In accordance with my consideration, I referred to an older dream in which she had seen a woman dancing and exhibiting herself, and told the patient that she would like to show herself in a state of sexual excitement but that she reckoned with disappointment because she feared too much intensity. Then she would complain to me about my not having enough time for her.

Reaction. This was 100% right, and there were no *buts*. She added that she thought about a dream and her anxiety about giving birth.

Dream. She saw a pale child, the baby of a girlfriend from school who had always looked bad. (In the dream it was clear that the woman had too often had intercourse during pregnancy, injurying the child.) A man put a small boy on a elephant, between its ears, and she was very afraid that something would happen to him.

Associations. She said she knew that a woman should not have any intercourse the last few weeks before giving birth. The elephant's ears made her think of a woman's labia. There was something to her anxiety regarding pregnancy and giving birth, namely about losing something.

Consideration. The familiar topic of injury and loss returned again. I thought about the fantasies the patient had had during defloration and about her fear that her vagina would tear further and further open. She did not experience anything new in a child; it did not provide any new experiences. She thought most of all that something fell off (the boy between the ears/the labia). I puzzled about the equating of child and penis. The child does not augment her self-image, but it falls off. Why?

Interpretation. She had the impression that she would be injured while giving birth and would lose something. The small boy was where the elephant's trunk is, i. e., it was as if the boy would lose his trunk/penis. She had the impression that she had lost something compared to her brother, namely a penis, and she feared the injury could increase by giving birth.

Reaction. She could not recall such an idea with regard to her brother, but said that it was clear to her how much she was preoccupied by the thought of being injured while giving birth and of losing something. She was disturbed that she still had such thoughts and dreams despite the fact that she knew better.

Her anxiety about losing something was further clarified in a later session, almost without me making any contribution.

264th Session

Although she had really wanted to talk about the office opening that was due to take place in a few days, another topic forced its way out. It was one we had talked about a few sessions earlier, namely the idea of losing or dropping something. She said she had had a horrible dream about it.

Dream. A string of pieces of liver came out of her vagina. She was horrified, desperate, and full of anxiety, and stooped down to feel what it was and to pull the chain of pieces out of herself. Then she dreamed about a woman who wanted to give her mother such a piece of liver, which her mother refused.

Associations. The patient repeated her description of her horror and revulsion. This was followed by descriptions of the anxiety she had about losing a child during pregnancy. She thought about the noteworthy stooping position she got into to overcome her anxiety. And the patient had in fact frequently gone into a stooping position to relieve her anxiety. She would not be entirely on the floor, but half on the tips of her toes and resting her buttocks on her heels. The way she overcame her anxiety was similar to how she touched her genital region. The patient concluded about her dream that she obviously was afraid of losing control down there. "Yes, it's true, I was always afraid of bleeding to death during my period."

In passing, she mentioned that she had been able for the first time in years to eat at the same table as her husband. This was a positive change that must be seen in connection with the working through of various anxieties.

265th Session

After yesterday's session she had been very happy; her husband had sent her flowers via Fleurop but without sending a message. But now she was disturbed because she had had a ridiculous idea. She thought about exchanging a pair of shoes she had bought the day before. The idea had crossed her mind that it would be nice to drive to the train station with a patient she had met at the ward and who had a car. Now she was disturbed by the idea and had feelings of guilt toward her husband.
Consideration and Interpretation. In my interpretation I took into account that the patient spent some time at the ward before the session. In passing I noted that the patient she had referred to had shown an interest in her for some time. I pointed out to her that she was acting as if she had not done anything to encourage him.
Reaction. She said she had to admit that this was the case.

I responded by pointing out that this was the reason she avoided sitting opposite a man on a train. She then admitted how good it made her feel for the man to be interested in her.
Consideration. This was probably a displacement of transference. The patient she referred to was an older, married man she assumed had known many women. She had earlier complained several times that her husband was so boyish, lacking paternal features and experience. She transferred incestuous desires to this patient.
Interpretation. In a relationship with an older, more experienced, fatherly man - through a sexual relationship with me - she sought the confirmation she had not received earlier because, as she had dreamed, her father only had intercourse with her mother. Now she had guilt feelings for having these desires, which she tried to suppress.
Reaction. She said this was 100% right and, besides, her husband was sometimes fatherly.
Consideration. Since the patient's incest anxiety kept her from letting her desires become part of her relationship to her husband and their only expression was split off, their marital relationship had become impoverished, i. e., unconsciously she kept her husband at the level of her brother.

In her *response* to my corresponding *interpretation*, the patient added that this must have been the reason that she had not been able to have sexual contact with her husband for such a long time.

275th Session

The patient assumed (correctly) that she had just met my wife in the hallway of the hospital, and had become very upset and would have like to have run away. She said it was not any of her business to be here now and to talk about personal things. In response to a question, the patient added that in comparison to my wife she not only felt empty but also small. People often think she is a single, 17-year-old girl.
Consideration. The patient experienced the coincidental meeting oedipally. She felt guilty for her incestuous desires and warded these guilt feelings off by, on the one hand, pushing them into the sphere of symptoms, and on the other saying of herself that she was much too small. In this way she erected a wall against her incestuous wishes.
Interpretation. The patient had recently dreamed about a woman who was pregnant and was in my room. I interpreted that she thought she could not be the one, thus telling her mother, so to speak, "I don't have an illicit relationship with my brother/analyst."

The patient picked up this line of thought. We spoke about another form of behavior she used to hide her desires. The analyst should be the seducer and have the say, such as in setting the time for the sessions. The subject was once again a visit to see her mother. I told her that she was not coming to me now to get a rest at her mother's and to let her know that she was small and helpless and was not going to the man (the analyst as father).

She picked up this idea and said yes, but also that she could not imagine anything more beautiful than to visit her mother with a baby. She had even had this fantasy toward me, namely to pay me a visit with her husband and the child they desired and she hoped one day to bear.

Follow-up. The positive identification that the patient slowly formed with her own sex diminished her anxieties about being pregnant and giving birth. It is highly probable that this also made it easier for her to conceive. For the record, Beatrice X has been healthy for some 20 years and is the mother of several children. All the important data for judging her case to be a success are positive. The patient has remained free of anxiety and is leading a satisfied and happy life with her family.

8.4 Acting Out

As we have explained in detail in Vol.1 (Sect. 8.6), the traditional understanding of acting out has undergone a significant transformation in the last few decades under the influence of object relations theories. The current theory of technique takes a different view of both the phenomena referred to by this concept and their origin. Acting out and the related phenomenon of acting in are especially good means for demonstrating the consequences of the polarization between classical insight therapy, with its emphasis on interpretation, and the therapy of emotional experience. This polarization goes back to the controversy between Freud and Ferenczi that psychoanalytic practice did not pay sufficient consideration to experiencing. Cremerius (Cremerius et al. 1979) called for analysts to surmount this polarization by asking "Are there *two* psychoanalytic techniques?" The attitudes to the phenomena traditionally referred to as acting out offer a good opportunity to attempt to integrate these divergent and one-sided approaches.

The phenomenology of acting out is very diverse, yet as soon as we go beyond a descriptive phenomenology in psychoanalysis we encounter the question as to the functional status of individual acts. Since this status consists of individual and dyadic aspects, it is necessary to examine the acting out, whether performed in analysis or outside it, within the context of the momentary transference and countertransference processes. Its function can be either benign or malignant. The patient who caught a glimpse of the analyst's wife while searching for a female identification figure demonstrated her ingenuity in overcoming a fantasized deficit; the patient we described in Sect. 2.2.4 destroyed the basis of therapy by constantly prying into the analyst's private sphere. In that regard we also discussed the fact that the patient's behavior was partially dependent on the analyst's personal situation and the particular form that her therapy took. Since examples of what is customarily called acting out can be found in numerous other places in this book, here we will restrict ourselves to describing two examples of "acting in," which at least since Balint's description of the new beginning has lost its negative meaning.

First Example

Ingrid X came to her first session after the three week Christmas break and began by making the statement that she wanted to show me something. Without waiting for an answer, she went to the couch, knelt down, and began to spread out a game of tarok. I was taken aback, and she asked me to sit on the stool next to her. She placed the cards the same way they were on New Year's Eve. She said she had rediscovered our understanding of her life history in the cards.

We examined the individual cards, considering many details, and she explained which of the figure's features led her to have which ideas. At the center of attention were trophy cups, which either were full and stood for life, or were knocked over and symbolized unlived life. She was particularly touched by a figure in which she saw herself depicted as a lonely hermit.

At the core of her self-interpretation was her mother, who would not give her a sealed cup, who did not seem to begrudge her anything.

After the patient had explained these details, I felt that she expected me to make the one or other supplementary comment. I was supposed to participate in this summary of what we had already achieved. Then she seemed satisfied, packed the cards together, and laid on the couch.

If there were a catalogue of the unusual situations that have occurred in the career of an individual analyst, then this experience would be part of mine. Unusual for me was especially the matter of factness with which everything happened. For me to have refused and cited a rule as the reason would have done more than hurt her feelings.

The patient then described a dream rich in facts. The first image referred to my office, and was followed by other scenes, alluding among other things to a love affair that ended recently. While telling me about her dream, she commented that in the dream she was attempting to put an estate into order.

Without relating the dream to our relationship, Ingrid X continued, describing how she had spent Christmas with her husband. They had had to cope with the familiar problems. The patient's need to provide as complete a report about her holidays as possible and to tell me about them made me pause. The wealth of details she had mentioned led me after about a half hour to point out to the patient that she wanted to bring her experiencing along and had started the session by telling me about the unusual item she had brought along. This led her to reflect about what was happening.

P: Yes, it's important to me. To bring them along, to tell you everything. By the way, I also do this when I'm not here, speak with you and let you take part in what preoccupies me.

She then described that she had been able to continue the dialogue with me on her own for about two weeks. At that point this inner relationship seemed to have ended abruptly. It was not without pride that she told me that, together with others (friends and acquaintances), she had managed to continue this kind of self-communication.

In this connection I had to think of a question - which I asked the patient - namely whether there was a temporal connection between the loss of her inner relationship to me and the game of tarok. She confirmed that there was; this insight was a surprising gain for each of us. We concluded that the loss of the inner relationship was compensated by her retreat to a magical level. The world of the tarok game took the place of the absent analyst, and was used at the transition from one year to the next to cope with our common past and the future that awaited us. Our understanding of her desire to inform me about the result of this card game constituted a link between the period before the holiday interruption and that in front of us. Ingrid X recalled her emotionally important relationship to her violine teacher, to whom she could always bring anything she wanted. If she had practiced enough, there had always been enough time left for her to show the teacher her interesting books or her new pair of roller skates. Her vivid description of this consoling experience led her to recall the painful memory that her mother, who had been very involved in her career, had not been there enough. For numerous reasons, however, the patient had been in a position to find satisfactory substitutes for some of her chronic disappointments regarding her relationship to her mother.

Our understanding of the acting in on the basis of her own life history led to the statement that we were in a kind of violine teacher relationship. In reaction to the long separation, the analyst (I) became the disappointing, unavailable mother, and then, in the role of the violine teacher, had to make it possible for the patient to bring something playful along. He especially had to be able to appreciate her ability to find substitute solutions, which the patient was justifiably proud of. These solutions can fail, however, if the disappointment is too strong. As an example she then mentioned that her father-in-law had not made the effort to find a present that suited her, simply giving her an art book he had received from some company for Christmas. In this example she was able to feel her longing for personal attention, which was hidden behind her previous opportunities for coping.

The game of tarok can be viewed as an attempt - successful in this situation - to replace the loss of the inner object "analyst" by turning to a nonpersonal stage on which she could see a summary of our previous labors. The break mobilized a negative mother transference: Who or what is the filled cup that her mother (the analyst) did not begrudge her? To ward off the associated affects, the patient was able to take advantage of an idealizing mother transference in the form of acting in, in order to communicate her feeling of loneliness ("the lonely hermit").

Second Example

Despite his successful career and his numerous interests - making him into someone everyone in his large circle of friends enjoyed talking to - Theodor Y felt lonely and insecure. His outward appearance did not correspond to his negative self-esteem; he considered himself to be completely unattractive.

His father had died in the war, and his mother had had to work hard to enable several children obtain a good education. In addition to their poverty, however, his mother's depression had been a burden on the patient's childhood and adolescence. He became really aware of his homoerotic inclinations after puberty. He came for therapy after his homosexuality while under the influence of alcohol had created a social crisis.

In the 350th session he anxiously recalled an experience that had occurred about 15 years before and after which he had increased his efforts to make homosexual contacts. He had been together with a woman for several months and had had a good sexual relationship with her. He had been planning a trip with a friend, and his girlfriend had been disappointed and enraged that he had not wanted to take her along. While on the trip, he had found out to his consternation that the two of them (his friend and his girlfriend) were going to marry. The patient had completed the trip with his friend as if nothing had happened. This description came as such a surprise to me that I spontaneously said, "You didn't even have any harsh words with your friend." In my countertransference I had put myself in his position and expected him to react jealously, without taking into consideration that such a triangle offered numerous kinds of gratifications which would make the absence of normal jealousy comprehensible.

He came to the following session much earlier than ususal. He was outraged over the smell of stale air in the room and stormed to the window. There was a short verbal-averbal confrontation during which he pushed the window wide open. For a while we stood close together. Since it was very cold outside and although he was right about the air, I soon said "That's enough; now we can close it."

Theodor Y immediately began speaking about the subject of yesterday's session. While listening I noticed that I was still preoccupied with the initial scene, which he did not mention again, and wondered if there was a connection with the subject the patient was talking about.

A: [After a while] I think I've hurt your feelings, both in the last session and just now again.

P: [Vehemently] No, no, I simply need fresh air.

A: Judging from what has just happened, perhaps you felt criticized because of the matter with your friend.

Even at this second attempt, the patient was not convinced, but turned the tables:

P: I think it's rather that your feelings are hurt and you are mad because I'm denying you your stale air.

He spoke for a long time about aggression and evil as such, before turning to the current situation.

P: And now I'm even contradicting you and feel terribly anxious because I'm afraid that you are very mad at me. Here I can sense that you're the clever one .... I'm anxious now, and am afraid of your aggression ... or of mine? .... If you aren't so perfect? .... Yesterday you said, "Very interesting." The important analyst is interested in me, or ... yes, what is "psychologically" highly interesting is what you're actually interested in.

This was followed by a longer monologue, before he finally paused.

P: Am I gabbing it to death?

A: It really seems to me as if you had taken over my role as well, and in that sense you have out gabbed me.

P: Yes, somehow I guess I'm afraid. [Pause]

A: I wanted to tell you that I assume I made a mistake yesterday, and that is the reason I have referred to how you've acted today – you've never come in that fiercely before.

Once again Theodor Y denied there was any connection between the two starting points of my construction and got lost in general philosophical thoughts. Toward the end of the session I attempted once again to inject a consideration into the dialogue.

A: I would like to ask you to listen to it one more time; it might be that you disagree completely. I think that I see something that's impossible for you to see at this time. Perhaps your hurt feelings are also related to my comment about "very interesting."

This statement had the immediate effect of calming the patient, even though he had a dubious look on his face when he left.

After the session I had to ask myself what the meaning of the smell was that led him to tear open the window. Is the fact that my interest in him is "only psychological" really what stank?

Theodor Y began the next session with a conciliatory offer:

If you manage to convince me about what you felt yesterday and said, the business with the window ... then I'll have learned something. It seems typical to me. And because you said it was significant. And because I didn't notice it.

A: If you ask me like this, are you curious now, or are you still concerned about yesterday's disruption and want to conform now?

P: No, I don't think so. I thought that you're waiting to see what happened .... So what can you show me? I'm an idiot. I can't get it. Still, it's true, my anxiety has decreased ... I tear open the window, and then you close it, that tells me something ... The result is a lot of confusion, insecurity, a disturbing scene.

A: You didn't talk about it like this yesterday.

I gave this interpretation with the positive intention of emphasizing the positive in the development of his thoughts from yesterday to today.

P: Yeh, yesterday I couldn't know everything, notice it, and say it at the same time. Theodor Y thus reacted promptly to a hidden critical aspect of my interpretation.

A: Yes, you're right about that.

P: So, I'm an idiot.

I wondered if he was now accepting my latent criticism. I decided to make another clarifying statement about yesterday's incident.

A: I realize now that it made you feel much more insecure than I had thought or perhaps even could have known.

P: Tuesday's session was about my friend. When you criticized me for not having had it out with him, in that situation, well I felt like a fool.

Theodor Y now mentioned an anxiety that had been a less obvious burden yesterday, and the confusion that was associated with it. I thought of the title of one of Fassbinder's movies, "Angst essen Seele auf" (literally, anxiety eat up souls [sic]).

A: Anxiety isn't just there, it also destroys, it keeps you from reaching your potential. Even in speaking. Anxiety devours souls.

P: Good .... Yesterday morning, at work, before the session here, it was just the same; the secretary told me to get lost. It was horrible. They're all stupid .... And I'm the little boy who doesn't understand. My boss, too; he's stupid. And me the little boy, not reaching my potential .... Really a vivid description, that anxiety devours souls. There is a strong similarity between the scene at work and the scene at the window, the same anxiety. Good God, you're right. If you had seen me at work. My little helpless boy's soul caught in the web, naked and exposed and pitiful. You'd have been overcome with pity, "The poor .... "

A: Me, out of pity, and you out of a feeling of shame.

P: [Baffled] Feeling of shame? Perhaps I'll manage via a round about way. Who am I? My analyst has the same feeling toward me that I had toward the secretary. She was very frightened, pitiful when I finally beat it. And then I think that I want this and that and you've just got to keep your mouth shut .... Then the old officer's attitude comes through, with rage, outwardly hard, etc., but it doesn't help.

In my thoughts the patient's wish to submit to his friend and his girlfriend was linked with the current transference situation; in each he was just left standing there. He was not able to be a rival or to argue because the betrayal had struck him so deeply that he was paralyzed. My comment that he had not confronted his friend was in the same vein. By criticizing him, I "castrated" him.

A: Perhaps we could say that everything happened yesterday because you felt yourself criticized. That would be an answer to the question you raised at the beginning of the session, about what I can tell you today.

P: Yes. [Longer pause] If I don't confront things, then it's a lack of masculinity. That works. That hits me where it causes me to act. Just as you observed, and how I acted here yesterday with the window and coming early today and this morning at work. People get nervous if you tell them the truth. Sensitivity, that's it. But what is truth?

Theodor Y began holding an intellectual excurse about the question of truth that became incomprehensible. He was probably looking more for the *emotional* truth.

P: It's true that my feelings are unclear, yet accurate is my sensibility, my vulnerability. That's true. And that I'm not a man .... And the link between the feelings is the decisive item. It has to rhyme. That's healing. The fact that it rhymes reestablishes a whole. You could play a role in it. [Long pause] That I couldn't see it? Now I'll take a look at what happened at the window from your perspective.

Theodor Y reconsidered the scene at the window.

P: At the window I really felt castrated. Because you set me a limit. I made such a big deal out of it, yesterday I didn't notice it .... But that's no reason for you to close the window right in front of me. It's all true. My inflated masculinity, the aggression. I would kill to prove myself as a man. I want to have my way, even murder if I had to .... I'm not feeling any better now .... I can feel my solar plexus. Yesterday I had real pain and was all confused .... Then you say once again that I'm a hypochondriac.

This was a statement that was typical for the patient, half ironic, half serious. He always thought that the other person would realize the seriousness of the situation despite the veil he put around it and although he tried to protect himself from it.

A: I believe that I should now try to give you some help.

P: Can you?

This was another ironic question. Behind it I sensed disbelief and amazement.

A: You would be a hypochondriac if we couldn't understand why you feel castrated. You are not a hypochondriac if I can understand that it's your distress that causes you to have such thoughts. It's better if you can feel the acknowledgment in this distress, that you feel yourself to be so small, castrated, or whatever the right word is for it. Acknowledging this would be the help. Then you wouldn't sink so far, resorting to murder or suicide.

The patient was then able, in associations that moved him very strongly, to accept my (the analyst's) capacity to tolerate him and to set his own limits, and in this way turned to the working through that awaited him (Bilger 1986).

8.5 Working Through

8.5.1 Repetition of Trauma

The polarity into catharsis and working through has been carried over into the dispute about the relationship between experiencing and insight. In our opinion the polemics of this dispute become superfluous if we assume that one aspect of the analyst's skill is to link the present with the past in an affectively significant manner. In such moments the traumatic experience can be repeated under new and more favorable conditions, enabling the patient to actively master what had previously been governed by passive attitudes. Freud described this in the following general terms:

> The ego, which experienced the trauma passively, now repeats it actively in a weakened version, in the hope of being able itself to direct its course. It is certain that children behave in this fashion towards every distressing impression they receive, by reproducing it in their play. In thus changing from passivity to activity they attempt to master their experiences psychically. (Freud 1926d, p. 167)

In the following we excerpt a few sections from a course of treatment that Jiménez (1988) has provided a comprehensive documentation for, and comment on it. Our goal is to show how the trauma is repeated in transference and describe the roles catharsis and working through play. The analyst in this case facilitated the patient's recalling of the traumatic experience and its subsequent working through by making a literal reference to the homosexual seductions by his father; this created a realistic and distanced attitude in the therapeutic relationship. After this turning point the patient widened his capacity to distinguish between his lived experiences with his father in the past and his new experiences with the analyst (Strachey 1934).

Treatment Report

Peter Y, a highly educated 40-year-old man, visited me at the advice of his priest because of the sexual and affective difficulties he was having with his wife. In the first sessions he spoke a lot about his general dissatisfaction with life. He had had traumatic experiences with his alcoholic father, who had homosexually seduced him several times while the patient was 11–13 years old, practicing oral sex (fellatio) on him. The father-son relationship was limited to perverse episodes since the father was almost always away from home on business and the seductions occurred regularly when he returned home during this period of time. The patient spoke about these episodes surprisingly objectively in the initial interview, immediately adding that he was not homosexual but did suffer from premature ejaculation, which was a danger to his marriage. He described the focus of his life history as being his inhibitions toward women, which were in contrast to his wealth of fantasies. He was almost constantly in a state of sexual excitement; this was a source of great torment, which he was only able to escape temporarily by means of masturbation.

What had motivated the patient to seek analytic help at precisely this time became apparent during the first sessions. The reason was his anxiety that he might repeat with his own son the traumatic experiences he had had with his father, i. e., that he might perform fellatio on his son.

Despite the severity of the disturbance there were no psychopathological indications that would have led me to suspect a borderline case. On the contrary, I came to the conclusion that it was probably a severe character neurosis.

At this point it is helpful to make a few remarks about diagnosis in psychoanalysis. We agree with Kernberg (1977) that a patient cannot be considered a borderline case solely on the basis of fantasies containing archaic elements. This would be just as unfounded as a diagnosis of a perversion on the basis of perverse fantasies. Descriptive psychopathological and structural aspects must always be taken into consideration. Many people would have to be classified as severely ill if only the contents of unconscious fantasies were considered, which would mean that the diagnosis would lose its most important function, namely that of making a distinction. Taking the formal aspects of unconscious fantasies, i. e., the structure of their contents, into consideration means to judge them in the context of the personality. The purpose in doing so is to detect their consequences on behavior in general and on the structuring of the therapeutic relationship in particular.

Reenactment of the Trauma in Transference

After the analysis had continued for about 6 months, which are not summarized here, the tension in the sessions gradually began to decrease. Peter Y was a good dreamer. His dreams and associations facilitated the task of understanding the transference and reconstructing his unconscious life history. The material provided insights into different layers of his identification with his mother and father.

The patient's sexual relationship with his father varied from one dream to the next, enabling me to gain insights into deeper layers. In one dream his mother showed him her breast in a very provocative way. And he also saw his girlfriend and mother lying on a bed, wearing makeup as if they were whores, and turned away from both of them. He saw himself living in a very dignified manner, like a bishop, going into a monastery, without responding to the requests of both women, who pleaded with him to change his mind. In the 192nd session, Peter Y described a dream containing numerous versions of his traumatic experience: "I was having sexual intercourse with my wife, but in a very unusual manner. I was masturbating into her vagina. At the same time we were kissing, and this was the really important thing. Each of us achieved an orgasm and ejaculated with our mouths into the mouth of the other."

The patient's recollections testified to his heroic attempts to escape from his distressing oedipal and pregenital sexual desires that were directed at his father and mother and to achieve peace in the monastery. Yet there his anxiety took on a new content, namely his fear of being seduced by other novices or by the priests.

At a deeper level, Peter Y's fixation led him to experience all interpersonal relationships as sexual provocations that disturbed everyone involved. The perverse acts and oral-phallic gratification during puberty increased his unconscious fixation to the maternal breast. For his unconscious fantasies I accordingly played the role in transference of the seductive parents. He rapidly switched between the paternal and maternal roles he attributed to me; this rapid alteration of symbolic interaction was facilitated by the confused division of his body image into self- and object representations.

The tendernous and kissing constituted the really important relationship in the dream mentioned above. Of course, in transference this was also a repetition that included all the compromises that had formed. At the level of symptoms, his premature ejaculation was an example of such a compromise. In transference the patient stimulated me into making interpretations by describing exciting dreams and putting words in my mouth, just as he had ejaculated into his father's.

Regardless of whatever other unconscious wishes Peter Y might have had, it was necessary to proceed from the fact that he was exceptionally confused and humiliated by his father's behavior. Gradually I was able to recognize that in regression the patient experienced my interpretations to be intrusions robbing him of his autonomy and forcing him to assume a feminine position. He was involved in an intense and sexualized verbal exchange that offered each of us narcissistic gratification, he by referring to significant dreams, to which I responded by making "brilliant" interpretations.

In addition to these fantasies, Peter Y exhibited other transferences. The rivalry with me was expressed in dreams with political and aggressive contents, about power struggles etc., and in acting out in transference. It was clear to me that by telling me about so many dreams the patient made it impossible for me to make detailed interpretations. I pointed this fact out to him numerous times, interpreting it as ambivalence. Furthermore, when I thought it was wise to interpret a particular aspect of a dream, he responded too quickly by saying "Yes, of course" or "Yes, that's true," only to continue his topic without showing any sign of being impressed. I was irritated that he did not reply to what I had said and felt his "yes, of course" to be more a sign of his desire to be pleasant or even to subjugate himself. This passive aggressive behavior corresponded to his character traits and enabled him to control the course of the sessions. Later it became evident that he had in fact listened to and remembered the interpretations I had made. Thus following a session in which he, as he later said, had the feeling that I had restricted him, he dreamed that he had attempted to drill a hole into the ground, using a heavy and sharp steel pole. Then a general came, claimed the pole was his property, and stuck it in his mouth, which in the dream the patient had interpreted to be a religious ritual. Yet even during the dream the patient felt a strong sense of panic because he had rebelled against those in power, and also felt enraged at the humiliation of having to tolerate the "pole" being put into his mouth. While he was still half asleep the pole changed into a penis.

Commentary. After the analyst and patient had discovered that both the act of interpretation itself and the contents of the interpretations had traumatic side effects, it was logical to view the general as the intrusive father (analyst), especially since the patient himself had made this interpretive identification while waking up. The patient's helplessness was thus repeated in transference, and the patient felt as little justified to resist the general as he had his father. Or is it more accurate to say that he never - neither with the general nor with his father - really *wanted* to put up any resistance? This perverse act provided a compromise satisfaction for a number of wishes and fantasies in one. To mention several aspects, his longing for his long absent father found a satisfaction in which his father made himself entirely dependent on his son. In ejaculating the patient himself became the general, and at the unconscious level used the mouth as a kind of cavernous opening with numerous meanings and also identified with the person sucking. Finally, the fact that there was a link between the patient's deriving pleasure from power and his rage at its misuse cannot be overlooked. His dependence on his father (and at a deeper layer, on his mother) and on instinctual satisfaction was tied to the misuse of power.

In contrast to this transference constellation and after intensively working through his difficulties, he described dreams in which a more realistic positive transference was expressed. In them I was pictured as a teacher patiently instructing his pupils. Predominant was, however, a homosexual transference with a rapid alteration of the feminine and masculine roles.

In contrast to the problems in the therapeutic relationship, the patient described his increasing satisfaction with his daily life. His capacity to work was raised by his greater sense of balance, and he successfully asserted himself against his boss. He noticed a reduction in his inhibitions toward women, and there was also an improvement in the disturbance of his potency.

Following this the patient started acting out sexually, which continued for a lengthy period of time and gradually assumed significance in transference. He began an erotic relationship to a girl who came to clean his house several times a week; this secret relationship was limited to extensive caressing, which as a rule ended in an ejaculation without emission. One purpose of this acting out, in addition to other unconscious meanings, was to relieve the burden from the homosexual transference with me. If the latter increased, the patient missed a session and excused himself subsequently, saying that he had been able to spend the hour alone with the girl at home.

During this period the homosexual transference always manifested itself as something that pursued the patient and that he attempted to resist. The repetition of these fantasies and their intensity led me to infer there was a strong fixation in the negative phase of the oedipus complex, which because of the traumatic experiences in puberty could not develop into a positive identification with his father.

In order to give the patient more support in overcoming the confusion of his identity, I changed my strategy of interpretation by contrasting the present, realistic aspects of our relationship with the positive and aggressive pregenital repetitions. My goal was to overcome the erotization that the patient sought. I now realized that frequently precisely those interpretations that especially moved him satisfied his homosexual fantasy. After interruptions the patient had unconsciously awaited the moments in which his father seduced him after returning home (he was only home for some 3-4 months a year on average). We had been moving in a vicious circle for far too long. We were an analytic couple in which the patient, with his dreams and associations, stimulated my interpretive work, the latter both satisfying him and also making him feel violated - a sadomasochistic circle. Whatever I said was to him a confirmation of my homosexual interest in him. When I realized this, I began to exercise more restraint and attempted to interrupt this vicious circle by frequently remaining silent.

After we had discussed this problem repeatedly, the patient described the following dream in the 385th session: "I wanted to pick up an important document in an office or maybe the results of a test in a doctor's office. I was surprised to discover it was a lawyer's office, and it a document from a court. I was surprised again because in reality it was the police headquarters. The chief submitted me to a rigorous interrogation while at the same time caressing me very tenderly. I ran outside and took a bus to get home, only to notice that by quickly getting in the rear door I had taken the wrong bus and was riding in the wrong direction."

The combination of the patient's associations and my considerations enabled me to make the interpretation that he had come to analysis looking for an attorney who was supposed to protect him from his father who seduced him and from his mother who made him feel disturbed. In the course of his analysis it had become increasingly difficult for him to distinguish between his new experiences with me and his childhood relationship to his parents. He claimed this was due to the fact that something which was completely hidden was being repeated in the present relationship and that it was very satisfying. Then for the first time in the analysis I called his father a homosexual and an alcoholic, which made him feel very disturbed and led him to recall a dream he had recently had. He saw a door that had many rusty padlocks and that definitely had not been opened for a long time. He associated a room used for storing bottled gas. I explained to him that he had just told me that it was difficult for him to open the door to his memory for me and thus to be frank about what had happened with his father because he was afraid of its very explosive contents. He then mentioned his immense shame and his anxiety about revealing to me his homosexual wishes and fantasies. The analysis had been going in the wrong direction because the "back" door had been *confused* with the "front" door, just as I had been with his father.

Commentary. We have emphasized the word "confused" in the analyst's report because it marks the turning point described in more detail in the following summary of the treatment. By distancing himself from the patient's perverse father and seducing parents, the analyst had distinguished himself through an act of judgment, which presumably clarified the confusion that had resulted from the traumatic experience and that apparently had not diminished as a result of the interpretation of the continued homosexual transference. The patient took the interpretations all too literally, at face value, presumably obtaining numerous satisfactions and both expecting and, probably, fearing that his relationship with the analyst would end the same way as that with his father. Yet the analyst had apparently passed his test, finally convincingly separating himself from the father. The effect of such clarifying assurances should not be underestimated. It is necessary to establish a position outside the repetitions to overcome such confusion. With regard to such *confusion* we recommend that readers turn to Sect. 9.3.2, where we cite a patient's criticism of an interpretive technique that failed to put the patient's new experiences with the analyst and the repetition into a balanced relationship and thus to interrupt the repetition.

The actual incestuous and homosexual abuse of children is the cause of serious traumatic experiences because it transgresses limits whose purpose is to guarantee autonomy. Such security is required for human desires and fantasies to develop, in order for children to be able to distinguish between inside and outside within the many layers of social reality. The sexual abuse of children by their own parents or other adults destroys this space, which is taboo for many good reasons. Oedipal and incestuous wishes and fantasies obtain their deep anthropological significance precisely from this taboo, i. e., from incest actually not occurring. Otherwise a hopeless confusion of the generations results which has catastrophic effects on the formation of the identity of the children and adolescents. As this case history demonstrates, a deep insecurity seems to remain after homosexual seductions or after father-daughter or mother-son incest. Afterwards everything seems possible. Real incestuous experiences undermine the child's confidence in a fundamental manner (see MacFarlane et al. 1986; Walker 1988).

Consideration. The dynamic of the session described above deserves to be emphasized because it was under its impact that I changed my therapeutic technique. In retrospect I believe that this change was not only the result of my reflection but also the result of a genuine working through by the patient, which took place parallel to the homosexual transference described above. My interpretation that Peter Y confused me with his father in transference emphasized the aspect of repetition or, in other words, the distortion that the transference caused because of its roots in the past. Yet I had the feeling that I had in some way contributed to the development of this transference constellation. The second interpretation emphasized the plausibility of the patient's perception in the sense elaborated by Gill and Hoffmann (1982), not the distortion.

In hindsight I believe that I could have stated much earlier or more clearly how this repetition in transference developed. In any case, the consequence of the emphasis I put on the difference was that from this moment on the patient's healthy features started playing a predominant role in overcoming the trauma. The fact that I showed myself to be a real person distinct from his homosexual father formed the basis of my attempt to interrupt the circular projective and introjective identification.

Commentary. The issue here is a fundamental one, namely how a psychoanalyst fulfills his functions to enable the patient to achieve change and to overcome traumatic experiences. In transference, repetition is one side of the coin and is labeled "similarity." In this sense it is completely plausible, accurate, and realistic that this patient experienced the analyst's efforts to gain influence as being intrusive or seductive. The other side of the coin is that the word "differences" must be taken seriously. It is not the discovery of *similarities* that leads out of repetition, it is the experience of *differences*. As we mentioned with regard to the confusion, this problem affects all of psychoanalysis and is not limited to one school. In the Kleinian school, the question of how new experiences lead to change, i. e., interrupt the circular processes of projective and introjective identification, was neglected for a long time. It is obvious that the therapeutic effect of a psychoanalysis does not consist in repeating traumatic experiences and creating circular repetition in transference, but in interrupting them.

Catharsis

The information literally gushed out of Peter Y during a short period encompassing four sessions (the 341st to 344th), when he, in great turmoil, described the sexual episodes he had had with his father. This was the first time he had mentioned his great longing for his father while he had been gone and how he had been happy about his return. He described how his father began to drink and became merry, how the tender touching began and the excitement mounted, which ended with the father kneeing in front of his son and sucking his penis until ejaculation. He described his conflicting feelings: the sexual desire, but also the anxiety, shame, the strong feeling of triumph upon ejaculating into his father's mouth, his later sensation of guilt, and his feeling of domination over his father. This report was very emotional, in complete contrast to the obsessive style characterizing the initial interviews. After this catharsis it became clear to me that the conscious recollections of these episodes that he had previously related were devoid of any and all feelings. He told how he, following an unspoken aggreement with his father, had kept these events a secret from his mother and decided after two years to end the episodes because he was feeling more and more insecure. He had the support of his priest. It then became clear to the patient that his image of an aggressive and actively seductive father was incomplete. He realized that his father was weak and an alcoholic and that he had established a secret collusion with him to their mutual satisfaction.

Overcoming Traumatic Experiences

The catharsis paralleled the patient's distancing from his father, which could also be seen in the changed nature of transference. Especially impressive was the fact that Peter Y managed to develop a relationship to his son that was free of anxiety. His new experiences in therapy made it easier for him to assume paternal responsibilities and to empathize with his son. He tried to find out how he had wanted his father to be. The erotization decreased, and his capacity for reflection - self-analysis - increased. The patient acknowledged my work and accepted what he had learned in analysis as something new. The sessions became calmer, and the patient reported fewer dreams. As a matter of course, I made fewer comments and interpretations. The patient also acknowledged his homosexual longing for his father, which stayed very strong for a long time, yet understood it was a substitute satisfaction and compensation for the lack of things that father and son had in common, with the accompanying depressive reactions.

The following dream was from this period:

P: I was walking on a street. An older gentleman was walking toward me, taking up all the space, so that I had to step off the sidewalk. I was carrying a gigantic, very long roll of wrapping paper under my arm. I walked further and noticed that somebody was trying to take it away from me from behind, and it was getting difficult to hold on. It was the older man who was bothering me from behind. I went into a house, opened the roll of paper, and saw a giant Christmas tree with every imaginable decoration and kind of lights. It was lovely and very impressive. The room that I was in had a small window to an adjacent room. I could see a couch and a man, apparently dead, lying on it. I was afraid. I took a closer look and noticed that he wasn't dead, but very ill; he was hardly breathing. I calmed down. I went even closer and saw that it was me. In the back portion of the room there was a priest who was holding mass from a very cluttered baroque altar. He was wearing a richly decorated cassock. There was a giant clock on the wall above the couch. It was a kind of cuckoo clock, and from time to time figures - wooden puppets like Pinocchio - came out, including bishops and generals, who made ridiculous gestures of submission, bowing and showing their reverence. I thought it was repulsive.

By analyzing the dream it was possible for us to approach the patient's inner, live core; he was still breathing although he was almost dead and inhibited by the roles he had adopted. Almost all of his associations to this part of the dream belonged to the topic that Winnicott referred to as the "false self" and that had become the patient's second nature. In the dream he had also submitted to me, the analyst. In my opinion this dream was very useful in terms of a reconstruction, yet it seemed especially interesting to me because of its significance as an indicator of the psychoanalytic process. The history of the patient's therapy was recorded in the layers of the dream. Three parts can be distinguished in the dream. The first part presented the period of the analysis in which the patient felt disturbed by the interpretations; he felt they were an attempt to destroy his phallus from behind. In the second part the patient unfolded, at a deeper level (inside the house), his triumphant narcissism. This probably corresponded to the period in which he found satisfaction in transference as well as to the period in which he discovered the little window - the significance of analysis for him - which offered him access to a part of his self. This part was repressed and contained an "inner world" of identifications that had been grafted on and of religious idealizations; at the same time it was also the seat of his more lively qualities. Especially interesting here was that in the part corresponding to the third area of the dream, in which even deeper inner features were expressed, the analyst was represented by a cuckoo clock that gave the time and expressed, one after another, the various roles that the patient had played in the course of therapy.

Peter Y reported a decrease in the enduring sexual arousal that used to plague him. The frequency of his compulsive masturbation also decreased and was limited to weekends and other interruptions of therapy.

Commentary. In the course of therapy the patient's attempts to cope with his traumatic experiences and to change from being passive to being active became more and more successful. Freud's understanding of this essential component of the effectiveness of analysis, which we referred to at the beginning of this section, can also be expressed in the theory of projective and introjective identification if the latter are taken to represent communication and interaction. The turning point in the case presented here was characterized by the joint discovery of patient and analyst that both the contents of the interpretation and the act of interpretation itself had unnoticed and unfavorable side effects. The confusion was facilitated by the analyst's therapeutic technique, and the patient experienced the therapeutic relationship from the perspective of his traumatic experiences with his father. The patient managed to make new experiences after this "confusion" had been clarified. After two years of seducing each other and letting oneself be seduced, the analyst was finally in a position to understand the meaning of the repetition of the trauma in the analytic relationship. The work in this time provided not only indirect satisfactions via the partial repetition in transference, but also prepared the way for a catharsis and for the patient's working through.

8.5.2 Denial of Castration Anxiety

After having hesitated for two years, Arthur Y decided to enlarge the region he covered as a salesman by expanding into an area that a colleague had neglected for a long time. The lack of contact to customers in this area had caused the sales there to be far below average. Arthur Y was convinced that it would be possible to increase the sales in this region several times over without any great effort. Despite the general dissatisfaction with the easy going - even lazy - colleague, who was also a drinker and had become a burden to the company, Arthur Y had hesitated for a long time to make a decision about enlarging his sales area. Pity and his scruples had kept him from taking action and blocked his ability to consider whether there were any solutions that might not harm or even ruin his colleague's career. His unconscious identification of expansion with sadistic destruction and his immediate shift to masochistic identification with the victim had long been in balance and kept the patient from being able to expand his field of operations or to become more successful. This sophisticated man had, for the same reason, also not been able to find an acceptable solution that satisfied his motto of live and let live.

The interpretive support I provided, which was directed at his unconscious equating of expansion and destruction, had enabled Arthur Y to become more successful and to overcome his inhibitions about enlargening his sales region, which he did without inflicting any substantial harm on his colleague. He had found a good compromise.

P: I don't feel anxious any more about getting ahead with this matter. It's connected with being potent, in the widest sense of the word. I have the suspicion that there are different ways of showing potency. One way to be potent is, after all, to be successful in an area where another failed. Am I making some kind of a shift? Then I could withdraw sexually even more from my wife. Nobody could be mad at me. Most importantly I'm the devoted father doing everything for my family.

A: The fact that everything is to the benefit of your family is a relief to you. Couldn't you get more sexual pleasure? Maybe something inside you - your ideas about purity and the boundaries of shame that you feel automatically - constitutes inhibitions keeping you from having pleasure.

P: That's the problem, namely that I'm really quite happy the way things are. I'm doing quite well, and therefore it's not worthwhile to tackle this issue. Who knows - I have the feeling-what's going to come and cause me to get all worried. I much prefer, a thousand times over, having my inner, emotional peace and quiet. I'm happy and satisfied and take pleasure from success, perhaps less pleasure from sex than may be theoretically possible, better than - I simply have some reservations - than letting everything get started again. I don't want to be exposed to the danger of emotionally falling as low as I was a couple of years ago. If I could choose to have a realistic increase in pleasure from sex combined with returning to my earlier state of anxiety, then I prefer things the way they are a thousand times over. Yes, I'm very shy about getting involved.

A: Why are you worried that things could become the way they were several years ago, that you could fall so low, that sex is a source of such distress, of more distress than pleasure?

P: In commercial terms, that I'd be making a bad deal in order to make a theoretically better one, which I don't really want because things are fine the way they are. That I'd be taking an uncalculated risk.

The thought of the risk made the patient go silent. He remained silent for several minutes until I continued:

A: So it's clear that you fear the distress of making a bad deal. The possibility of having more joy and pleasure is just theory.

The patient then made a comparison.

P: I'm sitting in a restaurant and eating a good meal. Somebody comes over and says he's a surgeon and that if I let him operate on me, he would operate on my tongue and put it in a bit differently, giving me more pleasure from eating. The operation is connected with the risk that my tongue might not grow on correctly and there might be terrible complications.

A: There are all sorts of terrible consequences one could think of if your tongue wouldn't grow on. This image is a radical expression of your distress, and I'm the restaurant's manager.

P: No, the surgeon.

Consideration. I obviously treated everything as if it were less serious because of a reactivation of my own castration anxieties. The surgeon, and not the manager, was obviously the source of danger. Although I immediately became aware ot this, later in the session I again played down the danger of a threat, using the word "snack" to refer to the witch's cannibalism in Hansel and Gretel.

A: Oh, yes, the surgeon, not the manager. I was thinking about the restaurant manager.

P: No, the manager is completely neutral; he just provides a good meal.

A: So the surgeon. Then it's understandable that you're hesitating. There's good reason. The surgeon who made this proposal.

P: It's not that far-fetched. I been through it dozens of times, for instance with Professor Z. I was having problems with my knee, and he seriously proposed cutting out bits of the bone because I'm slightly bowlegged and letting them grow back together straight, removing the bowleggedness and my problems. In the meantime I have hiked through all of Germany - without the operation. And Professor Z is a famous orthopedic surgeon. I just wanted to say that the comparison of the operation and my tongue isn't so far-fetched after all.

A: Yes, the comparison is very accurate. It's not far-fetched at all. Your comparison is even much better because it's linked with other things, with all the threats that were not directed at your tongue even though people talk about having a sharp tongue, but instead with the punishments affecting the organ of pleasure, namely your penis. Everything that might happen, all the stories . . . anxieties about contagious illnesses, injuries after masturbation, and other such things, with X and Y and others [references to several persons from his childhood and adolescence].

P: I just observed something interesting on me. While you were mentioning this list, the thought went through my mind that I hadn't been told what some parents tell their sons, namely that if they grab down there then it will get very big and then it will be cut off. I thought of this example, and while I thought about it, my recollection changed. I'm completely sure now that my grandmother said something of the sort to me. It's resurfaced in my memory.

A: Your momentary experiencing might be involved, so that you first established some distance by saying that it hadn't happened to me. First you negated it. First you established some distance to it, and now you are much closer to it.

Commentary. It is instructive that Arthur Y was able to recall this forgotten disturbance and threat with the help of distancing, i. e., a lessening of his anxiety. He may have adopted this tactic from the analyst without noticing it. The analyst had first, because of a countertransference, minimized the dangers in order to be able to later acknowledge them.

P: Parents use the threat to make their children afraid. Is it still being used? [Analyst confirmed.] Yes, it's nonsense. It puts a boy in a dilemma if he takes everything seriously. On the highway just now I was driving behind a truck filled with pigs. One pig stuck its snout out the back, and I thought, "You poor pig, you don't have a chance to escape." The difference to humans is that the poor pig wasn't aware of what was coming. It may have been afraid, but it didn't know where the truck was going. A pig's emotional life is probably different from a human's. The pig's hopeless situation reminded me of certain situations in my own life where I felt the same way. I was worse off than the pig, because it doesn't know what's coming.

A: You were worse off, but you also had another chance, by saying just a moment ago that people tell such stories but that you were never involved. First you denied something disturbing, to save your snout, your tail, your penis - "I'm not involved." And then, after you achieved some security, then it became possible, I think, for you to consider it conceivable or probable that it might have happened to you, too. The denial lessened the anxiety, just like your knowledge that your penis is still there. That's one part of your memory, that it gets big, and pleasure is the reason you get punished.

Commentary. This exchange is exemplary, with regard to both therapeutic technique and the theory describing how anxiety originates and can be overcome. An individual's anxiety is linked with fantasies, which is the reason that all neurotic anxieties, by definition, originate as expectations. It also creates space for protection and defense mechanisms, which is the object of the analyst's interpretation that proceeds from the security the patient had gained. Starting from a secure position, it was thus possible for the patient to cope with his anxiety because he knew he had rescued his penis.

P: Yes, when a child's penis gets hard, he can't hide it if his pajamas reveal its shape or if he is half naked.

A: Or the morning erection, which is a natural phenomenon, the "water stiffness," which is linked with the urge to urinate.

P: I've just thought of something else. I can remember it very precisely. When I was a young boy, maybe 4 or 5 years old, I wore shorts and had the habit of reaching up my pants' leg. There was a picture of me, a snapshot that showed me with a small girl in a sand box. The picture was enlarged and put up on the wall. I can still hear my grandmother say, "Look there, so that's how you do it. You have to stop doing that, otherwise . . . ."

I'm not as sure about my memory of her saying that as I am about my doing it and about the photograph that was on the wall. I don't know if it was right for the picture to be enlarged and put up. It disappeared long ago, but I can still see it hanging there. And there are a lot of feelings attached to the picture and my memories of my grandmother. It would be better not to have to talk about it because I don't want to have to go through these years again.

A: These bad memories are very closely tied to pleasure. You can't imagine that pleasure could be separated from the inhibitions and anxieties. The anxieties connected with the touching seem to come back first, before the pleasure. If your wife wants more from you, if she desires you, then it is closely linked with distress and danger, and then you experience your wife both as a little girl and as your grandmother, who turns into a witch. When your penis gets too big, then it is chopped off. Just like with Hansel and Gretel, only there it was a finger, a fat finger.

P: Yes, I know, people attempt to interpret so much into these fairy tales. Why can't the fairy tales be left for what they are?

A: Yes, of course.

Commentary. The analyst agreed with the patient, and probably precisely for this reason the patient did not cooperate in playing down the danger.

P: [After a long period of silence] It's completely logical. Hansel is locked in the cage and gets a lot to eat and gets fatter, and the witch can tell from his finger. Very fat people have very chubby fingers. It can be left at that. And then we're back at the beginning again. Everything can be left the way it is.

A: Yes, leave everything the way it is to avoid being exposed to the danger depicted in the fairy tale, namely exposed to the danger of becoming the witch's snack.

P: Yes, but snack makes it sound too pleasant.

A: Yes, I just played down the danger and that is surely inappropriate. But the consequence was, after all, that you were able to make it clear how horrible it was. You emphasized that everything should be left as it is. Yet part of the story is how Hansel and Gretel deceived the witch about the fattened finger.

P: Yes, by sticking out a thin stick.

A: Yes, it was dangerous. And you hid your penis. Maybe you've continued hiding like this by hiding from your wife and from yourself, too. And then there's less pleasure. There is an automatic inhibition.

At the start of the next session Arthur Y was silent.

P: It took a while for me to make the transition. It's a completely different world in here. I read a newspaper article a few days ago. Just by chance I glanced at a picture of a fox in a trap; its paw was caught in it. The article was about the cruelty of the devices used to catch animals. Many of them end in a wretched way, and hunters use the innocent word "trapping" to describe this cruelty. "Trapping." Even while I was reading, I thought that this story was going to make me worry a lot. I can sense the feelings again that I thought I had long overcome. Now I feel immensely better, and for a long time I've meant to ask how safe I am against having a relapse, a word I don't like. The word brings back all the misery that I played down in my memory, in my experiencing. The feeling of despair comes back immediately.

A: I don't think it's a coincidence that you're asking about it. You can certainly recall how miserable it was to be the prisoner, just like the fox who is a victim. I think your distress is connected with the topic of our previous session. You are worried that I will set a trap for you, and pose a danger to you if you become more involved in sex. You described a horrible image about a tongue that's operated on, cut off, and doesn't grow back together right.

The patient claimed he had "forgotten" the entire scene and asked "Was it a dream? No." I reminded him of his fantasy about his tongue that was operated on and sewed on incorrectly or would not grow together at all. The patient recalled the surgeon, but the object, the part of the body that was to be operated on was completely gone.

A: There is a terrible danger, and I believe that the story about trapper, who enticed you to leave your hiding place, continues this topic.

The patient reminded me that I had played down the danger to Hansel in the fairy tale.

Commentary. We would like to draw the reader's attention to the unconscious defense processes that can be deduced from omissions and displacements. The organ, the penis or its substitute (the tongue), was omitted. It remained vague what the intentions of the surgeon were. The action was interrupted. The patient was then able to recognize the playing down with reference to the analyst and, by means of this objectification, to cope with it.

The analyst interpreted the closing of the trap as a symbol of his castration anxiety. The scenes from the last session were repeated, including especially the denial and the function of distancing himself from his anxieties. The patient spoke once more about the photograph, which probably served to constantly show him what he was not supposed to do.

P: Yes, that's the way it is after being liberated from anxieties and compulsions. Yesterday I visited my new region, and there are some very scenic spots. I particularly liked one hotel, which I've noted down as a place to stay on future business trips. Earlier I would never have had the idea of stopping at such an establishment. Yet I'd like to bracket out the sex. I would really prefer to act as if it weren't there. I even avoid my wife when I feel that she's going to make an advance.

A: I presume you avoid a number of things and then don't have the pleasure that might be possible.

P: Yes, I would like to do without desire.

A: You aren't committing yourself to a new sacrifice. It's more like with a salamander; people say salamanders lose their tails when they are in danger. You've created a sense of security like the salamander's, who's gotten past the dangers. You express your concern that there might be more desire. To me your concern that symptoms might return if you had more desires is an indication that there are a number of things still latent within you.

P: Yes, and that's the reason that I mentioned sex. Otherwise I would simply accept the restrictions.

A: Your wife is your reminder. What does she remind you of? A distressing seduction?

P: No, of a demand that I can't meet. To me it's an unreasonable demand, a ... [long silence]. I have the fewest inhibitions after I've drunk some alcohol.

The patient came to speak of the proximity of the sexual organs to the organs of defecation. This was how he explained his shyness.

A: You're reminded more of the shameful and humiliating situations, of how you dirtied your pants every day, not of the relieving expelling, but of the humiliations.

The patient had the idea that the cleansing really had to be done in advance and prevent spontaneous desire. "Complete lack of desire is the best protection against every kind of sexual involvement and the distress that comes from it." Precisely in marital intercourse, which is not inhibited by any restrictions, complications, or conflicts and in which sex has been quasi-legalized, his inner warning lamps lit up particularly strongly. This comment convinced the patient that he had internalized conflicts and anxieties of his childhood and that they now began showing their effects, even though he knew better. In their otherwise happy marriage, intercourse was a disturbance and premature ejaculation or anxiety about impotence were frequent, although his merry wife gave him encouragement and he himself did not have any conscious scruples. Yet he could not do anything against his revulsion and shame. The patient summarized his concern in the words, "Whoever gets himself in danger dies as a result."

8.5.3 Splitting of Transference

The purpose of transference splitting is frequently to find suitable objects for desired identifications. At the same time, this splitting can also result from a defensive goal, namely to keep identifications from occurring or being stabilized by rapidly switching from one object to another.

Recently Clara X had made up a story about a hermit who lived on a mountain and who was supplied with the goods he needed by a woman who lived in the valley. To get some relief, this woman had frequently sent a younger girl up to the hermit. The patient represented herself in this "coveted" creation.

The patient talked about this story and the hermit with a friend she spent an evening with. They departed, wishing each other sweet dreams. Laughing, she told me that she really had dreamed about something beautiful. The next morning she had not been able to remember the dream immediately. Bit by bit the patient developed the following dream image:

P: It was a big family reunion. You were there, and for sure my previous therapist, Mrs. Z. There were a lot of people there with whom I'm acquainted and who I somehow feel to be my spiritual family. And my real brother was there. All of us wanted to fly to my home town by helicopter, to visit my parents. We waited for the helicopter for quite a while, but since we weren't in a rush I managed to have a pleasant conversation. We traveled together, and there was plenty of time to talk. I also talked with you; we were standing at the window and looking out. You were to my left, and the character of our conversation was different than here - a little more ironic, a little more playful, with lots of allusions. My father would have said teasing. You came a little closer and nudged my shoulder, just like my father could have done. Trying to turn me on, in a friendly way, but perhaps also a little pushy, like children can be when they try to push each other off the road in a game.

In response to my questions, the patient provided additional information to her dream report, especially regarding the meaning of the phrase "turn on." The patient emphasized the friendly nature of this contact, yet it also contained an implication of aggression. The patient knew the colloquial connotations of the word, but in the dream it was not disturbing. She recalled her dealings with boys during puberty, which in hindsight did not seem repulsive, bad-mannered, or unpleasant, and she said literally, "That is one of the levels accessible to me, just like earlier when I roused myself to look for contact with boys my age. I wasn't able to make eyes at them or to flirt. Whenever it was possible I attempted to make body contact in some tomboyish way by suggesting some small game." Then she turned to speak about her husband. "I'm always on the lookout for some wonder weapon to draw my husband out of his reserve."

I established a connection between the past and the present by pointing out that her old and her new families were together and visited her home town. Clara X said jokingly that it showed how much of a family person she was.

P: I really like being right in the middle of things. It's a feeling that I don't have in my current family, I mean with my husband and child; I don't feel secure and protected. I can feel a strong centrifugal force, but also the compulsion, a coercion, that I'd better stay there. There's an immense tension between the two forces. In the dream I thought I was at the right spot. On the other hand, in the last few days I've recalled how the funny story about the hermit continued. Well, the coveted girl went up to the hermit, hugged him, looked at him, and said, "What should we do now?" At this the hermit stood up and excused himself. "I can understand what you mean, but unfortunately I can't help you at the moment. I've just realized that I have missed a lot in the last twenty years." He then left his mountain and moved into the old woman's hut. The young girl turned right around, went home, and found herself a lover from the neighborhood and spent the night with him. The next day she walked up the mountain and set fire to the hermit's hut, burning it to the ground. You might say, well, he doesn't need it any more.

I made a reference particularly to the young girl's hurt feelings. The patient responded that this was the reason she quickly looked for someone else, but wasn't satisfied with the substitute. He was simply a substitute. I then interpreted the transference aspects of the story.

A: It seems logical to assume that you've portrayed me as the hermit and your earlier therapist as the old woman who had sent the hermit supplies for years, and your therapist did have her office on a mountain.

In making this interpretation I had not taken into consideration the fact that the patient definitely did not view her earlier therapist as an older woman, but identified with her and through this identification had fantasized a positive outcome of the oedipal rivalry. A friend of the patient's said that it was possible that the hermit would accept the young girl's offer and she would move into his hut.

P: "And what would the old woman do now?" my girlfriend asked. I just laughed, and without thinking about it promptly said that she would get rheumatism. I was absolutely certain that the older woman would later suffer from this chronic illness, and only afterward did I remember that my mother had actually suffered from rheumatism for years. In that moment it was clear to me that my mother was the older woman, the way that I saw her or the way she presented herself to me. "I sacrificed twenty years of my life and put off my own goals and desires, and then my own daughter threatens to have a fling with the man I took care of, the hermit." Yet my mother would never have been able to aggressively have her own way.

I then focused on the issue of aggressive rivalry, especially with regard to her own inhibitions that resulted from her sympathy from her mother. As a consequence of them, she was not able to openly express her own qualities of a young girl. The patient in fact felt inferior to her own daughter. She summarized her situation in very moving terms.

P: Yes, in the story I'm both persons, first the old woman and then the young girl, and even today I don't know for sure who I really am.

A: You looked for a solution that could lead you out of your dilemma, namely not to be either one and instead be a tomboy, or spiny, or covered by a shell like a turtle.

P: Yes, I decided not to be a woman. I considered it the best solution for the entire family for me to step back and stay there.

I pointed out to Clara X that her girlfriend had encouraged her to have a beautiful and exciting dream and had given her the advice to enjoy something before falling asleep. "Yes, she approved of my consumption of candy." We then went on to talk about the table manners at her girlfriend's and at her own house, especially about the difficulties of coordinating the needs of the children with those of the adults. (One of the patient's symptoms was that she secretly ate candy at night and, as she herself said, had shifted the satisfaction of her needs in that direction.)

In connection with the patient's dream the topic shifted to the question of how difficult it was to create a prosperous, cozy, and enjoyable atmosphere at home and that this difficult task should not be left entirely to the wife and mother. The patient went on to complain about her husband, who rejected her requests that the two of them eat out or go out alone some time. She was most able to enjoy herself, aside from her displacement to nighttime, when she was together with her girlfriends. Excusing herself for using the fashionable word "frustration," the patient complained the denial was not her greatest source of despair, which was rather the fact that her husband or men in general complained that everything was her fault. She vigorously complained about her husband's lack of understanding, and that he said her problem was responsible for everything; on the other hand, he was unwilling to contribute anything toward uniting their divergent interests.

While acknowledging the real difficulties, I pointed out that she had required a long time to be able to admit her own needs and that there might still be many ways to convince her husband - just like the hermit - that he should try a different approach. At the end of the session the patient despondently remained convinced that everything was in vain. She said her husband simply took her to be a monster and something unnatural, and that she therefore wanted to at least free herself from constantly feeling guilty and for being ashamed of her own failures.

It was obvious that this name calling had hardened the attitudes of the patient and her husband, and that they were becoming increasingly alienated from each other. Just as obvious was that the patient obtained relief by attacking her husband, who for his part considered her to be all the more a monster. In a concluding interpretation of the transference I emphasized that everyone was involved in determining how much room for maneuvering there was, both in the primary family and in the fictitious one (the analytic family, i. e., her relationship to her female and male therapists). In the story about the hermit she had made the discovery that he too was not immune to her wooing.

In the next session the patient referred back to her dream.

P: In the last session you said something that was very important to me. I mean that I felt pity toward the old woman. I had said that the woman got rheumatism. Yet I experienced her like I did my mother, who sacrificed herself for her family for twenty years, denying her own desires and longings. At the same time, as her daughter I felt so attached to her that I did not want to struggle against her. Or how should I say, well, I would have felt it unfair and mean for me to puff myself up and force her out of the nest. Then you said something along the line that this was the reason it was particularly difficult for me to accept the competition with my daughter. I want to ask once more whether you really think that we're competing. I see it that way, but I can't help thinking that it's completely ridiculous. And yet it always comes back.

Clara X gave a, as she described it, ridiculous and banal example of how she had become upset at her daughter's being proud of being able to get dressed faster than she could.

I reminded her of the solution to her conflict that she had arrived at out of sympathy - her compromise to be neither the one nor the other but to have found a third way, the nonfeminine and tomboyish way.

P: That's right, but it's a step too fast. It's tremendously important to me for somebody to understand me. Even that would help me to be a bit more gentle in the ridiculous struggle that I have each day with my daughter. How much is innocence and how much doe she do on purpose? It's extremely difficult for me to separate reality and what I notoriously do wrong. Is it always like that?

A: Do you mean the rivalry between mothers and daughters?

P: Yes, it sounds brutal. Worst of all is the firm belief that it just can't be, for God's sake. Out in the open everything is very harmonic, but under the table we can't stop kicking each other in the shins.

A: Yes, in the open you can't compete and be rivals. You're struggling for having and possessing and out of envy. This envy is one side of your rivalry. Another is who is faster at making themselves pretty.

P: Yes, as an adult I have so many more possibilities, much more room to decide. Yet, on the other hand, I view everything as if I had a much worse starting position and had to give her a powerful shove; but then I feel sorry again. It's probably related to the fact that when I was young I actually trained myself to do without and limit myself. This was a good approach at home, to be neither the one nor the other, not to oppose my mother but to stay a step behind her and to behave like a tomboy. In this way I got quite a bit of approval from my father. He approved of having such an uncivilized son, half a son. In some hidden way I was thus able to get his support and interest. He probably would not have been able to do much with a vain, pretty little daughter; so it was a fantastic solution for me, and I was very good at learning to act that way. So I'm not too amazed that I can't get any further.

Stimulated by a letter from her brother, the patient then turned to the question of female creativity. Her brother had touched on it, mentioning in passing that he had frequently fantasized about what it would be like to be a woman. Clara X said it was probably the opposite of a woman's wish to play the male's sexual role once and was quite natural. Yet what common family experiences were involved?

P: I assume that he made the same observations I did, just from the perspective of a son. I mean, my brother suffered from the fact that our mother viewed herself to be a victim, as if there was no joy in life. As if she could not have done anything but spend decades taking care of the hermit.

The patient sighed and then noted questioningly that I had related myself to Ms. Z, her previous analyst, in the last session.

A: Both of us were depicted in the dream. Yes, Ms. Z lived here on the mountain for years. Of course, it's not clear what the relationship was, whether it was out in the open or out of sight.

P: To me it looked different. I don't consider Ms. Z to be an older woman but a young woman who is independent in every regard. She was here but then became independent. She did not take the sacrificial route like the old woman did; no, on the contrary, she is happy go lucky, like a snotty little brat.

Clara X identified with her previous analyst, who had made her own way. She related details from correspondence with her, one of which was about a painting by a Pre-Raphaelite depicting the Annunciation (see Sect. 2.4.7). The painting was shown in a book on "the crazy sex." Immaculate conception is a hot subject for people who, like the patient, want to avoid sexuality.

P: I thought that it couldn't be true. Mary, her entire body and facial features were those of a young girl suffering from anorexia and she stared with an astonished look into the future that had been imposed on her. "Help, I'm supposed to be a mother. I don't want to, not at all." Fear and anxiety. When I wrote to Ms. Z that I wanted to draw this picture, she wrote back asking why I didn't draw a different figure, one of a woman sitting in bed and looking into the future and exuding confidence. Well, for the first I stopped drawing.

A: Yes, you could draw your future and your picture as you wish. Things don't have to continue as they are forever.

P: My husband is still deeply resigned to it.

The patient described her attempts get closer to him and also how strongly she was still dominated by a subliminal aggression. The session ended with a story she told about a couple getting together and trying to make their feelings fit together. This showed that the transference was centralized after all.

8.5.4 Mother Fixation

Heinrich Y was a 35-year-old man who had suffered since late adolescence from depression, which severly incapacitated him. It had led him to undergo a four-year supportive psychotherapy while a student. Most closely tied to his mother, Heinrich Y was a bachelor living in his parent's house. He largely denied having a positive image of his father. Although he had lived in another city for several years while attending a university, it was only at home and from his mother that he found the complete care and attention that he demanded.

Heinrich Y was the fourth of five children and in his opinion had always been the least favored. Distinct inferiority feelings had even overshadowed his childhood and puberty. From his comments about his earlier therapy I concluded that he had been able to find security and support from the directive technique employed by the older and religious female psychotherapist. As also demonstrated by the present report, his ambivalence remained suppressed.

At the time of our therapy, the patient was again living with his bigotted mother, who admired him, took care of him, and also controlled him by helping him to plan his dates with women. She patiently bore his repeated outbreaks of depression. The stable character of this neurotic living arrangement could also be seen in the fact that a colleague had expressly told him a few years before that psychotherapy was essential. An offer of analysis at that time had foundered on his ambivalence. The patient had instead had hypnosis and homeopathic cures, each of which had satisfied his passive expectations and had effects that were short-term in nature.

The ups and downs of his moods were closely associated with admiration and confirmation; if the latter were lacking, his mood was in danger of switching to depression. The fixated behavior he displayed toward his mother provided him security; he was always able to obtain her attention and care. His conscious motives for living in his parent's house were both laziness and the opportunity to repeat his chronic complaints against his father. Because of his pronounced hypochondric nature, he forced his mother to base their daily meals on the particular color of his morning bowel movement.

His contacts outside his family were limited, being restricted to people who had to satisfy specific desires. They were primarily women with whom he enjoyed recreational activities; he rejected any further-reaching claims they might make. At the same time he was looking for the "woman of his life," one who united all the desirable features spread among his various contacts. He had professional contacts to men, but shyed away from permitting closer friendships to develop.

The crisis that led him to seek treatment was precipitated by his anxiety that he might have made a girlfriend pregnant and be held responsible. His initial attitude was characterized by great insecurity and distrust, which went so far that he refused to pay for therapy. After several months I managed to overcome his doubts to the extent that the external conditions for an analysis were finally established.

Several months into therapy (86th session) Heinrich Y referred to the factors that had radically changed his life recently. He mentioned, among other things, his relationship to his analyst. Since he had met me, he had for the first time had the feeling that somebody was there for him, that he was welcome, and that he could speak. This praise contained an element of anxiety that his warm feelings might have something to do with homosexuality.

At first I calmed him, saying that trust and homosexuality were two completely different things. My motive was to emphasize the differences in order to be able to better expose his unconscious identifications. My plan worked. He said he was afraid that things might go further. "I can't give you a hug," something he would have liked to have down at the beginning of the session. He said this development had started about Easter, i. e., a number of weeks before, when after a vacation break he came to the first session with the feeling of going to his lover.

I had noticed the increase in his positive feelings in the past weeks, but had not interpreted them. I now suggested that he give me a more precise description of his anxieties.

P: I mistrust myself about whether my feelings are entirely gentle. I sometimes fall in love with boys [apprentices he met at work], from a distance, especially in ones who look like I did as a boy, especially with blonds.

At this point he stopped and was silent for a longer period of time. I inquired whether he had recalled something that he was particularly ashamed of.

P: Well, just a thought, one I've had frequently but always pushed away immediately. If I could fuck a real ass some time, that would be a fantastic story.

A: Yes, what would be so fantastic?

P: Naturally I'd be the one who was active. My partner could be either a man or a woman; in either case, I don't want to see the front. Only the movement would be important, just this in and out. I'd finally have a sphincter that would take tight hold my penis.

Later in the session he disparaged the role of women, warding off his castration anxiety, by criticizing their "limpy holes," which he was afraid of falling into. This was the reason the other fantasy - the encircling snugness - exerted such an unbelievable fascination on him. Yet he had always brushed this thought away quickly whenever it came to him because, he said, it was impossible to speak with anyone about it.

A: When at the beginning of the session you told me about your moving feeling that you have found something new here, namely somebody who is there for you and listens to you, then this probably also meant that you can tell me about such fantasies without being rejected.

The patient then felt secure enough to tell me for the first time about his masturbation practices, which he preferred to having intercourse with women because he could stimulate himself precisely where it was most pleasurable. His glans was somewhat too sensitive, and he liked to stimulate himself on the shaft of his penis. The fantasy of using his hand to imitate a sphincter was particularly stimulating for him.

Important with regard to my considerations about how to proceed was that I let him have the active role and did not offer any deeper interpretations, such as that his comment about "limpy holes" might be based on a terrifying fantasy about being consumed (castrated) by a woman. At the end of the session I therefore only emphasized that he had kept these thoughts to himself until now because he was insecure about whether he would be rejected.

The patient began the following session by telling me a dream about a ski course, which he had had after the previous session.

P: While skiing we were in a group led by a woman, who told us that we were all incurably ill. She expected us to drown ourselves in a lake. I was afraid of dying and said that I didn't want to die. I managed to move over to one side, and all the others followed her command and drowned. I saw their heads in the water and called out to them, "I'm sure I'll find somebody who can cure me. You can die, but I want to live." I then fled to the other shore.

This woman reminded him of "Emma," the pejorative name he gave his earlier therapist. She had once told him that she had had a patient who had killed himself in her waiting room after four years of therapy, probably to keep him from doing something similar. At the time he had thought, "I'll kill myself to show the bitch that she's incompetent." He added that his wish to kill himself had been strong at the time, but that he now wanted to live, not to die. He said he was also somehow mad at me for not having immediately begun therapy following the preliminary interview. Then he distanced himself from the strong affect of his criticism. With decisiveness, he referred to the thoughts about committing suicide that he had had in the period before therapy actually began. Over and over again he worked himself into a tirade against me, making me responsible for his condition at that time. He said I should have offered him more hope during the preliminary interview; he had wanted more carrots, as it were, although he himself knew that it would only hold on for a couple of days.

At this point I managed to redirect his attention to the expectation he had in his dream of being saved. He immediately picked up this reference; yes, he was looking for a savior, someone to rescue him. He recalled that the passage "You might die, but I want to live" stemmed from a psalm that he prayed three to five times a day. He had chosen his earlier therapist because of her Christian orientation, but then felt that she had exerted substantial moral pressure on him. She had, he admitted, helped him get through a difficult period while he was at the university - like an admonishing teacher - yet she had also morally extorted him, saying that if he did not forswear his dirty fantasies, he would end in a terrible way, just like the other patient before him.

Heinreich Y then associated that he had been together with a girl the day before and they had been affectionate in public. Out of pure excitement, he had developed a large swelling in his upper arm. He felt he could uproot trees, while girls would be much too weak to do so.

With a view to the homosexual element of transference that was developing I gave the following interpretation. He hoped that I would be strong enough to survive the boxing match with him that might come of his stored power. The patient laughed heartily and freely. Clear traces of tears were visible in his eyes when he departed.

By means of my interpretation I turned the passivity of a dream looking for a savior into the active position of a son looking to conquer a spot of his own in the world via a test of strength with his father. My interpretation followed the consideration that the patient's derogatory, frequently clownish self-representation was rooted in his attempt to defend himself against strong feelings of rivalry, in order for him, in the position of the helpless boy at the mercy of the castrating mother, to find a masculine identification with his father. The analogy to the boxing match was supposed to express this, a test of strength at the limits of playful reality and encircled by the boxing ring. The fantasy about his preferred form of masturbation that he detailed in the previous session - a powerful sphincterlike ring on the shaft of his penis - also contained a conflict with homosexuality and pleasurable body feelings.

In the following sessions it became clear that the patient spoke to me by first name in his inner dialogues, using a form of address that is used for small boys. He compared his own powerful athletic figure with my own and did not believe that I would be up to a physical confrontation. He used the actual difference in size, being himself the largest, to disparage his hated father. In the first phase of therapy the patient had created the image of him as being a weak and worthless do-nothing. After the war, when the patient was 6 years old, he had not managed to reestablish himself in his own profession. He had not managed to provide sufficiently for the family, working only at part-time jobs.

In terms of therapeutic technique the point was to indicate what "the other shore" was that the patient was looking for in order to liberate himself from the powerful, caring, and consuming clasp of his mother. This theme was discussed again in the further course of the therapy. It became concretely clear how situations in which he was enclosed in an encircling space represented for him the pregenital mother, with whom he had to maintain contact and who, in the form of interchangable idealized women, determined his social life. This was again shown by a dream, which was about a grave danger. The immediate precipitant for this anxiety was that the patient had decided, after 18 months of therapy, to leave home and look for an apartment; he even made concrete plans to build a house of his own.

The patient's first comment was that I had closed the curtains (to protect the room from the sunlight). "When I'm able to close the curtains in a house of my own, that would be wonderful." Then he described his efforts to find an apartment, which was turning out to be difficult. He said that although he was increasingly beginning to react to things allergically at home, he did not want to leave in anger, but simply to become independent. He added that he had recently had two very funny dreams about being in danger. He then described the following dream.

P: I was carrying a backpack and walking through an underpass, accompanied by an Italian woman. She told me to be careful: "There's a gang; they're going to attack you." The woman was gone as I left the underpass, and then two men did come up to me. The one tore my backpack away from me and tossed it to the other one. I wasn't able to defend myself. It's terrible; in such dreams I'm always the loser.

His first association was about the Italian woman. Heinrich Y had frequently told me that the woman of his dreams was a black haired beauty with smoldering eyes, like the woman in a picture hanging on the wall of his parent's living room.

P: Where does it come from? It's happened so often recently; I have an exact mental picture of the dream. As long as the woman is there, nobody does anything to me. None of the bad guys does anything to me. Yesterday I went hiking with a woman I recently met, and I happened to think that there was always a woman present every time I've been tested. It's obvious that I can't cope with life without having a woman nearby. What does the backpack mean? People take my things away from me again. [He then came to speak of his fantasized future wife.] I believe I have to reach an agreement on maintaining separate property, or even better, for my wife to pay me rent. Maybe the two bad guys are also my tenants.

I asked about the underpass.

P: Well, it's just a bunch of nonsense. But yes, the underpass; I think I remember my duties, and next year is going to be a difficult one. The people might be the decisions I have to make in connection with the building. Ever since I was a child one of my important tasks has been to ward off thoughts that might be unchaste. I see in thoughts the danger of eternal damnation. You can have unchaste thoughts in a fraction of a second, a cardinal sin. If you die at that moment, then you're damned for all eternity. That's especially bad. And here it's really bad because I have to, or at least can, say everything. In the evening I often have to think, "Boy, at work today you really said some things. Who's going to use it as a trap for you?"

A: Your associations to the underpass could be nonsense or unchaste.

P: [Laughing] Yes, I immediately have to think of something, put it in, the cunt, go into a deep hole where there are a lot's of dangers waiting. The woman in the dream told me not to be afraid. Maybe when I have the right woman some time, I won't be afraid any more and can go into the hole without getting worried.

A: Maybe there's an unchaste side to the backpack, too.

P: [Laughing] Well, the young boys, they might have been about 14, maybe the young boys were a symbol. Perhaps they took my bag away from me. [Long pause] Today I'm again having doubts about the work here. It costs so much; my money is just running away – DM 77 for you and DM 30 for the time it costs me, making a total of DM 107. I believe I'm looking for arguments against our work here, to cut back. When the days start getting longer again, I'll have to cut the Friday session. Maybe the underpass means that I can't see any light in analysis. Maybe you are the woman and the underpass means that I have to submit to you. I think that it's no different here than in other places; I'll always prefer to submit in order to really be on the safe side and be sure that everything will be alright.

A: That means that I'm supposed to protect you against the bad guys, against your own bad thoughts.

P: Yes, hold off the unchaste ideas, yes that would be real nice. The only dangerous thing here, that's really the only evil. I think I'm really proud of myself, that I got something out of the dream. I'm really overwhelmed.

A: How old were you when you were a bad boy and had unchaste thoughts?

P: Oh, I used to be radical in fighting off everything. No, that's not quite true. Naturally I used to read some things secretly, for example about artificial insemination. It always gave me a hard-on. Once I even saw a naked breast. When I was 18 I read a book and it only said that two people had slept together. Boy, was I excited. Of course, I mentioned it during confession. So crazy, I was an ass, ruined my life. I'm 35 now and haven't managed to live yet. Thank God, it may not be too late for everything.

A: Is everything really still in the sack, in your backpack?

P: Well, I feel so impotent, as if somebody had stolen my bag. I'm generally incompetent. Of course, I cope with life, but not in the way I think about it; there I'm impotent. I had imagined doing so many things. [Pause] I've got a lot on my mind. I think I'll stop this stuff with the girlfriends. I don't want to tell you anything; I'm so ashamed. My new girlfriend congratulated me for not having married Rita. They know each other. I think I feel ashamed toward you. You're sure to really criticize me now. Saturday I met one in A.; I really made her fall in love with me. That was Berta, and Sunday I was with Claudia. I think all these contacts to women just cause me a lot of trouble; sometimes it's a real struggle to keep them apart.

A: All these contacts to women give you the feeling that there's still something in your backpack.

P: Yes, it's a kind of protection for me. As soon as there are more, then it starts, and they try to get my backpack. And that's why I'd never get married in winter. It would take the last energy I have, and going skiing is still my greatest love. Then I simply wouldn't have any strength left in reserve. [Pause]

A: You feel ashamed because you're also afraid that I will condemn you here.

P: Yes, a while ago it was very strong, a little less now, but I still have thoughts that I can't immediately talk about. For example, right now I see the cross section of a vagina. It's a fantasy that overwhelms me, that really takes hold of me, and the more I do against it, the clearer the image is. I remember that a teacher once distributed booklets on sex education. One picture in it showed the genitals in union. I have the booklet in a cupboard that I don't use much. Sometimes I happen across it, and then I get it out and look at it. I want to see something like that some time, really be there, like going back and forth. That's why I like to stand in front of the mirror and jerk off because I have the feeling I can really see it in detail. It's just important that it isn't simply gone. There's this constant feeling with women, the feeling that I lose sight of it. I once told Rita that she should do it with her hand, I preferred it that way, because then I could see everything. Watching is really important. I'm just split. In fantasy I would really like to have a good fuck, really going in and out, but in reality I can't take my eyes off it.

A: You become afraid when you lose sight of it.

P: Yes, when I lose sight of something, then I lose control of it. I got a hard-on that Claudia admired, but as soon as I wanted to put it to use it's gone. I think it really has something to do with anxiety. If I could only trust the girl. Maybe, when I really have a woman I can trust some time, then it will be alright. I'm sure it's not because of the fear of having a child; I don't think so any more.

A: You're really very ambivalent to women. On the one hand there is this anxiety, and on the other in the dream the woman was the one providing protection.

P: Yes, it's really funny. On the one hand I want to have one and can't trust her enough. I think I have a great need for success. I see my increase in energy as a measure of the therapeutic success. I only have strength in the chest, too little in my head and too little below my waist. I simply don't have the juice. I just had the idea that as soon as my house is finished, I'm going to get a sandbag and start boxing.

Commentary. If we consider the beginning of the session from the patient's perspective, we can assume that he experienced the office as being restrictive, and with reference to the dream it was logical to equate the underpass with the analyst's office. He needed the eye contact to the analyst to control any possible aggressive acts. Consequently, the interruption of his eye contact led to the activation of various dangers, resulting - in transference - in his fear of being ruined financially. However, his subordination also protected him from his anxiety of loss, with is multiple determinants. In analysis he experienced the anxiety localized in his penis, over which he had visual control, in his relationship to his analyst, and it was there that the numerous nuances of the subject of separation in transference were unfolded and worked through.

8.5.5 Commonplace Mistakes

Technical mistakes are inevitable. They play an important function in the process that A. Freud (1954, p. 618) referred to as the reduction of the psychoanalyst to his "true status." By admitting his mistakes, the analyst facilitates the elimination of idealizations.

By technical mistakes we mean all the deviations that an analyst makes from the middle line formed during the respective dyad and that ideally is extended from session to session without any substantial digressions. Important is the fact that we define the middle line dyadically. Based on his experience with an analyst, each patient develops a certain feeling for the customary *atmosphere* he expects in the sessions. Since the analyst's behavior is guided by rules, after a short while the patient can sense which attitude the analyst has to this or that subject.

An exchange of opinions takes place in the psychoanalytic dialogue. It is customary for misunderstandings to occur occasionally and for them to be clarified and overcome. The mistakes an analyst makes are, in contrast, facts that cannot be corrected but have to be acknowledged, and their *consequences* interpreted if at all possible. Mistakes, in particular, make it clear that the analyst's capacity for understanding is limited by his personality and his incomplete knowledge. This makes something of the analyst's true status visible. Malpractice, in contrast, implies deviations that lead to lasting damage as certified by a court.

The relationship between *therapeutic alliance* and transference must be taken into consideration when mistakes are evaluated. There is general agreement that the therapeutic alliance should have reached a degree of sufficient stability for realistic perspectives to be predominant despite the fact that fluctuations might still occur, especially during the termination phase.

In the psychoanalytic dialogue the interplay between transference and countertransference is rooted in the emotions and thoughts the analyst and patient have - whether mentioned in the dialogue or not - about emotional and cognitive processes, some of which are accessible to self-perception. Now we have to consider what the psychoanalyst contributes to the patient learning in the course of time to recognize his true status. As we can see from the memoires of Lampl-de Groot (1976) about her own analysis, Freud facilitated this process by making the interplay between the transference neurotic and "normal" aspects of the relationship apparent from his behavior. Such conspicuous differences are today probably only offered by a small number of psychoanalysts. It is therefore all the more important to look for other means that can lead to the elimination of idealizations.

We can no more expect a more realistic attitude to develop on its own and to appear as a phoenix out of the ashes of the transference neurosis than we can for the transference neurosis itself to develop without the analyst doing his part. The predominance of the therapeutic alliance in the later phase of therapy, as assumed by Greenson (1967), is process dependent inasfar as this shift takes place if the analyst has taken preparatory steps in the direction of termination when suitable themes are being discussed. Very appropriate in this connection are interruptions for vacations because they contain everything in miniature that is related to separation and its working through.

We would now like to describe two situations that are suited to clearly indicate the consequences mistakes can have. They intensify fluctuations between transference and working alliance that ultimately point to the separation at the termination of therapy.

The first point consists of the last session prior to a vacation interruption and the first session afterwards. This interruption occurred during a phase of treatment in which the patient had repeatedly raised the issue of *termination.* I did not feel that the transference neurosis had been worked through to a sufficient degree for me to have already started thinking about terminating the therapy. In my opinion it was important for Dorothea X simply to consider the topic itself. In the last session prior to the break we talked about whether she would still be dependent on being able to locate me mentally, i. e., whether she would be potentially able to reach me, at least in writing, in an emergency. I was uncertain, and the patient realized it; I showed my uncertainty in not telling the patient where I would be but, after hesitating, adding that I could be reached via my office - "in an emergency" - and would be in the office once in the middle of the break. In contrast to her earlier states of severe depression and anxiety neurosis, I judged that in the current situation she would hardly have a need to contact me; yet I was still uncertain, and this uncertainty led me to make a compromise offer. Dorothea X did not need to contact me during the relatively long vacation break, and came to the first session rested and free of symptoms. While greeting each other I responded spontaneously to a hidden allusion she made to my vacation by expanding on a comment she made about the nice weather to refer to my vacation as well. For the moment I acted without reflecting on what was happening, and my spontaneity stimulated the patient to make comparisons to the last session prior to the break. She compared my momentary spontaneity with my previous pausing to contemplate, and on the basis of this comparison she drew conclusions about how sick or how healthy she thought I felt she was. As I thought more about this problem, was silent for a longer period, and did not pay attention to her subsequent comments, she sensed my mental absence. She interpreted my distracted silence as a withdrawal that she feared she had provoked because I had taken her comments about the session prior to the break to be criticism.

I explained to Dorothea X the reasons for my contemplation and my being distracted, telling her that I did in fact have to carefully consider whether it was necessary or therapeutically useful to give a patient my vacation address. She responded by mentioning a series of other observations, all of which indicated how important it was for her to participate in my evaluation of her condition because she gained self-confidence from the confidence I placed in her ability to take stress. By acting spontaneously and naturally, I had transformed *her* image of me as a overly worried psychoanalyst into one that was more accurate; my spontaneity, she said, made her healthier. The more confidence I placed in her by reacting "naturally," the more confidence she said she was able to gain in herself.

Many topics take on special importance at the termination of a therapy. Dorothea X had noted with great and visible disappointment that she increasingly viewed me more realistically although she ardently tried to ward it off. This process of normalization was further eased by several other mistakes and an incident in which, in her opinion, I "really bungled" something. This bungle was that I had advised her to soon go for an examination when she thought that she was pregnant, something she both desired and feared, and as a widow and mother of grown children could not imagine – among other reasons because of the danger to the child from a pregnancy at her age. In her opinion a conception could have taken place as early as several months before, and time was precious if an abortion was necessary. It turned out to be a false pregnancy, and the changes her body had undergone were typical of one. Although I had not overlooked the wish aspect and the hypomanic happiness she showed while describing her condition, she had unconsciously taken my comment about the urgency of a examination to be a step preparing for the abortion of the (transference) child. It was impossible for me to make up for my bungle. She herself became aware, however, that her false pregnancy was a misguided and vain attempt to make up for an earlier abortion. Her longing at this time was directed toward having a harmonious relationship, which came true inasmuch as her friend would have welcomed a pregnancy if it had occurred in a different phase of life. That this phase was gone for good was something the patient became painfully aware of. My mistake thus contributed to her achieving a more realistic attitude to her life.

I had lost a gem from my crown by not understanding her deeply unconscious desire. Yet there were several other situations that contributed to deidealizing my role. A topic must be mentioned in this context that arose during the termination phase and that had a connection to an earlier situation in therapy. While we were playing through the termination of therapy at that time, the patient had asked me about the role that aggression played. She understood me to say that aggressive topics might reappear at the termination. I could not recall making this statement, but I had obviously caused a misunderstanding that – while uncorrected – continued to be my "mistake" because such a statement would have to obstruct the termination and put a taboo on aggression for a patient who suffered precisely from the anxiety she might hurt someone's feelings and was constantly striving to compensate. The patient had in fact drawn the consequence from my mistake that she could not be aggressive because she would then enter the phase of termination and no longer be in a position to offer compensation for the damage she inflicted.

In this context a unique resistance manifested itself. It consisted in the patient consciously raising other topics for discussion; although working through these topics had a high therapeutic value, the patient brought them up in order to avoid or postpone aggressive transferences. She described "typical ways women are nasty" and mentioned numerous examples for how the envy and hypocracy of woman bothered her. At the same time she developed a deep longing for harmony and togetherness with a woman. By this time the patient had become aware of her ambivalence toward her mother and the neurotic repetition associated with her without being able to admit the full extent of her longing. The defenses still active in her were demonstrated by an exclamation she made in one session, "If only I were a little lesbian!" She changed after I immediately replied, "In that sense, we're all a little lesbian."

By these means aggressiveness was avoided in transference and shifted to her relations to women. It could also be said that the patient displaced her mother transference, acting it out or discovering it in her relationship to the women she knew.

Working through her ambivalent relationship to her mother ultimately provided the basis for an increased capacity to be more aggressive in transference, as demonstrated by the following example. Dismayed and with intense inner suffering, the patient experienced, for example in her clever manipulating, especially while shopping, that she was much more her father's daughter than she had wanted to believe. She was tortured by the fact that she had unconsciously adopted his petty figuring, which she found repulsive. In order to overcome this form of behavior and to be different from her father, she had incidentally always insisted on paying a portion of the costs for therapy herself. She did not submit any claims to the insurance company that would have covered all the costs, instead only submitting claims to another insurance organization that only covered part of the expenses, leaving her to pay approximately DM 40 herself. This self payment amounted to a financial burden that her family was able to bear without it requiring any substantial sacrifices of her or her family. The patient experienced the fact that she bore part of the costs as an expression of her independence in her relationship to me aw well as toward her father. Her inner tension between her intention to have a free and generous attitude toward money and, on the other hand, her father's superego dictate to be frugal and her own inclination to petty figuring was clearly demonstrated by a delay in preparing a bill; the delay might have led the insurance organization to refuse to make its payment in full. This additional burden would have been too much for the patient to bear, and the "father" in her would have won over her autonomy.

Her observation about how I reacted to her comments about my mistakes further increased her insight. She noted that I made great efforts to avoid making mistakes, and I naturally acknowledged that misunderstandings do occur and that they were my responsibility. My verbal admission of my mistakes was, however, apparently accompanied by an ideal of flawlessness. Dorothea X wanted a psychoanalyst who was sovereign in human matters but who could also give an averbal signal that mistakes were part of the trade and a part of life. As a matter of fact, this patient did open my eyes to the fact that my own ambition kept me from accepting the fact that mistakes are commonplace events, and from being able to deal with them in a more magnanimous manner. Dorothea X sought a role model for magnanimity, in order to be able to gain a new, i.e., more magnanimous, attitude to herself.

8.6 Interruptions

From the point of view of diagnosis, it is logical to consider whether interruptions precipitate typical separation reactions, regardless of whether they are more characterized by anxiety or by depression. From the point of view of therapy, however, it is decisive that the analyst provide assistance in a manner that contributes to increasing the patient's capacity to gradually master such reactions. We therefore recommend that the analyst also consider measures to bridge interruptions.

Example

Clara X came to the last session before Christmas.

P: In the last session a person has either got nothing to say or . . . or something important on his mind but that he can't remember. [Silence] I simply don't want to tackle the topic of separation. I have the impression that I've always evaded it. Sometimes even by getting sick. I'm sure it's connected with my anxiety toward emotions.

A: Your anxiety about emotions you can't control . . . leads you to avoid some painful things, but not merely painful things. The less filled with emotions, the more intense the pain of separation turns out to be. And avoiding emotions causes separations to be more painful than they would have to be; it leads to a feeling of deprivation, an issue we talked about in the previous session. We're talking about the provisions for a journey.

Consideration. Various ideas were combined in this interpretation. I presumed that Clara X was in a state of chronic and all-encompassing privation because of her eating disturbance. In connection with temporary interruptions or even the final separation, a patient's longing to obtain compensation for the deficit increases. At the same time, at some level of consciousness some kind of balancing takes place. Although anorexic individuals attempt to deceive themselves by appearing helpless to themselves and others, in some corner of their mind they are completely aware of their great longing for their hunger to be satisfied. The limitation of one's needs, even when this takes the extreme forms of abstinence, is an attempt to avoid all the disappointments that in fact do frequently accompany an increase in unconscious longings and desires. My interpretation was thus based on the assumption that it is easier for a patient to separate from the analyst if his vital needs are satisfied. The pain of separation can in this case also grow: "All desire seeks eternity, deep, deep eternity" (Nietzsche, *Thus Spoke Zarathustra*). In this regard the metaphor of "provisions for a journey" is a paltry offer for bridging the gap despite its numerous connotations.

Clara X drew my attention to the fact that I had frequently spoken of provisions for a journey prior to interruptions, something I had not been aware of.

A: My favorite words cannot simply produce the provisions for a journey.

The patient wondered whether she had ever had the experience outside of therapy that provisions had helped her get over a separation. Long silence, sighs. After about three minutes she asked what a person could do to cope with separations, adding that one method was to think about the reunion.

P: What do you have to say about it?

A: To reunion? You're thinking of the reunion, of bridging the gap and continuing, and of the new beginning as a link. A reunion provides perspective.

P: Unfortunately I can't find any perspectives. January 12th - the next session. By then I will have forgotten all my good resolutions for the new year. At any rate I hope you don't show up with your leg in a cast [she knew that I was going skiing]. And I hope that you have something of your vacation. Maybe you'll even get a tan. [Then she asks directly] Are you going away together with your wife, or alone in order to be able to think without being disturbed?

A: Hum, what would you prefer?

P: [Laughs out loud] You're not going to plan your vacation according to what I prefer.

A: It's important to know what you prefer. You're probably ambivalent, making it not very easy to answer. To have the peace and quiet to reflect and write would probably be easier if I weren't distracted by my wife. From that point of view you would probably prefer to send me on vacation alone.

P: Perhaps I'm thinking along a different line, about your wife most of all. Maybe it would be boring for her if your thoughts took posssession of you; it would be monotonous for your wife. Then it would be better to stay here and work. Let's say, my tendency in your wife's place would be to go along for a week after the holidays, for relaxation and skiing, and then to leave you to yourself for another week and in that week, who knows, go somewhere. If you have something meaningful to do, to do something for yourself, to visit friends.

A: That's a very wise solution, thinking about my wife in this way, and meaning the best for me and her and yourself. Because it also means that I would have eight days to dedicate to thinking intensively about you.

P: I wasn't assuming that you would think about me; I asumed that you would think about your patients in general.

A: If I think about my patients, then that includes you too. That you weren't thinking about yourself most of all is connected with the fact that you, how did we say it once, are afraid of your uncontrollable emotions and desires.

P: I'm not so sure about that. The situation is a little different. If you reflect while one of us is gone, well it's something that makes me feel rather uneasy. [Two minute pause] Maybe I'm afraid that you'll reach some final decision and I can't say anything about it.

A: Oh, perhaps because you'd be excluded.

P: Parents think about how to raise their children when they aren't around, and make decisions.

A: And that is why I said that it's important whether you benefit from it.

P: Simply the fact that it happens like that would be a denial of my rights, even if it did benefit me. [She continued ironically] Yes, that's how it always is, everything is for the child's own good, and it's still a disconcerting idea.

A: The idea is disconcerting, but you also often have some thoughts of your own, about me, between sessions, and I'm not there either.

P: That's something I avoid.

A: Because you'd take possession of me without my being able to say anything. It's eerie. You experience very intensely that I take possession of you in my thoughts and control you and deny you your rights. Obviously an important reason for you to avoid thinking about me or anything else that belongs to me.

Commentary. The analyst assumed that the patient had such intense claims to possess him, keep him, hold on to him, take possession of him, to deny his rights, that she - via projective identification - was afraid that the analyst also had control of her. In the patient's language this was that her rights were being denied. The issue was the control of oral impulses, which however cannot be so complete as to prevent disturbances from being felt. On the contrary, the more aspects of one's self that are denied and return in projection, the larger the anxiety about being overwhelmed orally from the outside, i. e., by the analyst. (On introjective identification, see Sect. 3.7).

P: The other item, the one that's eerie, is . . . is this wondering. I know it from my mother. It went in the direction of masochistic doubts about everything she might have done wrong, in the direction of guilt feelings and pessimism, sorrow and so forth. I don't like it. And now I'm going to say a outrageous sentence. A mother is supposed to believe in her children and that means in herself too. That doesn't mean that you won't make any mistakes; that's not the point. It's the anxiety, the doubts about what will happen that really makes life miserable for her. That's also what I think of in connection with this wondering, that it could go in this direction, and I don't want it to happen like that. I could imagine that for you primarily negative things come out when I talk about my ideas like this. Most of all you think that she just can't stop talking about cardinal sins, she'll never manage to stop smoking, and she won't manage with the eating either, so everything will stay the way it's been, and otherwise she may talk about the good fairy at the junction, and then she's up and ready to make her own way, drags a breakfast up here and wants a child, and a couple of weeks later has decided she doesn't after all. And then she hangs around for a while. You just can't really understand her. Everything is very immature, and otherwise there's the feeling, yes, what is there then!

A: And now our reflection has come to a very satisfying conclusion.

P: [Laughs loudly] At the moment I don't think so at all.

A: Well, for me it has, namely the conclusion that I've understood why you don't want me to think about you, and why you avoid thinking about me. Because you are so terribly anxious of taking possession, of denying my rights, of not worrying about what I want, what I think, but that you want to take possession, uncontrolled. Now I've also understood why it's so difficult to stop smoking, because stopping would be very sensible for your health, but it's logical for psychic reasons that you can't stop doing it because you concentrate all your desires in it.

P: With the taking possession, there's something to it; I'm afraid so. Dominating and possessive, I'm afraid of it. How much of it is true and how much is my fear?

A: Both. You are like that and you are afraid of being much more tyrannical that you really are, because everything is locked away in the basement, where the potatoes are rooting, driving lascivious roots. In light they would turn green.

Commentary. The supportive and encouraging side of this interpretation seems to be based on the view that the libidinal forces rampant in the dark might take on an eerie shape and then actually become dangerous for more than an individual's preconscious premonitions. A consequence of this is that evil and destructiveness are dependent on development, i. e., are variables that depend on unconscious defense processes, as we explained in Vol.1 (Sect. 4.4.2). It was Freud's opinion "that the instinctual representative develops with less interference and more profusely if it is withdrawn by repression from conscious influence. It proliferates *in the dark*, as it were, and takes on *extreme forms of consciousness*" (Freud 1915d, p. 149, emphasis added; a correct translation might read, "... as it were, taking on the form of extreme expressions").

P: But when I go down into the basement, then I'm seized by immense horror; I close the door again right away. You can't look at those things. Once in a while I take a peek. Well, toward you I can't feel it; I have a block, but in the family I notice it occasionally. I really can't judge how far I do it and how much it's my desire once again because I would actually like to have the say about it and have everything under control. The mother of the brigade. What I say is how it's done. I'm completely shattered if I don't get my way. When I take a closer look, then everything gets confused. First I get enraged, and then I withdraw, and usually I withdraw before I get enraged, because of my fear that I might become enraged. But why do I have to smoke if I'm possessive?

Consideration. I recalled the sensations I had from smoking and stopping.

A: You've got something in your hand and take it inside you. You inhale, absorb it. At this point you can finally be greedy and desirous and give up your block.

After this there was a relaxed silence that lasted about five minutes. The patient said "merry Christmas" upon her departure, and I returned the good wishes.

Commentary. The last interpretation probably provided relief and led to relaxation. The analyst encouraged the patient to achieve oral satisfaction even though it is located at the level of a substitution. Yet such substitute satisfactions are vital to the severely ill and contribute to easing separation reactions. Transitional objects facilitate the bridging of gaps.

9 The Psychoanalytic Process: Treatment and Results

Introduction

Some of the psychoanalytic treatments presented in this chapter go back to the form of systematic case study we mentioned in Sect. 1.3. Nostalgia is not the reason that we refer back to therapies that are long past; the reason is that the long follow-up periods are an excellent basis for discussing the *outcome of therapy*. The research into the process and outcome of psychoanalysis that we have initiated in Ulm has developed out of our experience with systematic case studies (Thomä 1978) and the investigation of interpretative actions (see Sect. 8.3); the results of this research have motivated us to adopt a new understanding of the psychoanalytic process (see Vol.1, Chap. 9). More is expected of this research than we can present in this textbook, which for didactic reasons must have a broad clinical basis and include a large number of different cases. The combined research into the process and outcome of psychoanalysis with respect to individual cases, which we and others have propagated, is still in its infancy (Grawe 1988). If we were to describe such cases in the necessary detail, then this textbook would consist of only one of them.

The important therapeutic changes in cases other than those presented in this chapter can be followed without any great effort by reading the individual cases referred to throughout the book in sequence (see the index of patients at the beginning of the book). In addition, Sects. 5.1–5.3 contain descriptions of typical excerpts of an analysis, selected with regard to a series of dreams, and Sect. 6.3.1 contains an excerpt of an analysis prepared for a referee within the peer report system of applying for health insurance coverage.

This chapter begins with a section entitled "Anxiety and Neurosis;" we know of no better place to discuss this important topic. This section (Sect. 9.1) provides the reader a survey of the psychoanalytic theory of anxiety, which is followed by the case studies in which anxiety played a central role (Sects. 9.2–9.5). Since neurotic anxieties play a significant role in every treatment - even where they are not openly manifest among the primary symptoms - anxiety constitutes an important general indicator for evaluating the success of therapy. It has furthermore proved necessary for us to discuss several central concepts of the general and specific theories of neurosis. Thus following the presentation of a case of neurodermatitis (Sect. 9.6), we discuss nonspecificity (Sect. 9.7), regression (Sect. 9.8), alexithymia (Sect. 9.9), and the role of the body in the psychoanalytic method (Sect. 9.10). Finally, in Sect. 9.11, we invite the reader to confront the problems involved in preparing a systematic psychoanalytic case study.

9.1 Anxiety and Neurosis

We will now provide a short survey of the theory of anxiety, before turning to several specific forms of anxiety. Although we argued the necessity of a differentiated consideration of affects in Vol.1 (Sect. 4.2), we are justified in focusing on anxiety in this section since many affects have an anxiety component. As Freud (1926d, p. 144) once summarized, anxiety is "the fundamental phenomenon and main problem of neurosis."

In making a diagnosis, analysts usually proceed from the specific nature of the anxiety manifestation. One important criterion for differentiation is the more or less close link of neurotic anxieties to a particular situation. Anxiety neurosis is characterized by free floating anxiety, which seems to appear for no apparent reason and is therefore experienced as inevitable, uncontrollable, and potentially fatal. Both the concept of anxiety neurosis and the first complete and still valid description of its symptoms stem from Freud, who distinguished in diagnosis between the syndrome of anxiety neurosis and neurasthenia. He used the term "anxiety neurosis" to refer to this syndrome "because all its components can be grouped round the chief symptom of anxiety" (Freud 1895b, p. 91). Among the bodily disturbances that occur in an anxiety attack are, according to Freud, cardiac dysfunction, cardiac palpitation with arrhythmia, tachycardia, breathing disturbances, nervous dyspnea, sweating, trembling and shaking, attacks of diarrhea, and locomotional dizziness. Characteristic of anxiety neurosis are that it is manifest in attacks and is accompanied by hypochondriac expectations.

Frequently one component of the syndrome assumes a predominant role in the patient's experiencing, and it is not unusual for the anxiety to be tied primarily to one symptom (e. g., the tachycardia, nervous dyspnea, sweating, or diarrhea). The syndrome of anxiety neurosis and the numerous manifestations of its components afflict a large number of the patients who come to analysis. Among those described here are Beatrice X, who suffered from a breathing disturbance (Sect. 9.2); Christain Y, whose primary problems were arrythmias and sweating (Sect. 9.3); and Rudolf Y, who had diarrhea when he was overwhelened by panic attacks. There can be no doubt that anxiety is the fundamental problem in every neurosis and in the psychic component of the genesis and course of many somatic illnesses.

It is instructive to demonstrate the changes that have occurred in the last hundred years by referring to the complex of symptoms called anxiety neurosis. During this period of time our knowledge of the somatic correlates of anxiety – i. e., the physiology, neuroendocrinology, and neurophysiology of anxiety – has increased substantially. On the basis of epidemiological, neurochemical, and therapeutic studies of anxiety illnesses, the American Psychiatric Association's classification (DSM-III, 1980) subsumes under the term "anxiety disturbances" a series of psychic disturbances such as panic attacks with or without agoraphobia, social and simple phobias, compulsion, and posttraumatic stress reactions. This classification attributes a dominant role to the special subgroup "panic attacks" as a prototype of other anxiety disturbances. For example, in the most recent revision (DSM-IIIR, 1987), agoraphobia was not viewed as a subform of the phobias, but primarily as a consequence of previous panic attacks, which have led to avoidance behavior. Of interest to the psychoanalyst here is the fact that the diagnostic criteria for the newly defined subgroup "panic disturbances" are largely the same as those Freud described for anxiety attacks in 1895. In his first description of anxiety neurosis Freud also viewed agoraphobia as a consequence of such an attack of anxiety. On the other hand, the physiological understanding of anxiety that Freud (1895b) had considered the basis of anxiety neurosis and panic attacks was submitted to a revision in psychoanalysis long ago. One reason was the discovery that free floating anxiety merely appears to occur for no reason. In anxiety neurosis it is possible for a wealth of nonspecific and unconsciously perceived danger signals to precipitate an anxiety attack because of an increased disposition for anxiety resulting from an individual's particular experiences. This discovery led Freud, in his epoch-making study *Inhibitions, Symptoms and Anxiety* (1926d), to revise the psychoanalytic theory of anxiety. One important passage reads:

Real danger is a danger that is known, and realistic anxiety is anxiety about a known danger of this sort. Neurotic anxiety is anxiety about an unknown danger. Neurotic danger is thus a danger that has still to be discovered. Analysis has shown that it is an instinctual danger. By bringing this danger which is not known to the ego into consciousness, the analyst makes neurotic anxiety no different from realistic anxiety, so that it can be dealt with in the same way. There are two reactions to real danger. One is an affective reaction, an outbreak of anxiety. The other is a protective action. The same will presumably be true of instinctual danger. (Freud 1926d, p. 165)

The advance in Freud's explanatory model consists in the fact that the anxiety reaction was traced back to a danger situation:

We can find out still more about this if, not content with tracing anxiety back to danger, we go on to enquire what the essence and meaning of a danger-situation is. Clearly, it consists in the subject's estimation of his own strength compared to the magnitude of the danger and in his admission of helplessness in the face of it - *physical helplessness* if the danger is real and *psychical helplessness* if it is instinctual .... Let us call a situation of helpless of this kind that has been actually experienced a *traumatic situation.* We shall then have good grounds for distinguishing a traumatic situation from a *danger-situation* .... The signal announces: "I am expecting a situation of helplessness to set in," or: "The present situation reminds me of one of the traumatic experiences I have had before. Therefore I will anticipate the trauma and behave as though it had already come, while there is yet time to turn it aside." Anxiety is therefore on the one hand an expectation of a trauma, and on the other a repetition of it in a mitigated form. Thus the two features of anxiety which we have noted have a different origin. Its connection to expectation belongs to the danger-situation, whereas its indefiniteness and lack of object belong to the traumatic situation of helplessness - the helplessness anticipated in the danger-situation. (Freud 1926d, p. 166, emphasis added)

Anxiety, as "the fundamental phenomenon and main problem of neurosis," demonstrates its central position in the psychogenetic and psychodynamic explanation of symptoms. The latter arise in order for the subject to avoid specific danger situations - signalled by the increase in anxiety - and the helplessness (trauma) associated with them.

Despite the far-reaching revisions, many ambiguities in the psychoanalytic theory of anxiety have remained, as a survey by Compton (1972a, b, 1980) convicingly demonstrates. Freud never repudiated the idea of anxiety as transformed libido. Rank's theory of birth trauma, although rejected as an explanation of neurotic anxieties, continued to serve as a model for the pathophysiology of anxiety. Freud went on "to overemphasize energies which from the start had interfered with the development of a psychoanalytic theory of affects" (Compton 1972a, p. 40). We agree with Rangell that anxiety, "which is *always* a signal of the *danger* of *psychic* trauma, is always a reaction to its presence" (1968, p. 389, emphasis added). It is the imminent and present danger which causes a panic attack or a state of free floating anxiety. Unconscious motives can be regularly discoverd by the psychoanalytic method.

Waelder (1960) criticized that the term "anxiety signal" does not precisely reproduce the sequence of endopsychic events. He postulated that fear or anxiety does not constitute an essential element in the sequence "perception of danger-adaptive reaction," and rather that a "danger signal" is biologically necessary to precipitate certain reactions. According to Waelder, this signal does not need to consist of a sensation of anxiety; he suggested that one speak of a danger signal instead of an anxiety signal because in this sequence the sensation of anxiety is not or not yet contained in the signal itself. The fact that the awareness of psychic or physical sensations of anxiety increases to a degree that makes it impossible for the real or imagined danger situation to be avoided sheds light precisely on chronic states of neurotic anxiety. The reason, according to Waelder, is that in these states there is a constant danger signal together with an incapacity for active coping.

Expressed in terms of behavior theory, the danger (threat) elicits an emergency reaction (Cannon 1920). The evaluation of the danger leads to either escape or attack, depending on the anticipated relative strengths of the threat and what is threatened. Anxiety and anger are the emotional correlates of escape and attack and have, via feedback loops, motivating power. A danger signal can thus trigger either an anxiety signal or an aggressive affect.

The difference between *real* and *psychic* helplessness is blurred in anxiety attacks, creating a ongoing trauma whose effects are cumulative. The paralyzed and blocked action potential thus gets stuck, so to speak, at the stage of the unconscious schema, where purposive action is dedifferentiated. Repeated defeats also stimulate the blocked unconscious aggression that, in the sense of Freud's instinctual danger, now even leads to an increase in anxiety. It is thus no coincidence that the affect physiologies of anxiety and of aggression are very similar.

If the analyst proceeds from the phenomenology of the anxieties described by the patient, the dangers seem to be clear. The anxiety about becoming insane is a condition whose many aspects reflect all the subsets of feeling and acting that the patient himself experiences, ranging from the "insane" loss of control to the disintegration or destruction of his previous identity or self-esteem. What the anxiety neurotic is ultimately afraid of thus seems to be clear: the destruction of his existence, which in his experiencing can either take more the form of his social ego or of his body-ego, i.e., his body image.

Even at the phenomenological level, there are discrepancies in how members of this large group of patients experience their conditions. These discrepancies constitute a starting point for the psychoanalytic method. For example, a distinguishing feature of the feared event is that it does *not* occur. Whoever is afraid of becoming insane or dying from an infarct does not experience such a fate any more frequently than is statistically probable. Indeed, these anxieties even seem to speak against the actual manifestation of a psychosis or an infarct. Yet such statistical data are not convincing to the patients themselves or only have a short-term effect. Important is the observation that anxiety neurotic patients are quite able to bear real dangers and that they - aside from their imagined anxieties - have no greater anxieties about dying than healthy individuals do. It is thus not true that anxiety neurotics think, to use everyday terms, that they are more important than they really are or that they, because of a pronounced narcissism, cannot accept the idea that life is finite and death inevitable. Precisely because an individual cannot fully anticipate his own death, at most experience it in his imagination and by analogy, the end of life remains a secret that is the object of speculation and fantasies. Every thorough examination of an anxiety neurotic consequently discloses that the anxiety the patient experiences about *dying or being destroyed* expresses a disguised *anxiety about life.* This opens psychoanalysis an access to the origin of helplessness, according to Freud's theory of anxiety, and to overcoming it with the help of therapy. In therapy the anxiety about death or the loss of one's physical or psychic existence (e.g., anxiety about cardiac arrest or a psychotic loss of control) is transformed into biographical situations of danger and helplessness that the individual was originally unable to master and that he now, under more favorable conditions, can overcome. A sequence of events regularly occurs in therapy that permits the analyst to draw conclusions about the origin of neurotic anxieties. The neurotic anxieties about dying, whose numerous manifestations have become symbolic for being left alone, loss, and destruction - and which the affected individual submits to in disturbing passivity - can be dissolved into life-historical elements and reintegrated. During this process there is usually not a linear reduction in neurotic anxieties and their transformation into weaker real dangers that can be experienced and overcome in the therapeutic relationship. In fact, anxieties that have multiplied to become symptoms can reach extreme intensities in transference. Part of the analyst's therapeutic skill is to apply technical rules in a way that the transformation of anxieties linked with symptoms into an interactional context promotes the patient's well-being and cure. The following general rule may aid in orientation: The more severe an anxiety disorder and the longer it has undermined the individual's self-confidence, becoming an anxiety permeating every aspect of existence, the larger is the potential for interactional anxiety to be rekindled in the therapeutic relationship. We agree with Mentzos (1984) that the anxiety about dying that is experienced by the anxiety neurotic develops on the basis of displacements and other unconscious defense processes, which in therapy can be traced back in the opposite direction.

In summary, we would like to emphasize that a linkage is established between anxiety, as an affect, and the helplessness that can occur in typical danger situations. A central place in Freud's theory is occupied by the anxiety about object loss or the loss of the object's love, i.e., separation anxiety; castration anxiety is a special instance of this and therefore subordinate to it. A *depressive* reaction often predominates in object loss (see Sect. 9.3). The common denominator of anxiety and depression is the helplessness toward losses that are real or experienced psychically. Häfner described these observations, which can be explained in psychoanalytic terms, in the following manner:

If we proceed from the manifest anxiety disorders, such as panic attacks, generalized anxiety syndrome, or agoraphobias, then we also, depending on the severity of the anxiety syndrome, come to the 40%-90% of those affected who have already been through one depressive episode or who are also suffering from depressive symptoms.... Anxiety, as I have previously tried to demonstrate, has something to do with the threat of dangers. Anxiety can have something to do with losses, being left alone, or more universal threats to one's own existence and what is of value to it. One of the reasons for the frequent joint manifestation of anxiety and depression probably consists of these elements of a threat to one's existence, which differ only marginally. The connection between the two can be sequential; the transition from severe panic states to generalized helplessness and depression is an example of a process that takes place rapidly. A slower transition from anxiety states to depression is frequently encountered in the course of severe anxiety disorders, in which the anxieties spread through several spheres of life, block activity and self-security, and sometimes lead to a continued increase in the helplessness an individual experiences. (Häfner 1987, p. 198)

It is essential from therapeutic perspectives that the danger signals corresponding to a specific helplessness be recognized; just as important, however, is to find forms of coping that lead out of the helplessness and extend the patient's scope for action. Just talking out loud may help the person groping in the dark, enabling him to gain reassurance of his self.

The psychoanalytic theory of anxiety in our opinion not only explains a complex phenomenology extending from the apparently empty existential anxiety to psychotic anxieties, but also clarifies the points different therapies proceed from. This makes it all the more surprising that - to use a phrase from Hoffmann (1987, p. 528) - an "overly rushed biologization of human anxiety" was accompanied by the conception of a biologically rooted anxiety disorder that disregarded the knowledge that psychoanalysis and psychosomatic medicine have compiled on free floating anxiety for almost a hundred years. Margraf et al. (1986) mentioned that until recently no particular significance was attributed to Freud's complete clinical description of anxiety attacks. D.F. Klein (1981) and Sheehan and Sheehan (1983) have designed biological models of the anxiety attack; in these models the biological arguments merge in the concept of "panic attack." According to them, the apparently *spontaneous* manifestation of the anxiety attack differs qualitatively from the anticipatory anxiety that can be found in phobias. Another distinguishing criterion for these authors is the difference in response to psychopharmaceuticals. Tricyclic antidepressives and monoaminooxydase inhibitors seem to be more effective for panic attacks, while benzodiazepine derivatives induce a symptomatic improvement in anticipatory anxieties. These authors have presented a biological model of endogenous anxiety and panic attacks without ackowledging that these anxieties occur in reaction to *unconsciously* feared precipitants that as such are inaccessible to the individual concerned yet are amenable to successful analysis. A drug therapy of anxiety that is limited to the somatic symptoms and ignores psychic causes has also been the object of strong criticism by behavior therapy, as shown by the controversy between Klein et al. (1987), Klein (1987), and Lelliott and Marks (1987).

The anticipated influence that the worldwide spread of the DSM-III system may achieve in this regard is a cause for concern. In current psychiatric research, primarily biological hypotheses are being considered for the origin of panic attacks. This has resulted in a primacy of psychopharmaceutical therapy for anxiety disturbances, as opposed to psychoanalysis and behavior therapy. Insufficient attention is being paid to the psychodynamic precipitants and psychological factors of anxiety attacks. A very large number of patients are thus receiving one-sided - and consequently inadequate - pharmacological treatment regardless of whether it is possible to demonstrate that the anxiety attacks have psychic precipitants. This is the case although anxiety disorders exhibiting a more or less complete manifestation of the syndrome described by Freud belong, together with alcoholism and depressions, to the most common psychic illnesses. In an anxiety attack a biological pattern rooted in a personal disposition manifests itself when there are situative precipitants. It is a conspicuous feature of medical history that the central significance of Freud's description of anxiety neurosis, as a pathophysiological syndrome, has been rediscovered while the psychic conditions for its origin and course have been neglected. Even beta-blockers only alleviate the somatic symptoms constituting an important aspect of the manifestation of anxiety, such as cardiac palpitations. We agree with Häfner that the psychic processes leading to anxiety states as a rule cannot be overcome by a drug therapy:

> The most that can be achieved is that the blockade of severe anxieties enables the affected individual to successfully use his own capacities to cope with anxiety. Chronic states of anxiety, especially anxiety neuroses, require psychotherapy. (Häfner 1987, p. 203)

The overreliance on tranquilizers in treating psychic disorders can be seen, for example, in the fact that tranquilizers are taken by about 10% of the population of the USA, that they rank third among prescribed drugs, and that the value of their annual sales in the FRG amounts to DM 240 million.

In fact, the symptomatic effectiveness of tranquilizers has not been demonstrated to be statistically significant precisely for patients with neurotic disorders and symptoms of anxiety and depression. The patients treated with placebo in these comparative studies also showed clear improvements, particularly in long-term treatments. This demonstrates the significance of the general therapeutic factors that enter into treatment via the doctor-patient relationship and the psychological and psychotherapeutic orientation of therapists (Kächele 1988a).

A disposition to anxiety reactions, which is often referred to as a trait, can be transformed into an acute state of anxiety by a multitude of danger signals (see Spielberger 1980). In extreme cases, almost every stimulus can precipitate an anxiety attack and turn, if left untreated, the free floating anxiety into a chronic condition. At the other end of the spectrum, even if it is not possible to draw a firm distinction, are the phobias, which only precipitate anxiety when there is a circumscribed stimulus or specific situation that the patient can avoid. Greenson (1959) reported that diffuse anxiety states resembling anxiety neurosis are manifest at the beginning of many phobias, in which a secondary linkage between the anxiety attack and the associated situation is drawn by means of causal attribution. The individual is free of anxiety insofar as he avoids the phobic object, e. g., the spider, snake, mouse, open square, bridge, or airplane.

A distinction is commonly made between a diffuse and undirected anxiety and the fear related to a concrete danger. This distinction has, as Mentzos (1984) has emphasized,

> lost in significance in ordinary language because the word anxiety is also used with regard to a concrete danger. Yet it still seems sensible to differentiate between more diffuse, less organized, undirected, somatic anxiety reactions, on the one hand, and more structured, organized, desomatisized, and clearly directed reactions, on the other, even if in practice it is not always possible or desirable to draw a sharp distinction between anxiety and fear. In the fewest of cases is it possible to proceed from either this or that; on the contrary, there are countless nuances in the continuum from diffuse anxiety to concrete, directed fear. (Mentzos 1984, p. 14)

An anxiety that first appears in a specific situation may later possibly be precipitated by other, similar situations. This stimulus generalization takes place to the degree that avoidance behavior increases as a result of negative reinforcement. Avoidance in turn increases the anxiety about a danger situation, which can be an additional reason for the disproportion between the observed precipitant and the severity of the panic attack.

Disproportion here means that the patient reacts psychosomatically as if he were in great danger. If the conscious and unconscious ideas that anxiety neurotic patients have about threats are taken seriously, then there are good reasons for the manifestation of the anxieties that are freely floating and only appear to lack an object. The threats experienced by the anxiety neurotic are so overpowering because he cannot avoid the situation precipitating the anxiety; destruction is thus ubiquitous. To common sense, the person suffering from anxiety only imagines dangers that either do not exist in reality or are greatly exaggerated. Modern clinical diagnostic procedures contribute to this mistaken attribution by frequently detecting minimal deviations that are incorrectly considered to be its cause or a part of the anxiety neurosis instead of an equivalent or correlate of the anxiety. Doctor and patient then believe they have found a specific cause, which can result in temporary relief when therapeutic measures are undertaken. Yet the disappointment is all the greater when the removal of the node in the thyroid or some other treatment does not achieve the desired results. There is hardly another clinical condition that is so frequently misdiagnosed by modern medicine as anxiety neurosis and its multifaceted forms.

Countless *circumstantial diagnoses* based on symptoms such as eye flutter, sweating, and trembling serve to maintain the patient's distress and reinforce his anxiety. Diagnostically it is often difficult to find the (psychic) precipitant of the somatic equivalent of the anxiety, and accordingly it is impossible for the patient to find relief by avoiding the precipitating situations, as the phobic patient does. Since the individual with cardiac neurosis or heart phobia cannot distance himself from his heart as if it were a spider, this syndrome belongs to anxiety neurosis, but at the transition to hypochondric states. The term "heart phobia" is therefore inaccurate phenomenologically and psychodynamically. Bowlby (1973) has also suggested a clinically convincing manner to differentiate the phobias, which Hoffmann (1986) has recently drawn renewed attention to. The agoraphobic is not afraid of the market square but lacks in this situation the person providing security, i.e., a "regulatory object" (König 1981). Richter and Beckmann (1969) also described a differentiation for cardiac neurosis. They described two types, distinguishing between their reactions to separation anxieties. As a result, there are substantial differences in the therapeutic difficulties posed by anxiety disorders and their subforms.

Psychoanalysis relies on the healthy elements of an individual's personality even more than somatic therapy does. The more severe the anxiety disorder, the smaller the space from which the patient is capable of mastering, with the analyst's assistance, the conditions of the anxiety that are rooted in his distant past and revived in the present. If the patient is extremely insecure, it is essential that the analyst employ supporting measures to strengthen the patient's position to the extent necessary to ensure that the patient can reflect on his situation and perform trial actions. Verbal relief is often insufficient in states of acute anxiety and agitation, making it necessary for tranquilizers, antidepressives, and beta-blockers to be used against the concomitant somatic symptoms. Essential is that this supportive use of medication be included in the *psychoanalytic* plan of treatment and be subordinate to it (see Benkert and Hippius 1986; Strian 1983; Wurmser 1987).

The more diffuse and free floating the anxiety, the more difficult it is to master it. In such cases it is therefore important to work with the patient to discover where the anxiety is transformed into object-related fear, in order to gain a sphere in which to overcome the patient's helplessness. This psychodynamic process goes hand in hand with a phenomenological differentiation between anxiety and fear. The more successful one is in objectifying the anxiety and recognizing what the patient is afraid of, the greater the opportunities for mastering the perils of the object that originate in the patient himself.

This differentiation has had great significance in the psychoanalytic theory of development because maturation is defined there as the change from diffuse anxiety to concrete fear. Consequently Mentzos, despite his reservations against a sharp differentiation between anxiety and fear, argues

> that one [should] proceed in developmental psychology from a tendency toward maturation and thus, for example, consider diffuse, somatically experienced, and apparently unfounded anxiety states in adults to be a regressive reactivation of ontogentically earlier modes of anxiety, or at least assume there has been a disintegration of a later, more mature pattern of anxiety. (Mentzos 1984, p. 15)

We agree with Mentzos that the capacity to control anxiety is an indicator of ego maturity. Knowledge of the prototypical fundamental anxieties of children thus facilitates the diagnosis of neurotic anxieties in adults.

In conclusion we would like to mention several principles of therapeutic technique that have shown their value in the psychoanalytic therapy of anxiety disorders, regardless of severity. Essential is to promote the patient's capacity for integration as opposed to the stimuli precipitating anxiety. The statement that precisely the severely ill anxiety neurotics suffer from ego weakness says nothing else than that the threshhold for emotions is lowered and apparently banal desires appear as "instinctual anxiety" and precipitate a danger signal resulting in anxiety. The technical consequence of this description is complete reliance on the analyst's function as an auxiliary ego. Chronic anxieties lead to a loss of self-confidence and self-security. In his function as an auxiliary ego, the analyst can contribute to the patient's capacity to extend his sphere of action by providing encouragement in the form of acknowledging what the patient is still able to accomplish. This direct and indirect support must be underpinned through the specifically psychoanalytic tool of interpretation. Self-security and self-confidence grow, for example, to the degree that "superficial" anxieties, which Freud referred to as social and superego anxieties, are eliminated. Proceeding from the surface into the depths is a tried and proven therapeutic technique, which we have discussed in the introduction to Chap. 4. Of course, following this rule achieves little if at the same time concomitant acknowledgments of the patient's remaining capacities are carefully avoided out of a false understanding of the rules of neutrality and abstinence. Coping with neurotic anxieties is eased if we take advantage of all the possibilities offered by the mastery theory of therapy.

In severe, chronic anxiety neurosis with panic attacks, distressing defeats have continuously raised the *unconscious* potential for aggression so high that there are hardly any harmless wishes left. For example, the anxiety that one may die from a heart attack is unconsciously frequently linked with aggression that is directed precisely against the people that the patient relies on for protection. The resulting dilemma would obviously be reinforced, to the disadavantage of therapy, if an analyst proceeded to interpret anger on the basis of this connection. Helpful interpretations are oriented on the patient's capacity for integrating affects. The patient's self-confidence grows in the relationship to the analyst if the latter provides suggestions from the position of an auxiliary ego. Ambivalences always have the effect of increasing anxiety and should therefore be called by name where they are accessible to the patient. In accordance with this, the patient increases his capacity to distinguish unconscious fantasies, which in light appear less sinister than they do in the dark of the night.

We encounter anxiety, which constitutes the fundamental problem of all neuroses and their gradual resolution, in numerous examples in this volume. Moderately severe anxiety neuroses - all those suffering from the syndrome Freud described, which includes the cardiac neuroses - are very accessible to psychoanalytic therapy. Long-term follow-ups verify enduring treatment results, even for very severe anxiety neuroses (Thomä 1978).

9.2 Anxiety Hysteria

Anxieties and hypochondriac fantasies about one's body are a frequent and at least sporadic manifestation accompanying the hysterias described by Charcot and Freud. The contents of the anxiety provide a secure access to the patient's experiencing and also indicate that physiological deviations are the equivalents of affects. In this regard the analyst must pay special attention to the patient's fantasies and *private theory* of his illness; it is otherwise impossible to recognize that, for example, nervous breathing difficulties are the somatic equivalent of an anxiety neurosis.

Hysterical symptoms - as originally meaningful achievements and fragmentary actions - should especially be expected if unconscious portions of the *body image* are incompatible or contradict the *physiological regulations.* Most important in the process of *conversion* is that incompatible fantasies are displaced within the body image. The concept of *displacement* refers to a mechanism that plays an important role with regard to the development of hysterical and phobic symptoms in both the theory of dreaming and the theory of neurosis. Compromise formations are formed in dreams and in the genesis of symptoms by means of displacement, and psychoanalysis--as the psychopathology of conflict - has demonstrated its clinical effectiveness in the therapeutic resolution of these compromises. One reason for our emphasis on displacement is that this process is helpful in comprehending both the unconscious fantasies about body image of the individuals described below and their production of dreams and symptoms. The presumed transformation of energy, which Freud linked with the theory of conversion, is an obsolete hypothesis. Readers who first wish to gain information about the theory of conversion and body image should turn to Sect. 9.2.1.

Symptoms

At the beginning of treatment Beatrice X was 24 years old, had been married for 2 years, and did not have any children. For some 8 years she had been suffering from cramped breathing accompanied by a feeling of constriction and severe distress. These symptoms appeared for the first time in the year of her father's death, who died from a chronic cardiac disorder accompanied by difficulties in breathing. Her condition, which was diagnosed by an internist as a nervous breathing disorder, had worsened for about 2 years, making her fear that she would suffocate. She incessantly coughed and cleared her throat throughout the entire day (nervous cough). During her honeymoon her anxiety increased so much, particularly while eating in the company of her husband and then also in the presence of others, that the patient had had to eat her meals alone ever since. Her symptoms were accompanied by abstruse fantasies about her body: terrible experiences of emptiness; she thought her thorax was empty and no air went into it; thought she was too weak to breathe and that the air escaped as it does from a porous ball. Then she would feel as if she were a steel pipe. Coitus was impossible due to vaginismus.

Beatrice X frequently squatted, since she somehow felt safer crouching on the floor. It was intolerable to her for an empty space to be in front of her or "to be empty in front." She therefore sat completely cramped while driving. Countless incidental acts betrayed her great inner distress. She found support by playing around with whatever objects were at hand. She controlled herself and her surroundings.

The following information, reported by the patient at the beginning of her analysis, deserves to be emphasized with regard to events preceding her illness:

From the age of two until 15 the patient was in the habit of masturbating by making a jumping sliding movement her mother referred to as hopping. Her mother's prohibitions made this hopping into something evil. Her own old anxiety about having injured herself reappeared in her later symptoms.

The patient avoided hopping on her father's knees. The revival of incest desires in puberty brought forth stereotype dreams. In these dreams something terrible always happened between her and her father, and she woke from an orgasm. A rewarding daydream recurred frequently during a long period of time, namely that she had a blister on her lower arm that a doctor had to open. This frequent fantasy was accompanied by great pleasure.

She had practiced her oedipal incest desires in games with her brother. He had wanted her to stroke his penis, and used all his effort to maintain his self control. That he did not twitch a muscle made him into a model of masculine self-control that others should imitate and made him an example of "control." After these controlled satisfactions the patient went into the bathroom to have cold showers. Her mother must have had some premonition because she separated them. The patient later believed that her parents never had intercourse since they did not sleep together.

In hindsight the patient dated the onset of her breathing difficulties back to when she was 15 years old, the year she successfully suppressed her self-gratifications (i. e., the hopping). The patient was overcome by her first severe anxiety attack after she had met her future husband; their relationship became more intimite about a year before they married. At first the patient was afraid to have intercourse, and she and her friend initially limited their contact to mutual stimulation and gratification, which however was more intensive than her experiences with her brother had been. The patient's hysterical somatic symptoms became more severe following her first anxiety attack and particularly following their honeymoon. Beatice X's symptoms belonged to those of the syndrome of anxiety neurosis. The addition *anxiety hysteria* is justified because of the primarily oedipal sexual contents of her anxiety, yet the pejorative meaning of the word "hysterical" makes it advisable for it not to be used in any correspondence or in discussions with the patient or family members. To discontinue using this traditional term in scientific discussion, however, would amount to a cover-up. Hysterical mechanisms and contents are pathogenic factors that continue to be frequent in anxiety neurosis.

In this treatment report, prepared about 30 years ago, the focal points of therapeutic technique are related to specific assumptions about psychogenetic relationships. The systematic description of this treatment covers more than a hundred closely typed pages. The successful psychoanalysis lasted about 350 sessions in all. For external reasons Beatrice Y twice had to be admitted for in-patient treatment; during these periods six sessions were held each week. In the interval and afterwards the patient came an average of twice a week until she was cured. Beatrice X has remained essentially free of symptoms since then, leads a harmonious family life, and has several children. She has coped very well with the burdens of life.

To make the sequences stemming from later sessions more comprehensible, we would like to mention that a multifaceted transference neurosis was formed during the first period of in-patient treatment. The patient's dream language was rich in symbols, which provided an immediate access to her still infantile sexual theories and to the hysterical disturbances of her body image and the anxieties that were associated with them. Her dream metaphors were unusually closely connected with her unconscious body image and its different layers. Reversing displacements, i. e., referring to these "transferences" (in Greek, *metapherein*) by name, played an important role in transforming her unconsciously disturbed postural language.

Analysis of Beatrice X's imitations led to specific questions about the psychogenesis, for instance about the significance of her unconscious feeling of guilt, which was gratified by her punishing herself by having the same symptoms her father had had. Everyday excitement and the observation of accidents made the patient become violently agitated because they reminded her of her father's illness and death. After his death the patient had continued her father's illness with her own symptoms, her shortness of breath and her anxiety. By means of these symptoms she had maintained ties to her father, who had long suffered from heart disease and shortness of breath.

The similarities in the symptoms, specifically the shortage of breath, had even been noted by her family doctor, but the patient had not caught his allusions to it. It often takes a long period of preparation for insights into such imitations rooted in unconscious identifications to be made *therapeutically* productive. Of course, the process of making a patient aware of unconscious identifications that can find their symbolic expression in hysterical symptoms is facilitated when the patient practices the imitation of particular features in his own body.

After long preparation the ground had finally been paved in the 123rd session for the patient to understand an imitation. The patient disclosed her longing to be linked with her father in conscious fantasies. The pain and mourning that were linked with her separation from her father were revived. She became certain, by means of a *transferred idea*, that it is possible through symptoms to maintain a relationship for a long period of time and despite a final separation. She then referred to her gift for observation, but only after making many apologies and revealing a bad conscience that even she found suspicious. Finally after making many reservations, Beatrice X made derogatory statements about my peculiar manner of walking and how I moved my arms arrhythmically.

Beatrice X had pantomimed her observations for herself outside the session. This attempt at imitation became a significant event in the attempt to recognize her unconsciously anchored identifications and the concomitant affects. Her derogatory comments about me took the same line as her old feelings of guilt toward her father. In this session she cried passionately for the first time.

The following later observations are relevant in this context. In her associations she first mentioned something external, namely that I had talked to her earlier in the ward to make sure that the session was actually at 5 p.m. She said I had looked tired and tried to get me to cancel the session. This was followed by the following series of associations that are instructive for the genesis of her symptoms and my comprehension of them. Her father had often been tired and, especially in the years of his illness, hardly in a condition to have his meals at the table. He was asked to, and he made an effort. I gave the following interpretation: You were obviously afraid then that something could happen to your father while eating; as short of breath as he was, the potatoe you gave him might mean his death. Today you wanted to prevent me from also becoming exhausted, and possibly weakened or even suffocated, from the things you served me.

Since there had already been an allusion in the session to an earlier dream about hedgehog meat, I incorporated this allusion into my interpretation and told her she was afraid of giving me something harmful, such as the hedgehog meat with its spines, which would not agree with me. (In this earlier dream she had regretfully given someone hedgehog meat.)

The subject of her *identification with her sick father* was further resolved. This problem can be illustrated with regard to one small detail in transference. Beatrice X requested that the window be closed, but called this wish horrible. Interpretative work led to her father and the fact that he had been constantly short of breath - so that the window had to be kept open - and to tension at meals, which increased as his condition worsened. In hindsight the patient had the feeling that her father simply could not take it any more. I offered the interpretation that she was now anxious that I could not take it anymore, either, with the window closed and being very exhausted.

The other line of interpretation was her anger at her father, who was only concerned with business. At home the family had to be careful not to disturb him, but precisely at meals there was conflict. Beatrice X herself was a mediator, the one who could not bear the conflict and her parents' talk about divorce. The previous night she had had a dream, namely that the firm was ruined. She had walked with her mother through the destroyed building and said that everything her father had build up was ruined. In transference she showed similar feelings, concerns about me, and the criticism that I did not care for my own family either.

Displacement Downwards and Upwards

We would like to supplement our theoretical comments about body image and displacemnt by describing a clinical example in which breathing constituted the starting point with regard to symptoms.

Two Dreams. The patient, in great desperation and anxious horror, saw herself surrounded by numerous little men, as if they were rubber dolls. These little men exploded one after another. The patient tried to find some support and held on to a rope that somehow hang from the sky.

In the second dream she was on a bridge together with numerous other onlookers. The main action in the dream was a shark hunt. From the bridge they could see how a shark that tried to fight itself free was drawn into a small boat. Although it swung its tail back and forth, it was killed by a spear thrust into its belly.

Since Beatrice X, as she recalled in this connection, had previously dreamed about a rope on which she had been drawn down into the depths, the relationship to this earlier manifest dream content was established first. In the previous session we had really jumped from one topic to another, familiar items being considered without any profit. I established a connection between the explosion of the little men and her anxiety that a condom might rupture. These ideas led us to talk once again about her compulsion to control.

I silently assumed that that her anxiety about such a rupture might somehow be linked with her castration anxiety. I considered this hunch all the more because we had discussed the unusual positions she took on the couch. She was always a little diagonal, because in this position she had the feeling that she had better control of the situation.

Her comments about her posture stimulated me to fantasize that she had obviously overcome her castration anxiety by using her body as a phallus, as Lewin (1933) had described. Peculiar was, however, that her anxiety was that she would get less air when stretched out than when she was stooped over a little. At this point she became aware that her playing with her body served to discharge excitation. We talked about her masturbation being her attempt to overcome her feeling of emptiness by touching.

With regard to the fish dream, I interpreted her inclination toward taking revenge on me (analyst) by alluding to the fact that she took revenge on the fish – i. e., the penis that tried to force its way into her, just like the rocket in another dream. In this connection the patient had recalled an earlier dream in which she drove into a path that was too narrow. Her recollections and transference fantasies could not be linked to unconscious oedipal conflicts.

That evening Beatrice X continued her self-analysis and at the next session admitted that she had kept an important association to her dreams to herself. She said that according to her feelings the bursting of the little men definitely had to interpreted in connection with a series of fantasies she had had before, during, and after her defloration.

Next she surprised me by giving a precise description of her honeymoon trip, the first night, and the following day. On the second day she had gone swimming with her husband in the sea and had felt that – as she said – there was a hole in her and could not control what went in or came out. These were the words she used to describe her body feeling after her defloration, and I added: "When you went into the sea, you had the fantasy that water could enter your vagina, just like air when you were outside." This meant, in her dream language, that a fish (penis) could also enter her.

Beatice X actually believes up to this very day that her vagina continues to rip further and further apart. In this connection she recalled an earlier dream. The notches in a fly's wings she had dreamed about were, according to her, definitely the kind of tears that happened during defloration.

The patient now added that she then had the desire - which she found completely incomprehensible - not to eat together with the other guests. This disturbance thus also began shortly after her defloration, at the same time her breathing disturbance became more severe. She immediately sensed that this was an *upward displacement*. It was the attempt to exert control where it was possible by means of her voluntary muscles, to at least close the "holes" there.

The interpretation of the fish dream led further. The patient talked about her revulsion at fish, which she had felt since her honeymoon. She also had an aversion to the smell of fish, which resulted from the analogy between the smell of fish and that of ejaculation, which now became conscious.

I also interpreted her aggression toward her husband, telling her: "You had pain, felt hurt, and therefore took revenge on your husband and his penis. In the dream you had him kill the shark; in reality you often hack up your husband."

In the previous session the bursting of the little men, the rubber balloons - in an association she mentioned that the entire matter was like the bursting of soap bubbles - had led to a different allusion that was initially not productive. I had the thought that the bursting represented a still unclear association to the pleasurable fantasy in which she had had a blister on her lower arm that a doctor had opened. The patient could not recall whether she had then thought that something had been in the blister. The idea did not go beyond an allusion.

In the 131st session Beatrice X did not mention this "blister" again immediately, not until after she had talked about her vacation, referring to the fish dream and associations about eating fish. She started this line of thought by saying that although they had stayed at a good hotel, she had discovered a mouse in the bathroom, which then disappeared. She fantasized that the mouse might have hidden in the toilette. The night after this she had a very repulsive dream.

P: I had a bowel movement. In it there was a large fish.

The patient had already had the idea that she produced something to demonstrate her independence. I interpreted that she had something in the dream that otherwise entered her, not leave her. After this interpretation she recalled the dream she had had the previous night.

P: I had a blister on my nose. A man came who opened the blister with a pin, but what came out was that I had the same kind of pin hidden in the blister.

This dream seemed to fit her dream about her anal excretion of a penis. I summarized the patient's associations in a transference interpretation. She then said that she would very much like to read my notes to finally know what I thought about her; she often asked herself what I would write after a session. The interpretative work proceeded as follows. The secrets she presumed were in the report were probably precisely the hidden item - the assumption that I did not think much of her as a woman - and she now thought that she had to attach a very high value to the hidden element. I interpreted her private revenge as the unconscious idea that I, just like her husband, wasted her beautiful associations, her bowel movement, her money, and her ideas in order to make a beautiful project and to become an ever greater person, architect, and analyst, while she believed she had to sacrifice everything and always ended up empty handed (an allusion to the pen with which I wrote and her husband used in becoming a successful architect and to it as a symbol for a penis).

Her nervous cough has disappeared almost entirely. In the past few weeks she has been able to eat together with her husband for the first time since their honeymoon.

Their sexual relationship has become more satisfying, and she pays less attention to contraception, even though her anxiety about conceiving and bearing a child has increased.

Summary. Our goal in describing the two excerpts from this analysis of anxiety hysteria is to let the reader take part in a partial resolution of symptoms. Both the patient's unconsciously anchored imitation of her father's symptoms and the displacement from bottom to top were partial causes that were resolved, resulting in a significant improvement in the symptoms they had caused. The fact that symptoms continued to exist is an indication that other unconscious conditions were active. And in fact other anxiety contents then moved to the focus. Birth anxiety took the place of some earlier symptoms; i. e., there was a change in symptoms (see Sect. 9.5). Noteworthy is the alloplastic structure of her new anxieties in comparison with her previous hypochondriac anxieties. It is always a positive sign when it is possible to ease the autoplastic representation of conflicts, i. e., their far-reaching internalization, which is implied in the differentiation between autoplastic and alloplastic processes that goes back to Ferenczi (1921).

In Sect. 8.3 we describe the resolution of these neurotic anxieties and present a *sequential protocol.*

9.2.1 Conversion and Body Image

Anyone who accepts Darwin's description of emotions, which has retained an exemplary character for modern theories of affects (see Vol.1, Sect. 4.2), does not have to face the problem of conversion - i. e., the hypothesis that psychic energy is transformed into physical energy or excitation. To reach a diagnostic and therapeutic understanding of many functional syndromes, it suffices to view them as an unconscious expression of emotions. The expressive meaning of hysterical symptoms is *not* restricted to sexuality. Freud attributed *conversion* to Darwin's principle of the "overflow of excitation" (Freud 1895d, p. 91). In the case history of Elisabeth R., he wrote, for instance, "All these sensations and innervations belong to the field of 'The Expression of the Emotions', which, as Darwin has taught us, consists of actions which originally had a meaning and served a purpose" (1895d, p. 181). Many such examples of symptoms in which, for example, aggressive impulses find unconscious expression can be found in Freud's case histories.

It is not necessary to resort to the assumption that there is a conversion of psychic energy into physical energy for us to comprehend that hysterical symptoms are, according to Freud (1895d, p. 133), unconscious fantasies that have become visible in disguised form. The *causal* assertion in this sentence is retained even without the expression "through conversion" (such as a *transformation* of psychic energy into physical innervation). Hysterical symptoms and many functional syndromes are fragmentary sensory or motoric acts that, because of defense processes, are expressed only partially (pars pro toto). The ideational component, i. e., the idea and the goal, is no longer accessible to the patient himself. This is the basis of causal and prognostic criteria for clinical validation.

The mind-body problem, which cannot be resolved empirically anyway, can be ignored just as can the related "mysterious leap from the mental to the physical" (Freud 1916/17, p. 258). Hysterical symptoms are rudimentary and originally meaningful events and as such their psychophysiology is no more mysterious than are purposive acts (Rangell 1959). The fact that psychoanalysis took the theory of conversion to mean the transformation of one form of energy into another is a particularly clear demonstration of how far astray it has been led for decades by the economic principle (see Vol.1, Sect. 1.1). The psychoanalytic method based on Freud's psychological theory is itself completely sufficient to understand the language of hysteria and to explain the formation of symptoms:

By carrying what is unconscious on into what is conscious, we lift the repressions, we remove the preconditions for the formation of symptoms, we transform the pathogenic conflict into a normal one for which it must be possible somehow to find a solution. All that we bring about in a patient is this single psychical change: the length to which it is carried is the measure of the help we provide. Where no repressions (or analogous psychical processes) can be undone, our therapy has nothing to expect. (Freud 1916/17, p. 435)

Hysterical symptoms and a group of functional ones prevent affects from completely expressing themselves. A part represents the whole. In such conditions, the sick individual lacks most of all a means of gaining access to his intentions. These are, to quote Freud's words, "kept from conscious processing." The essential fact is that the disruption caused by repression - the necessary causal condition (Grünbaum 1984) - can be reversed by means of *interpretations*. The situation is different with the symptoms of physical illnesses. Alexander, back in 1935 (p. 505), wrote: "It is a methodological error to attempt to interpret psychologically an organic symptom which is the end-result of an intermediary chain of organic processes." This view agrees with Freud's clear methodological guidelines about physical disturbances that cannot be interpreted symbolically (Freud 1910i, p. 217), which brings us to the modern theories of action and affects, and to the view, following Christian, that:

From the perspective of a theory of action, the symptoms of conversion hysteria constitute the actual genesis of a fantasy. Also important is the outcome of the fantasy, namely precisely not the outcome of a natural and normal action but the realization of abbridged opportunities to act in certain scenic simplifications. The following comparison may make this clearer: Complete scenic realizations of body language are embodied in dance theater, where scenes are depicted in body language, but in an artistic manner. The hysterical enactment is, in contrast, more primitive and unartisitic; it is somewhat theatric, which is precisely not artisitic. Freud also noted this reduction to a primitive fantasy in conversion symptoms .... The symptoms are both a substitute for actions that would otherwise have to be carried out (substitute or fragmentary acts) and expressions of the unconscious conflicts (representative acts). (Christian 1986, p. 81)

The sexual revolution and Freud's teachings have made substantial contributions to making the hysterias and anxiety hysterias that were so widespread in the nineteenth century, and whose symptoms Charcot could have patients reproduce and enact in the Salpetrière by means of suggestion, become so rare in today's society. On the other hand, the same symptoms of anxiety hysteria continue to exist in the "functional syndromes," the increasingly subtle diagnosis of which continues to mount pressure on modern medicine. The disturbed patient - who cannot know that his symptoms are expressions of unconscious emotions - insists that the physician repeat the diagnostic examinations to exclude a hidden and possibly malignant illness. Frequently the result of these examinations is some harmless deviation from normal that, because of its ambiguity, can become the source of new disturbances and lead to measures that are entirely inappropriate for alleviating the patient's neurotic anxieties. The precise reason for this follows from the structure of these anxieties and the development of a vicious circle in which helplessness, hopelessness, and anxiety reinforce each other. We describe these connections in the excurse on the central role of anxiety in psychoanalysis in Sect. 9.1. One of the most fundamental facts Freud discovered was that an unconscious intention is directed at an external object or at its image, and that the latter can be imprinted onto one's own body (or self-image). The specific unconscious fantasies themselves vary from case to case. Analysts are well advised, however, to presume that impulses that have been warded off, i. e., aggressive impulses that have become unconscious, are present in *all* dysmorphophobias, that is in all body image disorders in which the patient subjectively experiences some deformity as being present although in fact it is *not* (Sect. 5.5). This regular observation can be understood if one realizes that in identifications the shadow of objects that have been given up also falls on the *body image*, to modify Freud's well-known metaphor. In this process, a fight in which an imagined or real injury is inflicted on the opponent (the "object") is portrayed on the individual's own body image, by the individual putting himself partially in the other person's place. This process can be the basis both of simple imitations and of mystical participation, for instance, in the suffering of Jesus on the cross.

Because of the fundamental significance of *body schema* and *body image* in our overall understanding of illness, we discuss this concept in the following section (see the comprehensive description given by Joraschky 1983). The concept of body schema was coined in neurology and used by Pick and Head as a general concept for describing bizarre body perceptions by patients with brain lesions. Head referred to body schema as the frame of reference for body perception, i. e., for spatial orientation and posture. Body schema was defined by him in neurophysiological terms: Man's use of the schema is not a psychic process but takes place at the physiological level (as described by Joraschky 1983, p. 35). Schilder (1923) initially also followed Head's definition, but this creative author later made a special contribution to extending this concept to the subjective experience of one's body, i. e., to the psychic spatial image originating from interpersonal interaction. We will simplify the issue by orienting ourselves on Schilder, who consistently integrated psychological and psychodynamic results into the theory of body schema and who referred to the concept "body image" in his later book *The Image and Appearance of the Human Body* (1935).

From body schema to body image – these key words emphasize the discoveries Schilder made, which have proven to be extremely fertile in psychoanalysis and psychosomatic medicine, even though Schilder himself is rarely cited and this although, according to Rapaport (1953, p. 7), he was one of the most widely versed thinkers in the history of psychiatry. For just this reason we want to cite several representative passages from his largely unknown article "Das Körperbild und die Sozialpsychologie" (Body Image and Social Psychology) from 1933. We will emphasize those of Schilder's views that are of special relevance for therapeutic technique. For example, body and world are correlated concepts:

The consciousness of substantiality, the three-dimensional image we have of ourselves, must be acquired in just the same manner as our knowledge of the external world. It is continually being built out of tactile, kinesthetic, and optical raw materials .... The subjectively exprienced body image thus becomes the map of the instinctual impulses. (p. 368)

Schilder gave a brief description of a patient who felt her body had fallen into separate pieces. This was correlated with impulses to tear others into pieces. For Schilder, the desire to be seen is just as original as the desire to see.

One's own body image has very much in common with the body image one has of others. When we construct our own body image, we are constantly attempting to find out what can be assimilated into our own body. We are no less curious with regard to our own body than to that of others. When our eye is satisfied, then we want our touch to be satisfied too. Our fingers force their way into every orifice of the body. Voyeurism and exhibitionism have the same roots. Body image is a social phenomenon, but the human body is never quiet, always in motion. Body movement is either expression or action; it is the body of a person with passions and motives. (p. 371)

After describing a neurotic symptom, Schilder made the summarizing interpretation that the patient plays the roles of numerous people in his actions. He saw this as an example of the fact that:

one's own body image contains the body images of others. Yet the latter must be given in the patient before he can merge them into his own body image. At one and the same time he lives in his body and outside of it. We have our own and the other body image at the same time. Body image is not the product of an apersonization of the body images of others although we assimilate portions of them into our own body image. It is not a product of identification, either, although such identifications might enrich our own body image .... The body image is never at rest. It changes according to the situation. It is a creative construction. It is constructed, dissolved, and rebuilt. In this constant process of construction, reconstruction, and dissolution, the processes of identification, apersonization, and projection are of special significance .... Yet social life is not only based on identifications, but also on actions, a precondition of which is that the other person is a person with his own body. There are two conflicting tendencies. The one assimilates the other person into one's own ego by means of identification and related processes; the other, no less strong and original, sets and accepts the other person as an independent unit. This social antinomy has the greatest of consequences. (pp. 373, 375)

Schilder's vivid language probably reminds everyone of various facets of their own body image. The constant interaction between one's own body image and that of the other person naturally goes far beyond a comparison according to aesthetic points of view. The relationship of nearness and distance is also part of this social antinomy. Proceeding from clinical observations, in just a few pages Schilder provided an overview that emphasizes the social psychological dimensions of the development of body image. Emotions, expressions, and fragmentary acts, in the sense of hysterical symptoms, are thus constantly in a close relationship to an aspect of body image that is more or less unconscious.

The body image is formed in conjunction with the development of the neurophysiological body schema and unites a wealth of representations of conscious and unconscious ideas. These representations can coincide, compete, or even disregard body functions as they are laid out physiologically. Because of its numerous layers, the body image can be compared with a painting that has been painted over repeatedly so that on one and the same canvas there might be paintings that match - or that do not. In this metaphor, the canvas would be the foundation or the neurophysiologically formed body schema, or in even more general terms, Freud's body ego. Incidentally, the individual, as the painter, is and remains a part of his body image because he is linked throughout his life to what has been drawn in, and because the relationship between idea and image can be dominated by either productive or destructive tension.

9.3 Anxiety Neurosis

Christian Y suffered from such an unusually severe anxiety neurosis concomitant with paroxysmal tachycardia that a long period of in-patient treatment in a department of internal medicine had been necessary. In the preceding years his self-security had decreased substantially. Any banal stimulus, even minimal atmospheric fluctuations, in either the literal or the metaphoric sense, could suffice to increase his anxiety and cause a heart attack. The patient was incapacitated, unable to leave the hospital, and dependent on its support.

The patient had difficulty maintaining his composure during the diagnostic interviews. He described how he had been tormented by insecurity and anxieties for years. He said he had a deep mortal anxiety, was lethargic and depressed, and only continued to live out of a certain feeling of duty toward his parents. For a long time he had planned to commit suicide. His security was just show; he was only able to bear his anxieties and their somatic consequences in or close to the hospital.

An anxiety neurosis with a narcissistic personality structure was diagnosed. The analyst gave the following chronological description of the previous history of the patient's symptoms:

The patient grew up the oldest son in a large family, preceded only by two substantially older stepsisters from his father's first marriage. His mother was overanxious and overcaring, had a special attraction to her oldest son, and was a dominating figure. His father was a successful physicist and for professional reasons had been away from the family for several years during the patient's childhood; even later he was not present very often.

Preschool Period (Age 0–6). Numerous strong infantile anxieties. The patient grew up in the absence of his father and developed a very strong fixation on his mother. This fixation became more intense over the years because of his anxieties about being in darkness and being alone. Father returned when he was 3 years old. His infantile anxieties increased in connection with dreams in which the patient was punished by a man's evil glances or was threatened with physical abuse (with a pair of pliers).

Age of 6–12. A pronounced school phobia improved under his mother's care; for a long time she walked with him to school and did his homework.

Age of 12–22. Death of his beloved grandfather from heart failure. Clinical examination and treatment of the patient for "cardiovascular disturbances." The diagnosis he remembered – "he had a weak heart" – was accompanied by the recommendation that he be spared physical exertion. This marked the end of a short phase of athletic and physical activity, which changed into passivity and dependence. Starting from the age of 12 the patient was in treatment by numerous doctors for his feelings of anxiety and cardiac disturbances.

The extreme maternal care was linked to the patient's acceptance of her ideals. The boy therefore became excessively well behaved and overconform and restricted his curiosity and activity extremely in order to retain his mother's love. His rivalry to his two younger brothers was suppressed. His school achievement remained far below what it might have been on the basis of his above-average intelligence. He concealed his disturbed concentration and capacity to work by easily achieving average results because of his high intelligence. As long as he reached his goal without any effort, he felt well, but even the slightest stress led to unpleasure and anxiety and shattered his fragile self-esteem. Although the patient had always been well liked because of his good upbringing, he could not remember any phase of his life in which he felt satisfied with himself in any regard or was able to get a feeling of security from an interpersonal relationship.

During puberty he had tried very hard to overcome his fixation on his mother. He was incapable of competing in athletic events. The fact that he had to quit just before winning was typical of his behavior pattern.

The patient attempted, in conscious decisiveness, to free himself of his mother's ideals, without being able to be happy about his successes with girls. His friendships had a narcissistic character and, just like masturbation, gave him more feelings of guilt than satisfaction. He lost the last rest of his self-security when a girl rejected him. This insult led to decompensation and heart anxieties he experienced as an irreparable physical handicap.

Christian X had to interrupt his education because of his symptoms and is incapacitated.

In retrospect we can see that the analyst in this case incorrectly judged the severity of the illness, paying too little attention in adjusting technical rules to the fact that Christian Y was still in the late adolescent phase of development. Since the problem of power-powerlessness is particularly delicate for this age group, the therapeutic technique should have be more characterized by "cooperation as between partners" (Bohleber 1982). In addition, the analyst's therapeutic technique – when the analysis was initiated some 20 years ago – led to immmanent mistakes that had unfavorable consequences. For instance, it was too early to recommend that the patient reduce or stop taking medication. Better cooperation between the physicians treating Christian Y would also have contributed to raising his self-security and reducing the number of defeats leading to a further loss of self-security.

The following aspects of the external features of the course of therapy deserve mentioning. The analysis began 20 years ago and was completed after more than 10 years and a total of about 1400 sessions. Christian Y required in-patient therapy for more than 18 months because of the severity of his anxiety neurosis. Starting with the 320th session he was able to continue the intensive therapy of five sessions per week while residing in a halfway house. After a while he was able to walk to the consulting room and was no longer dependent on the protection afforded by a taxi, which could have rapidly brought him to a hospital if necessary. After three years of treatment Christian Y was able, despite his continuing inhibitions, to start a professional career in another city. At this point, the frequency of therapy was gradually reduced. Thus of the 1400 sessions, 600 were during the first three years and the rest were spread over many years. This case thus includes a long follow-up period. Christian Y is today over 40 and has been successful professionally for years. He founded a family and is a happy husband and father, although he does still complain about a certain lack of self-confidence.

We describe four examples from this analysis. In the following section we present the 203rd session, from the phase of in-patient therapy. In Sect. 4.3 we described, in the context of displeasure as id resistance, the 503rd session in which his lethargy and incapacity to work reached their zenith. Finally, in Sects. 9.3.2 and 9.3.3 were refer to two excerpts from the phase of termination, to which Christian Y provided in retrospect an instructive commentary.

9.3.1 Separation Anxiety

The intensity of the underlying problem of separation is clearly demonstrated in the following excerpt with regard to a precipitating situation. This example shows the analyst's attempt to clarify the patient's conflicting needs and desires.

Prior to this session the patient had told his parents about his dependence on them during a weekend visit. He had never noticed this feeling in such clarity before. His parents had left with friends for a few hours, and the patient felt the urgent demand for them to stay there, to be there for him, and to take care of him. In the hospital three doctors gave him intensive attention, especially since it was difficult to control the degree of his tachycardia attacks with beta-blockers. At this point the patient, probably as a consequence of the analytic therapy, was ambivalent toward the drug therapy; he seems to have identified with the opinion that the analyst openly articulated that he should attempt to get by without medication. At the same time the drug treatment provided the direct support he did not receive from the analyst.

The patient had acute symptoms when he came to the session.

P: I feel queasy again, I have this . . . terrible agitation, shortness of breath, not really shortness of breath, that's exaggerated, but not enough air and heart problems. I haven't taken any medication because you didn't want me to, but . . . I'm not sure what it is, but . . . well, what could it be. [Pause] While I felt this queasiness, several times I felt the longing for you to be with me, and then I realized that I was angry at you, at least I thought I realized it but I couldn't admit how strong it was. Somehow I'm angry at you. [Pause] Well, it's funny; right now I can't think any more at all, and the symptoms are gone, too. All that's left is the annoyance that I was so uncontrolled, and the anxiety that I have somehow offended you.

A: But that is an anxiety that is obviously much weaker than the other one. Are the symptoms really gone now?

P: Hum, yes.

A: That shows that there's a very close connection between intense anger and your symptoms.

P: Yes, and then, whenever I feel as bad as this morning, then I have the desire to scream out loud for somebody. I always have to pull myself together to keep from screaming. Somehow not to be left alone or something like that is what I can think of.

A: And that's precisely what is was: the closed door and "Do Not Enter." Is he going to make me wait a quarter hour again today?

P: Well, I wouldn't have managed to wait this time. I called for the doctor and asked him; I felt so terrible. Now I have intense palpitations again, pounding, not fast . . . . And it must be these moods that I feel when I leave you or home. I apparently inflict all of my indignation on myself. But why can't I learn that it's nonsense?

A: Yes. Because you don't scream and yell and shout at me that way, and I'm the one who leaves you. By not acting that way, you feel more secure, because you think that I would otherwise leave you for sure.

P: Maybe it makes me feel calmer or amazed that you didn't make a face. I didn't think that there was anybody here in the room with you, or I wouldn't have knocked.

A: Yes, you've experienced that I'm not mad. That means that the anger you felt before knocking didn't have any terrible consequences. And then your anxiety goes away a little. Yes, he's not indignant after all, and then the symptoms are gone, the anger is gone, and nothing very bad happened.

Commentary. The sequence of events demonstrated that the patient had already been upset when he came from the ward. Before he came, he had obtained the assurance of the doctor there that nothing could happen. When he arrived at my office, he saw the sign "Do Not Enter." He experienced this moment as if he had been abruptly left alone, and became angry in reaction, but the anger could not reach its goal and got stuck in his symptoms.

Decisive was that the analyst himself mentioned the precipitating factor, the closed door, and the consequences the patient feared. He took the patient's place in verbalizing his aggressive fantasy and named the reason the patient could not shout and scream. Of course, this first step did not solve the problem, although it did clearly demonstrate the problem to the patient for the first time. This can be seen in the further course of the session in which resistance developed against the further assimilation of this insight that was primarily spread by the analyst.

P: Now I'm beginning to feel the anxiety again because I don't know if I can understand what you just said, I mean that nothing happens when I'm really mad.

A: Well, you understood it just a moment ago.

P: Yes, but, hum . . . apparently I know it but I'm still not entirely convinced of it.

A: Yes, you would like my friendly presence to give you reassurance every minute.

P: Yes, that's what I constantly told myself down below [in the ward], that nothing would happen if I'm angry. But that doesn't provide any relief.

A: If I'm not there, you get angrier, and you'ld like me to give you reassurance - which in turn just makes you angrier - that I'm there and my posture and friendly expression show you that it's true.

P: Yes, and in this way the whole matter is simply shifted.

A: What do you mean "shifted"?

P: Well, now it's not the anger itself that gives me a headache, but the question of the certainty that nothing will really happen. You've told me and showed me often enough: Nothing happens.

A: Yes, but maybe something else is involved too. Although you would like nothing to happen, this makes me the know-it-all we talked about yesterday. It would be unbearable if I never forgot myself, never lost control and showed that I have feelings, too.

P: Well, I'm in a bad predicament.

The patient was caught up in a dilemma that is fundamental for the maintenance of neurotic processes, a phenomenon which Strupp (1985) has referred to as the "maladaptive vicious circle." When intense negative feelings are directed at the primary role model, the anxiety is focussed on being left alone. Yet fulfillment of the resulting desire that the other person should always be friendly and unchanging only provides confirmation that the difference between child and mother is irreconcilable. This insult precipitates new aggressions, which in turn have to be pacified by desires to cling to the person. How can such a patient be helped out of this predicament? In this case the analyst first explained the dilemma once more, saying "Whatever I do, it's wrong. If I were friendly, it would be terrible; if I were unmoved and less friendly, it would also be terrible." He then suggested that the patient himself inquire whether he sensed an indirect gratification from passively asserting himself in this predicament. The analyst apparently had the psychodynamics of secondary gain from illness in mind and described this conflict to the patient in order to provide him relief. Although this interpretation is theoretically well grounded, it is far too far from the patient's experiencing to provide him any support. It is easy to understand that the patient then fell into a sullen mood, and what followed were long pauses. The attempt to reestablish the faltering dialogue proved difficult and unproductive, the patient growing increasingly angrier and madder that once again nothing new had happened.

To counteract the patient's fantasy that his aggression led to object loss and being left alone and to shorten the weekend interruption, at the end of the session the analyst offered the patient an additional session on Saturday, which he gladly accepted.

After a longer pause, the analyst cleared his throat.

A: Hum?

P: Well, I haven't thought of anything I haven't already said. As long as I'm not completely convinced that you are still there, that my doubts are going to make me afraid again. I have . . .

A: a good means to finally move me to do more for you than sit here and just say something, especially on Friday when the weekend is approaching, to really do more.

P: Yes, but all I can think of is anger. It's the same as before. The anger that I'm alone, always left alone. Or maybe I haven't understood you; maybe you wanted to show me something else.

A: No, it's nothing new, but that's just the point, that nothing new happened again, just words once more.

P: Then there's apparently nothing else to say about it. I'm useless, angry about it, that's all.

A: Useless? I don't know. You're angry.

P: Yes, and I can't even show it. I'm probably even pretty angry, but I talk so suspiciously indifferent.

<u>Commentary.</u> The unproductive period seems to have been overcome. In this session the analyst determined what the affect was, using the differentiation - which in our opinion was too weak - between "useless" and "angry." The anger affect was now directed straight at the analyst and could be accepted by each of them. An important turning point in this session was the acknowledgment of the fact that it was a Friday session - this was a noteworthy point in view of the fact that the patient came to therapy five times a week and spent the weekend alone in the

hospital. For the patient's unconscious experiencing, it was the analyst who left him for the weekend, and the patient was therefore more than justified in being mad at him.

A: Well, you're also glad that the anxiety you had when you came in is gone. It's Friday, after all, and you would like to leave with a positive feeling.
P: Well, we had agreed that it's nothing terrible for me to have an outbreak of anger.
A: Yes.
P: On the contrary, it's welcome.
A: You're not entirely convinced.
P: See, and that was the point. Why aren't I convinced, and how can I convince myself of it?
A: You don't want to convince yourself of it. The point is that you want me to convince you.

Commentary. In this transference interpretation the analyst gave one reason the patient held on to his anxiety. The patient refused to accept autonomy, struggling to maintain the dyadic situation in which he was pampered: It was the other person, not he himself, who was supposed to convince him, so that he would always be the winner because the task of convincing him would, like the labors of Sisyphus, always be in vain. The point was to move the patient to relinquish his infantile demands. In the following exchange this position was tested with regard to the role the ward doctor played for this session:

A: So you called the ward doctor to ask whether you could go, whether he thought that you would make it alright, or why?
P: No, I just didn't know which way to turn, no, very simply. I couldn't even march halfway down the hall [in the ward], because I was already so afraid and because of my heart problem, too.
A: And you still didn't take anything?
P: But you said that I shouldn't take anything.
A: Yes, but I didn't mean it unconditionally; you know that.
P: Yes, sure.
A: It's important that you didn't take anything for my sake. I don't know whether you can really manage. Perhaps it was a test of whether you can believe me enough that you can try it?

Commentary. The idea of a test brought up the patient's ambivalence: should he place more trust in the ward doctor or blindly obey the anaylst? Was it an unjustified sign of trust, or was he testing the analyst's reactions by involving the ward doctor. Here the analyst seemed to place too much faith in his words.

P: Hum, I would be too afraid. Perhaps, but it seems strange to me. Well, I was really afraid of messing something up. And now I'm starting to feel bad again.
A: Yes, it's getting to be the end of the session, so it's probable that . . .
P: . . . the anxiety is coming back.
A: And your longing to take more with you is increasing.

Commentary. Christian Y received a bonus in the form of an extra session on Saturday, and in this sense he was able to take a lot more with him. After consulting with the analyst in question, it seems probable that he made the patient this special offer because he felt he had not been up to par in this session. Christian Y did in fact get drawn into a situation of conflicting loyalties with regard to his two doctors, and suffered a defeat while attempting to reduce his medication to do the analyst a favor. According to the psychoanalytic theory of anxiety, this repetition of helplessness was a renewed traumatic experience. The analyst's last sentence also did more to promote the patient's helplessness than to overcome it because the feeling of impotence increased when the patient's longing to take more grew without him being able to get it by means of his own action. Several aspects of separation anxiety were worked out convincingly, but a certain helplessness seemed to predominate on both sides about how the patient could escape his dilemma.

9.3.2 Termination Phase

After this analysis had lasted over 10 years, the primary purpose of the termination phase was to correct mistakes that the analyst had made on the basis of false diagnostic and therapeutic conclusions. Although these conclusions are specific to this particular case, we are concerned with reproducing typical problems that the analyst traced back to his understanding of technique, i. e., to the one he had some 20 years ago. Christian Y's criticism had not only put some things right that had gone wrong during the treatment, but it opened his analyst's eyes for systematic mistakes.

The following is not a restrospective reconstruction of the course of this analysis. In an analysis that is still in progress, the focus must always be on the current moment and on the task of arriving at therapeutically effective insights by means of new forms of exchange and reflection.

In retrospect Christian Y expressed the suspicion that the purpose of my interpretations of the positive transference was not only to change his image or fantasies about the past, but also to invite him to clothe me in his fantasy wishes and, consequently, to confuse me with another. Almost literally he said:

P: I've suspected from the beginning that you're attempting to change the past by using this figure of the "other," which you've given form in various questions, that is to reverse my memory of my mother, which is predominantly negative, and to put her in a positive setting. A patient is in a terrible situation. As a result of the *confusion* that you probably call *transference*, he's the dumb one. For example, he relates his expectations of love to you, and if you go off talking, then I may know intellectually that you don't love me but I'm in danger anyway of making something out of it in my fantasy. I've never claimed that I've never been loved or can't be loved in the future. You've obviously misunderstood that. On the contrary, my mother poured enough love on me for several lives. But whatever might have been important to me or is important now was bracketed out. I don't have anything but the old rejection. The confirmation I was looking for with regard to sexuality and aggression was missing, and that's why I'm afraid of everything that I'm worried about.

What followed was a clarifying exchange of ideas resulting in the statement that the patient was not what he wanted to be, rather a kind of false image of his self. Yet his anxieties did not permit him to want and be more of what he wanted, which was the difference to what his mother had made out of him.

Commentary. This exchange reminds one of Winnicott's false and true self. It must be emphasized that the patient's elementary anxieties made it almost impossible for him to make a spontaneous movement that he could have experienced as an authentic act related to his true self.

Christian Y then came to speak about the phase of therapy in which he had been sitting.

P: Seeing you keeps or kept me from losing control of my fantasy. And then it's not as easy for a confusion to happen.
A: Not just that you lose control of me, but of you yourself.
P: What's meant is clear.

Commentary. The analyst had let himself be led in the earlier phases of therapy by the idea that the patient's mother - who had treated him as her favorite during his father's long absence--could not have had a purely negative attitude toward his vitality. Now it turned out, however, that Christian Y had taken the interpretations that the analyst had made in this direction as an attempt by the analyst to transfigure the past, specifically as a kind of corrective restropsective illusion, i. e., a kind of self-deception. His suspicion was aroused by all the cautious, subjunctive interpretations intended to stimulate his reflection, such as whether it might not have been the case that his aggressive or libidinal impulses had sometimes been received postively. He said such interpretations might animate him to accept some confusion and self-deception, i. e., to be healed through illusion.

The significance of the propositional nature of the subjunctive case as used in psychoanalytic therapy deserves some comment. For many patients its use has a positive outcome. The subjunctive case is a verb mode that makes it possible to refer to something that does *not* exist. This verb form is thus specific to something that is solely imagined, and has been called by the author Arno Schmidt "an internal revolt against reality" and "even a linguistic vote of mistrust against God: if everything were really unimprovable, there would not be any need for a subjunctive." The role of the subjunctive in the works of Lichtenberg combined, according to Albrecht Schöne (after Schneider 1987, p. 296), destructive potential with productive energy. It is thus no wonder that the subjunctive case enjoys great favor in the language used in psychoanalytic therapy and that expressions such as "what would happen if ... ," "I could imagine that ... ," and "wouldn't it be possible that ... " are preferred to the indicative mode of expression, which specifies what is or should be. Our intention in using the subjunctive case in this propositional sense is to revive the possibilities that have become unconscious.

For people who are inhibited and restricted by compulsive superego formations, cautiously applied hints can provide encouragement that otherwise leaves them sufficient room to make their own choices. Caution is appropriate in order not to evoke resistance. An altogether different situation is that of the large group of patients in whom borders are easily blurred and who therefore are desperate for security and seek clear statements of verbal support. Christian Y belonged to the latter group; he, incidentally, demonstrated to his analyst that the subjunctive case has a destructive potential if it does not have a strong partner in the indicative case. In this connection it must also be mentioned that the patient had memorized and retained his analyst's comments for a long period of time, something the analyst had misunderstood as idealization.

Very slowly it became apparent that his mother's extreme emotionalization had made him very suspicious of positive feelings. He therefore sought a sober and clear form of language and, from a distance, a confirmation of his thoughts and actions in order to successfully partially identify with the analyst.

The patient was angry and said that he had often tried to convince me of how important clear and direct confirmation was to him, to overcome his catastrophic shortage of self-esteem.

He said he was hardly interested in my personal circumstances, but was in the thoughts I had about him. He drew my attention to how important it was for him to become familiar with the context in which my interpretations arose, in order to become familiar with my feelings and thoughts about him.

P: I've always accused you of sitting behind me and having a lot more thoughts than you tell me, and that leads over to another point. I've always been much more interested in what you think but don't mention. You give some interpretations. You expand on some of my fantasies or develop your own, using some images. I don't want it, never have; I've tried to make it clear to you that you aren't permitted to do it. I want to know the notes you jot in the margin, as it were. I don't know what to confuse or transfer means. It's my opinion that it's very different from what a healthy individual normally does, and then I'm afraid, when I confuse you, that you'll make yourself come alive in my fantasies by stimulating some of them. That's not reality, but reality is what I want. When you use metaphors, then I get suspicious. I suspect that you want to suggest to me that this is a part of real life.

I agreed with the patient that insight into the connections that formed the basis of my interpretations would in fact make possible a critical examination, especially when the two sides of an issue were discussed in the dialogue. Out of the world of my thoughts that were open to precise discussion, he was particularly interested in my positive ideas about his sexuality and aggression.

In fact, the theoretical basis of many of the interpretations I made in the course of this therapy was that the patient's neurotic anxieties stemmed primarily from his anxiety about object loss or a loss of love. Christian Y intensely criticized this line of interpretation.

P: I'm enraged; you said I was afraid of losing my mother's love and that this fear kept me from believing that some sign of affection was left and not everything lost, despite the anger. I took this to be encouragement to vary the image of my mother that I had in my head, the old monument, to make a better mother appear, and I told you each and every time that I'm not going to let you change my past, regardless of whether my mother was really so evil or whether she just seems so evil because I'm so angry. To me it's clear that she rejected this and that, and I'm not going to let you alter it.

A: So, if you were to vary something, then you would be lying to yourself.

P: Yes, then I'd be lying to myself, and I've accused you over and over again of inciting me to deceive myself.

A: But isn't it possible that you're still liked despite your being angry and that there hasn't been a total loss of love? Even though it is asking too much for you to receive affection the same moment that you are inflicting pain.

I then explained to the patient that anxiety about object loss was the consequence of unconsciously active anger.

A: I thought that you were afraid that your anger was so intense, so powerful, that everything would be destroyed and every affection would cease, because in real life the person attacked usually strikes back. And there would be a fight in which you would be destroyed, and it would be too much for me and I would give up and stop.

P: You know, I have a completely different conception, that I don't suffer so much from this or that interaction of anxiety and anger etc., but that my illness is a *deficit*. It's true that my fear has decreased since I've become more aware of how unlimited my anger is. It's become clear to me that the anger inside me is not sufficient to trigger a catastrophe, and here I have the freedom, in the sense let's say of an extended fantasy, to talk about anger or be angry. I know that nothing will happen, but what I don't learn is how to feel satisfied with the anger. In the meantime I've got rid of my more-or-less intense anger, or at least diminished it substantially, but sorrow has taken its place and I've cut off the sorrow branch.

Christian Y then talked about pleasure in speaking and that the point was to link his pleasure to the tree [as a metaphor for himself]. I asked him how he thought he could counter the *deficit* he had just referred to again. He returned the question, saying that this was my field and he did not have an answer. He said it was clear to him that it could not take place via an alteration in his memory. After a long pause I admitted my helplessness as to how this deficit could be overcome today. I pointed out to the patient that he had corrected something, namely my thoughts and actions with regard to therapy.

A: Is it possible that my acknowledgment of the clarity of your criticism might contribute to overcoming your deficit? You've achieved and experienced an increase in self-security toward me.

The patient immediately weakened my comment:

P: I'm always concerned about my relationship to the external world.

A: Yes, and above all about acknowledgment, and I've just given you one.

Commentary. This working through was continued in the subsequent session and in the long termination phase. The consequence of the fact that the analyst had discouraged this patient, who was intelligent and interested in his thoughts, from posing abstract thoughts - for example, clarifying the significance of the concept of ambivalence in discussion during the session - was particularly disadvantageous. The patient had drawn the conclusion from this that everything that had to do with abstract thought and analytic thinking was simply taboo for him. In violating such taboos he felt the anxiety that he was doing something forbidden.

A: It was an outright mistake not to give you more information about my thoughts.

P: Yes, it's often hard to envisage the consequences.

A: Yes, but it had the consequence that it hindered your efforts to become familiar with my way of thinking and to understand connections.

P: Another consequence was, let me put it this way, that I thought you were acting insincerely because I assumed that although you say what you think, you didn't tell me everything you thought.

Commentary. This was the reason for the patient's continuing mistrust. Warmth, tolerance, and empathy made him suspicious. The patient admitted that, also for practical therapeutic reasons, it was essential for the analyst to select from a number of possible thoughts and comments. The subject of self-security and the fact that his deficient self-esteem was a basis of his anxieties again became a focus of attention.

P: I've tried to tell you that tolerance and such things don't really help me. To confuse you with someone else can't be genuine. For me it's just a kind of extended fantasy, nothing real. The real thing would be to reach out to outside reality or to what you're thinking; I can genuinely relate to that. There it's possible to avoid the danger of confusion or clarify what's happened. Yes, in that regard I'm terribly curious; I want to know.

A: Yes, my views, opinions, thinking differs from that of our parents. Something new and different is involved.

Then Christian Y began to speak once more about the difficulties that result form the confusion, i. e., from transference. He had a vivid recollection of a session from long back in which he was very enraged and I had answered in an irritated voice.

P: That was an enormous disappointment; I was mad for once and then you let me have it again. I still haven't really understood how my confusing you with someone else can have something to do with something coming from you if you aren't affected at all. Yet I've taken some of the actions you use here to be a kind of advanced bridge head that you work from, even if you as a person are far behind it and your actions are still very difficult for me to predict. And I don't really care about what I know about you. What's important is the question of trust and being able to follow what's said.

A: Yes, yes, because – to be brief – I am I and you are you; my goals don't have to be the same as yours.

P: We have to find the things we have in common somewhere else. Since I've been thinking about the question of confirmation, I've tried to force you into an *eccentric position*, so that you're no longer the one being confused but that you could say something about what I'm doing. Then I might be able to find some kind of reinforcement. But for reasons unknown to me you've avoided it. When I talk about anger, then you're still very similar to the one whose toes I'm stepping on. I know that this is a problem that's hard to solve, but if you would say something in that third position, I might be able to draw some gain from it if I could identify with what you say. That depends on your taking a stand and not talking in some disconnected manner and leaving it up to the patient to imagine what your opinion is. I still assert that you don't express yourself in what you say because it's always related to the patient's horizon.

I referred approvingly to the "eccentric position" that the patient invented, and mentioned its advantages.

A: It makes it easier for you and me not to have the great anxiety that would be (and was) present in confusions if you feared and expected that I would react exactly the same as your mother, father, teacher, or somebody else. Repetitions have repeatedly taken place in your life, i. e., confusions.

P: Just look, if you remove the anxiety, the anxiety of punishment and the such, the questions that remain concern the consequences of the punishment.

Commentary. This was a reference to the consequences that the internalization of his experiences had in his persisting superego and social anxieties and the subsequent behavioral difficulties associated with his intense loss of self-security and self-esteem.

The issue was then whether an eccentric position would keep the analyst from reacting sensitively to, for example, aggression and insults. The patient, who was a keen observer, had been able to detect during the period of analysis in which he had been sitting a lot on the analyst's face that confirmed to him the maliciousness of his aggression.

A: The eccentric position made it possible for me to bear the pain and tolerate your actions.
P: But you know that I don't have any logical reason to step on your toes or hurt you in any other way.
A: But I've done some things to you. I've missed a lot of things. I've overlooked some opportunities and I've made mistakes. Your recovery hasn't been optimal, and you still can't do what you want and be entirely satisfied.
P: Well, it would depend on the mistake, I've told you that before, and second you can't inflict any more damage than I brought with me in the first place. And I haven't made any complaints. The problem is only the eccentric position; I swear to you that I wouldn't accept anything [that is not logical], it triggers a multitude of anxieties because I don't consider the confusion to be something genuine. The point is that an original, good feeling about anger cannot be produced. Anxiety and rage cannot be reduced, and the good feeling makes it easier to bear the real anxiety. It's a question of the inner balance, but what I'm striving for is to produce a good feeling. The good feeling, you mentioned it once, but it comes up far too little in the therapy. Since then I'm the only one to have mentioned it.

The patient criticized the analyst for not assuming the *eccentric position* more clearly and for behaving more like someone making a supreme sacrifice and acting as if he tolerated it, which however made it possible for the patient to be angry during the sessions. The patient instead demanded clear statements that the analyst expressly approved of his sexuality and aggression and that they reach a consensus at this level. The patient then drew the following conclusion:

P: Then I could identify with what you say, but not because you yourself are the object, which moreover is allegedly what I'm looking for. I felt this to be dishonest.
A: So I've become an object of confusion. By offering myself to you as an apparent object from an eccentric position, I was unable to show you sufficiently that you yourself also have an eccentric position to this apparent object.
P: Yes, maybe you can say it that way.
A: We're linked and identified via the eccentric position, and that might lead you to better recognize it in little things or to have more inner security and authenticity.
P: Might be, yes, inasfar as we clearly distinguish what is confused and what is real.
A: At any rate, today I've better understood how important the eccentric position is in establishing some distance to the confusions, repetitions, and mistakes, and thus in finding confirmation and security.

Statement by Christian Y

After the analysis had ended, Christian Y generously provided a detailed statement to the reports cited in Sects. 9.3.2 and 9.3.3. His instructive comments were based on the original transcripts, i. e., the protocols were still uncommented when he read the transcripts. In retrospect, he wrote:

At the beginning of therapy I welcomed what I've referred to all these years as confusion because I considered it to be therapy's mode of functioning. It was not until later that it took on a negative accent. That was related, in addition to my clumsiness, to the way you handled it. At the time I had the impression that the confusion did not come about on its own, but that you had forced it. You had talked about a "relationship." I always firmly rejected it because I take it to be something interactive and despite my best efforts simply couldn't imagine confusion to be interactive in any way. You really confused me when you said, "it's genuine too." For me the confusion ended at the back edge of the couch. At first I took sentences such as "why not think that you are still being loved when . . . ," "you can't believe that you are still being loved if . . . ," and "perhaps the other person is not as limited as you think" to be allusions to think more "positively." Well, as a matter of fact, I didn't-rationally - have such a low opinion of my goals as my earlier experiences had made me think. As simple considerations, your statements did not go far beyond my own thoughts and were not very effective. So that couldn't be the reason. Then I developed a comparison. I imagined that a "healthy" person lying on the couch and talking about himself would probably confuse you in a "positive" way. I also thought that the figure of the other person, the choice of subjunctive or passive voice, etc. was supposed to help me simply repole my negative fantasies and expectations in the confusion, to confuse you now in a "positive" manner. Symbolically I thus thought that you wanted to move on the screen onto which I projected the confusion in order to achieve change. Now and then you spoke about the rehearsals that I undertook against you. I can't understand it like that. I think that verbal actions, even if they are expressed with all the fundamental and accompanying emotions, are merely copies of the image that the patient has made of you. It's not even a trial action. For this reason alone I was always skeptical when you related yourself to my actions toward you. I was, for example, a little suspicious when I was angry and you wanted to suggest to me that you tolerated my anger. You tended to react in unusual ways when the topic was transferred love or sexuality. I want genuine answers in response to genuine questions.

Of course, the eccentric position cannot be on the periphery because this would make it impossible for the analyst to assume the human significance that is an essential prerequisite enabling him to balance the influence of older figures. This is thus a kind of critical distance that makes something new possible and that also prevents an impenetrable emotional confusion from developing, i. e., a mishmash without boundaries.

9.3.3 Confirmation and Self-Esteem

In the psychoanalysis of Christian Y the analyst had refrained from providing direct confirmation for two reasons: first, in order not to influence the patient, and second, on the assumption that his positive attitude toward the patient's sexuality and aggression was obvious and did not require explicit mention. Christian Y demonstrated convincingly, however, that the subjunctive mode of speech left many things open and that he consequently had not felt he had received confirmation. The patient then went on to describe his professional success.

A: Naturally I've always been pleased by your successes, but I didn't mention it in a manner that would have been immediately obvious to you.

P: Yes, you weren't able to help me as much as you might have because you only described circumstances and assumed that my new self-esteem would develop all on its own. But what good are my changed ideas about myself if I can't anchor them somehow. [Long pause] You once told a joke about a psychiatrist who had a patient who thought he was a mouse but ended up agreeing with the psychiatrist that he was wrong. But if the cat doesn't know that I'm not a mouse any more, then I stay afraid of the cat. The joke in this joke is obvious, I mean what good is the rapport between in here and out there? What I call a confusion [the word that Christian Y used to refer to transference] is not limited to people who are sick or to here, but a general principle of life. Man perceives his environment from a certain perspective. [The patient described this by referring to photographs showing snow in very different colors.] Snow is white, but it's not always white. The color depends on the lighting. Everything I experience is black in me because my parents ruined everything I saw. It's hard for me to experience situations anew without support from outside because they're organized according to the old perspectives and I just can't simply replace them.

Christian Y was very excited - which I pointed out to him - while he described the different colors snow could have.

A: Were you the photographer who used the picture to show the spectator that you know better, that you can show me something too and that you see it more precisely and sharper or at least that your view of the matter is definitive?

P: No, I felt insecure because I thought that it was a silly comparison.

He traced his difficulties in being self-confident back to the absence of positive images.

P: You see, I have difficulty being self-confident because I don't have any positive images of myself. Whoever is self-confident out there has positive images of himself, and he is naive. If he's put into a situation in which he looks bad, then he still relates more to the positive image he has of himself. But I just can't do it; I've had these thoughts for a long time but haven't mentioned them. For me it's an arduous mental feat, an effort to keep things together when I'm confronted by some difficulties. [Pause] For example, if I can't be very aggressive but am confronted by others' aggressiveness, then I have difficulties with colleagues who put themselves in the limelight.

In the previous session Christian Y had told me that he would like to attend another vocational course and had a goal. Having a goal was tremendously important for him. He expressed his pleasure that I explicitly approved of his plan, but was at the same time disappointed that I had not previously approved of his goals.

P: You usually stay neutral, and that's made me terribly angry for a long time. I guessed that you don't want to make any firm comments for scientific reasons.

A: Although it was clear to me that people, especially the ill, need goals, I didn't pay enough attention to the fact that it is not only important for the patient to set goals but that it's just as important for the analyst to confirm them or to make it possible for the patient to anchor them by providing encouragement. I now see the necessity. It's essential for me to express myself clearly, and then you can disregard it if you want to.

P: That's what I've always said. Otherwise freedom would become a feeling of being lost; that would be the only time you could enjoy your freedom. And to be honest, I can't get a picture of myself as I'd like to be; on the contrary, just thinking about it triggers so much anxiety that I have to stop immediately. I've been moaning here for years, am afraid of sex and aggression and other things, afraid of change, but what I want to be is something I don't know either. The normal person doesn't become what he is on the basis of what he was given, but by interacting with his environment, doesn't he?

A: Yes, exactly.

P: When you act in a neutral manner, then I'm deprived all the more of the environment that I didn't have with the old figures, at least not in the desired manner.

A: Despite all the friction and the aggression, there's no foundation that you can use to distinguish yourself.

P: I don't like my memories of the period when I was so aggressive here; I don't like them. I want to get my way, and actually I want to be furious out there and aggressive in a sensible way; what I expect from you is – now I've forgotten what I wanted to say. I would like support enabling me to show it when I'm in a situation out there. [Pause] A few days ago somebody was talking about psychoanalysis and said that neurotics suffer from a limited capacity to act, but not in my case. I have numerous reactions at my disposal. What I suffer from is that none of the ones that appeal to me seem to me to be right or suitable. The other description seems to me to apply more to compulsives.

The interview then turned once again to photography and imaging.

A: You're a passionate and very good photographer, and photography is a source of your sharpness. You're a very precise observer. Yet you don't want people to become aware of it; it has to stay subliminal. You're so good at your job because you're critical and a precise observer. It's also the source of your anxiety, namely that somebody might notice how sharp you can be. And in hindsight that is why it is so disagreeable to you that you were very sharp and aggressive to me. You don't want to act so uncontrolled. It should be well done, a well grounded aggression. And that is why this is such an important process of clarification, that I can now tell you, and honestly have to tell you, that your criticism was well made. So it's important for your criticism here to be accepted as true and accurate, but there isn't anyone who can't react in an uncontrolled manner.

Commentary. Christian Y made many astute and sharp-sighted observations about the analyst, particularly in the period when the treatment was conducted in sitting, as he wished. At that time he had seen expressions of sadness and irritation on the analyst's face, which he registered as a renewed rejection, as the opposite of encouragement and pleasure at his aggression, a subject that filled later phases of treatment. Without a doubt, the change in position and the opportunities that accompanied it contributed to the growth of the patient's self-esteem.

P: I recall it as a terrible period; I was so aggressive, and then you made this sad face. As a child I was unable to look at my father's face. He was a bogeyman, and children cried when they saw him. I was afraid of him too; he had a very dark face, dark hair, and glowing green eyes – he was a nightmare. I wasn't able to look you in the eyes either. After a while I managed, when I departed, but I only acted as if I had looked at your face and didn't even see you because I was so afraid of your face. The second thing is that I assign you a certain predominant role so that nothing from outside, none of the old problems, can bother me. I can't discuss everything I want to do with you anymore.

A: As you rightly say, it's easier to identify yourself if there's a clear difference and no mingling.

P: When you say you're happy, well that's more than I demand of you. I've never said I want something great. I'm satisfied with a positive sign. I'm not after something absolute that exceeds all limits, and when I referred to the distance between you and me, then I didn't mean that I'm afraid of closeness. I only didn't want any mingling in the original sense. I thought that identifications were also possible if there was some distance. It is possible from a distance; there doesn't have to be anything personal, and when you're happy it's not for show but real - it simply moves me. Without being overwhelmed by confirmation, I've always emphasized that my mother's position might have seemed so negative to me because it inhibited me and not just because of her overwhelming feelings. Confirmation for me can thus be more emphatic without getting too strong. A few weeks ago I said I felt some anxiety about what you might say to me, but that was simply my uncertainty. If you say that you're happy, then it moves me but doesn't make me anxious.

Commentary. Their mutual pleasure did not stem from latent homosexuality, something which had upset the patient in earlier phases of the treatment.

Change is easier if it involves factual matters or goal-directed work, while interpersonal contact outside therapy poses more difficulties because a patient frequently still has the feeling of being unwelcome. Christian Y described this condition with regard to the problems he encountered playing tennis. When he won, he would almost apoligize. His anxiety that playing aggressively would make him unwelcome caused him not to hit the ball powerfully and cramped his style. He correctly assumed that he would improve his capacity for concentration if he could be more aggressive. His anxieties impeded the transformation of his intentions into purposive acts.

A: Well, perhaps you can find some satisfaction in the fact that your arguments have convinced me, and in that regard you've reached a goal. Of course, I naturally regret that I expected you to take this round about route and that I put some obstacles in your path. But who's happy about the mistakes he makes!

P: You know that I don't want to even consider such ideas. You're supposed to be the one who's happy when I can do this or that, but you're not supposed to be the one that I have a share in because it reminds me too much of the confusion. And I know too little about it to say that you've made a mistake or that we're taking a detour. I just say that I don't like something and defend myself without being able to say whether I'm right.

A few sessions later Christian Y described a dream that accurately symbolized his condition. In it he was in an airplane that was airborne, and he had overcome a nascent anxiety by recalling his increasing certainty that he could rely on the footing he had found. He had already interpreted his dream, namely his increased confidence in the foothold he had. He summarized his identification with me and emphasized once again how important it was for him that I had taken a positive stance toward his sexuality and aggression. He would not have been satisfied with some atmospheric or tacit agreement. He said he required clear confirmation. For a long time we were then concerned with the difficulties he encountered making his new self-confidence reality outside therapy.

In the course of the session I interpreted his passivity as an attempt to assert his self and protect it against his mother, who on the one hand exhibited hysterical outbursts and on the other expected her son to follow clearly defined forms of behavior, i. e., forced a kind of "false self" on him. This assumption made it seem logical that he had withdrawn and adjusted to her values. At the same time the patient felt that he was actually very different, and claimed he had always wanted to be different, from how he had to appear to be.

The patient was still suspicious of my attitude toward his sexuality. Once again he was unable to continue to talk because he was ashamed. Later he managed to overcome his shame, which apparently was connected with his recollection of earlier sessions.

P: I simply want to, I can's say why; it's strange. I just want to [Pause] . . . I have to turn around; perhaps I'll get where I want to be, namely that here . . . when I demand it of you, I want confirmation. It's a kind of model for something I want out there. I want something from others, and this wanting is awfully problematic for me because I . . . at home I learned that you shouldn't want anything from others if at all possible, and should try and influence them. And especially out there, what I want is to get confirmation from others; that's something that's extremely difficult for me.

A: And then it's clearer where the confusion has just arisen. It was the moment you made the intense demand that I pay attention to you in a particular manner. I satisfied your wish, expectation, longing, and intense demand by saying, "Yes, that's what's important," which I didn't offer in a general way but in a very concrete one. So I did satisfy something.

P: That makes me feel anxious because I . . . .

A: You were confused because you could finally satisfy it.

P: Another idea is tormenting me. I would like to refer to the image of Jacob and the angel that you once mentioned. In a sense, my ideas are too insignificant to get this blessing.

A: Hum.

P: Aren't they?

A: Hum. [Pause] I believe you're using this thought to protect yourself against the overwhelming liberation represented by being blessed.

P: Yes, of course, that too.

A: Hum.

P: Because precisely the confirmation was missing and I had the impression that you were drawing my attention to something else; in a sense I had the impression that all of that wasn't anything for me and I'd just have to learn to live with the limitations. Just like earlier when someone said that I was too small for everything.

A: Hum.

P: Don't know. At the moment I just can't say. I've always assumed that you possess what I'm looking for, but that something has kept you from telling me what it is.

Christian Y recalled that he had asked me about my attitude to sex in the very first interview. In essence I answered that it was less important what *my* attitude was than that *he* reach clarity about his own. He took this comment to be a rejection, i. e., he experienced a lack of confirmation.

My therapeutic attitude at the time was exactly as described by the patient. One aspect of my style of treatment was that I gave evasive answers as a matter of principle. It was only the subsequent correction of my attitude and technique that led to the change which the patient, in his dream, referred to in this session and in other sessions and which made it possible for him to be successful and largely free of anxiety in both family life and business life. It is very probable that the analysis would have taken an different course if I had made an identification possible in the first sessions by offering *confirmation.*

It would incidentally be a mistake to believe that the patient had been particularly curious about *my* sexuality at that time or later. He was only marginally interested in my private life, much more in my attitude to the extent that it might help him establish a positive identification with a value system independent of his mother. At the same time he wanted *distance*. This presumption is a hypothesis supported by many statements the patient made. In today's session, for example, the patient had mentioned the shame he felt from the confusions, i. e., from his transference fantasies.

The following excerpt is from the patient's written evaluation that is mentioned above [Sect. 9.3.2].

I started from a simple assumption, which in principle I still adhere to. You showed me how I had adopted the attitudes of the older figures, had identified with them in a deleterious manner. At first I was mad at myself for having been so dumb. I have to add that I am convinced that the suitability and willingness to identify is expressed to very different degrees in different people; I consider myself to be one of those initially more dependent on it and inclined to do it. This mood soon changed, making room for some hope which has remained until this day. I then came to understand the features I had adopted as being a great chance to identify with suitable role models and to gain definite self-esteem. I expected you to react correspondingly, which took a long time coming. The absence of oppotunities for identification led me to call my condition a deficit. In this context I am sure I usually spoke about wanting to be loved and not being loved; what I meant, naturally, was not a momentary desire, but the old one from childhood. Not being loved was the focal point for my identification with my mother. I kept describing this starting point in my attempt to find some way out. It has become clear now that I don't need "love." The problem was "another solution." Deficits cannot be overcome by simply describing them. The separation from old figures, the liberation from them, does not put anything in their place. My goals in life out there are very varied. I profit immeasurably more if, with your support, these real goals gain in value. I don't understand why the discussion of my goals should be in the least bit less important momentarily or why the meaning I let you assign to it should be a trace less immediate than "direct verbal expressions." None of the intensity is lost, and the interview is not less personal as a result. Your options are unlimited; aggression and sexuality can be easily included without it being necessary to resort to some padding, artificial interpretations, and awkward intermediate steps. If it is possible to reach "agreement" at this level, it's always clear what and who is meant. Giving me a generally positive attitude does not in itself have a "mutative" effect. To me it seems to be necessary for you to take a stand. Just a little sign is enough; I think that just indicating a tendency is helpful in itself, if certain conditions are satisfied. You only relate warmth, tolerance, and a positive attitude to the presence of sexuality, aggression etc. in the patient, and of course empathy at their being the way they are. Massive changes in the patient are facilitated if the analyst, in addition to understanding, can also show an iota or minimal dose of identification with the patient - which of course is not supposed to alter the doctor. The old is discarded, and the new takes its place. Sympathy alone doesn't help me much; you stay "extinguished." What's decisive is a tiny bit of "life." The liberation from the old figures is thus a process that is largely free of mourning, because their positions are not empty but pleasurably filled. Even leaving from you is easy after the goal has been reached. The difficulties are somewhere else. People are what they are not only on the basis of predisposition, but also as a result of their interaction with their environment. Because of my lack of experience I have regularly felt that I am crippled, underdeveloped, and stunted, and have described myself in these terms. I have not had a suitable interaction with my environment. It is most difficult to make progress in analysis if there are "blind spots in my soul." The precondition is then that the analyst intervene and construct in a special sense, which probably contradicts the traditional conception of therapy. I have not really managed to convince you of the necessity of changes in this direction. On the other hand, I admit that I have come a long way and have probably reached quite a bit with your assistance. It hardly needs mentioning that I am grateful to you, especially for your flexible stance to this quite demanding and occasionally very trying patient.

Commentary. We would like to make a few comments here because of the fundamental significance of Christian Y's comments about transcripts from the termination phase of his treatment. We want to refer to the technical mistakes he complained about. The analyst always managed to make good for his mistakes, at least to the extent that a severly ill young man who had not been able to leave the hospital and had been nearly immobile both intellectually and physically had become able during treatment to reach both his personal and professional goals. Christian Y's criticism stems from the last phase of psychoanalysis, when patients frequently take stock. It thus seems logical for a patient who, despite numerous satisfactions, suffered from a deficit - seemingly and paradoxically because of his excess of maternal love - to conclude at the end of treatment where he came up short. This argument provokes another, and in no time we would be enbroiled in a very far-reaching discussion, which could only be conducted and grounded in an empirical case study that takes the form of a combined study of the course of treatment and of its outcome, such as is being undertaken by Leuzinger-Bohleber (1988). So let us return to the analyst in this case and accept his judgment that his technical mistakes were not only due to diagnostic error and to some aspect of his personal equation. In the analyst's words,

I began the psychoanalysis of Christian Y in accordance with the understanding of the psychoanalytic technique I had at the time, i. e., of the theory and practice of transference, countertransference, resistance, and regression. With regard to the subjects discussed in these two segments, I learned very much from Christian Y and from other patients with similar disturbances, and I believe this has been of great significance for my current conception of the psychoanalytic technique. In the course of time I have become convinced that philosophical and social psychological theories about the role that confirmation plays in the interpersonal development of self-esteem can be productive for the psychoanalytic technique. Düsing (1986) has evaluated the works of Fichte, Hegel, Mead, and Schütz with regard to these problems. Although she did not establish any connections to the theory of psychoanalytic technique, it is obvious from her study that different psychoanalytic conceptions about the development of self-esteem and the role of confirmation have their roots deep in intellectual history. This philosophical knowledge of man is now supplemented by empirical results on the existence of intersubjectivity between mother and child from birth on. [We pointed to the convergence with the interactional conception of transference and countertransference in Vol.1.]

Of course we cannot simply make, for example, Hegel's famous interpretation of the relationship between master and slave or his philosophical discussion of the mortal struggle for confirmation the subject of therapeutic interventions. Similarly, we cannot simply incorporate Mead's social psychological interpretation of the role that the significant other plays in the constitution of self-esteem into therapeutic technique [on this issue see Cheshire and Thomä 1987]. There are far too many ways that humans look for acknowledgment, which in turn has a wide range of implications. For instance, Christian Y looked precisely for confirmation other than that mediated by the glance in the mother's (or analyst's) eye, to refer to Kohut's metaphor for narcissistic mirroring. With the aid of an eccentric position he wanted exactly the opposite, namely to overcome the confusion in order to find himself in his own different nature. Christian Y sought mutual confirmation, which is avoided in the customary psychoanalytic neutrality. My positive comments about the patient's criticism during the termination phase and even earlier were based in my conviction, which fortunately also acquired a therapeutic function. The dialogues reproduced here represent great moments inasmuch as they point beyond the individual case and can contribute to the resolution of fundamental problems in psychoanalytic technique. The polished language and level of abstraction should not distract from the fact that both emotionally and existentially there are extremely important values at stake. Christian Y managed to verbalize this and thus, together with my agreement, to delimit his world and his self. It could have probably happened much earlier, yet at the beginning of therapy I did not know better.

9.4 Depression

Dorothea X, a 50-year-old female patient who suffered from depression accompanied by states of anxiety, had undergone unsuccessful pharmacotherapy for years. Her symptoms grew out of her mourning the death of her husband, who had died after a brief illness. She developed hypochondriac anxieties about dying just as her husband had, from a carcinoma that was discovered too late. The unconscious identification with her idealized late husband and the continuation of her internalized ambivalent relationship to him in the form of self-accusations followed the pattern typical of depressive reactions. Dorothea X lived withdrawn and hidden, in a literal sense - she pretended to have oversensitive eyes to justify wearing sunglasses and hiding behind them. Although she believed she had to take care of two of her grandchildren one day because of a daughter-in-law's chronic illness, she was afraid that her own illness made her incapable of doing so. This concern increased her suffering, yet also made her feel obliged to stay alive and not to succumb to her thoughts about committing suicide.

The Psychoanalyst as Transference Object

Working through the patient's depressive identification with her late husband had led to some symptomatic improvement and reestablished her capacity to relate to people, initially to me as her psychoanalyst, i. e., her transference object.

In transference Dorothea X tended to mother me in a friendly manner. At the same time she idealized my equanimity, as when she said "You are as calm as I've always wanted to be." The point at which her previously mild positive transference suddenly changed occurred accidentally. At a late afternoon session, which was not her customary time, she encountered a tired and exhausted analyst. An comment she made about my being tired, which I confirmed, precipitated agitation motivated by her irrational concerns. She suspected a serious illness was the reason for my exhaustion and felt that I could not be burdened with any further stress. The previously benign mothering took on exaggerated forms. Her symptoms disappeared almost completely, yet this was connected with her self-reproach that she would never be able to stop the treatment because she then would not have the opportunity to constantly convince herself that nothing serious had happened to me. She felt she at least had to be constantly ready to provide me some form of compensation. At the same time she accused herself of burdening me by continuing the treatment; she once again made herself guilty at the very time she was discovering old feelings of guilt.

Dorothea X's irrational concern about me as a transference figure facilitated the process of working through her unconscious ambivalence, which derived from the idea that she had been the cause of her mother's severe hypochondria. The loss of blood at her birth had been almost fatal for the mother, and for years this had been taken to be the reason for all of her mother's complaints. This background must be taken into consideration in order to understand the fantasies about death and rescue that were the central ideas in the patient's childhood.

While we, under the protection of a positive transference, succeeded in clarifying the negative and aggressive aspects of her thought and behavior, the defensive character of her idealizations became increasingly evident. It became apparent that the maternal role, which she too had fulfilled toward her late husband, who had been dependent on her, was ideally suited to hide her sexual needs and to satisfy them in a regressive manner. In mothering her husband she had been the one who, under her skirt, had worn the pants in the family, which provided additional satisfaction. She had also made a substantial contribution to his successful career.

I looked for a fitting opportunity to focus on the very human side of her transference figure. This was in vain because although the patient realized intellectually that I must have weak spots too, she did not really want to be aware of this fact.

There was a typical form of the interaction between idealization and disparagement. The patient acknowledged on the one hand a comment to the effect that I used my knowledge with her own good in mind, and on the other disparaged my remarks as narcissistic self-confirmation. The patient had to close this line of thought with a comment excusing me, which she did by tracing this "lack of concern" to some presumed terrible experiences I had had. For a long time, however, these disparaging thoughts remained as inaccessible to interpretation as her idealizations were.

Deidealization and Perception of the Real Person

A second turning point in this treatment occurred after Dorothea X had seen me race past her in my car. Her description of the circumstances, location, and time removed all doubt about the accuracy of her observation. Yet she attempted to suppress this knowledge and avoided verifying her observation by closing her eyes as she walked passed my parked car. For her, the large horsepower of my sports car did not fit her image of the calm and apparently undynamic psychoanalyst.

Her accurate observation on the street led to a lasting disruption of her idealization. After intense inner struggles about whether she dared find out for certain, i.e., whether she dared look at the car or not, Dorothea X finally decided to eliminate all doubt. She realized that her analyst was one of those men who was guided by irrational thoughts when choosing a car. Her attempts to find a justification and explanation for my behavior only led to temporary compromise relief. The aspect of reality introduced by the car took on numerous meanings: it represented and symbolized everything from power and dynamism to carelessness and waste. Finally the car became a true sexual symbol. The patient's agitation increased to the degree to which she recognized her idealization of her transference figure. In her transference figure she sought not just the satisfaction of her own needs, but especially *herself*, i.e., her own dynamism, which had been submerged by her idealization and mothering.

The primary goal of my interpretive work was to show Dorothea X that she had delegated significant parts of herself to me and the car. The return of her vitality was initially linked with great distress since she had had to learn to control her temperament in many regards during her long marriage. She managed to win back her energy and activity and integrate them as a consequence of the progress we made in working through the "delegation" idea. While working through the unconscious meanings, the course of the treatment was uncomplicated.

Both of the turning points in this therapy were precipitated by realistic observations that Dorothea X had made about me. My confirmation of her observations lent substance and conviction to my interpretations. In the first episode we traced her exaggerated concern about my tiredness back to aggressive components of transference. It is questionable whether an interpretation of the unconscious fantasies contained in the observations would have had the same effect. Would such an interpretation not instead have contributed to raisng doubts about the patient's capacity for perception, as if the analyst had not been tired at all and was therefore vulnerable?

In the second episode it was another realistic observation that offered her the chance to overcome the polarization of idealization and disparagement and that led her to approve my having - the previously denied - masculine qualities and to integrate her projected parts into her self-conception.

Epicrisis

Some three years after the termination of therapy Dorothea X wrote in a supplement to a questionaire specifically designed to examine the consequences of interruptions during therapy:

I answered all the questions immediatedly after receiving the questionaire, for me a sure sign of how much I still felt a close tie to psychotherapy and to my psychotherapist. The greater the distance to the last session, the more benefit I can derive from the treatment. For example, I've just now come to understand many of the therapist's ideas from that period and know how to handle them. I am thankful for every session of therapy in which I learned to live a bit more light-heartedly and happier.

Some time before the termination of my psychotherapy I rehearsed, laughing and crying, all by myself for the hour of separation. This game became so unbearable for me that I requested that the therapist announce the last session as quickly as possible. And I also clearly felt that the time was ripe. Afterwards I felt free--not happy and not sad - just waiting. I continued to live as before and had many mental conversations with my ex-therapist. I have never considered returning to therapy. The circle had closed. I knew that it was a good and productive period for me. In therapy and from the therapist I studied how to live better and more freely and rehearsed it. I then had the firm will and fairly secure feeling of being able to master life outside.

9.5 Anorexia Nervosa

Reconstructing Its Genesis

We have taken the following reconstruction of the origin of anorexia nervosa from a case history that has already been published in full (see Thomä 1967a, 1981). Although it is not a trivial matter that this reconstruction of a psychogenesis still retains such vitality after almost 30 years and that the problems posed by identification and identity in anorexia nervosa which are the focus of this reconstruction have in the meantime been acknowledged by all the schools of psychotherapy, we would like to emphasize something else. We want to familiarize the reader with the termination phase of a psychoanalysis, because in the eighth and ninth phases of this treatment there are hidden signs that in hindsight turned out to be significant regarding symptom substitution.

Henriette X's symptoms first appeared when she was 16. Her premorbid body weight of 50-52 kg (110-115 lb) fell to about 40 kg (88 lb). At the beginning of psychoanalysis three years later she weighed 46.3 kg (102 lb). Amenorrhea and obstipation had been present since the beginning of the illness. During the psychoanalysis, a total of 289 sessions in two years, the patient's weight increased to 55 kg (121 lb), her period returned spontaneously after an absence of nearly four years, and her obstipation improved.

In order to provide insight into several important psychodynamic processes in this case we proceed from the precipitating situation, which is intimately related to an asceticism of puberty as it has been described by A.Freud (1937).

Henriette X used to blush when boys looked at her or when a subject related in any way with love was mentioned at school. The developing erythrophobia was a symptom that tormented her. She had had the feeling that she was the master of the house (see Freud 1916/17, p. 285) until something happened that was beyond her control. She discovered that she could make her blushing anxiety disappear by fasting in the morning. The blushing ceased with her loss of weight. In the course of the psychoanalysis this process was reversed. Her recovery of her ability to blush was accompanied by the old conflicts that had previously led to her asceticism and by the fact that she recognized them and was able to overcome most of them.

It turned out that Henriette X blushed because she was embarrassed when someone looked at her as a girl. This summary focusses on the anxiety that accompanied this involuntary act and her ego's defense mechanisms. The important question is why her erythrophobia was so intense that it caused her to limit her nutrition for years and to reject her body, which was accompanied by isolation. In the following we give the analyst's attempt to provide a survey of this patient's psychodynamics.

1. The description that the patient had felt like the master in the house prior to the blushing refers to a peculiarly structured ego ideal. She wanted to be a boy, not be looked at as a girl. This desire to be a boy had been anchored in her particularly firmly by elements of her environment. She had grown up without a father, an only child, together with her mother. Her mother was a widow who projected her image of her husband onto her daughter, who was intellectually precocious and acted as an advisor and partner to her mother. In other words, the patient was forced into a "masculine" role. The family circumstances strengthened those features in the patient that are not inherently masculine or feminine but are primarily exhibited in Western society by men, such as independence, firmness, and vigor. She set the tone and was accustomed to her mother doing as she wanted. This circumstance was partially responsible for the fact that the patient hung on to the misapprehension of an "omnipotence of ideas" (Freud 1916/17, p. 285).
   The patient was also the active person in her long friendship with another girl. As long as she could play the role of the boy and succeeded in everything - she was an excellent athlete and pupil without having to work hard - her ego ideal was unimpaired. Her inner balance was disturbed until she reached puberty.
2. In the conflict between *not being able* to be a boy and *not wanting* to be a girl (in accordance with her ego ideal that was by now anchored in her unconscious), she reestablished a sense of security by adopting an asexual ideal. This is an example of the undifferentiated, primitive animosity between ego and libido or instinctual nature that A. Freud referred to in connection with the asceticism of puberty. The consequences of this patient's general rejection of libidinal wishes can be seen in her behavioral modifications in general and her disturbed eating behavior in particular. The

patient achieved an anxiety-free ego by denying dangerous aspects of external reality and repressing her own libidinal nature.

3. Hunger became the prototype of her bodily needs, and asceticism helped her to overcome her anxiety about the intensity of her drives.
4. Upon closer consideration, I differentiated this anxiety into its unconscious components, whose repression disturbed and inhibited the patient's thoughts and behavior. This led to, first, a limitation of the patient's capacity to enter interpersonal relations, second a disturbance of her capacity to work and concentrate and, third, functional disturbances. These consequences resulted from the different fates of the affect and mental representations of her unconscious impulses. The repressions were secured by means of anticathexes and alterations of her ego, as could be discerned in her behavior.
5. The following psychogenetic processes can be distinguished:
   (a) The avoidance of real satisfaction, retreat of the drive from the object, and satisfaction of desires in fantasy (daydreams about eating). This is already an attempt to avoid a danger that would be posed given an unrestricted and real satisfaction of drives.
   (b) It turned out that the patient's amazon behavior in general and the anexoria in particular were the result of the receptivity she warded off ("something comes in me") because food was unconsciously linked with fertilization. Revulsion and vomiting were related to sexual defense.
   (c) Oral gratification was unconsciously linked with destruction and killing. Her experiencing of eating was therefore restricted or burdened with guilt.
6. Her anxiety that the borders might be destroyed points to a longing for a relationship that is all-encompassing or transcends all differences. Since she felt anxiety about her ambivalence and destructive oral claim to totality, she repressed this longing and satisfied it in a regressive manner. From an economic perspective, the tension from the restricted nutritional intake was discharged in her urge to be active (excessive walks). The urge to move and be active also helped to purify her body and were thus a part of her defense.

Biography

Henriette X grew up as an only child and without a father. Two much older siblings had almost left home when she was born at the beginning of the war, in which her father died. It should be emphasized that a very close tie developed between her and her mother; her mother loved her more than anything else and let her sleep in her bed because the child otherwise fell into states of anxiety at night. From the perspective of the mother and other family members (a distant uncle who had a large family of his own took on an idealized father role), Henriette was a completely normal, happy, yet often difficult child who preferred to play outside than with dolls. She was intelligent and had a vivid fantasy. From early childhood she and Gusti were close friends, each of them playing a gamut of different roles. Of course, Henriette was not only the more inventive, but also frequently the active one, playing the "masculine" role.

School continued to pose no difficulty to her, and she continued to be one of the best in her class. Everything seemed to come easily for her. She was an excellent athlete, played piano well, and was gifted in learning languages. She was also one of the boyish leaders in her coed class, setting a tomboyish tone. She found complete satisfaction in her friendship with Gusti, which protected her against having to keep closer contact with the others in her class. Her relationship to the others consisted almost solely of competing in gym class. Henriette frantically attempted to maintain this constellation and detested her periods, which forced her to abstain from competition for days.

With the changes that took place in the class during puberty she gradually lost her position of leadership and changed her behavior, becoming quiet, fragile of character, and losing her desire to roam around. In contrast to earlier, when she enjoyed eating, just like Gusti, she now reduced her food intake and occasionally vomited. Her declining athletic prowess kept her from taking part in competition. At the age of 16 she had to change schools, taking a bus to one further away. This meant a separation from Gusti. The physical and psychopathological manifestations of her illness, which arose when she was 15, did not change during the following two years at the new school, at which point she came for treatment.

The Terminal Phase of Therapy

Eighth Phase of Treatment: Sessions 215-254

It was with some concern and also pleasure that Henriette X commented that the increase in her weight that she had achieved some time ago was accompanied by a change in her body feeling, adding that her muscles had become softer. Her concern resulted from sensations from her body, such as the pressure on her stomach when she wore a narrow skirt or belt. We were unable to understand a number of other, peculiar body sensations, but they appeared to us to be of significance for understanding the relationship between function and form, i. e., her disturbed nutrition and body image. The remarkable fact that many anorexics can maintain their body weights constant for years with only minimal fluctuations leads one to assume that food intake is automatically regulated by unconsciously signaled bodily perceptions.

Henriette X was just as moved by agitation that drove her to eat as by her perception of her body forms. In her states of anxiety she feared being overcome both from inside, by unknown instinctual dangers, and from outside. The unification of inside and outside, such as during eating and sexual intercourse, was the subject of the following dreams.

In the 237th session Henriette X mentioned a dream in which she had at first sought protection with her mother and then lay in bed with her analyst. There was a struggle, an injury, and bleeding. The important dream element in this context was that Henriette X was suffocated by the heavy beams in the ceiling of the room, which in the dream were acutally cookies. In further dreams (240th session) she once again had the sensation of suffocating, and in one of them had her period. Finally in the 245th session she dreamed about having had her period, which was partly white. In the dream the blood from her period, including the white parts, were mixed with food that she ate. Later in the dream she lay under a particularly beautiful girl and had intercourse with her. She did not have a sensation of a penis, but did feel the girl's beautiful body and see her well formed breasts.

Now it became clearer what the phrase "being married with food" meant; Henriette X occasionally used these words to describe her current condition. Her dream about the white color of some of her period and the mixture of her menstrual blood with her food depicted an unconscious fantasy that refers to self-sufficiency, parthenogenesis, and oral fertilization. The analyst interpreted the dream at two levels and - to be brief - in the psychic context viewed the white component in the one case as semen and in the other as milk. It was now also possible to better comprehend an earlier dream, in which a baby sucked at her genitals; she had unconsciously equated her excrements with food. The analyst referred to the narcissistic nature of the dream, in the sense that "I am strong and can do everything, both procreate and live from my own substance."

This autarky refers on the one hand to an anxiety about loss and death (nothing should be lost), and on the other to an attempt to overcome this anxiety. If this process is not restricted to the dream level but also governs behavior, then a situation develops that is apparently characteristic of many of those who refuse to eat. As a result of the maximal isolation caused by defense processes, nothing changes any more and the patient - even to the extreme of losing her life - retains her belief in her immortality, in a delusional manner. This paradox can be described by the following set phrases: "I live from my own inexhaustible substance and am thus not exposed to all of the dangers of an exchange that ultimitely lead to death. I am from nothing, and therefore not threatened by death." This denial enables the anorexic to be free of a fear of death. (Unconsciously, the person's own substance is identical with her mother's, so that the unconscious symbiosis appears eternalized in death.)

Fortunately Henriette X did not live in such autarky in reality, and with the help of other dreams we are also able to understand why she had been thrown back to its narcissistic nature. She had to ward off dangerous relationships, such as being overcome orally by cookies (displacement from bottom to top) and homosexual contacts, and the accompanying instinctual impulses. The object displacement of the dream image - e.g., the suffocating on the cookies - also corresponded to a peculiar body perception during association. Henriette X had the sensation that her tongue was swollon, and she reproduced the feeling of suffocation she experienced in the dream. The analyst took the swelling of her tongue to represent a displacement of excitation, and Henriette X feared that she might not be able to speak normally any more and would stutter. This fear disappeared immediately after the analyst interpreted the displacement as libidinal tendencies related to the mouth an the organ of articulation; in this regard he referred among other things to a homosexual dream. The patient commented that at this point she would have broken off the treatment if the analyst had been a woman because she would have been unable to speak with a woman about her needs for tendernous.

It is amazing that Henriette X managed to comprehend the analyst's interpretations, to place her initially seemingly unmotivated states of anxiety in the context of her experiencing, and to integrate them. She was particularly tormented by her aggression directed against her mother, which on the one hand helped her to ward off her desires to lean on somebody, and on the other was the result of frustration. Her feelings of guilt occasionally led her to be careless and get into very dangerous situations in traffic; also involved in this was the aspect of testing her skill.

To her own surprise the quality of her work at school improved, even in the sciences, even though she had little endurance - but when, then with great intensity - and in comparison to the others in her class she still did not work enough. Her choice of a profession created more difficulties. She wanted to keep all her options open and, moreover, as she ultimately realized, find a profession that would serve as a substitute for marriage and family. At a job counselling session she was characterized as being of above average intelligence overall. She made good for her lack of persistence with her great agility. She herself had already considered becoming an interpretor, and with her continued progress this choice of a carreer seemed to come naturally.

Ninth Phase: Sessions 255-289

Henriette X wanted to take advantage of the Christmas holidays to study hard, but it did not work out that way. For the first time she had fun at a party that she had organized together with her girlfriend Gusti. She was relaxed, enjoyed herself, and did not need to control herself. She was successful, admired by the boys, and courted in a friendly manner. She was not tormeted by impulses to kill. Yet she did not dare to go for a walk alone and occasionally had the feeling of suffocating.

Her relation to her mother had changed, and Henriette X regretted that she innerly was more separated from home. It was also obvious that she continued to ward off strong needs to lean on somebody, which had a peculiar effect on her dealings with children. Although she enjoyed playing with her nieces and nephew, she suffered from the impression of innerly not being free and uninhibited and of not having any realy contact to children. In her words, "I could have feelings toward children after all, now that I don't have any feelings toward my mother anymore." The only desire that seemed natural to her was to once have an intimate relationship, inconceivable in contrast the thought of bearing, feeding, and raising children. The analyst based his interpretations on the assumption that she could not have any feelings toward children because she would then partly identify with them, and precisely in identification with a child of her own she would experience infantile dependence. The interpretations were extended with reference to the above-mentioned dream about sucking and licking. The real problem expressed by both the patient's and the analyst's words was that of the interwoven nature of self- and object representation.

In the final phase of treatment Henriette X dreamed about suffocating her doctor. The dream contained some talk about love and lust. She associated a fantastic dream about a devil who waited for his victims before greedily devouring them. She also recalled that her 4-year-old nephew had once whispered to her while playing, "I want to tell you something very beautiful: I want to make you dead." The destructive force of her claim to love led the patient to ward off her desire to lean on somebody because in such a circumstance she would have been helpless against her own impulses.

Another fact that deserves mention is that on the weekend between the 258th and 259th sessions Henriette went dancing and fell intensely in love for the first time. A girlfriend commented, with satisfaction, "You're becoming normal."

The patient passed her final examinations at school without experiencing any anxiety or agitation. She also did not miss an opportunity to celebrate fasching (Mardi Gras). Her first intense love was replaced by a new fascination. One night she became enthusiastic about an "existentialist" boy, in whom she in many respects saw an image of herself. They discussed good and evil half the night, denying the existence of the latter. They also decided in favor of highly ascetic ideals and called every form of dependence on the body inhumane. These arguments did not, however, keep them from caressing passionately. During the brief period of sleep that followed, Henriette X dreamed about lying in bed with a young man and hiding him under the blankets from her mother. She subsequently had difficulty falling asleep, which resulted in part from the sexual arousal she felt every evening. Henriette then recalled that she had used to feel sexually aroused, but had rejected the feeling and had not masturbated.

The patient's experiences during fasching precipitated a dream which revealed one important root of her feelings of inferiority as a woman. Henriette X dreamed that a large number of small black bugs came out of her full and swollen breasts. This dream was motivated by her sensation of the boys' sexual arousal while dancing, which was autoplastically represented in the equation of breast and penis. The black bugs symbolized semen, making it something repulsive. The patient came to this interpretation practically on her own, especially since it now became clearer that she considered herself for ever unable to fulfill the role of a mother: breasts were supposed to procreate, not nurse.

The patient was excessively disturbed by a renewed difficulty to fall asleep that manifested itself during the final phase of treatment. Previously she would have resorted to a fantasy that worked promptly, but which was now ineffective. This was the idea of falling in a deep well. The explanation for this difficulty was that she experienced this "falling" to sleep both as something that overpowered her and as a regression into the security she longed for. It was characteristic that the patient now felt the anxiety about falling asleep during a session. That this letting herself fall was still burdened, via an unconscious linkage, with an aggressive and dangerous act was shown by a dream in which the patient fell over, paralyzed by a man's poison-filled pistol. A significant improvement in these symptoms was reached by a continued working through.

Henriette's treatment came to an end after she had finished school and was in good condition. Her period had come regularly for months. Her weight was 55 kg (121 lb) and the obstipation was significantly improved. Overall she showed a positive development. Yet with regard to her symptoms, it must be added that the patient still did not feel completely uninhibited while eating and took special pleasure in the last bite.

The analyst now felt justified to leave the rest to the vis medicatrix naturae, the healing power of nature, and to terminate the treatment. The patient wanted to pursue her education in another city. Arrangements were made for another 15 sessions, held some months later. Overall the patient's development had been positive.

The Problem of Symptom Substitution

Almost thirty years have passed since the termination of Henriette X's psychoanalysis, which provided important insights into the pathogenesis of anorexia nervosa. Her treatment produced lasting changes. We are completely justified in speaking about a cure because Henriette X has led a successful and full life, both privately and professionally, since completing treatment and because she has not exhibited any residual symptoms of anorexia nervosa. After graduating from college and starting a career that led her to spend some time abroad, Henriette X married the friend she had been living with for a long time.

Some twenty years ago she had a disturbing symptom, which led her to consult her analyst once again. She had rejected the intense desire that she and her husband had for children because of her neurotic anxiety that something might happen to their helpless children, and that she herself might do something to them. The patient, who had retained a vivid memory of her analyst, traced this symptom to the fact that in her psychoanalysis she had been separated from her mother too abruptly. Although she was completely happy with her husband and was grateful to psychoanalysis for her being at all able to establish a heterosexual relationship, among many other positive changes, she criticized the intensity of the treatment and the far-reaching changes, referring in particular to the abrupt resolution of her close relationship to her mother. She then went on to complain about another restriction of her otherwise active life - a light flight phobia - that she attributed to the changes caused by her treatment. In order to fly alone, she had to overcome her anxiety. She also blamed this inhibition on the analyst because he had contributed to her recognizing her dependence and thus losing the self-security she had had in her illness.

By acknowledging her complaints and thematizing them both at the relationship and transference levels, the analyst made it possible for the patient to undergo an intensive focal therapy, which for external reasons consisted of numerous sessions in a brief period of time. In the transference analysis the imaginative patient was able to relive her very aggressive feelings toward her mother and critically reflect on them. Since these aggressive feelings were manifested in a relationship she unconsciously experienced to be distinctly symbiotic, the patient could not be sure whether she was not referring to herself when she thought of her mother and any children she might have. She was anxious about the children she might have because the problems of a symbiotic relationship might be repeated for them. It was not difficult for the analyst to include her anxiety about flying alone in the focus of treatment, especially since the transference aspect was quite obvious. She could not face empty space without feeling anxiety because she still had an old bill to pay; having great trust in someone also means being very dependent and experiencing the related disappointments. The wide spaces represented a transference object whose reliability was cast in doubt by her own unconscious aggressions.

The patient's longing for an omniscient and omnipotent mother inevitably led to disappointments and aggressions that undermined the security she sought. Ultimately it was the unconscious process by means of which the symptom motivated the anxiety - as can be regularly observed with such symptoms - and was perpetuated by "external" confirmation, which has the effect of reinforcement. The symptoms improved in a short time as a result of the intensity of her experiencing in transference and of her insight.

Henriette X is now the mother of several children and has written her analyst about her family several times.

Several interviews were conducted about ten years ago in the course of a follow-up survey conducted by the analyst. They helped the patient to cope with a momentary stress situation. She had a particularly close relationship to her children, which made it difficult for her to bear the steps they took toward autonomy before and during puberty.

The issue of symptom substitution is raised by the phobic symptoms mentioned above which appeared some twenty years after the termination of Henriette X's treatment. The stumbling block is a comment referred to above that might be related thematically with the patient's later symptom. At the time the patient had said that it might be possible for her to have some feelings for children since she did not have any feelings left for her mother, but that bearing, feeding, and raising children was inconceivable to her. Based on our knowledge of the later course, we can now state that an unconscious constellation had remained that later brought forth a thematically related symptom.

Such observations contributed to the formation of the theory of symptom substitution and symptom displacement, which Freud (1937c) discussed in his late work *Analysis Terminable and Interminable.* The issue of symptom change is connected with a controversy between the psychodynamic schools of treatment and behavior therapy (Perrez and Otto 1978). Several comments about this are appropriate at this point in consideration of the course of Henriette X's illness. Taking into account the effects of so-called nonspecific factors in psychotherapy inevitably leads one to question the hypothesis that a treatment can be effective solely at the symptomatic level, because the motivations emitted by the symptom in a self-reinforcing manner remain linked with the earlier pathogenetic conditions. For this reason these conditions can be affected in some way even by treatment that is symptomatic and seemingly noncausal. Psychoanalysis has in practice neglected the dimension that consists of the course and secondary gain from illness, together with its repercussions on the underlying primary condition. It is not only with regard to the transference neurosis that the illness "is not something which has been rounded off and become rigid but that it is still growing and developing like a living organism" (Freud 1916/17, p. 444). A symptom displacement is only to be expected, on the basis of psychoanalytic theory, if important conditions of the origin of the symptom cannot be overcome by psychotherapy and continue to exert an influence. In the case of Henriette X an unconscious configuration survived, whose revival was precipitated in a particular situation and which became active again. A latent condition became manifest, preciptated by a thematically appropriate factor.

Since all neurotic symptoms are overdetermined, it is often sufficient to remove one of several conditions. The problem of symptom change thus amounts to the question of whether it is empirically possible to predict the conditions under which a configuration shifts from a latent to an active state, or to determine when the relevant links in a chain of conditions are actually interrupted.

The not insignificant difficulties involved in specifying the connections between latent dispositons and the probable future conditions of their manifestation seem to have contributed to the striving for a utopian solution, namely the destruction of all the pathogenic constellations that might become active in the future. Although Freud (1937c) demonstrated that such a goal is infinite, such utopias exert a great attraction. Paul Ehrlich's idea of one day developing a *therapia magna sterilisans*, i.e., a chemotherapy able to cure all infectious diseases with a single dose, corresponds to the utopia of resolving the disposition for psychopathological reactions by means of an interminable analysis.

We would now like to turn to the question of whether the *familial constellation* might have contributed to the origin of Henriette X's anorexia nervosa. This discussion will be exemplary in nature, providing a basis for different practical applications.

We will now summarize several of the peculiarities in Henriette X's family that had an affect on the formation of her inner world. Above we mentioned that in a certain sense Henriette X took the place of her father at her mother's side. This resulted in a very close tie between mother and child, the mother being able in her loneliness to find consolation in her daughter's company, which must have given Henriette X the feeling that she was very important to her mother. In the literature on family dynamics, the term "parentification" is used to refer to a situation in which a child takes on such a parental role (Boszormenyi-Nagy 1965). This is a kind of reversal of roles in which the mother or father directs desires to the child that were not satisfied in their relations to their parents or partner. They demand too much of a "parentified" child, forcing it prematurely into an adult role. Henriette replaced her father. We have described the difficulties this caused her in finding her sexual identity.

When Henriette X felt the desire to have children, she developed a neurotic anxiety that was rooted deep in her symbiosis. Later she actually sensed how her children's autonomy was a burden on her. The therapeutic work at this juncture was directed at resolving the parentification of her own children. In her close relationship to her children she attempted to satisfy her own childhood desires to lean on somebody that she had not been able to satisfy with her mother. This had been thwarted by her efforts to find autonomy and by her precociousness.

As the analytic treatment helped Henriette X to increasingly separate herself from her mother and to recognize her longings for dependence, and as she became careless in traffic because of her feelings of guilt about her aggression, Henriette's mother turned to the analyst. She was concerned that her daughter might do something to herself. In terms of family dynamics, the therapist was assigned the role of the father, which visibly relieved the patient. Henriette could transfer her worries about her mother to the therapist. At the same time the analyst was able to work out with the mother how the patient unconsciously attempted to assure herself her mother's attention in order to control her own strong desires for autonomy.

The family dynamics must be taken into consideration especially if a circular process cannot be interrupted by a change made by the patient. However we do not share Petzold's (1979) view that anorexia nervosa is the symptom of a family neurosis. The assumption that there are pathologic familial constellations which are specific for the origin of anorexia nervosa, other psychosomatic illnesses, schizophrenia, or cyclothymia may well prove just as illusory as the assumption of specific causes of psychosomatic illnesses (see Sect. 9.7). The adverse consequences of such a misjudgment are well known since the invention of the "schizophrenogenic" mother. Moreover, in an individual's experiencing the sense of cause is easily linked with guilt or at least with responsibility, which impedes or even obstructs any attempt to involve family members in the therapy because they feel misunderstood and perhaps withdraw completely.

The study of family diagnosis is still in its infancy. Research into the typology of psychosomatic, schizophrenic, and manic-depressive families (Wirsching and Stierlin 1982; Stierlin 1975; Stierlin et al. 1986) is burdened by so many methodological shortcomings that any assertion of causal relationships is dubious. Anderson (1986) has, for example, discussed such methodological problems with regard to the model of "psychotic family games" designed by Palazzoli Selvini (1986). We believe that a more modest goal is called for, also for reasons of theoretical plausibility; such a goal is for the family crisis precipitated by any chronic illness to be registered and included in the therapeutic scheme. Although Henriette X's family has to be considered incomplete, due to the death of her father, it still clearly demonstrates the "entanglement" between mother and child described by Minuchin (1977). This word refers to an extremely close and intensive form of interaction. Other descriptions of "typical families of anorexics" (Sperling and Massing 1972) also point to specific structural features in familial relations that appear to be typical. Meant are patterns of interaction that are identified *after* the manifestation of the illness. The approach of family therapy constitutes a supplement to individual treatment if it provides the patient the freedom to leave home and attain the necessary autonomy (Gurman et al. 1986).

It is misleading to act as if a child has no innate dispositions, space for individual freedom and decisions, or active participation. Despite a child's dependence, it does not simply react passively to its environment, but takes an active part in constructing it. This is particularly true of anorexics in puberty, who truly have a mind of their own.

9.6 Neurodermatitis

The repertoire of different types of somatic treatment for a chronic illness has usually been exhausted when a patient comes for psychotherapy. This fact, together with the study of changes during the analytic process, facilitates a *comparison of the case with itself* and thus the evaluation of the therapeutic efficacy of the new procedures, i. e., the psychotherapeutic ones. This constitutes a valid basis for single case study design, given that the only new factor is psychoanalytic therapy and that all the other conditions, particularly the patient's living conditions, are constant. This is a fruitful application of J.S. Mill's classical differential method in clinical research (see Eimer 1987).

First, it is necessary to name a few of the criteria that have to be taken into account in single case studies of this kind. The comparison of a case with itself is the most important basis for therapy research (Martini 1953; Schaumburg et al. 1974).

Ideally, the therapeutic interventions should be varied according to the etiological assumptions, with the goal of most effectively eliminating the pathogenic factors and symptoms. It is, thus, important to observe the course over a long period of time and note the alterations treatment brings about in the symptoms as indications for assumed structural changes (Edelson 1985; Wallerstein 1986).

In evaluating the therapeutic efficacy of psychoanalysis in the case of the neurodermatitis patient we would now like to present, it is necessary to distinguish three phases:

1. At the initiation of analytic therapy the patient had already had the illness for eight years. During this period the patient was treated regularly by a dermatologist and was often unable to work. Inpatient treatment was necessary four times because of a worsening of the skin disease (the total length of hospitalization was about six months).
2. The patient's external living conditions were unchanged during the 2.5 year period of analysis. The local dermatological therapy was continued as previously. The new approach consisted in the specific "influence" of psychoanalysis. It was possible to correlate the changes, improvements, and setbacks occurring during psychoanalysis to psychic processes. The patient's attitude to life, not his external circumstances, underwent significant changes. Since all the other conditions stayed the same, the changes brought about by analytic means can be considered the cause of the patient's lasting improvement and cure.
3. This thesis is supported by the follow-up; the patient has been healthy for the nearly 30 years that have elapsed since his analysis. He occasionally had light efflorescences, which did not require dermatological treatment.

Excerpts from the Case History

Over the years Bernhard Y's skin condition, which he called chronic eczema, had been the object of different diagnoses, including seborrheic dermatitis and atopical neurodermatitis. The patient had not told the doctors about his impotence and obsessive thoughts. The clinical records also made no mention of the events that precipitated the outbreaks of his illness. It was not until after ten years of treatment that the patient encountered a dermatologist who suspected a psychic factor and referred him for psychotherapy.

Course of the Illness

It is noteworthy that although the patient had suffered from rough and split skin since childhood and a rash near his mouth between the ages of 10 and 17, these symptoms disappeared after his initial separation from home when he served as a soldier. (His parents and siblings are healthy, and skin diseases and genetic predispositions are not present in the family.)

At the age of 20 Bernhard Y became ill (vomiting and loss of appetite), and the disappearance of this illness was immediately followed by an itching skin inflammation, which spread to his arms, breast, and back. The patient was unable to work and referred to a dermatology hospital for the first time in September 1948. A seborrheic dermatitis was diagnosed, and tests indicated that an oversensitivity to a particular brand of soap was the precipitating cause. The symptoms were improved by local therapy and radiotherapy to the extent that he could be released. Since then Bernhard Y had neurodermatitis; severe exacerbations made hospital care lasting numerous weeks necessary in 1950, 1951, and 1956. In the course of these clinical therapies detailed allergy tests were conducted, which demonstrated an oversensitivity to eggs. The patient had already detected this oversensitivity on the basis of adverse oral sensations.

Biography

Bernhard Y was raised according to strict Catholic tenets in a small town, where he attended elementary school from 1934 to 1941. He was an above-average pupil. He gave up his first choice of a profession (baker) because the work appeared too strenuous. After attending vocational school until 1943, he began an apprenticeship in a commercial firm, where he has worked to this day except for a short interruption at the end of the war. The patient had always been an especially conscientious person and was given his rigid moral code by his mother. As far as he could recall and particularly since puberty the patient said he had been shy and inhibited and had suffered from severe feelings of guilt. His long friendship to his later wife was primarily during the period he was ill, which added to his isolation. Under the impact of his mother's maxims and her warnings about the possible consequences of intimate contacts, the patient was inhibited and insecure toward his girlfriend, both physically and otherwise. Because of his skin disease he postponed sexual contacts for the distant future and thought about never marrying. He also feared that his skin disease was hereditary. He resisted marriage until the last moment, not deciding to marry until his wife assured him that she herself did not want any children.

Although the patient was frequently absent from work and had to restrict his contact to customers and people in general because of his itching exanthem, his reliability made him a valued employee.

Precipitating Situation

The latest symptom formation was preceded by a conflict at work. His boss and earlier master was a man who was particularly inaccessible and strict, and who left his employees in the dark about planned raises and such things. A new pay scale had come out, but the boss had not informed the patient about the raise he could expect. One day, while attempting to find the new pay scale on his boss' desk after work, his boss surprised him. He quickly thought of an excuse, which was a half truth, namely he was looking for a letter that had to be mailed. From this day on the patient was not able to work for several weeks because of vomiting and loss of appetite, and later was tormented by doubts about whether his boss would ever trust him again. Finally the patient talked about the matter with his boss, but without reestablishing the old relationship. The patient considered the fact that his skin disorder did not heal to be the punishment for his curiosity. Prior to this moment he had been able to maintain social contacts despite his intense inhibitions and inner insecurity; now in contrast, he was fairly isolated, a secondary consequence of his illness. The patient contemplated applying for an early pension for invalids.

Initiating Treatment

At the beginning of treatment the patient was unusually inhibited, seemingly having become an *alexithymist* (see Sect. 9.9) after having been ill and receiving somatic treatment for 10 years. That the therapy did not immediately founder on the initial resistance, such as has been decribed by V. von Weizsäcker (1950), was connected with the fact that the patient, despite being skeptical, sought help because of his difficult circumstances, and on the other hand had trust both in the institution and in me, a favorable prognostic sign.

The analyst's therapeutic technique at the time of this therapy was distinctly nondirective. He provided indirect encouragement, which facilitated dreams, associations, and self-reflection. The style of the protocols, dictated after each session, reflects this nondirective technique, compiling amost exclusively the patient's own thoughts. References to the analyst's feelings of countertransference, his considerations, and interpretations are sparse. Both for clinical and scientific reasons this type of treatment and preparation of protocols proved inadequate. Over the course of time they have undergone significant modification (see Thomä 1967b, 1976; Kächele et al. 1973). Although we are not able at this point to discuss the numerous conscious and unconscious reasons that dictated this therapeutic technique, we would like to refer to several factors that are important for the evaluation of the segments of treatment described above. Aside from the anaylst's own insecurity, he was concerned that his interpretations might have a "suggestive" influence on the patient. The analyst was still busy studying the misunderstanding regarding the differences between various forms of suggestion within the spectrum of psychotherapeutic and analytic techniqes (see Thomä 1977).

A lengthy first phase of treatment served to establish a viable working alliance, which the patient experienced as dangerous because of his intense ambivalence and deep-seated anxiety about punishment. A deterioration of his symptoms made him unfit for work, and his family doctor reported him sick for some two months. The patient tested his analyst's reliability and tolerance for criticism and aggression by obtaining negative statements about psychoanalysis from doctors and homeopaths. His retreat to home and into an incapacity to work, however, itself had adverse effects. Although he avoided intense psychic stress at work, he had only exchanged this for an increase in tension in his marriage, which he in turn attempted to avoid by withdrawing further into the autoerotic and autodestructive attention he paid his skin. The initially seemingly banal precipitating conflict situation attained, from the supplementary and corrective comments the patient made, a depth making his stress at work more comprehensible. At work the patient was constantly filled by the anxiety that his kleptomanic theft of penny sums would be discovered one day, a fear that strengthened his neurotic anxiety.

In his initial dream the patient had been held responsible for the loss of a key. It was not until much later that he was able to speak either about his thefts or about his impotence, which he initially had also not mentioned. It turned out that, contrary to his initial statement, his skin disease was not the reason that he had repeatedly postponed marrying or contemplated not getting married at all. After hesitating for a long time he finally spoke about his sexual problems, which he had not mentioned to any of the other doctors. As mentioned above, the patient did not decide to marry until his wife assured him that she herself did not want any children because she was too narrow and afraid that a cesarean section might prove necessary, as in the case of both of her sisters. They therefore agreed to lead a kind of platonic marriage. He feared he had so injured himself from masturbation that he had become infertile and impotent. Since his wife complained of pain, they could not have intercourse. After the patient learned to recognize his rationalizations of avoiding sexual contact with his wife, he experienced timidity, fear, and repulsion at the sight of his wife genitals as well as feelings of guilt and anxiety about his own aggression.

Overall it was clear that the patient suffered from severe hypochondric ideas about physical defects and resorted to magic means in his regressive attempt to overcompensate his defects.

The initial worsening of his symptoms can be traced back to his disturbing admissions in analysis. Even before treatment the patient himself had ascertained that changes in his symptoms had little to do with his somatic therapy, but much with whether he was left in peace and quiet. He felt he would have been best able to find quiet at home in early retirement if he had only stayed a bachelor and were not subject to tensions in his relationship to his wife.

His severe neurosis was accompanied by fantasies in which he had intercourse with a much older woman. For a long time his associations were too sparse to make the oedipal roots of both his inhibitions and his displaced desires visible. In his few dreams, of which he had only a fragmentary recollection, he saw himself, for example, walking arm in arm with a strange woman. In reality he was preoccupied with obsessive thoughts while walking on the street, especially with a compulsive counting of the passing cars and trucks. Whenever he went out onto the street, the patient decided which cars he would count on that day and how to evaluate the result. Through skilled manipulations he almost always arrived at a favorable number, even when he had previously chosen another; for example, if he had assumed that an odd number was adverse for a rapid cure of his skin disease, he manipulated the numbers until he could alter the adverse result. He usually consulted the number regarding the rapid cure of his exanthem or financial benefits, such as the amount of his future pension, unexpected income and so forth.

His magic way with numbers made him dream of financial benefits enabling him to lead the life of a pensioner and to be pampered by his wife. As long as his mother had survived, he had used this secondary gain from illness to be spared work at home, to be given preferential treatment versus his brothers and father, and to get their attention.

Skin Care as Regression

The patient spent several hours every day preoccupied with his skin; during this time he did not want to be disturbed. Although he did not say anything if his wife entered the bathroom, it irritated him and his criticism was displaced onto some other object, for instance that his shirt was not ready to wear.

The treatment sessions were also filled with his fairly monotonous and repetitive descriptions of his skin's condition. The patient had developed a rich vocabulary with which to describe his skin's different qualities. He even noted small differences - sometimes his skin was more chapped, once redder, occasionally scalier - that an expert would hardly have been able to detect.

He withdrew from his wife, retreating, as he himself said, back to his skin. His symptoms were one aspect of his interpersonal disputes, which expressed themselves in different ways and at different levels. He spoke about the "outrageous idea" that his wife might be the cause of his illness - his more severe skin disturbances had never actually disappeared since he had married and at times, e. g., during a vacation, he had observed that his skin became fairly good until the day his wife arrived. He wondered whether she emitted something poisonous or something that caused pimples, thinking of her vaginal secretion. His skin was, in general, the object of all of his moods; it was, so to speak, the organ of choice. When he was mad, he scratched himself; yet on the other hand he cared for his skin as if it were a object he loved.

These comments indicate Bernhard Y's regression to his body ego. The concentration on this theme in this case came almost automatically because of this patient's interweaving of subject and object and its significance for his therapy. His self-observations made it clear that his skin's condition - both its improvements and its aggravations - was very closely connected to the rubbing and scratching that, unnoticed and almost reflexlike, accompanied his hours of caring for his skin. The analysis of his retreat into the bathroom, especially in the evening, was at the focus of the entire therapy.

The description of this case can be organized around the questions the patient had to avoid for unconscious reasons - why he, having become impotent, had to avoid sexual gratification and what he was seeking in his autoerotic withdrawal. The patient gradually became aware that his behavior damaged his skin, yet he was unable to interrupt this vicious circle.

Viewing scratching simply as autoaggression is inadequate for both theoretical and technical reasons. Schur (1974; see Thomä 1981, p. 421), in particular, has pointed this out, showing that by acting this way a patient is seeking unconscious objects in himself with which he has maintained a link. In such regressions the self-reinforcing circular behavior strengthens the primary identifications and weakens the subject-object boundaries. In the course of the working through in this patient's analysis, his skin took on divergent object qualities or, more specifically, their representation (including of the transference relationship). Since to conscious perception these unconscious object images were sinister and a cause of extreme anxiety, the patient was able to achieve greater self-control by withdrawing, i. e., by loving and hating the object via his body, at the same time as avoiding any real contact, i. e., a real but extremely disturbing merging.

The patient was quite aware that the reason he withdrew from his wife into the bathroom, especially in the evening, was his anxiety about sex, a symptomatic manifestation of which was his impotence. Based on knowledge of his biography and the nature of the symptoms, it seemed reasonable for the analyst to assume that the oedipal situation was a barrier that led to regression.

The analysis alternated between focusing on the regression and on the oedipal factors that precipitated it. A first significant improvement in the patient's symptoms occurred when he overcame his impotence after reducing his oedipal feelings of guilt and partially overcoming his castration anxieties; at this point his strong anal fixation manifested itself again. He was aware of his feelings of guilt, which he traced back to the masturbation he continued practicing until he had overcome his impotence. His self-accusations were so strong that he wished he had died as a soldier.

During puberty he had been frequently disturbed by incestuous fantasies, and for many years struggled, ultimately successfully, to overcome his sadistic impulses. An immense castration anxiety had led him to hide his genitals under a protective cover. Even after he had overcome his impotence he was very frightened when his wife made sexual advances. He developed fantasies about how he could compensate for the loss of semen and the psychic damage he experienced. To cite from the protocol of one session:

The patient spoke about his oversensitivity. Despite everything, he still had reservations about whether everything would really turn out alright. An egg is life, man's semen, punishment for masturbation; eggs are the testes; peculiar thought that the skin could be irritated by one's own testes; he fantasized about swallowing his own semen, to keep from losing it or his strength. He had actually already thought about trying to do this, but was prevented by his revulsion. Another of his fantasies was to squeeze his sebacious glands and to use the secretion to treat his skin. Now he would have preferred to cover up his genitals and had an immense anxiey about losing them. He felt that looks alone meant that an attack, an intervention, would come. His body was supposed to belong to him and him alone.

In a long transitional period he described the unbearable tension he felt when he was unable to wash at the right time or take care of his skin. If it were impossible for him to withdraw, his agitation became so intense that it was not uncommon for him to think about suicide.

P: Although I'm able to postpone my skin care for a while, perhaps for 1–2 hours, the tension in me then becomes so great that most of all I would like to kill myself. Excessive skin care is like an addiciton, and then I'm able to make the rudest accusations against my wife, and I really have.

After the emotions and fantasies that had previously been tied to symptoms were unleashed, his various anxieties took on concrete forms that were accessible to interpretation. His magical thoughts and the compulsive anal rituals assumed a phallic meaning. One purpose of his phallic narcissism was to ward off castration anxiety, such as was exemplified by the following dream:

P: I was at the sports festival, taking part in both the high jump and the long jump, where I managed 7.80 meters. Uwe Seeler [a famous soccer player] was on the loudspeaker, and the women in the stadium were completely enchanted by his voice alone. A woman next to me moved as if in intercourse; just his voice made her have an orgasm.

In his associations, he thought it would be great if it were possible without intercourse, solely as a result of words. He wanted to be a famous athlete and jump so far that he would never touch the ground again. Having an immense penis, he said, would be the greatest of riches, being a male whore and injuring women. In his youth he had trained himself to suppress his sexuality, but also to realize his fantasies of omnipotence, in order to be like Uwe Seeler in his dream and fascinate women with his words. Then the patient became agitated and developed a momentary anxiety about being poisoned, which he immediately related to his skin infection - vaginal secretion could poison him.

Incidentally, in another phase of treatment this patient had expressed the desire to hear his voice once from the tape recorder in my office. He had never heard his own voice before. (Today I would presumably record the treatment, with the patient's approval, and surely not deny him his wish.)

His insight into the fact that he used his skin in place of objects and that his many nuances of pinching and scratching were his attempt to accommodate object-related feelings was facilitated by a dream that repeated itself in altered forms. In this impressive dream, the subject and object were exchanged - the one scratching and the one being scratched, the one applying the salve and the one being salved. He himself was the patient, but then he was not, after all; the features of the other person were not clear. In the transference I also had a part in this fantasized role playing in which the subject and object were exchanged. Regarding the origin, he remembered homosexual contacts and goings-on with his brothers. The longest period of time was filled by the fantasized exchange of ambivalent actions related to his skin. In another dream his damaged, eczematous skin was transposed onto a woman's breast. This transformation temporarily strengthened his anxiety about poisonous secretions from his wife. The anxiety decreased after he had retracted the projection of his own aggression, which had transformed the object into an evil object.

That projections of this kind are "only an element of a total identification with the object" is a fact that Marty (1974, p. 421) has described and given an anthropological foundation: "This intensive movement of total identification that allergy patients have with their objects is actually only a unalterable fixation, which is alive in each of us to a certain degree: the desire to be the other" (p. 445). It is definitely wrong to consider this process typical for allergy patients. Yet I do consider it possible that - *given* an allergy - the specific manner in which this patient cared for his skin and also his withdrawal, as it was caused by his illness, reinforced his unconscious confusion of subject and object. This was thus a retrograde revival of the undifferentiated phase that Freud described in the following way:

> The antithesis between subjective and objective does not exist from the first. It only comes into being from the fact that thinking possesses the capacity to bring before the mind once more something that has once been perceived, by reproducing it as a presentation without the external object having still to be there. (Freud 1925h, p. 237)

In this context it is possible to describe the development of the patient's oversensitivity to egg white. Although he was already aware that he had an allergy, even before he began analysis, he had noticed that the effects of the allergen on the target organ were very dependent on other factors. (He himself had noted that when he avoided all egg white he was able to detect even minute traces of them that accidentally got into a dish, by means of the taste sensations they stimulated, specifically a burning sensation in his mouth.) As already indicated, the patient had developed his own psychosomatic theory of his oversensitivity, in which some substances his wife secreted or transpired played a central role. Foodstuffs thus came to join the body substances he thought caused his disturbance.

The patient described, for example, his repugnance at having physical contact with his wife. He claimed she sometimes had a slight mouth odor, and he then used his skin as a pretext for not having closer contact. He said that he had a real anxiety about mouth odor; he would hold his breath when he passed by someone, or stay in back or pass by very quickly, to be sure to avoid the smell because exhaled air might be contagious.

His paranoid anxieties decreased and ultimately disappeared entirely, according to his degree of success in tracing his projections back to his own unconscious impulses. In this process, the dream in which he confused the subject and object took on a guiding function. In this context the patient had the following association: "Infect people with my disease, yes, that's what I want, first to wound them and then to infect them." His anxieties about injuring objects and himself were filled with contents from the oral, anal, urethral, and phallic phases of development. Initially the different contents were mixed together in his unconscious experiencing, which led to agitation and a worsening of his symptoms; then he became aware of the mixture, which made it possible for him to differentiate them and overcome his anxieties.

He wanted to gain sexual prowess by eating, using some powder, or taking one of various substances, e. g., a hormone or something for his testicles, but then was afraid that it might aggravate his skin. "I could annihilate all chickens to keep egg white from getting into food." Here his revulsion and hate were directed at eggs. He continued by associating about his fear that his testicles might get damaged. He became enraged by just thinking about his wife acting affectionately toward him and possibly making a sudden and unexpected movement - "touch my genitals." "It's an anxiety that almost has the same effect as pain." Incidentally, the patient's oversensitivity to eggs first developed in 1949, about 2 years after the onset of his illness, and he did not notice the burning sensation in his mouth after eating eggs until later. The allergy tests were conducted in 1950.

Whatever the conditions were that let the patient's latent disposition become manifest in this case, it can be seen in the course of treatment and in the case history that the patient's oversensitivity only played a subordinate role in the development of his chronic neurodermatitis. Much more serious were the meanings he attributed to certain "objects," such as his wife, as a result of which he developed an oversensitivity to them that continued until he succeeded in retracing his repulsion back to the indirect satisfaction concealed in it, recognizing it as pleasureable, and integrating it. It was then possible for him to give up his multifaceted withdrawal in favor of a less constrained relationship with his wife and his surroundings. In the last phase, exacerbations of his neurodermatitis became increasingly infrequent, to the same degree that his skin lost its character of being an autoerotic and autodestructive substitute object.

Epicritical Comments

The analyst's thematic concentration on regression raises various questions. Although the patient's daily routine was filled by such forms of experiencing and behavior, certain areas are underrepresented in this selective description and in the therapy. The analyst oriented himself on the psychodynamic processes, which exhibited a particularly close *situative* connection to the changes in symptoms. Since the issue was not to reconstruct the specific conditions of the regression and trace them back to fixations, the analyst emphasized the circumstances in the situations that governed the daily course of the disease. In repetition compulsion there are, of course, conserved causes at work, i. e., causes that have existed for a longer period of time, and from a therapeutic perspective special attention must be paid to circular self-reinforcement and the consequences it has on the primary conditions of symptom formation. Very different anxieties and (oedipal) guilt feelings - which, precisely because of the patient's skin symptoms, could be precipitated by situational factors at any time - intensified the regression and contributed indirectly to the aggravation of his symptoms.

If regressive processes of this kind exist long enough - and this patient had undergone unsuccessful dermatological treatment for eight years - then it is possible for externally directed intentions to become unconscious and affect the body feeling. At the risk of being misunderstood, we can describe this with the brief statement: This patient's life was limited to his skin. This simplification makes comprehensible the reasons that various psychoanalytic and psychotherapeutic theses about neurodermatitis and other dermatoses are accurate and can be useful in treatment. Regressions manifest the weak spots that - depending on the terminology in fashion and the technical and theoretical developments - belong to the psychodynamics of neurodermatitis and have a ***nonspecific correlation*** to it. This has been shown in the case of aggression (Thomä 1981), regardless of whether we refer to the sadomasochistic and exhibitionist features that Alexander emphasized, or to other averbal unconscious fantasies.

The guiding perspective in the presentation of this case resulted from the focusing on one form of regression. Yet guiding perspectives conceal dangers because they can be misunderstood as the special or even specific mechanisms of the particular symptoms. Such a thesis is not supported by the therapeutic experience with this patient. The following observations about the course of the illness during the analysis are relevant in this regard.

For both clinical and scientific reasons and in accordance with A. Mitscherlich's working hypothesis, it is important to pay special attention to the course of the symptoms as they correlate with psychodynamic events and changes in them (see Thomä 1978). For this patient, everything became a strain because of his withdrawal, anxieties, and feelings of guilt, and his skin was almost always also affected. The isolation of those conflicts accessible to therapy led to a reduction in the number and quality of "precipitants." The sequence in which conflicts open to resolution are worked out follows rules that differ from those determining pathogenetic significance. Because of this difficulty and because of the inadequate nature of the protocols of this case, it is impossible in retrospect to evaluate the clinical correlation more precisely.

The motives that had driven the patient into regression had been overcome when treatment was terminated. His symptoms had either disappeared or improved significantly. His relationship to his wife was and has remained satisfactory to each of them. For the first time the patient had confidence in his capacity of being able to structure his life in a meaningful manner. The neurodermatitis has not remanifested itself during the subsequent period of almost 30 years. Noteworthy is, however, that the patient has retained his oversensitivity to eggs, yet without his skin being affected.

Epicrisis

The clinical and scientific significance of the comparison of the case with itself is obvious. It reaffirms the causal significance of the psychogenesis without raising the claim that this patient's biographical data or that the insights gained in analysis into his conscious and unconscious experiencing are typical for neurodermatitis in general. The case history contains a description of several important preconditions of his symptoms. It was logical for the analyst to proceed from the regression linked to the symptoms and to focus on the effects of the rubbing and scratching that had become chronic in the self-reinforcing circle of events. The case history also demonstrates that significant causes of the neurodermatitis were overcome. It has never required any dermatological or other treatment.

On other hand, some five years after the termination of treatment the patient underwent an operation for a cataract on his right eye (his left lens was not affected). Since the lenses, just like the skin, stem from the ectoderm, the appearance of a cataract is an indication of a possible somatic source of his neurodermatitis. Finally, the patient underwent a successful plastic operation a few years ago for a clot in his right femoral artery.

The patient's private and professional life developed favorably and to his satisfaction. The couple had a son, and the patient went on to have a successful carreer. The patient attributed the curing of his neurodermatitis and the positive turn in his life to analysis, which freed him of severe guilt feelings and the anxieties that had restricted his life.

9.7 Nonspecificity

The psychosomatic research inspired by psychoanalysis, which was given a methodological foundation in the 1930s by Alexander's pioneering studies, was characterized by the *specificity hypothesis.* The results of decades of scientific effort support the following view: Regardless of the importance that psychosocial factors have for the genesis and course of somatic illnesses, it is rather improbable that there is a specific causality. The alternative hyposthesis - the assumption that psychic factors play a nonspecific role in the multifactoral constellation of conditions that cause illnesses - can, in contrast, be shown to agree with the available findings.

Related to the concept of specificity is a theory of causality that originated from our understanding of infections. A specific morphological change in tissue corrsponds to a specific pathogen, e. g., the diphtheria pathogen, the typhus pathogen, or the tubercle bacillus. Substances that are effective in countering pathogens are also referred to as specific. Thus the concept of specificity is double edged, referring both to the cause and the effects. Disposition, however, must also be taken into consideration, even in the case of infectious illnesses, in order to adequately comprehend the constellation of conditions. As we described in Sect. 1.1, Freud adopted in psychoanalysis the explanatory scheme that in principle is still valid in medicine, and in his theory of complemental series adapted it to the particular circumstances of mental diseases.

From today's perspective it was mistaken to mingle the scientific discrimination of necessary and sufficient causes with the concept of specificity. By the same token, the somatopsychic consequences, which in turn also have a causal effect on one's psychic state, were given inadequate consideration. Yet although it was a mistake to burden clinical research with the search for a typology of *specific* conflicts underlying somatic illnesses, this methodological approach has historical merits, as shown by its unbroken relevance. The multivariate approach that Alexander favored has remained part and parcel of psychosomatic medicine despite all the shifts in emphasis with regard to the variables studied. In Alexander's school it was postulated that the genesis and course of illnesses are governed by three groups of variables. One group of variables consists in a psychodynamic configuration that, together with the corresponding defense processes, is formed in childhood. The second group of variables refers to the precipitating situation in life, whether as a lived experience or a series of events immediately preceding the outbreak of the illness, that has a special emotional significance for the patient and in addition is suited to activating his central unconscious conflict. Finally, the third group of variables includes all of the somatic conditions, which Alexander took to mean a constitutionally or dispositionally determined "somatic compliance" (Freud) or "organ inferiority" (Adler). By renaming the "vulnerability" of the appropriate organ or organ system factor X, it has stayed too much in the dark, especially since precisely the pathophysiological and morphologic processes might be the ones that are responsible for the "choice of the symptoms."

Alexander et al. (1968) summarized their working hypothesis in a retrospective publication in the following manner. A patient in whom a specific organ or organ system is vulnerable and a characteristic psychodynamic configuration is present develops a corresponding illness if the circumstances in his life mobilize an earlier, unresolved, central conflict and if the resulting strains lead to a collapse of his primary defences. The correlation studies conducted on the basis of this working hypothesis showed that blind diagnoses and symptoms corresponded relatively well solely on the basis of knowledge about the psychodynamic variables. The studies conducted by Alexander and his students appeared to provide confirmation that forms of experiencing and behavior that can be traced back to endopsychic core conflicts are manifested more frequently than would occur by coincidence and that these frequencies differed for the seven illnesses that were studied. Alexander and his followers chose bronchial asthma, rheumatic arthritis, ulcerative colitis, essential hypertension, hyperthyroidism, stomach ulcer, and neurodermatitis as paradigms in their studies. These illnesses, referred to as the "Chicago seven," have a place of honor in the history of psychosomatic medicine and attracted so much attention that many physicians believed for a long time that both psychosomatic medicine and Alexander's approach were limited to these seven illnesses.

Psychic influences are conceivable and possible in all human illnesses, and for this reason psychosomatic medicine has never been limited to studying the seven illnesses named above. Initially the specificity hypothesis was applied and tested on these seven illnesses for several reasons, not least of all because of methodological and practical restrictions. Although we are today more inclined to assume that the relevant conflict constellations in these illnesses are nonspecific or variable, the seven have remained important paradigms in psychosomatic medicine, at least as far as it attempts to demonstrate correlations serving as the basis for further hypotheses and theories. Moreover, Alexander's specificity hypothesis never specified which side of the three-part model is the specifically determinative cause of pathogenetic conditions. The three groups actually consist of a multitude of individual features, which makes it necessary to employ a multivariate model and a corresponding methodology. One factor would only acquire "specific" weight in a very rare case, which is not to be expected in practice. Which of the postulated variables is decisive in selecting the organ that is affected remains an open question. It might well be factor X, the specific organ vulnerability (Pollock 1977).

Thus, improbable as it is that the specific cause of somatic illnesses can be found in certain conflict constellations or in Lacey's stimulus specificity (see Schonecke and Herrmann 1986), the fact that psychosomatic research was initially limited to a few illnesses has nevertheless proved to be productive in the history of psychosomatic medicine. Weiner (1977), for example, compiled a brilliant survey covering the six illnesses (without neurodermatitis) originally studied in Chicago, in which he described in exemplary fashion the problems that were of clinical importance and of relevance to research strategy in the 1980s. In retrospect it can be said that the research inaugurated by Alexander basically has a multivariate approach that can only satisfactorally describe the multifactorial etiological events if all the important variables are taken into consideration. A methodological consequence of the use of this general psychosomatic approach as a principle guiding physicians' actions is that the psychosocial factors influencing the genesis and course of somatic illnesses must be examined as thoroughly as possible and the patients be given psychotherapeutic treatment especially with regard to the consequences of these factors. As can be seen in Weiner's (1977) critical survey or in von Uexküll's (1986) encyclopedic textbook, the impact of psychosocial factors on the course of an illness can today be best assessed for those illnesses that previously served as paradigms. Despite all the complaints about body-mind dualism, psychosomatic medicine is also bound to a pluralistic methodology, which is frequently ontologized by materialistic or spiritualistic monisms and raised to an ideology (Groddeck 1977). For them, dualism is the evil factor (Meyer 1987).

Examples of such monism are, on the one side, Groddeck's all-encompassing spiritualism and, on the other, a materialism that identifies the neurophysiological substrate with mental and psychic processes. The autonomy of physical laws was overlooked in Groddeck's speculations, and in some areas of today's psychosomatic medicine psychic phenomena and their psychodynamics appear to dissolve into physiology. The history of the influence of the concept "conversion" shows how large the confusion can be. For instance, Lipowski (1976, pp. 11-12, emphasis added), in his influential survey of the state of psychosomatic medicine, advocated the view that "this area of research" - specifically that on "the interrelated neurophysiological, endocrine, and immunological processes and pathways whereby *symbolic* stimuli may affect any or all somatic functions" - that this area "has showed spectacular advances in the past decade or so, and it is now possible to bridge the so-called leap from the mind to the body." Lipowski added, "Without clear understanding of these processes, we are left with nothing more than correlation between specific events and *psychological* traits of the individuals exposed to them, on the one hand, and a given *bodily* dysfunction or disease, on the other."

Every physician who thinks in terms of psychosomatic categories emphasizes the qualitative autonomy of symbolic processes when confronting monists who equate psychic phenomena with the cerebral substrate. It is conceivable that the range of symbolic human activities that are tied to cerebral structures and functions influence all the processes in the organism down to individual cells. Yet to want to go from the recognition of physiological transmitter processes to psychic experiencing and symbol formation is a serious fallacy that is based on a fundamental confusion of different epistemological categories.

From a psychotherapeutic perspective, the studies by Alexander and his school have proven to be unusually productive. It is no coincidence that it was French (1952), a member of the Chicago research group, who was the first to introduce the concept of focus into the theory of technique. The significance of the here-and-now relationship was also made the center of attention there. Because of the different consequences of individual illnesses, it seems obvious that, for example, patients with a dermatological problem are more inclined to speak about themes dealing with exhibitionism. The fact that premorbid latent dispositions are activated and manifest ones are reinforced is, after all, an experience made in everyday clinical work. Furthermore, different realms of experiencing are associated with skin than with orality or with motility and restrictions of it. We emphasize the course of the illness and its circular consequences - in the sense of a self-reinforcing vicious circle - because it is here that psychoanalytic efforts can and must be focused. It is then possible to go from the somatopsychic consequences to the patient's experiencing without the manifestation of the particular resistances that appear to justify the assumption of specific "psychosomatic structures" (see Sect. 9.9). If the physician confronts the physically ill patient primarily by trying to discover psychic conflicts, i. e., in a broad sense to discover the psychogenesis of the complaints, then he triggers the reaction attributed to a patient suffering from a stomach ulcer: "But, Doc, my problem's im my stomach, not in my head." If the doctor proceeds from the physical complaints and pays serious consideration to both the somatic side of the body and the psychoanalytic discoveries about body image (see von Uexküll 1985), then he can effortlessly discover how patients cope with their illnesses. This is a means of accessing the psychosocial factors influencing the development of physical illnesses. It is always advisable to dwell on the momentary course of the illness for a long time, as we have described in Chap. 5 with regard to a case of wry neck. Psychoanalytic interviews seldom fail if the analyst orients himself on the fact that the physical complaints lead at least to a secondary complication of the unconscious fantasies associated with them. For example, heart anxiety restricts one's freedom of movement, and all complaints regarding the digestive tract lead to a sensibilization of orality, regardless of the significance of its role in the genesis of the disorder. In establishing a therapeutic relationship to patients whose complaints are somatic in nature, it is decisive that the analyst acknowledge the primacy of the body insofar as this is compatible with his methodological restriction to body image and with the fact that it is impossible for him at the same time to pay adequate consideration to the body in somatic terms. We of course agree with von Uexküll (1985, p. 100) that the psychoanalytic method, to the extent it can also move into the unconscious sphere of the body ego, can always only reach the different images or representations of the body and "does not catch sight of the body in its deeper dimensions that are in principle unconscious and that can never become the object of consciousness." Connected with this is the therapeutic range of psychoanalysis with regard to physical illnesses, i. e., the problem of the degree to which the therapeutic efforts regarding subjectively experienced body image have an affect on the somatic functions. The psychoanalytic observations that Rangell has summarized are relevant at least to an individual's subjective condition:

Thus there is no extensive psychoanalytic clinical report of an ulcer patient without observatons about the oral meaning of the gastric contractions or tensions, nor of a case of ulcerative colitis without an abundant reference to the incessant struggles around anality expressed in physical terms, nor of an asthmatic, or a neurodermatitis, without similar reconstructions of the symbolic distortions at various levels inherent in the multitude of physical and functional alterations ... In most cases, therefore, the resultant psychosomatic syndromes would be a combination of the organ-neurotic and the conversion processes. (Rangell 1959, p. 647)

In our opinion it is not just a coincidence that Rangell only referred to the kinds of cases whose symptoms can be linked in some manner to the suffering, acting, feeling, and thinking person. The skin and body orifices are, for example, associated with experiences that can be correlated with functions. The task that remains is to grasp the genesis of symptoms from the correlation with conflicts. Thus, Alexander did not assign a "meaning" to the morphological alteration itself, but he did assume there was a very close "emotional syllogism" between functions and experiencing. Even in his first studies (Alexander 1935) on psychosomatic illnesses of the digestive tract, it is possible to locate the conflict configurations in the "giving" and "taking" that were later designated "specific." Alexander observed that an ambitious person with an ulcer unconsciously identifies his repressed longing for love and help with the need for nutrition ("emotional syllogism"). This identification sets his stomach moving, which reacts as if nutrition were to be consumed or as if it were time for a meal. The conflicts of dependency that Alexander emphasized are repressed. Yet the ulcer itself does not express any symbolic meaning. Although Kubie's (1953) criticism of the specificity hypothesis has gained acceptance, the significance of Alexander's observations is not diminished if "specific" is replaced by "typical." The typical conflict constellations in Alexander's scheme did not constitute the specific factor in the sense of our understanding of infections because other etiological factors, such as the organ disposition, were also referred to as "specific." In the critical survey mentioned above, Weiner discussed a present-day pathophysiological classification of the dispositions in the illnesses studied by Alexander. The success of the multivariate approach was demonstrated particularly convincingly with regard to the etiology of ulcers of the stomach and duodenum (Schüffel and von Uexküll 1986).

From a psychotherapeutic perspective the distance between a focus - the theme of the interview - and the physical illness is initially unimportant. Decisive is rather that the patient gain confidence in the interview, i. e., that he accept it as being a means of therapy. The question regarding which bodily changes might at least in part have originated from psychic factors and might be reversed is completely open. Anyone who actually tries to reverse chronic somatic symptoms by means of psychotherapy will not lose touch with the real problems, which are due to the primary or secondary autonomy of physical symptoms.

9.8 Regression

In Vol.1 we discussed regression in connection with Balint's concept of a new beginning. Regression also played a prominent role in the conceptualization of the therapy for the patient suffering from neurodermatis. Precisely for this reason it is important to us to draw attention to the fact that we reject using an unlimited extension of the theory of regression as a pattern for explaining psychic, physical, and psychosomatic illnesses.

Even a brief consideration of the processes of regression indicates that the term refers primarily to a descriptive generalization. The concept of regression in its general sense means "a return from a higher to a lower stage of development - then repression too can be subsumed under the concept of regression, for it too can be described as a return to an earlier and deeper stage in the development of a psychical act" (Freud 1916/17, p. 342). In *The Interpretation of Dreams* Freud had already distinguished between topical, temporal, and formal aspects of regression. Freud first introduced Jackson's teachings about evolution and dissolution into his research on aphasia, and later put Jackson's views on functional degeneration to productive use in psychopathology. He later assumed "that particular regressions are characteristic of particular forms of illness" (Freud 1933a, p. 100). The concept of regression then goes beyond a descriptive generalization within the *explanatory theory* of psychoanalysis, obtaining an explanatory significance in connection with the concepts of precipitating conflict and fixation. In our opinion, this must be understood as an acquired disposition in the sense of an unconsciously anchored disposition (Thomä and Kächele 1973). Of note is the fact that the concept of regression refers exclusively to the explanation of *psychic processes.*

If, in contrast, fixation and regression are understood in terms of fictive *psychophysiological* categories, then the return to an earlier, unconscious level seems to be able to explain the development of both psychic and somatic illnesses. In fact, many theories in psychosomatic medicine since Groddeck's work have followed this assumption, even if this is not apparent at first sight.

It is not difficult for someone familiar with the subject to recognize a few patterns in this unlimited extension of the concept of regression. The common element stems from the psychoanalytic theory of defense, from which two theses about etiology can be derived. According to the first assertion, physical illnesses occur when Reich's character armor is reinforced and manifests itself somatically. Mitscherlich's two-phase repression goes back to the assumption of an existing character neurosis that is reinforced, so to speak, in the psychosomatic pathogenesis. Long ago one of us (Thomä 1953/54) published, very naively, a model case based on this idea without considering the fact that defense processes must be understood as *processes* and that even Freud, referring to repression, spoke of *afterpressure.*

The second widespread idea that has been derived for psychosomatic medicine from psychoanalytic theory is oriented on regression. Prototypical for it is Schur's (1955) conception that psychosomatic disturbances are connected with maturation and regression processes; he grasped the development of a healthy child as a process of "desomatization." According to Schur, a more conscious and psychic form of reaction develops through maturation, out of the undifferentiated and undeveloped structure of the newborn, in whom psychic and somatic elements are indivisibly linked with one another and who reacts primarily physically and unconsciously at this stage of development. Somatic forms of reaction diminish, and the child learns to react cognitively and psychically instead of somatically, i. e., through states of physical excitation. Schur associated this process of desomatization with the neutralization of instinctual energies by the ego. In the case of a psychosomatic illness, the ego is no longer able to cope with conflict situations by utilizing freely available, neutralized energy. Because of the anxiety associated with this, there is regression to the level of earlier patterns of behavior, i. e., to the level of the somatic form of reaction (psychophysiological or psychosomatic regression). Energies that had previously been tied down by the defense process of neutralization are released by the particular collapse of the ego and are expressed in an undifferentiated somatic manner corresponding to the stage of the regression. The particular shape of the resomatization, i. e., the choice of organ and the extent of the range of somatic reactions, depends on the infantile traumatic experiences and the consecutive fixations on the body's functional processes. Schur proceeded from the assumption that, in the course of ego differentiation during the process of physiological maturation, uncoordinated somatic processes are integrated cognitively and psychically, replacing the somatic reactions in the primary process with mental actions at the level of secondary processes. He viewed psychosomatic regression as a step backward, toward the original level at which the mind and body were a reaction unit that tended to discharge tension somatically.

The fundamental conception of this prototypical explanatory approach, which can also be found in the works of Mitscherlich (1967, 1983) and other authors, is the analogy or identification of infantile somatic-psychic forms of reacting with the psychosomatic form of reaction. Schur followed the psychological approach to neuroses inasfar as he viewed regression as the primary mode of the development of the illness and additionally included physical processes. The regression model is thus simply extended past the psychic level onto that of physiology. The specificity postulate is supposed to be satisfied by the familiar fixation hypothesis. It is typical for the theories formulated by many schools of psychoanalytically oriented psychosomatic medicine that the range of the particular approach is tested less from methodological perspectives than simply asserted with the help of dating the causes back into earliest childhood. If we do not let ourselves be deceived by the ingenuity with which new terms are created, then we soon recognize the uniform pattern in the assertion of the early (preoedipal) origin of psychosomatic illnesses, in which physiological laws are disregarded. It is amazing how false assumptions, with or without a dubious sense of reality, can continue to survive when authors avidly cite one another, or how secondary, terminological modifications can feign new knowledge. For example, Kutter (1981) raised Balint's *basic fault*, which was dubious even with regard to the etiology of neuroses, to the *basic conflict* of psychosomatic illnesses and contrasted them to neuroses. This makes patients suffering, for example, from one of the seven illnesses mentioned above into seriously ill borderline cases, which is compatible with neither the results obtained by Alexander nor our present-day knowledge. Kutter and others reduce the psychosomatic theory of illness to one fundamental condition, whose etiological primacy is even improbable in the theory of neuroses. The etiological theory that Freud created with his model of the complemental series has in the meantime assumed a complex form because of the multiplicity of psychic and somatic processes involved in the origin and course of every illness. It is out of the question that the basic fault constitutes the necessary condition for neuroses, i. e., that the latter develop out of it with the necessity of a law of nature, like an egg after insemination. This is also the reason for our criticism of Balint's conception of a new beginning, which we have summarized in Vol.1 (Sect. 8.3.4).

With the help of the assumption of a "psychophysiological or psychosomatic regression" and of the additional speculation that early traumatic experiences affect the psyche-soma unit, it appears to be possible to explain every severe somatic or psychic illness, from cancer to schizophrenia, from one vantage point. It seems to be possible to derive everything from the "psychosomatic structure." Bahnson, for instance, asserted in his *complementarity hypothesis* that

> In the somatic sphere the processes taking place resemble those in psychic regression (during neuroses and psychoses). If repression must assume the primary burden of the defense processes, instead of projection, then there is a shift of instinctual energy into the somatic sphere. Then we find a sequence of increasingly deeper somatic regression, from conversion hysteria to the deepest regression in the sphere of cell mitoses. (1986, p. 894)

Bahnson assigns the origin of malignancies to the deepest point of regression due to repression and, complementarily, that of psychoses to the deepest point of regression due to projection.

It is surprising how much fascination is exerted by the idea of psychophysiological regression, which was propogated by Margolin (1953) and which especially McDougall (1974, 1987) recently applied as the all-encompassing explanatory principle of psychic and somatic illnesses. The concept of psychophysiological regression, or at least the essence of the idea - although long ago shown to be untenable by Mendelson et al. (1956) - seems to be just as timeless as the hope for eternal life, and may even have its source in the latter. The search for meaning governs human life much more than scientific truths do, and part of it is the search for the interchangeability of body and mind, together with the idea of a concealed meaning of somatic illness that has been derived from psychoanalysis. On the basis of these assumptions one arrives at V. von Weizsäcker's principle of equivalence and the interchangeability of organic and psychic symptoms, which also amounts to a panpsychism in the thesis, "Nothing organic has no meaning." C.F. von Weizsäcker, in a discussion commemorating the 100th aniversary of the birth of Victor von Weizsäcker, the founder of anthropological medicine, stated unambiguously that one could not "assign each physical illness a psychic interpretation, which then takes on a scientific function in the interaction between physician and patient" (1987, p. 109). At that symposium, von Rad (1987, p. 163) drew attention to the panpsychism of anthropological medicine in the ideas of the interchangeability of body and mind and the security each finds in the other, and warned about the dangers associated with them. V. von Weizsäcker's philosophical ideas about human nature are, as von Rad documented by referring to several quotations from von Weizsäcker's writings (e. g., 1950, p. 259, 1951, p. 110), in fact dominated by the idea of a panpsychism, which from the very beginning has been a burden on the introduction of the subject into medicine. The scientific methodology of anthropological medicine is also in its beginnings. If bipersonality is taken seriously in therapy and scientific research, then all the problems characterizing the psychoanalytic paradigm are confronted. Clinical psychology has also been confronted by a paradigm change since the "cognitive revolution" of behavioralism (Bruner 1986). The contemporary attempts at integration, such as those presented by Wyss (1982, 1985), do not do justice to the comprehensive clinical knowledge that has been accumulated in psychoanalysis in this century.

To use the idea of psychosomatic regression - in whichever of its various but only apparently very different versions - as a basis for a comprehensive explanation of somatic illnesses leads to incorrect diagnoses and obstructs the development of more tenable theories.

The analogy of infantile psycho-somatic forms of reaction that are integrative in nature with somatic disturbances does not bear fruit, as we have demonstrated in Chap. 5 with regard to the example of wry neck. The physiology of the newborn is substantially different, as Meyer emphasized, from that of the adult:

> I would like to recall just one of the numerous differences, namely that of less functioning homeostasis. At the slightest infection newborns and infants have a body temperature of 39° or 40° C, they vomit at the slightest stress, they become exsiccated within hours. The only thing we do not find in the infant is an outright asthmalike or colitislike deviation that an adult might regress to. On the other hand, psychosomatic fever is unusual - the two cases that I have observed in 30 years did not result from physiological regression, but were residual stress consequences of herpes. (Meyer 1985, p. 54)

The infantile discharge of tension takes place through the body-mind unit because of the lack of cognitive forms of coping. In such integrative reactions characterized by the features of the primary process, the infant or newborn is in an animalistic phase of maturation. It is noteworthy that a psychosomatic illness does not occur in animals in the wild, only developing through artificially set conditions. In contrast to the infantile stage of development, events do not take place integratively in psychosomatic patients, i. e., not in the form of a body-mind unit; the characteristic feature of this form of disturbance is the complete lack of such a connection. Conceiving of psychosomatic decompensation as regression, understood as a reversion to infantile forms of the somatic discharge of tension, cannot explain the destructive aspect of physical illnesses.

The inclination of many psychoanalysts "to psychologize the physiological" (Schneider 1976) and their complementary inclination to disregard physiological laws when considering psychosomatic disturbances has led to a fatal stagnation. There is no mention of a differentiation between individual illnesses, rather the continued assertion of a seemingly holistic explanatory claim for "*the* psychosomatic illness." And there is no talk of a differentiation between acute and chronic illnesses, since many of the psychic features described in the course of chronic illnesses, such as the helplessness-hopelessness complex described by Engel and Schmale (1969), could after all be reactions of the sick individual to the somatic aspects of his illness!

9.9 Alexithymia

We made a reference to alexithymia when we said that the neurodermatitis patient behaved as if he were an alexithymist (p. 482). The term refers to the incapacity to "read," perceive, or express one's feelings.

The idea of psychophysiological regression, which was foreign to Freud's methodological manner of thinking, was also the moving force behind the description and explanation of alexithymia. This idea unites the countless fantasies that shift the source of somatic and psychic illnesses - ranging from cancer to psychosis - back to early infancy, i.e., to the time prior to the differentiation into psyche and body. At this age individuals allegedly develop with a so-called *psychosomatic structure* characterized by the particular absence of fantasies and mechanized thought (*pensée opératoire* or alexithymia).

Although considered a school, the authors counted among the "French school" of psychosomatic medicine have by no means a homogenous understanding of the concept "pensée opératoire." The processes of regression and fixation do, however, constitute the fix points in their ideas. De M'Uzan (1977) saw the lack of an opportunity to satisfy hallucinatory needs in childhood as being an important cause of the deficitary nature of psychic structure he believes characterizes the psychosomatically ill; Fain (1966) postulated a regression to a primitive defensive system of the ego as being the motor for the formation of somatic symptoms in psychosomatic illnesses; and Marty (1968) conceived of specific regressive processes (e.g., progressive disorganization, and partial and global regression). Marty (1969) traced the formation of somatic symptoms corresponding to these different forms of regression back to fixations originating from pathological humoral interactions between the fetus and mother, i.e., in the intrauterine phase. For these authors, this is the source of the clinical phenomena they describe. Operative thought is the "expression of an overcathexis of the most material, concrete, and practical elements in reality" (de M'Uzan 1977), which does not permit the patient any access to affective or fantasy levels, only creating images of the time and space relationship and thus a "bland relationship" to one's partner in conversation. They consider this the form of relationship characteristic of the psychosomatically ill. These French authors describe a tendency of such individuals to superficially identify with an object's features, a phenomenon they refer to as "reduplication." The patient thus makes an infinitely reproducible person out of himself; he grasps the other person only on the basis of his own model and has no comprehension of the other's individual personality.

Although Marty initially based his ideas on the assumption of intrauterine fixations, he later introduced a conception in which the origin of the primary fixation mechanisms responsible for the development of a psychosomatic disturbance was understood as being the result of the pathological interplay of death instinct and evolutionary process. Marty (1968) attempted with this idea to correlate the observed features of operative thought with the psychophysiological development of the individual. For him, human development is evolution that takes place under the influence of the life and death instincts. The proximity of these thoughts to Schur's concept of desomatization is obvious even though they are bound in a different theoretical framework. According to these authors, antievolutionary influences (caused by thanatos, the death instinct) disrupt the biological economy during the infantile development of the psychosomatic individual (evolutionary process, influenced by eros); although the pathological dysfunction is then eliminated, nothing can prevent these phases of development from continuing to be points of psychosomatic fixation.

It can be demonstrated for these French authors that they combine fragments of theories without integrating them and that they make no attempt to overcome the contradictions immanent in their theories in order to achieve a somewhat consistent theoretical model that is open to verification. For example, they assign operative thought to the sphere of the primary process, while they also discuss it as being a modality of the secondary process, with emphasis on orientation to reality, causality, logic, and continuity of thought processes (Marty and de M'Uzan 1963). This raises the question of how psychosomatic individuals then customarily demonstrate such a conspicuously high degree of social integration inspite of their functioning at the level of the primary process. The concept of reduplication has also not be refined sufficiently for it to be consistently related to the often mentioned observations of behavioral normalcy.

A new specificity assumption also guided the American authors who coined the term "alexithymia." They postulated a specific personality structure for psychosomatic individuals that - in contrast to that of neurotics - is characterized by alexithymia, the incapacity to express one's feelings appropriately in words. Sifneos (1973) has compiled a summary of the features he considers characteristic of psychosomatic patients: impoverished fantasy life with a sequential, functional manner of thinking, a tendency to avoid conflict constellations by acting out, a restricted capacity to experience feelings, and the difficulty to find the appropriate words to describe one's own feelings in individual situations. Although these authors (Nemiah and Sifneos 1970) initially proposed parallel psychodynamic, underdevelopment, and neurophysiological hypotheses, they later explicitly favored an idea borrowed from MacLean (1977), which is based on the assumption of a neuronal link between the limbic system (as the seat of libidinal and emotional processes) and the neocortex. It was thus possible for excitations to be directly discharged into the somatic realm via the hypothalamic-autonomic system.

These ideas stimulated intense empirical research, whose results however have been negative. Of 17 empirical studies to identify alexithymia as a personality feature, there were no indications for the presence of such a specific personality feature in psychosomatic patients except in the study by Sifneos himself and in two others by one other group of authors. The features measured by the other clinical groups and also demonstrated for control groups were, in contrast, verifiable (Ahrens and Deffner 1985). The retention of the idea of a specific psychosomatic personality structure, regardless of its particular form, has obstructed the further scientific development of a psychoanalytically oriented psychodynamic approach (Ahrens 1987). The intention of finding a uniform personality structure for the complex and diverse nature of psychosomatic disturbances constitutes a constriction contradicting clinical experience. The latter suggests the assumption that there are heterogeneous conflict constellations even for *one* psychosomatic symptom, which has also been shown in empirical studies (Overbeck 1977).

The most probable explanation is that all the important features of the so-called psychosomatic structure to which mechanized thought (*pensée opératoire*) and alexithymia are attributed are situative in origin. They are more likely to be the result of a specific manner of interviewing and the assumptions it is based on, than constant and etiologically relevant personality features, not to mention their alleged origin in the first year of life. Cremerius justifiably asked whether the verbal behavior that strongly inhibited the fantasies of patients - who, as mentioned in the published examples to document the diagnosis of lack of fantasy, confronted by a lecture hall in an unmediated manner and without any preparation in the guidance of the psychoanalytic interview - may itself not have been induced by this setting. His reference to the similarity of this style of speaking to the language spoken by members of the lower social classes also deserves notice. Ahrens (1986a,b) used a technique of content analysis to examine a sequence from an initial interview published by Sifneos and Nemiah in 1970, which they had employed as an example of alexithymia in psychosomatic patients. Over half the sentences the patient spoke in this sequence contained aggressive connotations that, however, the interviewer did not recognize or make the object of discussion and that, on the contrary, acquired a hidden resonance in the course of the interview. The authors thus projected the "problem of communication" mentioned in the title of their study into the patient and gave it the name "alexithymia," while bracketing out the problem of transference and countertransference. Other studies that compared groups of neurotic and somatically ill patients, using a differentiated methodological approach, came to results that contradict the idea of a specific psychosomatic personality structure since no differences between the two groups of patients could be determined (Ahrens 1986a,b). These results have been given little consideration; there is a very skewed ratio between the efforts to validate assertions in verifiable studies and the production of all-encompassing etiological fantasies.

It is quite obvious that we are challenging prejudices that can hardly be resolved or even weakened by the rational means of scientific validation. This raises the psychoanalytic question as to the motives that make such back-dating of the causes to a common matrix so fascinating and that protect them from reality testing - or actually provide this form of fantasizing a general immunity against scientific arguments.

Marty's hypothesis regarding the death instinct may serve as an example. An explanatory model is erected on hypothetical constructs that are inaccessible to empirical verification or even to the test of plausibility based on clinical experience. On the one hand, such speculation - in contrast to ideas and fantasies that can serve as a basis for scientific study and research - is bottomless; on the other, it governs therapeutic action without being able to provide a justification. Many psychoanalysts believe they can justify their speculation by referring to Freud's *drive mythology.* Freud's famous ironic and philosophical comment was,

> The theory of the instincts is so to say our mythology. Instincts are mythical entities, magnificent in their indefiniteness. In our work we cannot for a moment disregard them, yet we are never sure that we are seeing them clearly. (Freud 1933a, p. 95)

We attribute several different meanings to these sentences. Drives cannot be seen clearly because they are hidden in the biological unconscious. According to Freud, only their derivatives can be experienced psychically, namely inasmuch as they, as ideational or affect representatives, become conscious or can be deduced in a preconscious stage on the basis of symptoms. Drives share their greatness with mythical beings in the sense that they, just as the heroes in the personification of humans or gods in mythology, have effects. It is the latter that according to Freud's theory of drives must be identified scientifically. For instance, unconscious oedipal desires can thus be indirectly demonstrated clinically, at least in the sense of a relevant connection (Grünbaum 1984; Kettner 1987). In this Freud followed Mach's postulate about the theory of science; Mach did not deal with drive the question of what the essence of causative force, e. g., a drive, was, demanding instead that the causal connections be demonstrated by means of a systematic cause-and-effect analysis (Cheshire and Thomä 1991).

This theory of drives, just like many other theories, is imbued with the mythology of the natural philosophy going back to the early Greek philosophers, as Freud explicitly emphasized. This natural philosphy contains, in its dualistic views of love and hate, profound human knowledge giving meaning even to otherwise empirically false conceptions. There can hardly be any dispute about the fact that the goal Freud, an advocate of the enlightenment, pursued was not to promote a remythologization in the guise of false causal theories. Patients have a right, after all, to be treated on the basis of verifiable theories. There are two aspects to the view that the mythological mode of thinking must be replaced by theoretical explanation. First, the mythological element in subjective theories about illnesses must be clarified scientifically by means of causal explanations. Second, the liberation of scientific theory from mythological components is an accepted sign of progress. Once the distinction between theory and mythology is accepted, then there can be no objections to a recourse to a mythological mode of expression for the sake of a more vivid description. Freud made liberal use of it. If, however, the distinction between mythology and theory is ignored and the ontological language and naive realism of metapsychology are taken literally, then Freud's ideas are reversed into the opposite. Freud referred to metapsychology, which is supposed to provide the overall frame for explanation in order to incorporate magic, legends, fairy tails, mythology, and religion in a scientific *theory*, as a witch, and it is more than disturbing that this metapsychology has remained true to its traditional, witchlike nature.

The issue in Freud's model of causal explanation is of course not the mythical nature of drives, whatever they may be, but the demonstration of cause-and-effect connections (Kerz 1987). It is another matter that Freud's instinctual theory contains elements of a natural philosophy that has (re)turned into mythology.

Interpreting somatic illnesses satisfies man's longing for meaning, which grows in the face of incurable and fatal illnesses. The problem of death has, accordingly, become a starting point for private and social ideologies. Similarly, in animism, as Freud described in *Totem and Taboo* (1912/13), man attributes a soul to inanimate nature, creating for himself at the same time the belief in life after death.

This results not only in a universal tendency for man to take himself to be the measure of all things. Narcissism can become so intimately linked with a scientific method or a therapy that the latter seems to become universally applicable. Thus to trace the development of serious or fatal illnesses – such as mental illnesses or cancer - back to the beginning of life means to adopt the intellectual method of animism. In Freud's words, "It does not merely give an explanation of a particular phenomenon, but allows us to grasp the whole universe as a single unity from a single point of view" (1912/13, p. 77).

The division of medicine into separate fields and the inevitable, ever increasing specialization has created the opportunity for progress to be made in diagnosis and therapy in every field. Yet to the degree the specialization increases and as a consequence of the numerous threats to and complications of life, our longing for a unity and a whole also increases. Paradise is sought by fantasizing back: the loss of the whole after the Fall of Man brought time and death as well as knowledge.

9.10 The Body and the Psychoanalytic Method

The body is directly accessible to the psychoanalytic method via *bodily experience* without in this way becoming an object of medical examination. This means that it is important for psychoanalysts who have been trained as physicians, especially those active in psychosomatic medicine, to maintain their capacity to diagnose and treat somatic illnesses. Every specialist confronts the problem of how to maintain his general or specialized medical knowledge when he stops using it continuously.

In their capacity as specialists, psychoanalysts are confronted by the same general problems as all specialists are. General practioners have, as their title indicates, a wide range of knowledge, yet insufficient in any one field for them to act as specialists, while specialists, in contrast, lack the overview of general medicine that the general practitioner must have. A consequence of specialization and subspecialization is that experts constantly learn more and more about less and less. Yet this scornful remark is accurate only if the fact is disregarded that, regardless of how detailed intensive scientific study may be, connections continue to exist to major, fundamental problems that go far beyond the scope of a single discipline and require interdisciplinary collaboration. As we explained in Sect. 1.1, psychoanalysis is particulary reliant on an exchange of information with the other sciences studying human beings. Of course, this does not alter the fact that its method, insofar as it finds application as therapeutic technique, deals with the patient's psychic experiencing, not with his body. The comparison of methods need not be limited to the phenomena each leaves out of consideration; such comparisons must not lose sight of the fact that the individual is a unit. This results in diverse tensions, the consequence of which, in addition to of the methodological restrictions, is that the analyst only reacts adequately to the patient's holistic needs in his office in special moments. Tensions originate in the deficits between the desired, holistic, mind-body attention and reality. This thesis is based on the anthropological assumption that the human being is a unit that becomes immediate in holistic expectations, which he anticipates in conscious and unconscious fantasies and for which he constantly counts the deficit. This deficitary nature of man has long led philosophical anthropology to conceptualize man as a two-faced being who at one and the same time is characterized by an excess of fantasy. Dissatisfaction is consequently inherent, and is particularly great everywhere methodology brackets out phenomena or, because of man's obvious imperfectness, techniques are deficient.

Very intense and original holistic expectations are evoked in patients in pychoanalysts' offices; they point both to the past-as the lost paradise that existed prior to separation, trauma, or conscious awareness - and to the future - as a utopia. In our experience we can claim that "limitation proves the master," i. e., that the psychoanalyst earns respect if he is competent in employing the restricted scope of his method, despite the related problems this raises. At no time did this scope end at the frontier to the body, inasmuch as this is represented in conscious and unconscious experiencing as the *body image.* We refer the reader to Sect. 9.2.1 on "Conversion and Body Image" and emphasize that the origin of body image is one of the domains of psychoanalysis and that body image plays a decisive role in therapy. Psychoanalysts recognize numerous facets of body image by taking a patient's body feeling seriously. Yet this body image, including the unconscious and conscious ideational representatives united or in conflict in it, is obviously different from the *body* of modern medicine.

Psychosomatic phenomena affect the individual's subjective feeling, which in the form of body feeling is closely linked to body image. By proceeding from this domain of psychoanalysis, it is possible to recognize and possibly decrease the psychic effects on bodily phenomena. Difficult issues requiring the attention of different specialists raise problems as to integration and responsibility. We argue that the analyst should show a strong interest in his patients receiving the same care for intermittent or chronic somatic illnesses as he would want for himself or his family, because this adage leads to the best possible medicine. The role a medically trained psychoanalyst can play in an individual case depends both on methodological criteria and the analyst's evaluation of his competence. Taking somatic illnesses seriously, instead of psychologizing them in the irresponsbile manner of panpsycholigism, and working through the patient's subjective theory of his illness provide the psychoanalytic method great room for action. The care the analyst provides for somatic illnesses can go much further if he proceeds from the patient's subjective condition and body image than would be permitted by a wrongly understood principle of abstinence and neutrality.

It is in treating severe anxiety illnesses, borderline cases, and psychoses that analysts are most frequently confronted with the question of whether to prescribe psychopharmaceuticals. Even analysts experienced in pharmacotherapy hesitate to prescribe beta blockers or benzodiazepines for patients with anxiety neurosis. Their fear that the prescription might make it impossible to analyze the transference disregards the fact that a rejection might have even worse and lasting adverse side effects. Splitting medical functions among different persons can cause additional problems for some patients, particularly those already suffering from splitting processes. In a publication that has received little attention, Ostow made the followign correct observations:

But while such uniformity is desirable, it is essential only that all transactions with the patient be deliberate and controlled so that fantasy may be contrasted with reality. For example, no analyst will hesitate to offer a seriously depressed patient more assurance, more time, or more affection than he ordinarily does. Third, the administration of medication to a patient has unconscious meanings which can be analyzed as readily as the unconscious meanings of all the other contrived and fortuitous features of the therapeutic contact, such as disposition of the office furniture, the analyst's name, arrangements for payment of fees, an illness, an so on. (Ostow 1962, pp. 3-4)

This flexibility enables an analyst to treat very severely ill patients, even though Ostow's economic speculations about the mechanism of action of psychopharmaceuticals are untenable. Psychopharmaceutic medication must of course be viewed in the framework of analytic treatment, with special attention being paid to the problem of addiction. Many representatives of the biochemical school of psychiatry prescribe psychopharmaceuticals without paying attention to the genuine psychic source of anxiety (see Sect. 9.1). The lack of controlled studies makes it impossible to make a general recommendation as to who should prescribe medication in a joint treatment (see Klerman et al. 1984).

The tension between the holistic expectations of the patient, on the one hand, and the incompleteness, as manifested by specialized methods, on the other, can be put to productive use. The exclusion of the body, in contrast, seems to be taking its revenge on psychoanalysis, just as are excluded family members who seek an advocate among the family therapists. Yet for which body are body therapists the advocate?

The renaissance of the body in body therapy refers to *body image*, as can been seen in the informative book by Brähler (1988). Body image is also the object in Moser's (1987) enthusiasm for body therapies; a factor that has definitely promoted the spread of such therapies is the *exclusion* of the body in a particular form of psychoanalytic abstinence, which unfortunately is more than a caricature invented by Moser. We share his criticism, yet without drawing the consequences he does, for several reasons.

According to the experience of Benedetti (1980), Schneider (1977), Wolff (1977), and Ahrens (1988), and our own studies, patients with somatic symptoms develop an affective resonance and active fantasy after a period of treatment that are qualitatively and quantitatively comparable with those developing in the treatment of neurosis. The problems of therapeutic technique described by McDougall (1985, 1987) and Moser can therefore not be traced back to alexithymia. Of course, it would be logical to make at least an attempt at body therapy if there were a deficit in the preverbal phase of development that could be compensated. As Moser (1987) and Müller-Braunschweig (1988) have indicated, analysts should at any rate not let themselves be put off by the abstinence taboo, the rigid application of which was partly a sign of the times.

Theoretical considerations limit our willingness to expand our flexibility beyond certain limits. The success, or lack of it, of an analysis depends on so many conditions that it is impossible to blame the failure of the standard technique in patients with a "psychosomatic structure" on a hypothetical infantile disturbance. There is not even a consensus at the phenomenological level of diagnosis that goes beyond the agreement of an individual with himself, not to mention the differences of opinion regarding the reconstruction of the causal conditions. Moreover, our personal stance prohibits us from choosing a therapeutic step if we are convinced that the theory justifying it is misleading. Yet some helpful therapeutic steps stem from false theories. For example, it is conceivable that the action of a body therapist might work wonders if a patient has undergone severe frustration for years. This has little or nothing to do with traumas experienced in the first year of life or their compensation in such a fictive new beginning. What this proves is that it is damaging to frustrate a patient instead of providing him with the opportunity to cope with what he has been through. Regardless of whatever constitutes the curative effect, both the formation of deficits or defects in the self-feeling anchored in the body and their experiencing are a very complex matter. Finally, it is disturbing that the body therapist acts at an as-if level while allegedly at the appropriate moment doing paternal or maternal things to which he attributes a particularly realistic meaning. How does one go from the as-if level to deeper reality? Important are not solely the empirical contacts, among other things, but their significance as a sensory perception. To be specific, the issue is the body image, not the body (i.e, the object of scientific medicine), in the sense that only a wonder can help the latter by postponing death for a finite period of time if pathophysiological or malignant processes are present.

Where are the limits on the translation of body language into spoken language? "Symptom as Talk: Talk as Symptom" is a noteworthy heading in Forrester's (1980) book on language and psychoanalysis. Of course, *symptoms* and *talk* can have a dynamic all their own, independent of each other. Forrester thus correctly added, "Symptom as Symptom: Talk as Talk." He referred to the far-reaching ambiguity that has been an element of psychoanalytic theory from the beginning. We cannot consider both languages, that of symptoms and that of therapy, to be identical even though Freud discovered that a symptom can be an equivalent and take the place of a thought. The equivalence must be determined methodologically with reference to their interchangeability, which is excellently suited for determining in practice the therapeutic range of the psychoanalytic method - whose limits are where somatic symptoms defy *translation.* Although the symptoms of malignant disease can be described in words, they are *explained* with the aid of scientific concepts in the context of causal theories. For them, just as for many other somatic symptoms, translation cannot be employed to make them part of conscious experiencing in the sense that the symptoms might then be explained psychodynamically. Such somatic *symptoms* are not *symbols* for something else although the individual may attribute some *meaning* to his life, suffering, or death.

The following points of view should be observed in the diagnosis and psychoanalytic therapy of patients suffering from somatic symptoms. Patient and analyst often discover that somatic symptoms are involved in connection with, for example, situations of stress. The healthy individual then has a holistic experience. The manifestations of pleasure, sadness, and pain, to mention just a few examples, that are observable or accessible to introspection demand a circular description not specifying the starting point. The manifestation of physical pain at the same time a separation from someone dearly beloved is experienced does not in itself justify a statement about cause and effect. Correlations do not specify which side of a relationship is the dependent or independent variable or whether both are dependent. Of course, the demonstration of *correlations* is a precondition for clarifying the *causal relationship* of somatogenic and psychogenic conditions. We thus join Fahrenberg (1979, 1981) in pleading for a double consideration that is methodologically adequate to the emergence of the psychic manifestation (see Rager 1988; Hastedt 1988).

Higher life processes, i. e., the psychophysical processes linked to man's brain activity, can be described and analyzed in two different and nonconvertable (incomensurable and irreducable) reference systems. The one is not a secondary phenomenon, equivalent, function, or epiphenomenon of the other, but indispensable for the adequate description and complete understanding of the other. This complementary model of categorical structures shifts the ontological question to the sphere of the method of categorical analysis and excludes ideas about psychophysical isomorphism, simple reflective or dictionary functions, energetic interaction (psychic causality, psychogenesis, the assumption of mental influence on synapses or modules), and physicalistic-materialistic reductions. (Fahrenberg 1979, p. 161)

The *causal analysis* of the correlations between experiencing, behavior, and physiological functions make it possible to intervene systematically in causal relationships by distinguishing the different variables. It is in this context that the *psychogenesis* must be empirically shown, as in a *causal* connection, without reverting to energetic interactions such as are associated with conversion theory.

In diagnostic procedures the correlation between somatic symptoms and experiencing is usually dealt with in a one-sided manner. Since all somatic symptoms can have somatic causes, the diagnostic procedures to exclude potential causes are taking up increasing space in medicine. And since there are many potential causes, for instance, of pain in the groin that radiates toward the genitals or of pain in the upper abdomen, and they are investigated in different specialities, many specialists are involved. Frequently only minor deviations from normal are detected, which the patient, doctor, or both, dwell on and overemphasize. Since these attempts to find an explanation can be accompanied by advice as to therapy, it is not unusual for a vicious circle of hope and new disappointments to develop. Before this happens, as a consequence of a one-sided somatopsychic reading of the correlations, it is time to return to a holistic perspective, at least to approximate one. That we speak of an approximate return to holism might disturb the reader, yet the multitude of languages associated with methodological pluralism cannot transformed into *one* generally valid semiotic without a great loss of information on all sides. This is no more possible than a reduction of the psychoanalytic method to physiology or vice versa. It is therefore decisive that we at least approximately satisfy the insatiable longing for holism by making an *integrating evaluation* of the observations and results.

The involvement of somatic symptoms secondary to experiencing must be grounded *positively*, not just verified by excluding the other potential causes. The body language Freud discovered in hysterical patients was a hidden, unconscious form of expression that appeared to be independent of consciousness and take its course both blindly and arbitrarily. The grammar of feelings and affect, in particular, which can only be artificially separated from cognitive processes, follows rules whose discovery was a consequence of the psychoanalytic method. Freud's theory of a dynamic understanding of psychic life, which went beyond descriptive phenomenology, is characterized by its capacity to put symbollically expressed intentions into context and give them meaning. Even more important is the link of this theory to the *methodologically* grounded assertion that the experiencing and recognition of unconscious desires and intentions makes the symptoms disappear. As early as in his *Studies on Hysteria*, Freud wrote:

To begin with, the work becomes more obscure and difficult, as a rule, the deeper we penetrate into the stratified psychical structure which I have described above. But once we have worked our way as far as the nucleus, light dawns and we need not fear that the patient's general condition will be subject to any severe periods of gloom. But the reward of our labours, the cessation of the symptoms, can only be expected when we have accomplished the complete analysis of every individual symptom; and indeed, if the individual symptoms are interconnected at numerous nodal points, we shall not even be encouraged during the work by partial successes. Thanks to the abundant causal connections, every pathogenic idea which has not yet been got rid of operates as a motive for the whole of the products of the neurosis, and it is only with the last word of the analysis that the whole clinical picture vanishes, just as happens with memories that are reproduced individually. (Freud 1895d, pp. 298-299)

The oppostie is also true; just because of these interconnections - in which the pathogenic ideas are not isolated from another but instead mutually reinforce and support each other - the therapeutic work on one node or focus can radiate over the entire complex of the causal constellation. The therapeutic effect of the psychoanalytic dialogue thus spreads through the network of connections between the unconscious motives without it being necessary for each specific wish to be named individually or for each node to be resolved. We thus have a pragmatic guide at our disposal: the scope of the psychoanalytic method with regard to bodily phenomena does not end with its language because the therapeutic dialogue also realizes a nonverbal component.

The somatopsychic consequences of fatal illnesses have become an aspect of a psychoanalyst's experience since psychoanalysts have been confronted with therapeutic tasks while working as consultants in intensive care units and in psychooncology (Gaus and Köhle 1986; Köhle et al. 1986; Meerwein 1987; Sellschopp 1988). Of relevance here is also the body experience under the special circumstances of knowing or having a premonition about the nearing of death. With regard to the questions as to meaning that a patient poses the analyst at the end of his life, we recommend making a distinction. It is an obvious fact that psychoanalytic theory and its latent anthropology call for death to be acknowledged and are unable to provide consolation in the form of hope for fulfillment in the hereafter. The changes accomapnying fatal illnesses contribute to the dissolution of spatiotemporal borders, which probably can only be expressed via allegories, a form of language that both within and outside psychoanalysis employs metaphors of a return.

Such allegories provide the patient indirect consolation, for example by providing the subjective experience of security that makes the awareness of physical decline more tolerable (Eissler 1969; Haegglund 1978). The analyst, as every doctor, must respond as an individual who himself must confront the ultimate questions about the meaning of life and death. It seems very dubious to us whether analysts can provide better answers to these questions within the theoretical framework of the life and death instincts or that of object relations. We presume that analysts, as others, base their contact with patients in the throes of death on their personal attitudes about life and the world and use psychoanalytic theory, including its metapsychology, metaphorically and as a structure providing support.

9.11 Results

The starting point of the discussion about the outcome of psychoanalytic treatment was Freud's case histories. Fenichel (1930) reported the first systematic study of therapeutic results, performed by the Berlin Psychoanalytic Institute. This institute was conceived according to the idea, which Freud (1919j) also advocated, that health care, research, and teaching constituted a unit. Later the activities of most institutes became restricted almost exclusively to training. The studies Dührssen (1962) performed at the Berlin Central Institute for Psychogenic Illnesses had a far-reaching impact in Germany, specifically on the inclusion of psychodynamic and analytic treatment among the forms of therapy covered by health insurance (see Vol.1, Sect. 6.6); in practive, however, the systematic case history never gained widespread acceptance. In the meantime, research into the results of psychotherapy (see Kächele 1981; Lambert et al. 1986) has produced methodologically viable empirical studies about cases of intensive psychoanalysis (Bachrach et al. 1985; Bräutigam et al. 1980; Weber et al. 1966; Kernberg et al. 1972; Wallerstein 1986; Zerssen et al. 1986).

Many analysts defer research to institutions. Psychoanalysis had its origin, however, in practice, and Freud claimed there was an inseparable bond between research and treatment (see Vol.1, Chap. 10). In fact, therapist and researcher pursue different interests. The therapist requires security because his faith in his comments is an important element of any psychotherapeutic intervention (Kächele 1988a). It is his task to maximize positive evidence in order to maintain his capacity to act in the clinical situation. The scientist, however, is guided by a different interest. His task is to maximize negative evidence, i. e., to constantly question the results and their explanation, as Bowlby has emphasized:

> In his day to day work it is necessary for a scientist to exercise a high degree of criticism and self-criticism: and in the world he inhabits neither the data nor the theories of a leader, however admired personally he may be, are exempt from challenge and criticism. There is no place for authority.
>
> The same is not true in the practice of a profession. If he is to be effective a practitioner must be prepared to act as though certain principles and certain theories were valid; and in deciding which to adopt he is likely to be guided by those with experience from whom he learns. Since, moreover, there is a tendency in all of us to be impressed whenever the application of a theory appears to have been successful, practitioners are at special risk of placing greater confidence in a theory than the evidence available may justify. (Bowlby 1979, p. 4)

Many analysts appear to want to retain their security after the conclusion of a treatment since, as Schlessinger and Robbins (1983, p. 7) emphasized, there is an obvious deficit of follow-up studies among the wealth of psychoanalytic literature. They believe that a significant role is played by the defensive attitude of most analysts, such as knowing in advance what the result of a psychoanalysis should be, which obscures their perception for processes that do not agree with their traditional view.

We believe it is therefore important for a critical textbook of psychoanalytic practice to include comments about the nature of follow-up that is appropriate to clinical work. A critical examination of the consequences of an analyst's therapeutic technique is in the interest of his own expertise, the purpose of which is to promote the patient's well-being. This takes place during treatment, at the conclusion of treatment, and at one or more later points in time. Every analyst summarizes the severity of the symptoms at the beginning of therapy and makes conditional prognoses based on the patient's underlying psychodynamics (Sargent et al. 1968). These prognoses contain hypotheses about causal connections, and the conditional prognoses are corrected and extended in the course of therapy. Such an evaluation oriented on the oscillations during treatment enables the analyst to adjust his goals and strategies to the particular patient. At some point the analyst attempts to draw a realistic balance about the investment and return. This sober, economic perspective reminds one of the limitations on the modifications that psychoanalysis attempts to achieve.

Each participant, of course, attempts to take stock of the effects of treatment. The possible modalities are each for himself, both together, and by third parties (e. g., relatives). Since the issue of change is central during therapy, whether directly or indirectly, it is logical to jointly take stock during the final phase of analysis. In a favorable case, the analyst will hear that the patient is satisfied with the outcome, that the symptoms that led him to seek treatment have disappeared (if they have not been momentarily revived as part of the problem of separation), or that he feels like a new person because it was possible to achieve a substantial change of his character. Although patients seldom mention the capacity for self-analysis, which we discussed in Vol.1 (Sect. 8.9.4), they do describe the particular manner in which they internalized the analyst's functions, which are then partially continued in self-analysis. Genuine analytic use of this capacity is probably made by those patients who draw advantages for their profession from the treatment.

As a rule psychoanalytic treatment constitutes a large investment in time and money. The number of patients a practicing analyst can treat in some 20-30 years of work is limited in comparison to other fields of medicine. For this reason our knowledge of the later consequences of analytic interventions constitutes an important corrective for the psychoanalytic community, as described by Schlessinger and Robbins (1983).

Many analysts are reluctant to undertake follow-up studies of their patients because they fear a revival of the transference they believe has been dissolved. This concern is unjustified, for several reasons. It is known, since Pfeiffer's (1959, 1961, 1963) studies, which have been continued by Schlessinger and Robbins (1983; see also Nedelmann 1980), that the transference continues to exist in the patient's positive memories of the helping alliance, which are revived by follow-up interviews. If the course is favorable, those aspects of transference are resolved that can be segregated off as neurotic. Furthermore, the analyst continues to be a significant person for the patient, occupying a favored place in his experiencing. It is therefore easy for expatients to quickly find their way back to old modes of relationship and to reflect on this reactivation in follow-up interviews, whether with a third party or with the analyst. Although the idea of a complete dissolution of the transference has thus been refuted, it has not died out, but has led to a regular increase in the length of analyses, particularly of training analyses, since the late 1940s. Balint (1948) called them superanalyses. In our opinion they are linked with the thought that an intensive and lengthy analysis will resolve the transference especially thoroughly. In fact, however, the opposite effect, a vicious circle, seems to have resulted because the superanalyses have increased dependence precisely in analysts in training, reinforcing the neurotic elements of transference. In these analyses the idealization of the training analyst and the avoidance of realistic evaluations is particularly pronounced on both sides, causing each to go through a process of disillusionment after termination that continues for years and constitutes a not insubstantial burden on the professional community. The fact that this problem was recently the object of a detailed discussion must therefore be seen as a great advance (Cooper 1985; Thomä 1991).

We have to expect that follow-up studies will cause us to make substantial corrections to the conception that we acquired during the treatment itself. These corrections are of great value for the psychoanalytic theory of treatment because they can be either positive or negative (Kordy and Senf 1985).

9.11.1 Patients' Retrospection

Since we take the views of our patients about the consequences of our therapeutic actions particularly seriously, we have given a number of our patients the reports written about them and asked for their opinions. We have also received retrospective evaluations.

The following response is from Friedrich Y, about whom we reported in Sect. 2.3.1. He described his symptoms and impressions about the events in therapy. We have altered only those items necessary to ensure anonymity.

Looking Back at My Psychoanalysis

Symptoms

I was repeatedly confronted by my anxieties, by the energy it took to drive with the brakes on. Suffering: I could not openly express my anger and rage at colleagues or close associates, but only created a burden for my wife and myself. I avoided disagreeable meetings and parties, dances, and recreational events. I postponed difficult calls and visits. At work I often lost control of myself, went wild, became abusive, and once beat my wife. I often fled into the forest or into demanding too much of myself. I was unable to relax, calm down, or play with the children. I justified myself through what I achieved, putting my family second. I often had problems with my digestion and headaches, sore throat, and backache. My suffering grew. A friend of mine encouraged me to visit a therapist, someone he had also already consulted.

First Interview

I went: with the fear of being sent away, with complete frankness, almost self-exposure, aware that it was now or never, and with the strong desire: I want to ease the brakes inside me. I want more life. I want, finally, my life.

He took me. I get along with him. I want to get somewhere with him. He listened, very patiently. I said a lot, threw ballast overboard. He had something alive, experienced, generous, seductive. He wasn't pushy.

First Phase

With him I could let out my hate for my mother. She denied me so much life, beat me, oppressed me, forced me into being good. She ruined my father and misused me as his substitute. She used my bad conscience and religion to suppress my aggression and make me a weakling and cripple. At the same time I recognized that she perhaps did not have a choice, as the oldest daughter, having lost her father very early, having had a strong and energetic mother, and having been responsible for her sisters. She first suppressed her own life, especially after the death of my father. She had to struggle, be strong. And, she turned old, went from being the strong one to the weak one, from being the dominant one to the victim. Shameful time in her last two years; she was afraid of those near her, wanted to kill herself, and was a difficult patient for the family taking care of her.

In the last few years I was able to do something good for her, give something back to her. I could see what she had sacrificed for me. I saw, regretted, and was amazed by her struggle; I could help her in her weakness, helplessness, and occasionally unjustified anger. She died forty years after the end of Hitler's rule. (How had she lived then? We were never able to speak about it in peace. She always blocked it off, justified herself, gave excuses!)

Second Phase

What kind of a father did I lose, and what did I lose with him? He increasingly appeared in therapy behind my mother. I was never actually a son, boy, more a girl like my sisters. I did not have a male role model in my struggles, conflicts, self-assertion. Now I can work on my aggression.

I could stand up better at work, restrain myself, let myself be angry. I stopped hiding in groups, took responsibility, stood up to conflict. I stopped taking things or people as easy as I used to, and being so afraid of being hurt or hurting others. I've stopped hiding and am no longer ashamed about my being attracted to other women; I can handle it. I could more clearly feel where my wife suffered from me, felt overwhelmed or neglected by me. I became better able to accept conflict with her, coming closer to her in the process. I became better able to bear it if she were despaired. I could go to the limits and consciously restrain myself, of my own will, not because of a bad conscience or pressure. For example, my wife is more important to me than others are. Family is often more important than profession. Accepting something is sometimes more important than conflict "at any price." My sexual freedom together with my wife, in letting myself have something, is growing, also to the degree that my wife could do something for me. I became able to accept that my wife did something for herself, that she still needed time to get freer, to free herself from the burden that I had placed on her for such a long time. Even that she got mad after talking with me and the analyst. I was better able to accept my wife being weak and to accept that I have weaknesses too.

Third Phase: Termination of the Analysis

What I still wanted to work on: On the connection between the psychic and the body. Where do headaches come from, backache? How do I overcome illnesses? How could I work preventively, on the causes? One weekend something changed. For weeks I had had a sore throat after analysis, problems with my voice, difficulties singing, at work, speaking. I publicly stood up to my analysis, told others about it, and encouraged others to work on their problems. I stopped sweeping conflicts with close colleagues under the carpet, started defending myself, even being provocative. It was exhausting, to take the resistance and animosity. I got stronger, uncompromising in helping others, the oppressed, for example in letters against apartheid and racists. I didn't simply become enraged but actively fought, despite the risks, against "evil spirits" such as addiction, racism, fascism. I increasingly asked others, "Do you want to be healthy? If not, then I will tell you what your illness is, keep my distance, and not let myself get involved, especially in your neurosis." I would have rather cut out the rotten apple, cut through false appearances, cut open the festering ulcer - as the accomplice of the illness, the repression, the resignation.

How I Experienced My Therapist

He was usually patient. He could take silence. He could also be tough, not let loose. He often asked critical questions about "little" things, which helped me, things like gestures, greetings, forgetting a session, and saying goodbye. He made cautious reference to my dreams and often opened my eyes about their meaning. He initiated the separation, the end of therapy quite early (not too early fortunately, as I was once tempted). And even after therapy was over, he kept his door open for me. He encouraged me not to show him too much consideration (sometimes I wanted to "spare" him something, but he can take care of himself.)

When I managed to overcome my frugal habits, with his help, and to act more self-confidently, the price of the therapy wasn't a problem any more. I consciously decided to afford therapy (which was no big deal since most of it was refunded by the health insurance!), and am glad to have become so healthy, both psychically and physically.

This retrospective description was written a year after the end of the analysis. Subsequent events confirm that the patient had learned in his therapy how to make a decisive change in his life.

Therapeutic institutions desiring to follow-up a larger number of patients without resorting to an excessively complex methodology can employ a questionnaire devised by Strupp et al. (1964). Such a procedure makes it possible for the patient to make a retrospective evaluation of the success of therapy from various points of view.

In an examination of our own (Kächele et al. 1985b) we chose this approach to question a group of 91 patients who had undergone different types of treatment. On a scale from 1 to 6 (best to worst), the average grade for "the feeling of complete satisfaction with the therapeutic success" was 2.2. The obviously contrasting question of "Do you have the feeling that another treatment is necessary?" was given 3.1 and there were a wide range of answers, indicating a clear ambivalence. Although 36% of the patients were very satisfied and 27% satisfied - corresponding to the two-thirds rate found in many follow-up studies - a not insignificant number of patients were the view that they needed another treatment. In our opinion these apparently contradictory evaluations express a very differentiated view, namely that not all their goals have been achieved, but that everything was not possible. This idea clearly had an impact on the answers about the relationship between the cost and effect of the treatment, which were very favorable at 1.7. The capacity to admit the personal significance of one's own therapy in public is emphasized by the fact that 72% of the patients said that they would recommend that a close friend seek psychotherapeutic treatment if in need.

Of great practical significance is the outcome that the patient's evaluation of the therapist for the dimensions "empathy and acceptance" and "trust and esteem" make it possible to make a retrodictive prediction of the patient's satisfaction with the treatment. Even without elaborate research into the results of psychoanalysis, such a study confirms that the positive structuring of the therapeutic relationship is a necessary condition, although not a sufficient one, for the satisfaction with the outcome that both patient and analyst desire. The previously widespread and cynical argument that this esteem was only the consequence of the patient's financial sacrifice, which motivated him to believe idealizing self-deceptions, has fortunately been disproved by the introduction of health insurance coverage for psychodynamic treatment. We therefore proceed from the assumption that patients provide realistic information.

Aside from patients' attitudes, in whichever form they are obtained, is the question that every therapist must ask himself: Am I satisfied? This is a crucial question because it confronts the professional ego-ideal. The patient's subjective experiencing alone cannot suffice to satisfy the analyst; he also has to examine whether there is a tangible connection between the course and outcome of therapy, on the one hand, and, on the other, the nature of the genesis and resolution of symptoms and character traits according to the theory he adheres to. In his final reflections he will have to ask what his goals were at the beginning of therapy and which of them he managed to achieve. This perspective does not exclude the fact that the patient continues to be responsible for himself. The analyst, however, has to justify his methods and the outcome to himself and the professional group he identifies with.

The basis of the analyst's evaluation should be a comparison of his notes from the beginning of the treatment with those made at the end. Substantial modifications of the implicit and explicit goals of therapy are found particularly in therapies of long duration. We assume with good reason that it is inconceivable for an analysis to be conducted without some goal, and that psychoanalytic practice facilitates the view that the goal is a product of the process. It is a serious mistake to believe that analysts can maintain a distance to concrete goals linked with specific values (see Vol.1, Sect. 7.1). Bräutigam (1984) has presented a critical discussion of the modifications that goals have undergone in the course of the history of psychoanalysis, correctly referring to the fact that therapy-immanent goals - e.g., expansion of consciousness, affective discharge, regression - have increasingly gained in importance. In an effort to acquire the appearance of value neutrality, the expression "Where id was, there ego shall be" has been used to describe analytic work because it apparently provides an etiological, pathogenetic grounding for the therapeutic process. In the framework of the structural model this means that the ego gains better control of the id, which originally in the topographic theory was expressed as freer access to the unconscious. The psychoanalytic goal of structural change was linked to this movement from id to ego.

Since Wallerstein's (1986) profound reflections on the implications of the results of the Menninger Psychotherapy Project, the question of how "structural" change can be distinguished from behavioral change is fraught with problems, especially with methodological ones. The view cannot be maintained that it is exclusively the psychoanalytic technique that affords insight and achieves structural change. According to the definition that Rapaport (1967 [1957], p. 701) also supported, these structures are psychic processes that undergo change at a slow rate and that we hypostatize but that we can only detect in behavior and experiencing. We cite the following summary comments from Wallerstein's comprehenisve clinical review, probably the most comprehensive process study in the history of psychoanalysis:

> The treatment results, with patients selected either as suitable for trials at psychoanalysis or as appropriate for varying mixes of expressive-supportive psychotherapeutic approaches, tended with this population sample to converge rather than to diverge in outcome. Across the whole spectrum of treatment courses ... the treatment carried more supportive elements than originally intended, and these supportive elements accounted for more of the changes achieved than had been originally anticipated. The nature of supportive therapy - or, better, the supportive aspects of all psychotherapy, as conceptualized within a psychoanalytic theoretical framework - deserves far more respectful specification in all its forms and variants than has usually been accorded in the psychodynamic literature.... The kinds of changes reached by this cohort of patients - those reached primarily on the basis of the opposed covering-up varieties of supportive techniques - often seemed quite indistinguishable from each other in terms of being so-called "real" or "structural" changes in personality functioning, as least by the usually deployed indicators. (Wallerstein 1986, p. 730)

We prefer Freud's formulation in *Analysis Terminable and Interminable* (1937c, p. 250) in which he clearly described the operational goal of every treatment: "The business of the analysis is to secure the best possible psychological conditions for the functions of the ego; with that it has discharged its task." This makes sufficiently clear that the analyst should not lose sight of the distinction between goals in life and treatment goals, which Ticho (1972) has referred to.

Until now analysts have presumably done little to fulfill their tasks of discussing the goals of the treatment with patients at the very beginning. Many seem to fear the danger that the patient will then raise excessively goal-related demands that the analyst keep his promise.

9.11.2 Changes

Well, what are the goals of treatment and how do they differ from those in life? We would like to clarify this issue by discussing in detail the changes that one patient, Amalie X, achieved in psychoanalysis. We have evaluated these changes in numerous ways, since this case was studied particularly intensively in various projects within the framework of the study "Psychoanalytic Processes" supported by the German Research Council (Hohage and Kübler 1987; Neudert et al. 1987; Leuzinger 1988).

Since the patient accorded her hirsutism a prominent position in her subjective understanding of the causes of her neurosis, we begin by considering the status of this somatic disturbance, from which we derive the specific changes that constituted the goal. Hirsutism probably had a double significance to the patient. On the one hand it impeded her feminine identification, which was problematic anyway, by constantly revitalizing her unconscious desires to be a man. For her, femininity was not positively considered but rather associated with illness (her mother's) and discrimination (versus her brothers). Her increased hair growth occurred in puberty, a period when sexual identity is labile anyway. The appearance of masculinity provided by her body hair strengthened the developmental revival of oedipal penis envy. Of course, the latter must have already been at the focus of unresolved conflicts, because it would otherwise not have attained this significance. Signs of this can be seen in the patient's relationship to her two brothers, whom she admired and envied, although she often felt discriminated against. As long as the patient could fantasize that her penis desire was fulfilled, her hair growth corresponded to her body schema. Yet the fantasized wish fulfillment only offered relief as long as the patient managed to maintain it, which was impossible long term because virile hair growth does not make a man out of a woman. This raised the problem of sexual identity once again. It was on this basis that all cognitive processes connected with feminine self-reprentations became a source of conflict for the patient, causing distress and eliciting defense reactions.

On the other hand, her hirsutism secondarily acquired something of the quality of a presenting symptom, providing the patient with an excuse for generally avoiding sexually enticing situations. She was not consciously aware of this function of her physical disturbance.

Two demands can be derived from these thoughts that can serve as goals for a successful treatment. The patient would not be able to accept social and sexual contact until she, first, had attained a sufficiently secure sexual identity and overcome her self-insecurity, and second, had given up her feelings of guilt about her desires. Both points of this prognosis were confirmed. Amalie X significantly increased her capacity to establish relationships, and has lived with her partner for a longer period of time without being restricted by any symptoms. Her conscienciousness, which initially was often extreme, has mellowed, although the demands she placed on herself and those around her have continued to be very high. In discussions she has become livelier, showing more humor and apparently getting more pleasure from life. Can these changes be traced back to the fact that both of the causal conditions have demonstrably lost their effects as a consequence of her psychoanalytic treatment? We answer this decisive question in the affirmative although space prevents us from discussing the reasons in detail. The proof of structural changes requires detailed descriptions of the psychoanalytic process. We can say, in conclusion, that despite her virile hair growth Amalie X has found a feminine identification and freed herself of her religious scruples and feelings of guilt toward her sexuality, in accordance with the prognosis.

The results of the psychological tests, performed as a check on success at the beginning and after the termination of treatment and also as part of a follow-up two years later, confirmed the clinical evaluation of her analyst that the treatment was successful. A comparison of the profiles in the Freiburg Personality Inventory (similar to the Minnesota Multiphasic Personality Inventory) showed that the values at the end of treatment were more frequently in the normal area and less frequently at the extremes than at the beginning of treatment. This tendency had become more pronounced on follow-up.

Especially on the scales on which the patient had shown herself to be extremely (= standard value 1) irritated and hesitant (scale 6), very (= standard value 2) yielding and moderate (scale 7), very inhibited and tense (scale 8), and extremely emotionally fragile (scale N), the values returned to the normal area.

On a few scales the patient diverged positively from normal after treatment. Amalie X described herself as psychosomatically less disturbed (scale 1), more satisfied and self-secure (scale 3), more sociable and active (scale 5), and more extroverted (scale E). The standard value of 8 on scale 2 at the end of treatment deserves special attention because it expressed that the patient experiences herself as being spontaneously very aggressive and emotionally immature. At this point in time she may still have been anxious about her aggressive impulses, which she did not have such strong control over as at the beginning of treatment. On follow-up this value had returned to normal. The patient seems to have gained the security in the meantime that she no longer need fear an aggresive outburst. Conspicuous is also the extreme value on scale 3 on follow-up; Amalie X, whose desire for treatment was the result especially of depressive moods, described herself here as extremely satisfied and self-secure.

The values on the Giessen Test for the patient's self-image were within normal on all three testings. Beckmann and Richter, who developed this procedure, have commented about it that: "At its conception great weight was placed on experiencing how a proband describes himself in psychoanalytically relevant categories" (1972, p. 12). For Amalie X:

The more extreme values diverging from the normal range simply demonstrate the initial self-description to be relatively depressed (scale HM vs DE) and the concluding one to be rather dominant (scale DO vs GE). The profiles demonstrate especially a shift showing that the patient experienced herself after treatment to be more dominant, less compulsive, less depressive, and more permeable (opener, more capable of contact). On follow-up the profile of her self-image was completely inconspicuous.

Of note regarding the image that the analyst had of the patient at the beginning of treatment (Giessen Test of Imputed Image of Others) was that the analyst considered her to be more disturbed than she did. In his eyes she was significantly more compulsive, depressive, retentive, and socially restricted. In these dimensions the image attributed to others was outside the normal range. According to Zenz et al. (1975) such a clear discrepancy is frequently observed after the initial interview. This discrepancy disappeared at the end of treatment, when the analyst considered her to be just as healthy as she did. Somewhat larger differences persisted on only two scales, the analyst viewing her to be more appealing and desirable as well as more compulsive that she did.

The results of the psychological tests supported the analyst's evaluation, and those on follow-up confirmed the continued positive development in the postanalytic phase.

Process changes are also of great interest for a psychoanalytic theory of change; these are changes in how a patient can structure the psychoanalytic process (Luborsky and Schimek 1964). This question was studied for this patient within a project in which specific psychoanalytic criteria of change were registered with regard to the patient's reactions to dreams (Leuzinger 1988). To supplement the psychological tests, a theoretically informed content analysis was performed on verbatim protocols from the initial and concluding phases to determine how the patient's cognitive processes had changed during her confrontation with dreams. The wealth of individual results on the changes in cognitive processes confirmed the clinical and test evaluations.

The case study of how the patient suffered from herself and from her environment shows a course that is clinically instructive.

The patient's relationships were relatively constant in the first half of treatment. In analysis she was primarily concerned with herself and her inner world, as clearly demonstrated by the nature of the symptoms she described in the sessions. Erythrophobia, dependence on her parents, and sexual inhibitions keep the patient from actively confronting her environment. This phase of treatment seemed to be concluded around the 250th session; her suffering declined significantly. In the second half of treatment her suffering increased again. The treatment was molded by the intensive disputes with partners of the opposite sex, which was also particularly visible in the transference relationship. (Neudert et al. 1987)

The examination using "emotional insight" as a criterion of change also confirmed the positive outcome of this treatment:

If the first eight sessions of this analysis are compared with the last eight, then it can be seen that the patient's comments reflect her livelier experiencing. In contrast to the beginning, where she very frequently intellectually distanced herself from her current experiencing and fell into brooding, in the final sessions the patient submerged into her experiencing without losing the capacity for critical reflection. The conditions for a productive "emotional insight" were thus much better fulfilled at the end of treatment. (Hohage and Kübler 1987)

In the case of Amalie X we were able to demonstrate a large correspondence between change as described in clinical terms and as measured by psychological tests. Yet it is also important to realize that change is multidimensional and that its course is not always congruent in the different dimensions.

9.11.3 Separation

As we emphasized in the Introduction, the termination of analysis does not always take place according to a standard pattern. It is not unusual for therapy to lead to changes in lifestyle, which in turn lead to the termination. It would be a mistake to play external and internal reasons for termination off against one another and to equate the external factors with terminable analysis and inner ones with interminable analysis. On the other hand, a deep longing for the interminable seems to lead to the utopia of being able to achieve it. This mutual fantasy is expressed in the unrealistic conception of a normatively conceived phase of termination.

Kurt Y, a 32-year-old scientist, who was awkward, inconspicuous looking, friendly, and obsequious, sought treatment because of his impotence, which was a great strain on him. He had previously tried behavior therapy oriented on that of Masters and Johnson, which brought only short-term benefit. Even in the initial interview the patient himself traced his deficit in spontaneity, especially in sexual matters, back to his strict upbringing. For the first time he had established a firm friendship to a woman he wanted to marry and who, according to his description, went well with him.

In his work he was valued as a skilled experimentor and had an important position in the firm as a factotum; however, he had generally helped others to achieve successful careers while only attaining limited benefits for himself.

In the Freiburg Personality Inventory divergences from mean values were apparent especially on the scales for aggression (standard value 7), agitation (standard value 3), calmness (standard value

1), striving for domination (standard value 7), inhibition (standard value 7), and frankness (standard value 3). At the end of treatment his profile differed from the initial findings only on the scales for aggression (standard value 8), striving for domination (standard value 6), and inhibition (standard value 5). Of these, only the last amounted to a clinically significant change of two standard values.

On the Giessen Test, however, two scales indicated change in the patient. On the scale "uncontrolled-compulsive" he changed from a T value of 56 at the compulsive end to a T value of 39 at the uncontrolled end. A second impressive change was on the scale "retentive-permeable," where the patient moved from a T value of 58 to a T value of 42 in the direction of more permeable. Conspicuous was, however, that a distinctly negative self-esteem of T 30 only improved to a T value of 32.

The Rorschach test also showed only a minimal change at the end of therapy. The following statement is from the final report of the test supervisor:

> The patient responds quickly to emotional stimuli, showing different kinds of reactions to emotional situations. He can submit to partly primitive and elementary emotional stirring, while under other conditions he can put them to positive use by means of his intellectual controls and an increased awareness of reality. The compromises required by the latter prevent him from making full productive use of his high intelligence.
>
> If the affect controls mentioned above are inadequate, infantile spite and a disguised aggressive attitude appear that in a sense become independent. The numerous modes of emotional expression only become important when the situation has been clarified and does not appear dangerous. This clarification takes place primarily through a withdrawal to customary behavior and an intellectual, rational manner of coping. His coping with his often violent emotions is, despite everything, always linked with effort and frequently with anxiety and insecurity.
>
> He has great difficulty admitting to himself that he has needs for affection. He has a tendency to distance himself from other people, expecting only disappointments from them. The few opportunities for affective contact are alloyed with aggression, giving him the character of a fighter.

It is not difficult to discern from this summary evaluation of the Rorschach test that in comparison with the initial findings only the beginnings of structural change in the four years of psychoanalysis were detected on the tests. We would now like to list some of the clinically observed changes that we feel justify speaking of a substantial improvement in the overall picture of this patient's schizoid-compulsive personality. The fact that a man has his first intimite relationship at the age of 32 almost speaks for itself. It is not amazing that his sexual impotence was the consequence of a strict superego molded by archaic norms. His partial professional impotence must be seen parallel to this, consisting primarily in the fact that he can only be fully productive for others. At the time treatment was initiated, he had worked for years on his dissertation, which he managed to complete after working through the unconscious aggressive and grandiose fantasies associated with it. The latter were related in his preconscious with his fear that his boss might be usurped; this was unconsciously linked with his triumph over the modest achievements of his father, who had only advanced to be a medium-level civil servant in the post office. His sexual impotence was primarily caused by maternal introjections, which dictated a close tie between filth and sex. For long periods in therapy an unattainable goal for him was to submit to his pleasure as a precondition for having satisfying intercourse. It was only in the last year of his treatment that the patient permitted himself the desire to spend more than just weekends with his wife, seeking the everyday security and relaxed atmosphere that facilitated sexual pleasure.

Although the capacity to love and to work are the two pillars of the discussion of psychoanalytic goals, we should not overlook the fact that in consequence of the above-mentioned changes this patient experienced a number of seemingly minor enrichments in his life, such as being able to go to the cinema or to read something besides scientific texts before going to sleep. He was enthusiastic reading Stefan Zweig's *Sternstunden der Menschheit* one month before the end of therapy and compared himself to Goethe in old age, whose love as expressed in the *Marienbad Elegies* made it perfectly clear to the patient that "an old knotty tree can rejuvinate itself."

Measured against the ideal of the complete analysis, this treatment was painfully incomplete. The termination occurred primarily on the basis of the probably realistic estimate that Kurt Y would not go on for a career in science and would have difficulties at the age of 36 to find a suitable position. After a very long and tormenting search, an offer to become the director of a laboratory in a small town was the decisive factor in the decision to terminate the treatment.

In one of his last sessions Kurt Y talked about a question that was of importance to him, namely whether he would leave any marks on his current home town, specifically whether he had made a lasting impression on his analyst - a question he had carefully avoided until then.

He had always complained about his boss' favorites, the ones who knew how to ingratiate themselves, while he had only been able to formulate his love speechlessly, while sitting at the computer at night for endless hours. He concerned himself with the thought of whether it was not better for him to sacrifice such desires, since "it wasn't right to raise any unanswerable questions any more when you're waiting at the train station." Having grown up a single child, he had avoided the role of "siblings," i. e., fellow analysands, throughout the entire period of treatment and rejected any comments I made.

In the penultimate session he spoke about his experience with the Rorschach test. He only had a vague recollection of the tester, but he experienced the cards in an entirely different manner than at the beginning. He no longer felt anxious expectation, but the satisfying experience of having control of it and of playing with the cards. The "funny devil" gave him the idea that he could start painting, that he would especially like to paint autumn leaves in all their wealth of color. He added, "Previously, everything seemed gray in gray to me, but now I see colors."

Let us give the patient the final say, quoting several passages from his evaluation of the outcome of treatment in the last session:

P: Yes, I somehow think it was - also as far as my experiencing was concerned - I'm taking something with me. The sessions here, it was, well, I wanted to say it elegantly, but I can't find the right word. [Pause] Yes, I would simply say it was an experience, a real experience. Yes, I don't know any more what all has happened. Of course, I didn't always like it, but apparently that's part of its value. [Pause]

A: This experience, what might it have been? What was different here that you haven't been able to find in this way anywhere else? [Pause]

P: Well, I believe it was almost real - that here - when I came here to you, then I had the impression that I could get out of the corner I had fallen into. Yes, perhaps that's how to describe it, that I didn't really need to feel ashamed here, to feel ashamed about the corner I had got myself into. And that was appaently enough to get out of the corner. [Pause] And what does shame mean, I think that's part of it, too, that I managed to speak about it. Because you don't speak about shame, but withdraw and hide. I managed to interrupt the hiding here. Yes, speaking about it and thinking about it, experiencing myself - that was, I think, always one aspect of this, on the basis of which I was - on the basis of which I managed to crawl out of my corner. That was, how should I describe it, the tool, the machine that I used. [Pause] Well, it's linked with, I think, this day; it reminds me of the treatment. More specifically, I can't really remember the rooms, places, and persons. It's more your voice that stimulates me, yes, I'd say that it was the tool for escaping from the prison. Yes, it was really an entanglement of escaping. [Pause] An entanglement - I can recall it myself - that was impossible to undo. [Pause] Yes, I believe the most important fact was that I was given space here, in a figurative sense, space that I had apparently been seeking but that I hesitated to accept. And this space is perhaps a sign for it, for being able to talk about something.

A: And it seems to be a space that you had lost or that you perhaps hadn't known, in the narrowness, in the protection, in the limitations under which you grew up.

P: Yes, yes, well, I had at least lost most of it, and I don't even know whether I knew of it before. And now I've found more space with my wife.

A: Well, perhaps because you've had the experience here that you can make claim to it.

P: Yes, yes, that was, let's say, a long and arduous, I'd like to say an arduous discovery, a genuine discovery where I've gradually experienced that, yes, that I can make claim to this space. Perhaps, now at the very end, I would say that I can claim it, or something of the sorts. Claim, a word that sounds to me, when I think of the position I'm going to assume, I've told myself I can claim it, I tell myself I can claim the space. And no longer have this uncertainty when I have to be concrete; I will demand that I be taken seriously, and if I'm not, then I will be mad. And then I'll take it, I'll fight for it. I can demand that I act in my way, that I act the way I want to. That's come just gradually, almost at the end, that I've told myself where I could get used to demanding something and that's the same as that I'm entitled to it. [Pause] Yes, it's appeared just gradually. Yes, on the scale where I compare the beginning and the end, I can now lay claim to experiencing so much here. I'm no puppet on a string, no I'm not.

The patient was very emphatic in his denial that he was, after four years of psychoanalysis, no longer a puppet on a string. To this expression of the comprehensive and radical change in his self-esteem, we would only like to add the thought that such changes are tied to a rediscovery of pleasure in physical and mental activity. The puppet on a string served the patient, after all, as a metaphor for an inanimate toy whose movements are set in motion by someone else and from the outside.

10 Special Topics

Introduction

It is inevitable that the subject of this chapter must differ from that of Vol.1 (i. e., the relationship between theory and practice). The numerous examples we have given provide sufficient clarification of this relationship. Moreover, it is impossible for a clinical textbook to satisfy the requirements that the theory of science today poses to Freud's inseparable bond hypothesis about research and therapy.

In this chapter we will instead familiarize our readers with specific problems that are of great practical significance. The issue of consultation, covered in Sect. 10.1, is just one example. The subject of religiosity also deserves our special attention, both for therapeutic and interdisciplinary reasons (Sect. 10.3). Furthermore, as shown by the example of a "good hour," the participation of scientists from other fields in the study of the psychoanalytic dialogue leads us back to the hypothesis of an inseparable bond (Sect. 10.2).

10.1 Consultation

We distinguish, as did Szecsödy (1981), between consultation, which is a meeting in which colleagues meet as equals and one advises the other, as has always been the case when difficult diagnostic and therapeutic problems are confronted, and supervision, which is a learning situation within the framework of training. The process of supervison includes both overseeing and evaluating; participation is obligatory, in contrast to a consultation, which is voluntary. Three persons are involved in a consultation, namely the patient, the therapist, and the consultant. In supervision there is also a fourth element, namely an institution, i. e., the training institute whose standards are set and watched over by national and international bodies.

Because of his distance to the dyadic interaction between patient and therapist, the perspective of an outside analyst differs and in some regards is wider than that of the analyst providing the treatment. Since he is not entangled in the transference and countertransference processes, he is in a good position to make the therapist aware of the consequences and side effects of his feelings and thoughts.

A study of the complex issues of supervision and consultation that attempts to provide more precise answers to important questions than has been possible until now must utilize an approach that is both comprehensive and multifaceted. In this section we report on an excerpt from a study based on the following design. Ten successive sessions were transcribed. Between every session the therapist consulted a colleague experienced in supervision. Prior to the consultation the colleague studied the transcripts in detail and dictated his comments, which are included in the text and marked as such.

The colleague's comments demonstrate that, while the analyst bases his understanding and interventions on a strategy, the consultant himself relies on his own conception to view the interaction. In order to make the consultant's comments and suggestions more comprehensible, we will first cite several important passages indicating Szecsödy's understanding of supervision.

The supervisory situation will provide conditions in which learning can develop. To achieve such conditions is not easy and can be complicated by trainee as well as by supervisor. Parallel to the wish to learn and change, there is the fear from the unknown and a tendency to stay with the accustomed and to remian untouched by change.

There are many ambiguities in the supervisory situation:

- The trainee is a beginner, without much knowledge and/or skill. He has to be open and honest about this in his supervision as well as with himself. On the other hand he is expected to be an optimally good therapist for his patient.
- Another ambiguity stems from the fact that in the therapeutic relationship he is a "real person" with his professional and personal characteristics as well as a transference "object" for the patient. As a transference object he is placed in different and for him often foreign roles.
- Within the supervisory interaction, the therapist is reconstructing the process he is part of. He is also a trainee, who has to expose himself to the supervisor who aids, teaches and judges him.
- These positions for trainee and supervisor stimulate different emotions and reactions, both rational and irrational, conscious and unconscious. There is "a crowd present" in the supervisory room: a mentor, teacher, evaluator, judge, supervisor, future colleague, a staff member who is dependent on the candidate's acknowledgement and successful development, as well as the candidate himself who has to accept and carry a number of different roles.

The supervisor has to be prepared for and be aware of all these ambiguities and the problems these arouse. He has to work with them in different ways. The complex interaction between trainee and supervisor is influenced by many factors: the personalities of the patient, the trainee, the superviosr as well as how they are affected by the organisation they work in. (Szecsödy 1990, p. 12)

For change and growth to be facilitated, it is essential that the analyst create the necessary *space*. The figurative use of the concept of space refers back to qualities that Winnicott described with the image of an "intermediate area."

Since the goal is maximal frankness, it is logical that special attention in supervision and consultation is directed at the points at which the therapist impedes the development, either because of insufficient knowledge about the patient's specific disturbance or for emotional reasons, i.e., because of a situative or habitual countertransference. Szecsödy adopted the terms "dumbness" and "numbness" from Ekstein and Wallerstein (1972) to describe these obstructions.

The following presentation of the 114th session of Arthur Y's treatment has been enriched by the addition of information from other transcripts and supplemented with the consultant's comments.

Arthur Y began the session by telling me about an experience that was typical for him. He had recently discovered that he could get more space for himself by enlarging his study. In the process, he installed wood paneling. While doing this work he felt very insecure and thought to himself, "If I don't do a good job, I'll be faced by chaos." He used a fairly hard wood, and with some fantasy he imagined he could see the letter W in the grain. This gave him the idea, "Boy, turned around, W looks like M, M for murder, like in the movie M from the 1930s in which a man called himself M after he had committed a murder."

P: Typical! I was really terribly mad at myself. I managed to do everything right and then such nonsense, such an insane idea. Instead of being happy, I have to spend all my time thinking about whether I should replace all the panels. I just recalled that you're not going to be here next week. And I'm overcome by the feeling of being at somebody's mercy, the feeling of being left alone, because I can't talk about it with anyone else; they would just think I'm crazy.

Comment. The patient said that he had created more space for himself and that he then had encountered a danger. It is impossible for him to combine ties and independence. When he is mad at the analyst-father, for leaving him, his anger takes on murderous force. The analyst interpreted the symptom in connection with the patient's frequent changes in mood. Although the patient's happiness, enthusiasm, and pride at his good work increased, so did his critical self-evaluation and self-condemnation.

The analyst did not pick up the patient's remark about his feeling of being left alone, as was verified in the consultation. Instead of this, he focused on pride.

P: If it weren't the M, then it would be something else. It just completely ruins my satisfaction at having finished the work. I feel so much spite, am so mad! The panels stay where they are. I wouldn't think about doing all that work over again! I'm mad at this constant latent threat, which I've already experienced a thousand or ten thousand times.

A: This seems to be something new, what you've just thought about, I mean the increase in your rage.

P: Against whatever it is that keeps me from settling down.

A: Anger at what's confronting you.

P: That seems new to you? Haven't I ever talked about it before? Rage isn't anything new to me. I could smash the wood paneling to pieces.

A: That wasn't clear to me before.

P: For a second I think, "I'll take the panels down!" Then spite; "I wouldn't think of it!" I can't move everything that's ever made me feel afraid out of my way; I'd be busy forever trying to get things right.

Comment. Here the patient clearly revealed how he struggled against his previous maladaption. He wanted to retain his autonomy. He did not want to simply avoid things, he wanted to put his aggressive power to constructive use.

A: Yes, it's a real duel! A duel against the brutal superiority of this world, against the power of the oppressive object that's attacking you, that's directing your anger at being suppressed.

Comment. Although the analyst referred to the central issue by mentioning the internalized conflict (which the patient repeatedly had no difficulty in externalizing), in my opinion this was not the right time to make a historical generalization. The analyst should have worked through the rage in the relationship to himself.

P: Yesterday, despite all the chaos in my room, we were invited out. In the evening my son played the organ solo in the chapel. For 18 months now it's been a matter of routine for us to go with him and not to let him play alone. And for me it's an opportunity to hear how he's progressing.

A: And there's pride in sitting in the hall and being there when your son fills the space with music.

Comment. Another allusion to the analyst, who left and did not accompany the patient's progress. It would be important to know why the analyst put so much emphasis on pride. Is he proud of the patient or of himself? Is it a reaction to how the patient filled the space, e. g., found more room for himself and even wanted to fill the therapist's office?

P: This time it was impossible to go with him. We were invited out .... The point now in the back and forth of the feelings about tearing the paneling down or not is not really the work that's involved; the point is whether I let myself be conquered by my anxiety. Some time I'm bound to completely get over the problem with the help of analysis.

A: That's the one side, whether you let yourself be conquered or whether you're the one who's stronger. The other side, which may seem construed to you, is that your enemy is the benign one [a sadistic teacher at the boarding school] or a panel is the devil. So when you tear it down and smash it to pieces, then you're the winner. To make another big leap, it's a duel you're fighting with the panel, whether analysis helps or not. That you're mad at me, and when you leave today, mad that you haven't overcome it again and want to use the panel to beat me to pieces.

Comment. The patient spoke about his chances for coping with his enemies, such as anxiety and dependence. He was struggled for his autonomy, although he wanted to maintain his relationships. There is thus a conflict between his dependence and independence that is filled with spite and sadistic aggressiveness. The analyst took himself to be the object of rage. Why? It might be better to illuminate the patient's lack of autonomy by referring to the analyst's relative freedom (child-adult). The analyst can decide without any anxiety: He can go away and leave the patient behind with his anxieties. The question remains to be answered as to why the analyst did not pick up the patient's remark about the forthcoming separation.

P: I feel as if I were sitting in a trap, in a real dilemma, and time is just running out. If it weren't the paneling it would be something else. I don't really understand, suddenly feel anxiety, because I see this figure, somehow as if it were simply time once again to have a real dose of anxiety.

A: Or it's time to be mad, to feel the immense pleasure of being proud. Like the SS officer. [A reference to an event described in Sect. 8.3.] And then this pride contains something that is almost evil or cruel, an infinite arrogance.

P: Yes, I don't know. It seems to me that what you're saying today is so abstract, and that hinders me.

A: Yes, it is abstract. I've already hinted at one side of the matter, namely that when you are successful and are really happy, satisfied, and proud, that then the thought comes to you, "Well who is unsuccessful?" And it's followed by the thought that disturbs you and that you want to get rid of: that I'm the one who's helping you ....

P: Yes, are you finished already?

A: Yes, I'm finished.

P: It seemed to me [laughing] that you stopped in the middle of the sentence.

A: Hum.

P: Yes, for me it was - when I'm successful at doing something practical, it's bound up with astonishment. For a long time I thought I couldn't do it. And when I see it, I'm proud, but not very long .... And I can't remember anything of what you just said.

A: That the thought proves that I can't do anything.

P: [Laughs] And that is supposed to fill me with pride? I don't understand. I hung myself onto you, so to speak. If I compare you to a branch that I'm sitting on, well if it breaks, then I'll fall down. And that's supposed to fill me with pride?

A: Yes, that I can't finish anything.

P: But why is that supposed to make me feel happy? I can't understand it at all. What do I have from it?

A: Yes, like I said, it seems a bit construed to me, too.

P: I'm amazed that you can even have such an idea. That could only be true if I considered you a rival, that would be the only time I'ld be pleased to discover that you can't do anything. I come here to get help, the same as anybody who goes to a doctor. Nobody can be happy if he discovers that the person he has put his confidence in is incapable, a complete loser. I have the feeling that today we've got a knot somewhere.

Comment. The patient made an offer to the analyst that they determine how far the dialogue has progressed.

A: Yes, there's a knot, caused by my thoughts .... I didn't assume that your pleasure would come from denying my value as a craftsman. It's important to you that I'm good at my craft. That's not what I mean, but that there's an antagonism, together with an intensive struggle and rage, when you aren't begrudged the pleasure of your own success. And I tried to get involved in the struggle between you and the panels.

P: [Laughs a little] That sounds as if it's on the verge of insanity, the struggle between me and the panels. Maybe I'm just especially sensitive today .... Yes, it's awfully complicated, emotional life is. Yes, enjoy life, don't look for the thorns and find them. That's how you could describe my life.

A: Yes, when the thorns prick you, you feel pain, then get mad, and would like to tear them out and throw them away.

Comment. Most painful for the patient is: "It hurts to have to accept help. Angry and omnipotent, I want to destroy whoever leaves me and makes me painfully aware of my dependence." The analyst could work this out better, together with the patient. A good topic for the coming consultation.

The Consultation

We now give a summary description of the consultation, at the beginning of which the consultant said they should clarify how the analyst could best work with the patient's conflict (his struggle between autonomy and dependence). The analyst emphasized that he thought the session had been bad because he had offered too many intellectual constructions, with the intention of giving "the senseless symtom a meaning." He was dissatisfied because he had not managed to demonstrate that the patient wanted to deny the analyst success in their struggle. At this point the consultant reminded the analyst of a Freud quotation (1905e, p. 120) that he must have been aware of: "For how could the patient take a more effective revenge than by demonstrating upon her own person the helplessness and incapacity of the physician?" The two of them then reconstructed the course of events in this session and agreed that the "knot" - as the patient had referred to it - was the task for this consultation.

C: First I would like to hear, when you think back, whether are you dissatisfied? You made a knot - what can we do with it? Would you give your thoughts free reign to find out what you wanted to do?

A: Right now I think of – it goes well with a thought that I also had in the session – that one aspect of his overall desire and satisfaction is that he destroys what he has just made. Since the object becomes an enemy that he conquers, one part of this is that he first creates the object, but only to then ruin it.

C: Symbolically.

A: Yes, if I'm the one who suggests to him that he should let his anxiety work a little and try to delay his compulsive acts, then I'm the one who limits his pleasure.

C: The pleasure to destroy something.

A: Yes, and when he comes the next time, after he really felt good, he will have destroyed something again, and I obviously wanted to do something in order to ensure that the panels stay up and that he wouldn't destroy them. Today I wanted to give him some desire for satisfaction.

After the consultant asked the analyst to let his thoughts have free reign – which is not necessarily the same as free association, and more likely means thinking out loud in a relaxed atmosphere – the analyst discovered his part in the duel. By having done something, he also obstructed the patient. Instead of first letting things take their turn, he was interested in keeping the patient from destroying the panels. The analyst also assumed that he himself had a very strong interest in the success of the treatment. It was clearly apparent that the analyst had left his neutral position because of his desire to keep the patient from destroying what he had created.

In another step the consultant referred to the topic of being left alone, which he had noted while reading the protocol. It was obvious that the analyst simply had not heard this topic despite the patient's clear references to it, such as "left," "at someone's mercy," and "lonely." The confrontation with the material revived his memory but not the affective evidence that this might have been a dynamically relevant subject in the session.

A: I was simply on my own trip in the session. And after I had once gotten on it, I lost the flexibility to leave it again.

C: You started from the theory that he builds up his object over and over, only to destroy it. I see the following dynamic: The patient talked a lot about autonomy. You did not manage to present the subject of competition and success in a convincing manner; it appeared construed. Nonetheless your topic arose in the interaction and it led to an interaction. Instead of leading to cooperation and shared happiness at the success, it led to a duel. You didn't want to permit him to destroy what the two of you had built. But the patient felt left alone, as he illustrated with reference to his son, whom he did not want to let play by himself and yet had to leave.

A: Now I know why I didn't listen better: I was following another line of thought, not the one that he didn't want to let his son play by himself, but the one that he was so proud that he had to be there. In another sense, it also means that he cannot leave his son alone because he then loses his chance to participate in and identify with his son's success.

These comments confirmed the consultant's understanding that the analyst had reached this line of thought and stuck to it because he was just as identified with being successful in his therapeutic work as the patient was with his son. The result was the struggle between son and father and between patient and analyst. The consultant attempted, in the following excerpt, to demonstrate the potential of this view.

C: The idea of pride has both a positive and a negative aspect in a typical father-son relationship. They can be proud together, but they can also be rivals and react in the manner "I want to do it alone, just for myself. And I won't do it there because you always spoil my pleasure of having done it by myself."

A: Yes, there was a place where the patient said, "If I were like that, took pleasure in disparaging you, yes then I would be insane."

C: Yes, and then you said, "You have to use me as a good therapist." But if the patient experiences your success as exorbitant, then you will become involved in the struggle. I believe, to come to the heart of the matter, that we are working in different ways with the same image. I focus on the father-son dynamic: he killed his father and has to invent another one over and over in order to enable both of them to win if he feels well. But his desire for autonomy was filled with disappointment and anger when he was left alone.

A: The interesting aspect of our talk is the further development of my theory that although he had adopted our commandment, he felt anger and the desire to violate the prohibition. Now I'm curious whether he will tear down the panels or not. I hope I can be open for each outcome.

The course of this session made it clear to the consultant that a duel first took place until the analyst also responded to the other point of view. As a consequence of his desire to keep the patient from doing something, in order to feel successful himself, the analyst left his neutral ground and entered into a duel with the patient.

10.2 Theoretical Remarks About a "Good Hour"

The session following the consultation described in the previous section, the 115th, went so well that it immediately reminded the analyst of the concept of the "good hour" (Kris 1956). Elsewhere we have already published a comparison of the bad 114th and the good 115th sessions (see Löw-Beer and Thomä 1988).

We would like to draw attention to a special aspect of the following presentation. It has turned out to be unusually productive for both psychoanalytic practice and research if transcripts of therapeutic dialogues are examined by independent third parties, i. e., scientists from other disciplines. This can, first, put empirical process research on a solid footing. Furthermore, philosophers, for example, can study psychoanalytic texts, and the discussion between the social sciences and psychoanalysis is given a contemporary and objective starting point. Our psychoanalytic thinking and actions have substantially benefited from interdisciplinary cooperation in working with transcripts. The interpretation of a philosopher that is given below is an instructive example.

Object of the examination was a "good" hour. In order to understand what this means, it is first necessary to clarify what constitutes a patient's positive changes in a session.

The concept of a good session must be discussed from at least two perspectives. The first is to clarify what constitutes good interaction and the accompanying experiencing in analysis, for example whether the patient's insights and the analyst's interpretations complement each other and whether the patient feels understood (Kris 1956; Peterfreund 1983). The second perspective, which is our special focus of interest, is the curative change that is mediated by the interaction with the analyst. We must also ask whether unsuccessful interaction with the analyst - e. g., feeling not understood - can result in curative changes if the lack of empathy becomes the object of the dialogue.

It is possible to attempt to synthesize the different points of view on these questions once the differences are clear. The danger of an unreflected synthesis can be found in the literature, specifically if attention is only directed at the development of the patient's capacities that make a good session possible. Meant are the capacities for psychic integration, self-observation, and controlled regression. The article by Kris mentioned above does not avoid this trap completely, just as Peterfreund's comments are not entirely free of emphasizing qualities in patients that make adjusted analysands of them. It remains dubious, namely, whether the capacities that make a good session of analysis possible are identical with those necessary in ordinary life.

Attempts have been made to provide both descriptive and causal groundings of what is good and bad in sessions and what elicits relevant changes in a patient. Causal groundings must be taken with some caution, inasmuch as they are hypotheses that must be tested in other cases. Characteristic of a bad session is, for example, that the analyst disregards the patient's knowledge about his symptoms and suggests alternative interpretations. In a good session, in contrast, the analyst extends the patient's dealings with his symptoms in a manner permitting the patient to integrate disparate elements of his life history and to develop an emotionally and intellectually adequate perspective toward his own biography. Presumably, both the analyst's style of communication and his interpretations are relevant to the patient's positive development. A particular manner of communication, which we also call "dramaturgic technique," might be a valuable type of therapeutic action.

The following comments are based on the analysis of Arthur Y, who had suffered from obsessive thoughts since his youth. The most conspicuous aspect of his symptoms was his obsessive thought that he had to murder his own children, which appeared worse to him than dying. These obsessive thoughts led in a typical manner to defensive actions: "You will only be prevented from killing your children if you do this and that." Thus for a while he feared a cruel God, who could force him to murder his children if he were not obedient. In the patient's words, "As if God . . . were an officer in the SS . . . who, if I didn't greet him in the perfect way, might punish me with death or perhaps something even worse . . . . I would kill one of my own children, which would be worse than death."

The 115th session was a breakthrough session. In it the patient underwent a positive change that was spectacular. He came to the session feeling anxious and resigned, with the attitude of being a victim that was typical for him, and left it feeling liberated. Arthur Y found an almost poetic power of expression. His feeling of rage at having to bow to an evil power was previously limited to his symptoms; in the session his swaying between rage and powerlessness also came to be the decisive element in his relationships to persons of authority. His experiencing of this was extended from his symptoms into other situations in which it appeared appropriate. To use the analyst's words, "The patient has rediscovered his feelings." The analyst's hypothesis was that these were the conflicts to which the patient had reacted with pathogenic defense processes.

We summarize the session, concentrating on the aspects we believe facilitated the patient's development. We presume that the patient's insights into himself were not the cause of the change, but rather that the analyst's encouragement was vital in helping Arthur Y find emotionally appropriate reactions to situations of submission. The result was a particular form of insight, the patient acquiring an accurate understanding of his situation.

In the following scene the analyst acted like a director who prompted the patient to put himself into the roles that he recalled. He did this by extending dramaturgically the script, i. e., in this case the patient's recollections. The patient talked about a surgeon he had found unsympathetic and who had removed his tonsils under a local anesthetic. The patient had been afraid and constantly wanted to swollow; the doctor had barked at him to keep his mouth open.

A: Oh, there's so much blood.

P: Yes.

A: It makes you want to swollow all the time and makes you afraid of suffocating, as if you were up to your neck in water, or rather blood.

Consideration. I thought of the allusion to water because the patient had once been in a very dangerous situation and almost drowned.

A: The scalpel he used to cut you and to make you almost suffocate. That's how you experience it when the blood runs together back there in your throat. And if you spit blood in his face, then you have to fear that he'll get even angrier.

P: Yes, and to pick up this line of thought, how do you defend yourself in such a situation? An eye for an eye would be logical.

A: Yes, and there are the instruments, namely the scalpel or other sharp objects.

P: But you rule out such thoughts immediately.

A: They're also ruled out by the situation. The surgeon is just too powerful.

P: And then when you suppress it, so to speak, and suppress it over and over, then it just comes somewhere else - the scalpel. It even comes where - now I have an idea. If I were a 9-year-old boy and simply took the next object and shoved it through his face, then as a child I would expect him to finish me off.

A: If you take the scalpel he's using to cut you up.

P: So if I defend myself, then he'll finish me off, then it's over. Then it's over and I'm done for, just the same as what I'm still afraid of today.

A: Yes.

P: With the scalpel I would just end up the same, I'd be done for, finished, over.

A: Yes, and with the scalpel you're the powerful surgeon, SS officer, Hitler, etc., God the Almighty with the knife, and in the small children you yourself are a child; you're a victim.

P: Yes, yes.

A: But you don't mean your children, of course. You mean the immense power, but it's so terrible that nobody can point the scalpel at you, and this has implications for more distant, seemingly harmless things, such as you're not permitted to criticize the therapist, me.

P: I've understood you so far good, and you say "You don't mean your children . . . " but I mean Benignus, to use this to refer to everything vicious [the synonym he used to refer to a sadistic teacher, whose true name had a similar contradictory quality].

A: Yes.

P: My opponent, my enemy. I don't want to lose sight of the image that my anxieties in reality aren't about my children but about an enemy that I don't dare defend myself against. And when I let it pass review, then I can clearly feel that I have the same feelings toward you when you talk about increasing your fee, for example.

Arthur Y was then overcome by feelings of revenge and powerlessness. Although he had just been submissive in his attitude that he was a victim, he suddenly began, in dramatic monologues, to settle old scores with his various oppressors: his father, who had not attempted to understand him, but instead had punished him after a boyish prank and then gone away to war - never to return - without even saying goodbye; the patient would most of all have liked to attack him with a weapon. He would have liked to have his way with his sadistic teacher. He was mad at his mother from cheating him out of his childhood. Finally he attacked me, the analyst, because I had forced him to confess. He compared this compulsion, grinning, with the image of a dog that you have to carry to the hunt, i. e., he felt forced to do something that he actually instinctively wanted to do. He accused me of having provoked feelings of revenge in him that he could not satisfy. He made this accusation part of an impressive image of a man who could not even release his excitement by masturbating because he did not have any hands.

P: Yes, and here come all of these figures and become alive, and I get terribly mad about all of these years - who should I pay it off to? There's nobody there [mumbling]. I had the following thought. What's the use of getting horny somewhere if I don't, well if I don't have a woman or even two hands to satisfy myself?

What makes this session a *good hour*? What grounding is there for the intuition that it was a good session? What came of the breakthrough? In the following, we briefly discuss three important features of a good session.

An Improved Perspective About One's Own Past and Present

Prior to this breakthrough session, Arthur Y had been incapable of applying some values that were important to him to his own biography. He had held a view of his biography - rooted both in his intellect and, more importantly, in his experience - that was the opposite of his later ideal self-image. His later self-image conformed to the broad cultural consensus that both the patient and analyst accepted.

We understand a child who reacts to being mistreated by feeling intimidated and anxious, but when an adult goes through such oppressive situations we expect him to be indignant and mad at the persons who have treated him in such a manner. We believe that children should not be unnecessarily punished and not at all tormented, that we should let them have scope for playing, and that we should not force them to share our concerns. Arthur Y also shared these views and acted accordingly toward his own children. Yet for a long time he had been unable to grasp his own life history from this perspective. In the forefront was not only his rage and indignation at having been mistreated, but also the cries of the victim. As an adult he manifested this mentality of being the victim in an exaggerated form.

Even the mere thought that a person higher in the social hierarchy might criticize him precipitated the panic that he might be ruined. In the role of the person being addressed, he was incapable of distinguishing between arbitrary demonstrations of power and legitimate claims to authority.

The impression that this session embodied a breakthrough was due in part to the fact that Arthur Y not only complained intellectually about having been denied his elementary rights as a child, but that he felt himself deprived of his rights, experienced this as an existential loss, and reacted to it by becoming enraged. His emotional reactions became more appropriate, toward the past as well as in the present toward his analyst, both from his own perspective and from that of a third party. In the preceding sessions the patient had reacted several times in an outspoken, even panicky way toward the analyst. These situations were characterized by the dissonance between the patient's immediate judgments and his rational ones. Although he grapsed that the analyst's increased fee was not intended to ruin him, and that it in fact would not do so, he emotionally experienced the demand as a threat to his existence. The accusations he directed at the analyst in the good session were, in contrast, not the result of panic. He accused the analyst of coercing him into making a confession. Since he realized that he also felt a need to communicate, he added an ironic element to his criticism by including the image of a dog that had to be carried to the hunt, reaching a differentiated description of his relationship to his analyst. The patient's other criticism was also accurate, namely that the analyst elicited feelings of revenge in him without at the same time also being able to produce the original object of his hate. The image he used of a "horny" man who had neither a woman nor hands to satisfy himself was extremely succinct.

Liberation and Increased Freedom in Acting Toward One's Self

One aspect of liberation consists in the just mentioned *creative use of language*, in images that are condensed representations of feelings.

Conspicuous in the previous sessions was the patient's attitude that he was a victim. He felt persecuted, attacked, and at the mercy of a cruel God who might even demand that he kill his own children. The last session was dominated, in contrast, by his *rebellion against coercion*, rebellion against the unreasonable demands of the surgeon, his mother, etc. Such rebellion against coercion is one element of the idea of liberation. The patient did not want to submit to either an inner or an external coercion that he considered inappropriate.

Liberation is manifested not only in the rebellion against coercion, but also in the capacity to behave toward one's own condition, as has been described by Tugendhat (1979). The patient's capacity to reflect on the current dialogue situation developed in the breakthrough session. The patient succeeded not only in playfully putting himself in his childhood shoes, but also in reflecting on his role. He did not experience himself as a small child but as an adult who felt what it might have been like for a child to have been maltreated. The playful aspect did not prevent him from taking his biography more seriously than before. The patient's vivid description of every detail of various scenarios precipitated strong feelings in him.

He was filled with rage when he measured his own childhood against what childhood should be, but also with powerlessness because he had no alternative but to accept what had been. "What my father did was an act of insensitivity of the first order." He asked himself, "What can I now do with my feelings of revenge since the objects of this revenge are beyond my reach?"

In this session, in contrast to others, the patient was able to intregrate his emotional reaction to the setting of the analytic dialogue into his own comments. This was an example for the concept of reflection liberating from coercion. The patient articulated his understanding of his role in the analytic situation and in the process realized that he had submitted to a stereotypical expectation of a role, the role of the patient, in which he has to mention everything he thought of. He reflected on this now as being a coercion to confess, and asked himself whether he wanted to continue in this role, what he could do with the analyst, and to what extent the analyst was able to satisfy his needs. Asking these questions he abandoned the role of passively doing his duty, overcame the apparently prescribed forms of behavior, and acquired the capacity for distancing himself from his role.

Experiencing Symptoms as an Aid in the Formation of Productive Ideas

Arthur Y subjectively experienced his symptoms as part of a struggle against subjugation to senseless rituals that demanded a threatening and frightening superiority. In this session the patient used this subjective experience to describe his emotional state during his confrontation with his oppressors.

We would like to recall that the analyst had attempted in the "bad" session (see Sect. 10.1) to illuminate the patient's experience of his symptoms by referring to an analogy between how he experienced, on the one hand, his symptoms and, on the other, his life. He equated the patient's relationship to the wood paneling with that to his tormentors. In the good session he utilized the patient's momentary experience of his symptoms to emotionally revive his recollection of situations of suppression.

Dramaturgic Technique, or the Stage Model of Psychoanalytic Treatment

In Vol.1 (Sect. 3.4) we compared the events in psychoanalysis with those on a stage. According to the stage model, analysts and patients play roles and also keep an eye on themselves all the while. In addition to acting complementary to the patient's expectations, the analyst has the functions of a codirector and observer. The point is to test the roles that the patient did not adequately assume.

In the "breakthrough" the analyst cashed in on this program. At the beginning of the session described above, he directed his fantasy at making the patient aware of the bloody scenes in the tonsilectomy he described.

How did the analyst know about the bloody details of the patient's tonsilectomy, the overall impression of which moved the patient to put himself in the situation of a tormented 9-year-old boy? In fact, the analyst was not aware of the specific details, but he was culturally close enough to the patient to be able to imagine what had happened. In the stage model the vital issue is not to reconstruct the patient's actual biography but rather to understand, in this instance, how the patient *imagined* that a 9-year-old boy would have felt if he had been handled in that manner.

Analyst's Commentary. It is a pleasure for me that an unbiased outside scientist arrives at interpretations that are compatible with the stage model and even refers to *dramaturgic technique*. The tonsilectomy reminded me first of a tooth extraction I had had as an adult; so much blood collected in my pharynx that I felt as if "I were up to my throat in water." I intentionally use this metaphor that, as all allegories, covers a whole range of experiences. The metaphoric language of therapy promotes the intensity of experiencing. In this recollection I was still completely in control of myself, and at first did not give any sign to the dentist, who was concerned, because I wanted to push this extreme situation to the utmost. In other situations in childhood, however, I was just as powerless as the patient. No reader will have difficulty putting himself into a situation where there is a more or less frightening polarization into power and powerlessness. The psychoanalytic theory of the genesis of unconscious structures and dispositions facilitates understanding. Unconscious schemata of oneself, for example, find vivid representation in dream language. Explanatory psychoanalytic theory, however, leads us to expect that such representations conceal other self-images which find expression in action potentials, regardless of how split they may be from conscious experiencing. Where there is a victim, there is a perpetrator, just as masochism and sadism belong together. Knowledge of this enables the analyst to offer interpretations reviving repressed or split self elements that elicit associations in the patient. I consider the dialogic enrichment to be essential, although actually moving onto a stage and playing psychodramatic theater would make it difficult to formulate the respective interpretations. It may lie in my personal limitations - namely that I am often unable to grasp and interpret the meaning of a scene in relationship to unconscious motives and structures until I have had time to reflect on it in detail. I can accept Brecht's stage guidelines [mentioned below], and in this sense the term "dramaturgic technique" is accurate.

To clarify the analyst's approach, we can distinguish three ways of writing history. First, a simple chronicler restricts himself to saying what happened. A second historian may want to comment on historical events from his own perspective and thus pursues the goal of explaining history. The third approach is to imagine how it would have been to have lived during a particular period, which is the attitude that many authors and actors have.

The analyst enables the patient to pursue the last approach toward his own biography. In contrast to the historian, who does this on an experimental basis, and to the actor, whose role ends with the final applause, the patient inescapably suffers from his own life history, which dominates his present by means of the repetition compulsion of his symptoms. Thus viewed historically, the therapeutic situation is decisively characterized by opposite movements. On the one hand, the patient's present situation is a continuation of his past; on the other hand, analysis is supposed to help him revise his past in light of his present, at least inasfar as his past governs his life history (Marten 1983). The analyst does not suggest that the patient be the "little shitter" that he probably used to be and who could probably hardly imagine that he deserved to be treated better. The patient's task is to understand what it is like to be in the role of this tormented boy on the basis of the views he *now* has about how children should be treated.

With regard to his directing, the analyst has much in common with Brecht, who did not want the actor to conceal his own view of the character he was playing. If the actor plays a king, then he should not give himself and the audience the illusion that he is the king, but should rather play the role without ceasing to refer to it.

The advantage of dramaturgic technique consists in the fact that it promotes the application of the values to one's self that one has when judging others who are in similar situations. The indignation that was aroused in the patient was made possible by the fact that he had abandoned his previous attitude toward himself in favor of the one he quite naturally had toward his own children. This enabled him to view himself as a child who had been mishandled and cheated of his adolescence, just as he would see his children under similar circumstances.

This change in perspective cannot be achieved solely by means of dramaturgic technique, at the most for a brief moment. How should someone whose obsessive thoughts of murdering his own children play a tormenting role in his symptoms become indignant about a surgeon? How can he rebel against his childhood tormentors, even in his fantasy, given his broken self-esteem? It is thus necessary to supplement dramaturgic technique with interpretations that strengthen the patient's self-esteem. The analyst did this in this case by soothing the patient by giving him the intepretation that his thoughts of murder did not refer to his own children but were a sign of his rage at his enemies, both past and present. The corresponding passage in the dialogue was:

A: Yes, and with the scalpel you're the powerful surgeon, SS officer, Hitler, etc., God the Almighty with the knife, and in the small children you yourself are a child; you're a victim.

P: Yes, yes.

A: But you don't mean your children, of course. You mean the immense power, but it's so terrible that nobody can point the scalpel at you, and this has implications for more distant, seemingly harmless things, such as you're not permitted to criticize the therapist, me.

The patient's thoughts about murder had been displaced onto his own children because he had been incapable of risking these thoughts about the omnipotent force over him. This interpretation gave the patient relief, and he attempted to memorize it. It gave him a basis for confronting his tormentors. This interpretation, according to which he did not have to view himself as an evil person who deserved to be mishandled, consisted in two parts. The first said that the patient established identifications both as victim and as perpetrator. This was the reason that, when he became aware that he felt satisfied, he was overcome by the anxiety that he might destroy his children and, in the process, himself. The reason was that he was his own victim. He was the murderer of his double, similar to Mr. Hyde, who killed Dr. Jekyll. This part of the interpretation was the analyst's guiding thought theoretically, as we show in Sect. 8.2. The other part of the interpretation was used by Arthur Y. According to it, his thoughts of murder were actually directed at his tormentors, not at his children; they were merely displaced onto the latter because of his anxiety about confronting the power that dominated him.

We have three reasons for attributing a curative effect to this interpretation.

1. The patient expressed an awareness that the interpretation was significant for him. He himself considered it relevant. He was not satisfied with merely knowing about it and calling it helpful; he expanded on it and clarified it.
2. There was a thematic connection between this interpretation and the subsequent comments. The subject of the interpretation corresponded to the main subject of the session, namely the struggle against his enemies, the sadistic teacher, surgeon, etc. The substance of the interpretation was that his thoughts about murder were in truth directed at these enemies.
3. There was a substantive connection between the patient's development in the good session and this interpretation. It is plausible that it was impossible for the patient to be indignant about having being mistreated in childhood as long as he assumed he was thinking about murdering his own children. If he were capable of doing the worst thing he could imagine, then he would be so bad that he deserved having been mistreated. His childhood may explain that the potential sexual offender is a victim of circumstances. A precondition for the patient becoming enraged about mistreatment was that he had to value himself sufficiently to become enraged and reject his own experiences of having been mistreated.

Analyst's Commentary. Both theoretical and technical considerations motivated me to make this interpretation. I am convinced that Arthur Y did not mean his children as individuals but as symbols of his own powerlessness and helplessness. Of course, in his experiencing and especially in unconscious processes the concrete individuals cannot be separated from their symbolic meanings. In this sense the patient was also referring to his children and not only to their symbolic meaning. In order to be able eventually to differentiate between symbol and concrete individual, I employed a negation to enable the patient to achieve some distance, even if it only lasted a brief moment.

In his unconscious his children stood for his younger siblings, particularly for his younger brother whose birth had precipitated his humiliating behavior of dirtying his pants. There were numerous indications that his death wishes were directed at his brother and sisters. To return to the source of his aggressions naturally does not eliminate them or his concomitant feelings of guilt, but it does make it possible to understand the strange and sinister symptoms. In technical terms, a brief period of relief creates scope for reflection. Moreover, I assumed that the reason his obsessive thoughts were directed at his children, whom he loved more than anything else, was because this let him erect a nearly absolute barrier against the destructive impulses of hate that had been completely separated from his ego. This hate had accumulated since his childhood, and although it was split off it was precipitated by minor everyday insults. It was the hate of the completely powerlessness victim who was no longer capable of raising the slightest defensive impulse against his oppressor. It was only much later in the patient's life or enclosed in his obsessive symptoms that it was possible for him to reverse the sadomasochistic relationship. His children represented his own childhood powerlessness, and he could identify with the repesentatives of power and their cruel deeds, such as the children who made fun of him, with his mother and father, with the sadisitc teacher, with Hitler and the SS officers, and with the vengeful God, who considered absolute submission a sign of love and demanded such behavior.

In formal terms, the question that disturbed the patient was, "Do I think about murdering my own children?" This question has two connotations: first, are his obsessive thoughts directed at his children? and second, does he desire to kill his children? The first question must be answered affirmatively. The patient's obsessive thoughts and his verbal statements are related to his children. This is in fact what disturbed the patient. The second question was, however, even more disturbing to the patient. This is the question the analyst negated. His obsessive thoughts were not to be viewed as signs of a desire to murder his own children. The patient was not mistaken with regard to the persons who were the object of his statements, but he was mistaken with regard to the object of his desires.

Truth of the Interpretation

Were Arthur Y's desires to kill directed at his enemies and not at his beloved children? Did he displace these thoughts onto his own children because of his anxiety about his enemies' awesome power? The question of truth in the following is not related to the analyst's commentary but to the logical understanding of this interpretation, which the patient shared; namely he did not want to kill his children.

An interpretation appears more truthful if it, first, succeeds in putting a large number of motivationally apparently incomprehensible statements into a systematic and comprehensible connection (crieteria of coherence and rationality), second, is compatible with a causal hypothesis that has been well confirmed (genetic criterion), and third, is compatible with the best confirmed hypotheses of psychoanalytic theory. Applying these criteria in this case, there are many indications that at least one component in the formation of the patient's symptoms had to be sought in the fact that he wanted to protect himself against his murderous self-image. It could have been that he thought he was so bad that he had to fear he might kill the children he loved so dearly. The assumption is also justified that in his thoughts he confused the recollection of his siblings and the image of his own children. Yet transference of a certain relationship to other objects does not mean that verbal statements do not apply to the transference objects as well. In this case the analyst's interpretation did not make the patient aware of the fact that he equated his own children with his siblings. The important thought for the patient was that his aggression was actually directed at an external force.

Psychoanalytic Theory of Symptoms

Assumption 1. Symptoms are displaced and distorted gratifications of disapproved and repressed desires.

Assumption 2. People attempt with the aid of symptoms to cope with a traumatic situation.

Assumption 3. People unconsciously attempt to falsify their unconscious and pathogenic attitudes by means of their symptoms; this point can be subsumed under assumption 2. People attempt to cope with difficult situations by trying to falsify unconscious interpretations of situations.

The first assumption agrees with the analyst's commentary; in his unconscious fantasy the patient identified himself pleasurably with his tormentors, accepting their attitude. Assumptions 2 and 3 agree with the following explanation of the patient's symptoms: The patient wanted to hide the fact from himself that he considered himself so evil that he thought he could kill his own children. By resisting his obsessive thoughts about murder, he attempted to prove to himself and others that he was not this bad.

There are contexts in which the different psychoanalytic models of symptom explanation complement each other, and others in which they contradict one another. In this case they are complementary because "identification with the aggressor" can be interpreted both as an attempt to cope with a difficult situation and as an indirect gratification of destructive desires. The hypothesis here is that the defense mechanism of identification with the aggressor evoked a situation that was intolerable for the patient, which he attempted to cope with through the formation of his symptoms.

Symptoms have the function of concealing a negative self-image. This patient's thoughts about murder appear to be obsessive, pathologic, and isolated from his self-image (i. e., he defined himself as someone to whom these thoughts of murder were completely foreign).

Criterion of Coherence. Even the smallest of reasons made the patient feel guilty, as if he had been caught at something. For example, he was hard working and successful, but he regularly experienced panic when his boss called. The great majority of the stories in this 10-hour segment of his analysis were about the fact that he felt anxiety about being ruined or was spontaneously afraid of being responsible for something that was obviously not his doing, such as an accident at which he were merely a witness. He did not tire of demonstrating to the analyst and to himself that he reacted to minor events with unnecessary anxiety or guilt feelings. This might have had the function of showing that in reality everthing was fine except for his obviously irrational reactions, not to mention how he experienced his symptoms.

Another indication for the thesis of disturbed self-esteem was his attitude of being the victim, which the patient adhered to until the breakthrough. Although he was able to recall the never-ending disputes of his adolescence, he did so anxiously, not with anger. If a person assumes he is very bad, then he deserves to be treated accordingly; at the very least, such a person does not naturally assume he has a right to be treated decently. That, however, is a precondition for such mistreatment to elicit rage.

Genetic Criterion. There are also many genetic signs favoring the hypothesis about the patient's negative self-esteem. There is hardly any controversy that role acceptance is an important learning mechanism in socialization. It is plausible that the patient acted toward himself the same way others did, i. e., he internalized the negative attributions of others, which he encountered at every step.

In short, there were many indications that the purpose of his symptoms was to protect him from the conviction that he had murderous intentions and to prove that he was not as bad as he thought. This defense created a negative self-image. Unconsciously, the patient understood himself as being as bad as he had experienced his tormentors to have been toward him. He was even worse than they had been; he thought he was so bad that he could kill his own children. The development of his symptoms can be viewed as the patient's attempt to conceal this murderous self-understanding from himself and to refute it. He experienced his obsessive thoughts as if they had nothing to do with his own desires or self-images, and the successful resistance of the obsessive commands to kill as proof that the suspected impulses to kill were without substance.

If these hypotheses about his symptom formation were correct, then it would have to be grasped as the consequence and means of defense at a second level: The patient warded off the negative self-understanding formed as a result of his defenses. If only the immediate causes of the symptom formation are taken into consideration, then the interpretation would be false: The cause of the obsessive thoughts about murder would then not have been his displaced anger but the defense of his negative self-understanding. His understanding was negative, of course, because of the feelings of guilt associated with his anger.

Insight and Therapeutic Success

Just as the analyst suggested, identification with the aggressor was the defense mechanism that kept the patient from experiencing his anger in connection with his oppressors. Should we therefore conclude that the interpretation gave the patient false ideas?

Our discussion of dramaturgic technique leads us to draw different conclusions. We doubt that the goal of interpretations consists in making a patient *completely* aware of the causes of his symptoms. The goal is rather to concentrate on the cause that may make a curative change possible. The analyst must, in collaboration with the patient, provide him insights into his situation in life. Symptoms are defense products, i. e., inadequate attempts to cope with traumatic situations. In the case of Arthur Y, the patient's experience with his symptoms represents his cumulative experience of suppression and powerlessness in his life. Dramaturgic technique was used to put this experience back into the context of its origin, to give the patient the opportunity to finally confront the situations of suppression and unjust treatment in a positive, self-determined manner, instead of with defense. (On the question of self-determination and volition see Löw-Beer 1988.)

For this prupose it would not have been conducive to make the patient aware of a self-understanding that itself was a product of his defense, only providing a distorted image of his own situation. In his desires to kill his children he identified with the aggressors. He never had the self-confidence to develop anger and to resist the terrible force. The task of analysis was to enable the patient to face the situations of successive traumatic experiences in a nondefensive manner. The interpretation discussed above must be seen as a means for the patient to gain insight into his own situation. Such insight into his situation was a part of a curative change. The concept of curative change has been discussed in connection with acquiring insights, a sign that there is a conceptual connection and not merely an empirical one between therapeutic success and gaining insight into one's situation. Still to be determined is how successful sessions in therapy are related to living successfully outside therapy.

Acquiring insight into one's own situation means both a view of one's own situation that has been freed of defensive distortions and, in particular, an evaluative and emotional change. Arthur Y became mad at his oppressor in the breakthrough, and his anger was appropriate to the torment he had experienced. An evaluative change takes place only to a small degree, if at all, on the basis of a process of achieving awareness. It is also not based on an attempt to reconstruct real experiencing. One element of a patient's altered understanding of a situation consists in the inclusion of the values of the adult patient. This can be shown, for example, in Arthur Y's attitudes about childhood and adolescence. One thing he presumably suffered from was that his mother had shared her concerns with him. As a child he had probably not been aware of the fact that his mother had thus saddled him with the responsible role of an adviser, making him miss something of his adolescence, which he complained about in analysis. Presumably he did not know at that time that juveniles deserve a different role. Another example in this case was that although the history of his symptoms indicated that he had the impulse to kill his sadistic teacher, it was only as an adult that he understood the meaning of sadism and was able to judge how incorrect the teacher's behavior had been. It is an interesting question for further research to determine how much these evaluative concepts are acquired in analysis and whether they take the form of learning processes.

In a certain sense it is necessary to reconstruct the past on the basis of present values. It is, after all, impossible for individuals to voluntarily abstract from all their interests and evaluative concepts. But even here there are some differences in degree. The attempt can be made either to largely abstract from the contemporary perspective and to imagine what a person was like in the past, or to imagine how one would have reacted in a past situation on the basis of current views. The dramaturgic technique enacts the scenic presentation of conflicts from justified evaluative points of view.

10.3 Religiosity

Our Western civilization has been molded by ideas that are a mixture of Judeo-Christian religion with Greek philosophy and the classical Roman view of the world. Its ideas and expressions influence any individual's manner of feeling and thinking whether his education was religious in nature or not. Our language and our system of values are products of this cultural tradition. Every individual lives in a psychosocial reality whose subjective and objective components are mediated by society. A system of values, such as embodied by a religion, constitutes part of both the general and the individual comprehensions of reality because reality must be interpreted and always has been. Even the value system of atheists is largely the product of the ideas incorporated in the Ten Commandments. In our civilization, churches, as represented by their officials, mediate the contents of Christian religion. The traditional images of God have, however, always been influenced by individuals, depending on their personal experiences. People undergo change, just as does religion itself its image of man and God.

The critiques of religion that Feuerbach, Marx, Nietzsche, and Freud pioneered in the previous century embody a projection theory according to which man is the creator of all of his images of God. In the tradition of the Enlightenment, this critique aimed to abolish religion and to substitute atheistic ideas and ideologies for religious systems of interpretation and meaning, both for individuals and for society at large. Even nihilistic systems of thought are interpretations of reality.

The function of such systems of interpretation and meaning - that is, the function of religion, mythology, and ideology for the life of groups, societies, and peoples and for the individuals in them - can be examined in psychoanalytic terms. This is also true of the image of God that an individual has, both as it was given to him and as he has transformed it. It is not difficult to demonstrate that religious ideas fulfill various psychic functions. Pfister (1944), in his book *Die Angst und das Christentum* (Anxiety and Christianity), did this for the Christian religion, showing how one particular one-sided image of God, namely that of a vengeful God, promotes the development of neurotic anxieties. Previously, after Freud (1927c) had radically settled with every religion in *The Future of an Illusion*, Pfister (1928) had responded by reversing Freud's title - the illusion of a future - and accused Freud of succumbing to an ideology, namely that of science. For Freud, of course, this was an honor; his entire work was concerned with scientific enlightenment, which can only strive for preliminary truths. Has Pfister, a theologian, had the last word against Freud because new mythologies and ideologies have arisen since beliefs have been demythologized? Actually, Freud thought that man's capacity to soberly acknowledge realities was so limited that he gave wide room to religious consolations, especially to the belief in a life after death. In contrast to Nietzsche, in whose late works the phrase "God is dead" formed a central thesis, Freud was guided by the human longing for belief that provided support and consolation. According to his well-known description of the relationship between psychoanalysis and religion,

> If the application of the psycho-analytic method makes it possible to find a new argument against the truths of religion, *tant pis* for religion; but defenders of religion will by the same right make use of psycho-analysis in order to give full value to the affective significance of religious doctrines. (Freud 1927c, p. 37)

It has proved proper for analysts to stick to their own skills with regard to all problems of religion, and to use their method to examine the entire extent of the affective significance of religious ideas and the function of belief in the life of the individual within the different religious communities. In the process analysts often see the significance of *projection* for the creation of images of God. It was precisely this discovery of the projection of human fantasies of omnipotence in magical, mythical, and religious thought and experiencing that Freud, following Feuerbach, made the focus of his criticism of religion. Since we discuss these problems in the following case study in the section entitled "The Image of God as Projection," some introductory comments are appropriate.

The concept of projection and its grounding go back to Feuerbach in the nineteenth century. Schneider (1972), who is both a theologian and psychoanalyst, has described Feuerbach's theory of religion and critically examined the reaction of theology to it. Feuerbach provided a "critical, genetic" explanation of religion:

Religion is man's earliest and also indirect form of self-knowledge. Hence, religion everywhere precedes philosophy, as in the history of the race, so also in that of the individual. Man first of all sees his nature as if *out* of himself, before he finds it in himself. His own nature is in the first instance contemplated by him as that of another being. Religion is the childlike condition of humanity; but the child sees his nature - man - out of himself; in childhood a man is an object to himself, under the form of another man. Hence the historical progress of religion consists in this: that what by an earlier religion was regarded as objective, is now recognised as subjective; that is, what was formerly contemplated and worshipped as God is now perceived to be something *Shuman*... every advance in religion is therefore a deeper self-knowledge. (Feuerbach 1957, p. 13)

According to Schneider, Feuerbach traced religious ideas back to anthropologic phenomena that man was originally not able to recognize as being his own but projected onto his environment. Feuerbach conceived of religion, as Freud did later, as "the infantile nature of man," explaining it with the reference that a child perceives its essence in its parents. He therefore attempted to explain, for example, "the secret of prayer" with the fact that a child "finds in its father the feeling of its strength... and the certainity that its desires will be satisfied," concluding that "The omnipotence that man turns to in prayer is... in truth nothing other than the omnipotnece of the heart, feeling, which breaks through all the barriers of reason and overcomes all the borders of nature." In summary, he wrote that "The origin, true place, and significance of religion exist only in man's period of infancy... " (quoted according to Schneider 1972, p. 252).

Feuerbach sought the true essence of religion in anthropology. The larger part of his *The Essence of Christianity* is entitled "The True or Anthropological Essence of Religion." Freud extended this anthropological turn in the critique of religion by tracing religious and mythical ideas back to the infantile phase of life in an even more rigorous manner than Feuerbach had. The psychoanalytic critique of religion added important new dimensions - even according to Grünbaum (1987b), who referred to the example of belief in Immaculate Conception - by recognizing that taboos that develop during a person's life history are both the source of certain items of dogma and the basis for their plausibility. In this reduction Freud, of course, encountered a myth - that of Oedipus. His study of the origin of man's images of God and his discovery of projection thus led to his criticism of *revealed* Christian truth and, in a comprehensive sense, to demythologization, but also to a remythologization.

Psychoanalysis has contributed to this development in intellectual history in numerous ways, and here we will limit ourselves to mentioning just a few of these points. Freud outlined a *theory* of the genesis and function of myths, religions, and ideologies and created a method of investigation. As a representative of the enlightenment he conceived a reality principle that comprehended the world of facts and whose acknowledgment is a dictate of pure and practical reason. For Freud, science's view of the world leads to knowledge of the connections between facts and thus to truth, which in turn enables one to cope with life in a realistic manner. Facts are contrasted to imagination, and truth to illusion; the world of mythology and faith is molded by fiction and fantasy. This contrast between logic and myth can be traced back to early Greek philosophy (see Dupré 1973).

Proceeding from the reality principle, the process of mythology is primarily considered under the aspect of defense. Long ago Jones (1919) emphasized with regard to the prototype of defense (repression) that the related psychoanalytic theory of symbols employed a restricted concept of symbol. Psychoanalytic theory does not adequately recognize the overall significance of symbolic forms for human thought and action. Langer's (1942) critique of the psychoanalytic concept of symbol, in the spirit of Cassirer, has been discussed in the psychoanalytic literature, which has had a positive effect on the discussion at the theoretical level (Philipps 1962; Lorenzer 1970). The inclusion of the psychoanalytic concept of symbol in a philosophy of symbolic forms represents an extension of the psychoanalytic understanding of religious experience (see Braun et al. 1988).

Explaining elements of religion with reference to the infantile roots of emotional life has its strengths and weaknesses, as does every one-sided explanation. It is by no means necessary for religious feelings to simply disappear in the course of liberation from frightening infantile fantasies about God. It is also possible in the course of an analysis for new aspects of faith to arise parallel to the modification of those images of God that are filled with anxiety. A psychoanalyst is not competent to judge the *truth* of systems of faith. He can, however, proceeding from Freud's anthropological perspective, have an opinion about which items of faith are appropriate for an individual, i. e., harmonize with his essence, and which contradict it and are antagonistic to his life. Today all religions and world views have to accept the fact that they can be compared with regard to what they contribute to an individual leading a fulfilled life and to achieving a reconciliation between groups and peoples. Directly or indirectly, the psychoanalyst's critical attitude toward culture and religion influences the world view of his patients. Thus to the extent that values are a topic of discussion in treatment, psychoanalysis itself must be willing to accept the same kind of critical examination as has been directed at religion and secular expressions of faith since the anthropological turn. Such an examination cannot bracket out the way psychoanalysts act in their professional work and within the professional community, or the extent to which humane values such as those Freud adhered to are expressed.

In the following example the analyst did not shy away from tracing a patient's image of God back to projections. Although in doing so he was moving on "theological thin ice," he was only temporarily in danger of losing control. He stuck to the idea of negative theology, which he understood as saying that all human statements about God cannot, by definition, reveal his real essence, and that on the other hand it is also impossible not to make "any graven image, or any likeness" (Exodus, 20,4). This attitude is characterized by extreme openness toward all religious feelings. Whether an atheist is willing to discuss his repressed longing for his father, or a member of a sect is willing to examine the function of his belief in the beyond in connection with a presumed approaching demise of the world are technical questions that we cannot discuss here in detail. Decisive is that this openness exists, which makes it possible in principle for an analyst to treat members of all denominations.

Religious questions are encountered in every analysis at least in connection with the issue of guilt. It is often possible to restrict oneself to the genesis of *feelings of guilt* in connection with formation of the superego. Depressive patients, in particular, feel guilty without having done anything to warrant serious and real guilt. Confession and absolution do not reach where unconscious feelings of guilt have entered into a close connection with repressed intentions. It was with this category of patients that the role of the internalization of punishing parents and of the images of God copied from them was discovered. Theology and psychoanalysis meet at the transition from feelings of guilt to real guilt (Buber 1958).

Religious ideas are encountered especially frequently in compulsion neuroses. The psychopathological forms of compulsive defense rituals are related in numerous ways to superstition and magical thought. Anxieties and feelings of guilt, as well as the temporary alleviation provided by typical obsessive thoughts and compulsive acts characterize a syndrome that results in endless repetition of the same thought processes and sequences of events; in very severe cases normal behavor is hardly possible. Both the contents and the forms of compulsive neuroses lead one to compare the function of rituals in the individual's psychic life with those in systems of faith. From a psychoanalytic perspective the issue is to determine the influence that Christian faith and biblical stories exert on the neurotic anxieties of patients. Religious problems arise in psychoanalytic treatment primarily in individuals who have been injured by religion and its representatives, as the following example of Arthur Y demonstrates. The modification of symptoms is thus always accompanied by modifications of the images of God. An unanswered question concerns which religious feelings remain after infantile and magical thoughts lose their influence on thinking and emotions; there are differences of opinions on this issue between individual theologians and psychoanalysts (see Gay 1987; Küng 1987; Meissner 1984; Quervain 1978; Wangh 1989).

10.3.1 The Image of God as Projection

The excerpts of the case history of Arthur Y presented in Sects. 6.4 and 8.2 demonstrate that religious contents and motives played a dominant role in his compulsive symptoms. And apart from his compulsive symptoms, Arthur Y frequently confronted his analyst with religious questions about God's justness and the compatibility of the different images of God. The story of Abraham and Isaac became the sinister and incomprehensible example of sacrifice in which the patient was unable to discover any love. The following example stems from a late phase of Arthur Y's analysis, after he had already acquired a greater inner freedom. Because of the great significance of the problems discussed here, Sect. 10.3.2 contains a theologist's comments, entitled "The Analyst on Theological Thin Ice?" The title refers to a statement the patient made accusing *priests* of avoiding some topics to keep off thin ice.

The analyst's comments about his countertransference were clear indications of his insecurity regarding the problem of potential blasphemy. The "considerations" and "commentaries" were not added to this excerpt until after completion of the theologist's comments, which thus refers only to the uncommented excerpt of the session.

Arthur Y emphasized that he still had not come to terms with his own feelings of claiming power and force. For days he would feel excellent, and his condition would be incomparably better than it had been, but he wondered whether it might just be a forgetting (of anxiety). He had occasional relapses lasting seconds, minutes, or hours. He acknowledged that there had been great changes in the context of his anxiety; he had acquired a more secure basis for enjoying the pleasures of life, and he was able to be generous, not immediately imagining that economic ruin was approaching. He added, however, that his anxiety was still latently present.

Two major topics were still a source of distress for Arthur Y, namely force and sexuality. He came to speak of the Christian religion, asking how the daily struggle to take something away from others or even to ruin them materially could be reconciled with Christian ideals. A colleague had recently looked at him astonished as he had raised this question, and answered, "You can use your God-given abilities, and if they make you successful, then it can't be un-Christian." He had to admit that his colleague was right, adding that Christian forgiveness could not apply to everything. He said the idea of an existence free of force was not realistic and that pushing to get ahead could be observed everywhere in nature - every plant grew towards light and whoever did not keep up wasted away. His religious problems bothered him. He said it had been difficult for him to go to Communion at Christmas.

P: A few years ago I had the thought that if I didn't think of my anxieties when I took the host, then everything would be alright. After I had eaten the host the thought shot through my mind, "Murderer, chop his head off." I was thinking of myself. Then I managed to get my mind on something else and not to think about it any more. The same thing happened to me a few days ago; everything was calm and peaceful and suddenly I thought about the scene at the Communion.

The topic of religion continued to be at the focus of the patient's thoughts:

P: Christmas is the day of celebrating harmony, but just a few days later is Stephan's day, a gruesome history, the stoning of the holy Stephan, who was chased out of town. God even sent his Son to the Crucifixion to achieve reconciliation. My atheistic upbringing created the feeling in me that the world is cold and merciless, but the real world did not agree at all with my natural disposition. And after the Nazis were gone and mother sent me to church for opportunist reasons, I was surprised to encounter a world in which you are accepted and can even have anxiety. The old priest had understood how to guide me, but the pleasant experience wasn't continued at the parochial boarding school, where I ran into a terrible representative of God.

At the boarding school he had encountered two such representatives, one a repulsively ugly, homosexual seducer, the other a brutal sadist. He thought of Schiller's verse, "Shuddering, it crawled toward me, the monster crawled toward me - that's the impression the repulsive man gave me. This is how I developed the image of a diabolical God." He would have liked to recite several more verses from Schiller's *The Diver*, but did not in order not to create the impression that he wanted to show off how much he knew.

I pointed out to the patient that he referred to himself self-critically as some who boasted, when he wanted to say a few more verses, but interrupted this train of thought to avoid being one. I added that if he continued his story, he would come to the subject of power, and not only the power that affects him from outside, the representatives of his brutal image of God, but also to his own desire for power, which he then can use to assert himself against the strong force.

The patient then took the risk of approaching the monster that was in hiding by saying, "You can only face such monsters if you yourself have power, and then you're as powerful as people in power, murderers, such as God the Father who did not prevent his Son from dying on the cross."

Consideration. In a quiet moment the problem of theodicy immediately crossed my mind, specifically the defense of God against the criticism of also being, as creator of the world, responsible for all evil. Who is responsible for the evil in the world? And what about human freedom. Later I read about several suggestions as to philosophical and theological solutions to the theodicy problem. Yet at this moment I was overcome by a powerful countertransference, having to think of my own education. I sensed that the positive unconscious fantasy was behind the negative formulation that God "did not prevent his Son from dying on the cross." He had let him be killed, which means that in His omnipotence He Himself was the murderer. Overcoming strong inner resistance, I struggled against the accusation that I would commit blasphemy and thought, in my opinion also for the patient, his and my thoughts through to their logical conclusion, saying, "If you think these thoughts through to their logical conclusion, the God the Father killed His own son."

The patient was shocked and relieved at the same time that I had clearly spoken his thoughts.

P: You should say that to a priest some time. He would hit you over the head with his cross.

A: Thoughts of revenge come when you've been tormented. You didn't want to be like that, no vengeful God, no avenging God, and yet you do want to be like that, too. The priest would hit *me* on the head with his cross, as you said. Christ's sacrificial death is supposed to atone for and erase man's guilt.

P: Yes, that's hard to rhyme.

A: The son submits. Let not my will, but let thy will be done.

P: It's just natural to ask how something like this can fascinate and subjugate so many people for more than 2000 years. Anxiety and fascination. If the host had fallen on the floor, it would have been a catastrophe. Yes, it's impossible to touch the Lord God with your fingers. I would never have had the nerve to so in such a blunt way that God killed His own son. If I were to think such a thing, I would be punished. Then I would have to kill my own children. I've needed all this time to think these thoughts through to their logical conclusion.

A: Yes, if you had put my words into your own mouth, that is if you expressed your criticism yourself, if you became indignant about the subjugation you've experienced, if you rebelled against those in power, then you would be butchered like a sow [an allusion to a masochistic thought of the patient].

P: You told me once that you are protestant and had a Christian upbringing. How do you come to terms with saying that God is a murderer if you are Christian? How does that go together?

After reflecting for a long time, I gave an evasive answer: "What does Christian theology say about it?" I referred to the general theological statement that sacrificial death is the symbol of God's love. The patient was very relieved at having managed to talk about these thoughts that had repeatedly tormented him for a long time.

P: Should I be happy that I have talked about these ideas, or should I feel anxiety? I'm not satisfied with what you said.

A: Yes, you can't be satisfied with it.

<u>Consideration.</u> I could not think of anything else but to confirm that the patient was justified in feeling dissatisfied. I avoided the issue by generalizing it, because at the time I did not know how to proceed. At least I gained some room for making some therapeutically more helpful statements. My confirmation encouraged the patient to let his dissatisfaction motivate him to more intensive reflection. As a result, my evasiveness did not have any lasting negative consequences, as shown by the further course of treatment.

The patient then began to talk about the movies about Don Camillo and Peppone, a fictional priest and communist politician in a small Italian town.

P: Don Camillo talked with God as if they were equals. He carried the cross and talked with God or Christ as if from man to man, calling upward "Hold on tight!" when he wanted to use the cross to hit something. One side of God is similar to the sadistic teacher. The corresponding idea is, "Duck, keep down low, hide in the masses so that you're not conspicuous." It must have been that way in the concentration camps. A person was a little more secure if he didn't raise any attention. But that means crawling like a worm, lying flat on the ground or, even better, underground.

A: So, Don Camillo spoke with God as if they were equals and asked, "Why didn't you keep your son from being killed?" He wouldn't have said, "Why did you kill your son?" That would be an active deed. But the question of why God did not prevent the sacrificial death, this question even keeps theologists busy. According to the Bible, God's power extends over heaven and earth.

P: Yes, these thoughts are convincing, but you have to have the nerve to talk about them. I remember a radio play about a blasphemer who was threatened that he would be struck by lightening. And a little later there was a thunder storm. In the play this man trembled until it was all over, without being struck by lightening.

A: Many people simply don't dare to use their reason and think. Blasphemy is immediately followed by a bolt of lightening. You are punished by the mental bolt given to you by the all-powerful teacher - God in Heaven.

Consideration. My goal in this interpretation was to personify natural events and to create something in common between the different bolts, whether of lightening or of ideas, or to find similarities that could have common roots in the polarity of power and powerlessness. The comment about God as a teacher was an allusion to a sadistic teacher who had thrown bolts that, in turn, had caused a thunderous echo in the patient's compulsive neurotic ideas.

P: Yes, Don Camillo did something wrong. At the Crucifix he asked for God's forgiveness and promised not to smoke his cigar again, which was a great sacrifice. After he extinguished his cigar, the voice of God, from the Crucifix, said, "Don't just extinguish it, throw it away, don't put it in your pocket." And in fact Camillo had had the idea of smoking his cigar later on in his pipe, and was caught thinking about it - a funny story.

A: Yes, this God could have fun, but the other one, the cruel one, who met you in the person of your sadistic teacher . . . .

In the next session the patient spoke about the liberating effect the last session had had, even though he was shocked at my statements. He became more secure in talking about things that previously had been bracketed out. Yet something sinister remained:

P: The apocalyptic riders could come or, more simply, something could happen like in the boarding school, when a boy was beaten so badly that he later committed suicide. All of this was decisive in my development.

A: It's natural to forget the sinister, which is why everything in the last session seemed so new to you, as if you had never had such ideas before.

P: True, but you hadn't said it as explicitly before either. God, a murderer, the building ought to collapse.

A: You feel better not just because there hasn't been a catastrophe, but because I said the sentence. If God is angry and kills someone, then you won't be the victim, I will. I was the bad guy, the blasphemer.

P: Yes, you said it, but I was the reason, and that made me feel my anxiety. I settled down by telling myself that you said it, not me. It was only afterwards that I also felt proud. At first I was shocked and horrified. No, I was rather proud that I had gone as far as I did, and yet I'm still a little concerned that I brought you to say something blasphemous. I've known you long enough to know that I should take you seriously, and in response to my question about how you come to terms with it, you withdrew to a theological explanation. You didn't tell me your own opinion. To return to Don Camillo and his discussion with God about the Crucifix, Don Camillo asked, "What didn't you keep it from happening?" This question is much weaker. You just can't simply go and say such a blasphemous thing. I'm not the only one who would lose his breath; thousands would react just the same way. I told you the story about the host that I couldn't let fall on the floor.

A: Well, I'm responsible for what I said. And by taking the responsibility, I provided you relief.

P: I've observed myself a little more in the last few days. I noticed that I've sometimes attempted to avoid making visual contact. If I don't look at him or them, then they don't do anything to me. [Long silence] I'm not happy with one of your comments, namely that I don't risk something until you make the first move. As if you were taking something away from me that I thought I could have - a bit of courage. Well, you could see it a different way [the patient laughed]. You could say that I showed the courage to follow you after you had gone first.

A: Or to go in your own tracks.

P: I'd like to go back to the sentence and ask you directly, Don't you feel any anxiety about saying something like that? Didn't you really go a little too far? Did you lose control of yourself? Or is my memory fooling me? I can't imagine that I provoked you to go that far, so your emotions must have got the better of you; that would at least be an explanation for what you said.

A: Would it be eerie if you had so much power and provoked me to blasphemy?

P: Yes. I've just had the thought that I made a suggestion to a colleague, a manager, about how to solve a problem at work and he liked it very much. Why is it so hard for me to accept the fact that I can also have some good ideas? So, if I had the power to provoke you to make such a statement, I don't believe it would seem as sinister to me now as it would have before.

A: Yes, you did motivate me to make this comment. But I didn't lose control of myself. I'm in the company of many important theologians. It's a fundamental question of Christian theology to ask where evil comes from. Since God created the world, the problem is why he didn't prevent evil, that is, why he let it happen that his son was killed. I left out the intermediate step to make it clearer that an indirect or secondary act is also an deed.

P: I had the subliminal anxiety that it was impossible to speak about it and couldn't have any intellectual models for it. So, it's not only my problem. These contradictions don't only affect me, but thousands upon thousands of other people. Why isn't this issue a topic in church if everyone worries about it. Is it because priests don't want to go out on thin ice?

The patient began to speak about sermons that handle fundamental topics such as hate, love, reconciliation, and sacrifice, issues which had already been expressed in mythologies in the pre-Christian era. He said,

P:I'm amazed that people don't ask more often why they speak about a *dear* God. I might be able to answer this question from my own life history: They beat the desire out of me to ask critical questions.

With these thoughts a session ended that was memorable for both participants. It helped the patient to become able to integrate projected elements of his self.

10.3.2 The Analyst on Theological Thin Ice?

In order to provide a meaningful commentary to this impressive session, which seems to be a very condensed version of a problem affecting mankind, it is advantageous to examine the following five issues:

First, what do we learn in this vignette about the patient, his illness, and his progress in therapy, in connection with his biographical data?

The patient was pursued by his feeling of power and force, which was linked with his anxiety that he might do something to someone close to him. His fantasies of omnipotence, in which his own thoughts were attributed magical power, were turned around, making the patient the powerless victim who was destined, for example, to be ruined economically. He felt as if he belonged to two worlds, one in which he was accepted and could have anxiety, and another that was colored with sadism and sexuality and that he internalized via identification. Although he was "terrified about the envy of the Gods," he was now able to see that the scorned drive to have power was in himself. Yet his recognition of his own ambivalence was opposed by resistance that strove to achieve a clear distinction between the spheres of good and evil. In symbolic communication the analyst went first, taking the patient's place and saying the blasphemous thought about God's ambivalence. With this protection the patient was then able to approach his own ambivalence, which however cannot be logically connected.

By breaking the taboos, the analyst enabled the patient to discover "legitimate" possibilities for developing his own power in his life.

Second, what role did the patient's religious fantasies play in his treatment, especially against the background of his religious socialization? Did they facilitate his treatment, or were they used by his resistance? Which interpretative aids did he use himself, and which were provided by psychoanalytic theory?

Arthur Y apparently had the option of being able to express himself in myths. When he did, there was no difference between the outer world and his inner world, the ideal and the material coincided, subject and object were not separate. He felt as if he were the battleground of numinous powers that had to be kept separate at all cost. Everything was alright if he did not have to think about evil while he was being given the host during Communion, when his ambivalence was gone. Yet he still felt that this was no solution, and he sought for oppotunities for expressing his ambivalence. In passing he managed to say, "God, who accepted the Crucifixion of His Son for the sake of reconciliation." His image of the "diabolical God," the God who kills, reflected the dark side of his desire for power and force. He referred to the figure of Don Camillo as an aid in interpreting the dilemma of a God who is omnipotent yet also suffers; the irony is that he described a God who has humor and accepts the ambivalent qualities of his earthly representative, just as the patient was able to accept the fact that his analyst temporarily had the function of a substitute and to find new opportunites to use his own power.

The manifestation of mythical structures in relatively many situations in psychoanalysis is good reason to consider one of the fundamental problems of psychoanalytic theory, namely its "scientific" self-understanding in contrast to the "mythical" mental structures of many patients. Psychoanalysis, as a science in which "explanation" and "understanding" are linked in a unique way (Thomä and

Kächele 1973; Körner 1985, pp. 51 ff.), has itself contributed to a substantial revision of the intellectual climate, resulting especially in a new evaluation of the problem of myth in science. The hope that all mythology would be completely resolved by depth psychology, being traced back to the projection of unconscious desires and fantasies, has turned out to be an "illusion" (Pfister 1928).

Some philosophers today assert that "there is absolutely no theoretically necessary reason in science or philosophy" to reject myths (Hübner 1985, p. 343). "The myths that teach us very simply what constitutes a value are inevitable if human civilization is to exist" (Kolakowski 1974, p. 40). In contrast, the uncontrolled return of repressed myths, which has almost the strength of an eruption, is diagnosed as a weakness of our civilization (Hübner 1985, pp. 15 f.). A mythical element is hidden in numerous manifestations of our civilization (Hübner 1985, pp. 293 ff.). Furthermore, the chance has been described that conscious examination of mythical material can provide insight into repressed desires (Heinrich 1986, p. 240). There are many indications that remythologization is now taking the place of demythologization (Schlesier 1981; Vogt 1986). Following this small philosophical aside, we now turn back to the intervention strategy in this case.

Third, what did we experience about the analyst in his relationship to the patient and his religious ideas?

Initially the analyst apparently felt he was the advocate of "reality." He did not shy from taking a realitic standpoint. He attempted to use the idea of "nature" to mediate between the pompous and utopian ideals and conditions as they really exist. He probably feared that the two poles in the patient's ambivalence might break apart. He raised the latter to a new level by referring to the patient's mental wizardry, while at the same time drawing attention to the patient's own critical impulses toward it, which took the form of subliminal scorn and mockery. He used the patient's religious fantasy (the Crucifix as a weapon) to lead him to his own sadistic fantasies. He attempted to confront him with the scene of his "submission," to show him that rebellion is also punished by terrible penalties. He formulated for the patient the blasmphemous thought of an ambivalent God, but retreated to a general theological stance when the patient insistently asked how this could be made to agree; the patient was naturally not satisfied with such a response. He again approached the patient's ambivalence with the aid of a two-God theory (the God of Don Camillo and the God of the sadistic seducer), showing the patient his own hidden power, which he had used to provoke the analyst into making a blasmphemous statement. The frightening and isolating aspects of his ambivalence entered, on the one hand, in his identification with the analyst, and on the other in the general problem of mankind that could not be resolved by logic and for which there were no clearcut answers.

The analyst thus found himself in a dilemma of either putting himself and his own religious or nonreligious attitudes in the forefront, as an object of identification, or leaving the patient too alone by referring to the general problem of mankind or a "theological topography" that stayed at a very general level and for which the analyst had no responsibility.

What can help the analyst orient himself in such a dilemma, which has been neglected by both psychoanalytic theory and technique? It is a mistake to believe that mythical-religious images that are antagonistic to life will disintegrate of their own. Is the analyst left with the role of a nonparticipating observer who has to wait to see what develops on its own? This would certainly be a fateful misinterpretation of the inner dynamics of the therapeutic process. The analyst must also attempt to become aware of his own attitude toward the subject of religion in order to be able to handle his countertransference in the best interest of the patient. This is true even if he attempts to avoid as long as possible making a premature decision when a value conflict arises between him and the patient. I therefore ask:

Fourth, how is the subject of religion present in the analytic situation and in the interplay of transference and countertransference?

The structure of the scene described above is very strongly molded by the character of the substitute function and was interpreted by the analyst as such. As an auxiliary ego, he took the patient's place in stating the idea that the patient was still unable to verbalize. It contained the traits of the religious material provided by the patient. Yet to me it seems characteristic that here the transference was not molded by the image of his father (about whom nothing is said in this scene), but by that of the son who, although obedient (even he frequently withdrew to authority), also violated the taboo of his definite father with his blasphemous thoughts about ambivalence, which symbolized rebellion and indignation. To me, even the analyst's countertransference seems to be characterized by ambivalence. On the one hand, he saw himself as the representative of reality, while on the other he became so involved in the patient's religious fantasies that he attributed them a supraindiviudal realistic substance, which enabled the patient to feel linked with both the analyst and all of mankind. That the flash of a thought was not followed by one of punishment helped the patient to loosen the defense mechanisms of denial, isolation, and undoing and to experience his ambivalence.

This scene from therapy thus demonstrates clearly the ambivalence in religious fantasies. The fantasies were impressive reflections of the state of the analytic process. If a patient refers to religious ideas in treatment, then it is advantageous if the analyst has achieved a certain degree of awareness as to his own position toward these problems. He should have a clear understanding of the role that mythical and religious fantasies play in how a civilization understands itself and in its attitude toward its own intellectual history. Although the "enlightenment" hopes of the early psychoanalysts have not been fulfilled, this does not justify uncritically portraying myths as archtypical phenomena that are "ubiquitous, transhistorical, latently present, eternally returning [and that constitute] an inner bond between humans of all times and places" (Drewerman 1984, p. 165). Our insight into the historical transformations of myths prohibits such an understanding, just as some of Drewermann's other views are dubious for psychodynamic and theological reasons (Görres and Kasper 1988).

By assigning the concept "work" a central role in therapy and in the description of endopsychic events, Freud specified the decisive solution to the problem of the relationship between nature and history. Man's nature acquires its history by means of psychic work, and the psychoanalyst takes active part in these processes at both the individual and collective levels. Regardless of whether he wants to or not, he is inevitably involved in the "work with myths" that is considered to be such an urgent task (Blumenberg 1981, pp. 291 ff.). He should accept this responsibility with a greater awareness and willingness than seems to be the case at the present. This leads to my last question, which was the reason for examining this excerpt from therapy.

Fifth, why do psychoanalysts act so hesitantly toward the issue of religion, as if it were a taboo, and why is the violation of taboos such an important task for psychoanalysis?

Freud initiated the transformation of mythology into the psychology of the unconscious, and he was convinced that "a turning away from religion is bound to occur with the fatal inevitability of a process of growth" (1927c, p. 43).

The ubiquity of religious ideas, which take on more or less drastic forms in many analyses, is a reminder for us to concede these ideas their relative justification. They are after all an excellent means for expressing psychic realities that are very difficult to communicate in everyday language as it has been molded by purposive rationality. Of course, it is then necessary to make the effort of making substantive distinctions! The case discussed here obviously involves two different religious ideas. On the one hand, there was the attempt to isolate the sacred and the profane, separate good and evil, to treat them as absolutes and play them off against each other. On the other hand, there was the possibility, created by the idea of a substitute, to unite both sides of this ambivalent conflict; although this led to a logical contradictions, it provided the patient emotional relief and liberation.

For the patient's therapeutic progress there seems to be no doubt that the first idea inhibited him while the second apparently promoted his development. This implies a value, yet it is impossible to determine whether it is actually due to the results of psychoanalysis, or whether it has to be considered the result of the evolution of mankind's self-awareness and of religion as one of its means of expression.

The psychological comprehension of religion, which was in full blossom in the early days of psychoanalysis (see Nase and Scharfenberg 1977), has probably come to an impasse because the initial hopes for a complete transition to psychoanalysis were not fulfilled. Yet it did violate the taboo that mythical and religious ideas had to be respected at all times and places as the embodiment of constant and highest values. The unveiling of the ambivalent character of these values opened up the task of working them through, a task which Oskar Pfister - who has been forgotten by both psychoanalysts and theologians although he was a lifelong partner in Freud's struggles - pursued his entire life (see Freud and Pfister 1963). The psychoanalytic critique of religion has since taken on new forms and been further developed (see Scharfenberg 1968; Küng 1979, 1987: Meissner 1984), probably creating an entirely new situation compared to the bitter feuds during the infancy of psychoanalysis. The contribution of psychoanalysis to this new situation is, however, still unsatisfactory. The clinical excerpts that are the object of this commentary demonstrate very clearly that more such collaboration - which has already broken many religious taboos - is urgently needed.

References

Abraham K (1921) Beitrag zur Tic-Diskussion. Int Z Psychoanal 7: 393-396, quoted from Abraham K (1969) Psychoanalytische Studien zur Charakterbildung. Fischer, Frankfurt am Main, pp 64-68

Abraham K (1924) Versuch einer Entwicklungsgeschichte der Libido auf Grund der Psychoanalyse seelischer Störungen. Internationaler Psychoanalytischer Verlag, Leipzig

Adler A (1927) Studie über Minderwertigkeit von Organen. Bergmann, Munich

Ahrens S (1986a) Alexithymia and affective verbal behavior of psychosomatic patients and controls. In: Gottschalk LA, Lolas F, Viney LL (eds) Content analysis of verbal behavior. Springer, Berlin Heidelberg New York Tokyo, pp 207-214

Ahrens S (1986b) Experimentelle Untersuchungen affektiver Reaktionen bei psychosomatischen Patienten. Psychother Med Psychol 36: 47-50

Ahrens S (1987) Alexithymie und kein Ende? Versuch eines Resümees. Z Psychosom Med 33: 201-220

Ahrens S (1988) Die instrumentelle Forschung am instrumentellen Objekt. Kritik der Alexithymie-Forschung. Psyche 42: 225-241

Ahrens S, Deffner G (1985) Alexithymie - Ergebnisse und Methodik eines Forschungsbereiches der Psychosomatik. Psychother Med Psychol 35: 147-159

Aichhorn A (1925) Verwahrloste Jugend. Internationaler Psychoanalytischer Verlag, Leipzig

Albert H (1971) Theorie und Praxis. Max Weber und das Problem der Wertfreiheit und der Rationalität. In: Albert H, Topitsch E (eds) Werturteilsstreit. Wissenschaftliche Buchgesellschaft, Darmstadt, pp 200-236

Alexander F (1935) Über den Einfluß psychischer Faktoren auf gastrointestinale Störungen. Int Z Psychoanal 21: 189-219

Alexander F (1951) Psychosomatische Medizin. De Gruyter, Berlin

Alexander F, French T, Pollock G (1968) Psychosomatic specificity. University of Chicago Press, Chicago

Amsterdam BK, Greenberg LG (1977) Self-conscious behavior of infants. Developm Psychobiol 10: 1-6

Amsterdam BK, Levitt M (1980) Consciousness of self and painful self-consciousness. Psychoanal Study Child 35: 67-83

Anchin JC, Kiesler DJ (eds) (1982) Handbook of interpersonal psychotherapy. Pergamon, New York

Anderson CM (1986) The all-too-short trip from positive to negative connotation. J Marital Family Therapy 12: 351-354

Angst W (1980) Agression bei Affen und Menschen. Springer, Berlin Heidelberg New York

Anzieu A (1977) Review of Winnicott DW: Fragment d'une analyse. Payot, Paris 1975. Bulletin 11 European Psychoanalytic Federation, pp 25-29

Anzieu D (1986) Une Peau pour les Pensées: Entretiens avec Gilbert Tarrab. Clancier-Guenaud, Paris

Argelander H (1978) Das psychoanalytische Erstinterview und seine Methode. Ein Nachtrag zu Freud's Fall „Katharina". Psyche 32: 1089-1104

Arlow JA (1979) The genesis of interpretation. J Am Psychoanal Assoc 27: 193-206

Arlow JA (1982) Psychoanalytic education: a psychoanalytic perspective. Annu Psychoanal 10: 5-20

Arlow JA, Brenner C (1988) The future of psychoanalysis. Psychoanal Q 57: 1-14

Bachrach HM, Weber JJ, Murray S (1985) Factors associated with the outcome of psychoanalysis. Report of the Columbia Psychoanalytic Center Research Project (IV). Int Rev Psychoanal 12: 379-389
Bahnson CB (1986) Das Krebsproblem in psychosomatischer Dimension. In: Uexküll T von (ed) Psychosomatische Medizin, 3rd edn. Urban and Schwarzenberg, Munich, pp 889-909
Balint M (1935) Zur Kritik der Lehre von den prägenitalen Libidoorganisationen. Int Z Psychoanal 21: 525-543
Balint M (1948) On genital love. Int J Psychoanal 29: 34-40
Balint M (1965) Der Arzt, sein Patient und die Krankheit. Klett, Stuttgart
Baranger M, Baranger W, Mom J (1983) Process and non-process in analytic work. Int J Psychoanal 64: 1-15
Bartels M (1976) Selbstbewußtsein und Unbewußtes. Studien zu Freud und Heidegger. De Gruyter, Berlin
Beckmann D (1974) Der Analytiker und sein Patient. Untersuchungen zur Übertragung und Gegenübertragung. Huber, Bern
Beckmann D, Richter HE (1972) Gießen-Test. Ein Test für Individual- und Gruppendiagnostik. Huber, Bern
Beigler JS (1975) A commentary on Freud's treatment of the rat man. Annu Psychoanal 3: 271-285
Benedetti G (1980) Beitrag zum Problem der Alexithymie. Nervenarzt 51: 534-541
Benkert O, Hippius H (1980) Psychiatrische Pharmakotherapie, 3rd edn. Springer, Berlin Heidelberg New York
Bergmann P (1966) An experiment in filmed psychotherapy. In: Gottschalk LA, Auerbach HA (eds) Methods of research in psychotherapy. Appleton-Century-Crofts, New York, pp 35-49
Bernfeld S (1932) Der Begriff der „Deutung" in der Psychoanalyse. Z Angew Psychol 42: 448-497
Bernfeld S (1941) The facts of observation in psychoanalysis. J Psychol 12: 289-305
Bernstein B, Henderson D (1975) Schichtspezifische Unterschiede in der Bedeutung der Sprache für die Sozialisation. In: Bernstein B (ed) Sprachliche Kodes und soziale Kontrolle. Schwann, Düsseldorf, pp 22-45
Bertin C (1982) Marie Bonaparte. A life. Harcourt Brace Jovanovich, San Diego
Bettelheim B (1982) Freud and man's soul. Knopf, New York
Bilger A (1986) Agieren: Probleme und Chancen. Forum Psychoanal 2: 294-308
Bion WR (1959) Attacks on linking. In: Bion WR (ed) Second thoughts. Heinemann, London, pp 93-109
Black M (1962) Models and metaphors. Cornell University Press, Ithaca
Blarer A von, Brogle I (1983) Der Weg ist das Ziel. Zur Theorie und Metatheorie der psychoanalytischen Technik. In: Hoffmann SO (ed) Deutung und Beziehung. Kritische Beiträge zur Behandlungskonzeption und Technik in der Psychoanalyse. Fischer, Frankfurt am Main, pp 71-85
Blos P (1962) On adolescence. A psychoanalytic interpretation. Free Press, New York
Blos P (1970) The young adolescent. Clinical studies. Free Press, New York
Blos P (1983) The contribution of psychoanalysis to the psychotherapy of adolescents. Adolescent Psychiatry 11: 104-124
Blumenberg A (1981) Arbeit am Mythos. Suhrkamp, Frankfurt am Main
Blumenberg H (1960) Paradigmen zu einer Metaphorologie. Arch Begriffsgesch 6: 7-142
Blumer H (1973) Der methodische Standpunkt des symbolischen Interaktionismus. In: Arbeitsgruppe Bielefelder Soziologen (eds) Alltagswissen, Interaktion und gesellschaftliche Wirklichkeit, vol 1. Rowohlt, Reinbek, pp 80-146
Blos P (1985) Son and father. Before and beyond the Oedipus complex. Free Press, New York
Bohleber W (1982) Spätadoleszente Entwicklungsprozesse. Ihre Bedeutung für Diagnostik und psychotherapeutische Behandlung von Studenten. In: Krehci E, Bohleber W (eds) Spätadoleszente Konflikte. Indikation und Anwendung psychoanalytischer Verfahren bei Studenten. Verlag für Medizinische Psychologie, Göttingen, pp 11-52
Bolland J, Sandler J (1965) The Hampstead Psychoanalytic Index. International University Press, New York
Boor C de (1965) Zur Psychosomatik der Allergie, besonders der Asthma bronchiale. Huber/Klett, Bern/Stuttgart

Boszormenyi-Nagy I (1965) A theory of relationship. In: Boszormenyi-Nagy I, Framo LJ (eds) Intensive family therapy, vol 1. Harper and Row, New York, pp 33-86
Bowlby J (1973) Separation. Anxiety and anger. Hogarth, London
Bowlby J (1981) Psychoanalysis as a natural science. Int Rev Psychoanal 8: 243-256
Bracher KD (1982) The age of ideologies. Weidenfeld and Nicholson, London
Brähler E (1986) Körpererleben - ein vernachlässigter Aspekt der Medizin. In: Brähler E (ed) Körpererleben. Ein subjektiver Ausdruck von Leib und Seele. Springer, Berlin Heidelberg New York Tokyo, pp 3-18. English translation: Body experience. Springer, Berlin Heidelberg New York, 1988
Brandt LW (1961) Some notes on English Freudian terminology. J Am Psychoanal Assoc 9: 331-339
Brandt LW (1972) Mindless psychoanalysis. Contemp Psychol 17: 189-191
Brandt LW (1977) Psychoanalyse versus psychoanalysis: traduttore, traditore. Bedeutungsunterschiede zwischen psychoanalytischen Grundbegriffen im Englischen und Deutschen. Psyche 31: 1045-1051
Braun H-J, Holzhey H, Orth OW (1988) Über Ernst Cassirers Philosophie der symbolischen Formen. Suhrkamp, Frankfurt am Main
Bräutigam W (1954) Grundlagen und Erscheinungswesen des Torticollis pasticus. Nervenarzt 25: 451-462
Bräutigam W (1956) Extrapyramidale Symptome und umweltabhängige Verhaltensstörungen. Nervenarzt 27: 97-98
Bräutigam W (1984) Werte und Ziele in psychoanalytischen Therapien 1984. Z Psychosom Med Psychoanal 30: 62-71
Bräutigam W, Christian P (1986) Psychosomatische Medizin, 4th edn. Thieme, Stuttgart
Bräutigam W, Rad M von, Engel K (1980) Erfolgs- und Therapieforschung bei psychoanalytischen Behandlungen. Z Psychosom Med Psychoanal 26: 101-118
Brockhaus Enzyklopädie (1971), 17th edn, vol 12. Brockhaus, Wiesbaden, p 470
Bromley DB (1986) The case-study method in psychology and related disciplines. Wiley, New York
Brull HF (1975) A reconsideration of some translations of Sigmund Freud. Psychotherapy: Theory, Research and Practice 12: 273-279
Bruner J (1986) Actual minds, possible worlds. Harvard University Press, Cambridge
Buber (1958) Schuld und Schuldgefühle. Schneider, Heidelberg
Bucci W (1985) Dual coding: a cognitive model for psychoanalytic research. J Am Psychoanal Assoc 33: 571-607
Bühler K (1934) Sprachtheorie. Fischer, Stuttgart
Bürgin D (1980) Das Problem der Autonomie in der Spätadoleszenz. Psyche 34: 449-463
Cannon WB (1920) Bodily changes in pain, hunger, fear and rage. Appleton, New York
Cardinal M (1975) Les Mots pour le dire. Grasset et Fasquelle, Paris
Carveth DL (1984) The analyst's metaphors. A deconstructionist perspective. Psychoanal Contemp Thought 7: 491-560
Charlier T (1987) Über pathologische Trauer. Psyche 41: 865-882
Chassaguet-Smirgel (ed) (1974) Psychoanalyse der weiblichen Sexualität. Suhrkamp, Frankfurt am Main
Cheshire NM, Thomä H (eds) (1987) Self, symptoms and psychotherapy. Wiley, New York
Cheshire N, Thomä H (1991) Metaphor, neologism and "open texture": implications for translating Freud's scientific thought. Int Rev Psychoanal 18: 429-455
Christian P (1986) Moderne Handlungstheorie und der „Gestaltkreis". Ein Beitrag zum Werk von Viktor von Weizäcker mit klinischen Beispielen zum Verständnis psychomotorischer Störungen. Praxis Psychother Psychosom 31: 78-86
Christoffel H (1944) Trieb und Kultur. Zur Soziologie, Physiologie und Psychohygiene der Harntriebhaftigkeit mit besonderer Berücksichtigung der Enuresis. Schwabe, Basel
Colby KM, Stoller RJ (1988) Cognitive science and psychoanalysis. Analytic Press, Hillsdale
Compton AA (1972a) A study of the psychoanalytic theory of anxiety. I. The development of Freud's theory of anxiety. J Am Psychoanal Assoc 20: 3-44
Compton AA (1972b) A study of the psychoanalytic theory of anxiety. II. Developments in the theory of anxiety since 1926. J Am Psychoanal Assoc 20: 341-394

Compton AA (1980) A study of the psychoanalytic theory of anxiety. III. A preliminary formulation of the anxiety response. J Am Psychoanal Assoc 28: 739-773

Cooper AM (ed) (1985) The termination of the training. International Psychoanalytic Association monograph series, vol 5

Covner BJ (1942) Studies in phonographic recordings of verbal material: I. The use of phonographic recordings in counseling practice and research. J Consult Psychol 6: 105-113

Cremerius J (1977) Ist die „psychosomatische Struktur" der französischen Schule krankheitsspezifisch? Psyche 31: 293-317

Cremerius J (1981a) Die Präsenz des Dritten in der Psychoanalyse. Zur Problematik der Fremdfinanzierung. Psyche 35: 1-41

Cremerius J (1981b) Freud bei der Arbeit über die Schulter geschaut. Seine Technik im Spiegel von Schülern und Patienten. In: Ehebald U, Eickhoff FW (eds) Humanität und Technik in der Psychoanalyse. Jahrb Psychoanal, Beiheft 6. Huber, Bern, pp 123-158

Cremerius J (1984a [1966]) Schweigen als Problem der psychoanalytischen Technik. In: Cremerius J (ed) Vom Handwerk des Psychoanalytikers: Das Werkzeug der psychoanalytischen Technik, vol 1. Frommann-Holzboog, Stuttgart, pp 17-54

Cremerius J (1984b [1975]) Der Patient spricht zuviel. In: Cremerius J (ed) Vom Handwerk des Psychoanalytikers: Das Werkzeug der psychoanalytischen Technik, vol 1. Frommann-Holzboog, Stuttgart, pp 55-76

Cremerius J, Hoffmann SO, Trimborn W (1979) Psychoanalyse, Über-Ich und soziale Schicht. Die psychoanalytische Behandlung der Reichen, der Mächtigen und der sozial Schwachen. Kindler, München

Dahl H, Kächele H, Thomä H (eds) (1988) Psychoanalytic process research strategies. Springer, Berlin Heidelberg New York

Danckwardt J (1978) Zur Interaktion von Psychotherapie und Psychopharmakotherapie. Eine klinische Studie über die Wirkung von Parametern bei einer periodisch psychotischen Patientin. Psyche 32: 111-154

Deutsch F (1949) Thus speaks the body. An analysis of postural behavior. Trans NY Acad Sci Series II, 12(2): 58-62

Deutsch F (1952) Analytic posturology. Psychoanal Q 21: 196-214

Deutsch F (1959) On the mysterious leap from the mind to the body. International University Press, New York

Deutsch H (1926) Okkulte Vorgänge während der Psychoanalyse. Imago 12: 418-433

Deutsch H (1930) Psychoanalyse der Neurosen. Internationaler Psychoanalytischer Verlag, Vienna

Dewald PA (1972) The psychoanalytic process. A case illustration. Basic, New York

Dewald PA (1982) Serious illness in the analyst: transference, countertransference, and reality responses. J Am Psychoanal Assoc 30: 347-363

Doolittle H (1956) Tribute to Freud. Pantheon, New York

Drewermann E (1984) Tiefenpsychologie und Exegese. Walter, Olten

Dührssen A (1962) Katamnestische Ergebnisse bei 1004 Patienten nach analytischer Psychotherapie. Z Psychosom Med 8: 94-113

Dupré W (1973) Mythos. In: Krings H, Baumgartner HM, Wild C (eds) Handbuch philosophischer Grundbegriffe. Kösel, Munich, pp 948-956

Düsing E (1986) Intersubjektivität und Selbstbewußtsein. Behavioristische, phänomenologische und idealistische Begründungstheorien bei Mead, Schütz, Fichte und Hegel. Verlag für Philosophie, Cologne

Eagle M (1973a) Validation of motivational formulations: acknowledgement as a criterion. Psychoanal Contemp Sci 2: 265-275

Eagle M (1973b) Sherwood on the logic of explanation in psychoanalysis. Psychoanal Contemp Sci 2: 331-337

Eagle M (1984) Psychoanalysis and "narrative truth": a reply to Spence. Psychoanal Contemp Thought 7: 629-640

Eckstaedt A (1986) Two complementary cases of identification involving 'Third Reich' fathers. Int J Psychoanal 67: 317-328

Edelson M (1972) Language and dreams: the interpretation of dreams revisited. Psychoanal Study Child 27: 203-282

Edelson M (1975) Language and interpretation in psychoanalysis. Yale University Press, New Haven
Edelson M (1985) The hermeneutic turn and the single case study in psychoanalysis. Psychoanal Contemp Thought 8: 567-614
Edelson M (1986) The convergence of psychoanalysis and neuroscience: illusion and reality. Contemp Psychoanal 22: 479-519
Edelson M (1988) Psychoanalysis. A theory in crisis. University of Chicago Press, Chicago
Ehlich K (1979) Verwendungen der Deixis beim sprachlichen Handeln. Lang, Frankfurt
Eickhoff FW (1986) Identification and its vicissitudes in the context of the Nazi phenomenon. Int J Psychoanal 67: 33-44
Eimer M (1987) Konzepte von Kausalität. Huber, Bern
Eissler KR (1953) The effect of structure of the ego on psychoanalytic technique. J Am Psychoanal Assoc 1: 104-143
Eissler K (1969) The psychiatrist and the dying patient. International University Press, New York
Ekstein R (1981) Supervision hour 5: on the supervision of the supervisor. In: Wallerstein RS (ed) Becoming a psychoanalyst. A study of psychoanalytic supervision. International University Press, New York, pp 211-225
Ekstein R, Wallerstein RS (1972) The teaching and learning of psychotherapy. International University Press, New York
Engel GL (1975) The death of a twin. Int J Psychoanal 56: 23-40
Engel GL, Schmale AH jr (1967) Psychoanalytic theory of somatic disorder. J Am Psychoanal Assoc 15: 344-365
Erikson EH (1950) Childhood and society. Norton, New York
Erikson EH (1954) The dream specimen of psychoanalysis. J Am Psychoanal Assoc 2: 5-56
Erikson EH (1962) Reality and actuality. J Am Psychoanal Assoc 11: 451-474
Erikson EH (1968) Identity. Youth and crisis. Norton, New York
Etchegoyen RH (1986) Los fundamentos de la técnica psicoanalitica. Amorrortu editores, Buenos Aires
Fahrenberg J (1979) Das Komplementaritätsprinzip in der psychophysiologischen Forschung und psychosomatischen Medizin. Z Klin Psychol Psychother 27: 151-167
Fahrenberg J (1981) Zum Verständnis des Komplementaritätsprinzips. Z Klin Psychol Psychother 29: 205-208
Fain M (1966) Regression et psychosomatique. Rev Franc Psychoanal 30: 452-456
Fara G, Cundo P (1983) Psychoanalyse, ein bürgerlicher Roman. Roter Stern, Frankfurt am Main
Farrell BA (1961) Can psychoanalysis be refuted? Inquiry 4: 16-36
Fasshauer K (1983) Klinische und elektromyographische Verlaufsuntersuchungen beim Torticollis spasmodicus. Nervenarzt 54: 535-539
Fenichel O (1930) Statistischer Bericht über die therapeutische Tätigkeit 1920-1930. In: Radó S, Fenichel O, Müller-Braunschweig C (eds) Zehn Jahre Berliner Psychoanalytisches Institut. Poliklinik und Lehranstalt. Internationaler Psychoanalytischer Verlag, Vienna, pp 13-19
Fenichel O (1935) Concerning the theory of the psychoanalyic technique. In: The collected papers of Otto Fenichel, 1st series. Norton, New York, pp 332-348
Fenichel O (1941) Problems of psychoanalytic technique. Psychoanalytic Quarterly, Albany
Fenichel O (1945) The psychoanalytic theory of neurosis. Norton, New York
Fenichel O (1953) Respiratory introjection. In: The collected papers of Otto Fenichel, 1st series. Norton, New York, pp 221-240
Ferenczi S (1913) Stages of development of the sence of reality. Journal of Sexology and Psychoanalysis, pp 213-239
Ferenczi S (1921) Psycho-analytic observations on tic. Int J Psychoanal 2: 1-30
Ferenczi S (1927) Contraindications of the active psychoanalytic technique. In: Ferenczi S Further contributions to the theory and technique of psycho-analysis. Boni and Liveright, New York, pp 217-230
Ferenczi S (1927) On the technique of psychoanalysis. In: Ferenczi S Further contributions to the theory and technique of psycho-analysis. Boni and Liveright, New York, pp 177-189
Ferenczi S (1988) The clinical diary of Sandor Ferenczi. In: Dupont J (ed) Sandor Ferenczi. Harvard University Press, Cambridge
Ferenczi S, Rank O (1925) The development of psychoanalysis. Nervous and Mental Disease Publishing, New York

Fisher S, Cleveland SE (1968) Body image and personality. Dover, New York
Flader D (1979) Techniken der Verstehenssteuerung im psychoanalytischen Diskurs. In: Flader D, Wodak-Leodolter R (eds) Therapeutische Kommunikation. Scriptor, Königstein, pp 24-43
Flader D (1982) Die psychoanalytische Therapie als Gegenstand sprachwissenschaftlicher Forschung. In: Flader D, Grodzicki WD, Schröter K (eds) Psychoanalyse als Gespräch. Interaktionsanalytische Untersuchungen über Therapie und Supervision. Suhrkamp, Frankfurt am Main, pp 16-41
Flader D, Grodzicki WD, Schröter K (eds) (1982) Psychoanalyse als Gespräch. Interaktionsanalytische Untersuchungen über Therapie und Supervision. Suhrkamp, Frankfurt am Main
Fonagy I (1983) La vive voix. Payot, Paris
Forrester J (1980) Language and the origins of psychoanalysis. Macmillan, London
French TM (1952) The integration of behaviour. Vol I: Basic postulates. University of Chicago Press, Chicago
Freud A (1936) Das Ich und die Abwehrmechanismen. Int Psychoanal Verlag, Wien
Freud A (1954) The widening scope of indications for psychoanalysis. Discussion. J Am Psychoanal Assoc 2: 607-620
Freud A (1976) Contribution to plenary session on "Changes in psychoanalytic practice and experience: theoretical, technical and social implications". Reported by Shengold L and McLaughlin JT. Int J Psychoanal 57: 261-274
Freud S (1895b) On the grounds for detaching a particular syndrom from neurasthenia under the description "Anxiety Neurosis". SE vol 3, pp 85-115
Freud S (1895d) Studies on hysteria. SE vol 2
Freud S (1895f) A reply to criticisms of my paper on anxiety neurosis. SE vol 3, pp 119-139
Freud S (1896b) Further remarks on the neuro-psychoses of defence. SE vol 3, pp 162-185
Freud S (1910i) The psycho-analytic view of psychogenic disturbance of vision. SE vol 11, pp 209-218
Freud S (1912e) Recommendations to physicians practising psycho-analysis. SE vol 12, pp 109-120
Freud S (1912-13) Totem and taboo. SE vol 13
Freud S (1914g) Remembering, repeating and working-through. SE vol 12, pp 145-156
Freud S (1915a) Observations on transference-love. SE vol 12, pp 157-171
Freud S (1915b) Thoughts for the times on war and death. SE vol 14, pp 273-300
Freud S (1915d) Repression. SE vol 14, pp 141-158
Freud S (1916d) Some charakter-types met with in psycho-analytic work. SE vol 14, pp 309-333
Freud S (1916-17) Introductory lectures on psycho-analysis. SE vols 15-16
Freud S (1918b) From the history of an infantile neurosis. SE vol 17, pp 1-122
Freud S (1919a) Lines of advance in psycho-analytic therapy. SE vol 17, pp 157-168
Freud S (1919h) The "Uncanny". SE vol 17, pp 217-252
Freud S (1919j) On the teaching of psycho-analysis in universities. SE vol 17, pp 169-173
Freud S (1920a) The psychogenesis of a case of homosexuality in an woman. SE vol 18, pp 145-172
Freud S (1920g) Beyond the pleasure principle. SE vol 18, pp 1-64
Freud S (1922b) Some neurotic mechanisms in jealousy, paranoia and homosexuality. SE vol 18, pp 221-232
Freud S (1923a) "Psycho-Analysis" and "Libido Theory". SE vol 18, pp 233-259
Freud S (1923b) The ego and the id. SE vol 19, pp 1-66
Freud S (1925h) Negation. SE vol 19, pp 233-239
Freud S (1926d) Inhibitions, symptoms and anxiety. SE vol 20, pp 75-172
Freud S (1926e) The question of lay analysis. SE vol 20, pp 177-250
Freud S (1927a) Postscript to the question of lay analysis. SE vol 20, pp 251-258
Freud S (1927c) The future of an illusion. SE vol 21, pp 1-56
Freud S (1927e) Fetishism. SE vol 21, pp 147-157
Freud S (1930a) Civilization and its discontents. SE vol 21, pp 57-145
Freud S (1931b) Female sexuality. SE vol 21, pp 221-243
Freud S (1933a) New introductory lectures on psycho-analysis. SE vol 22, pp 1-182
Freud S (1933b) Why war? SE vol 22, pp 195-215
Freud S (1937c) Analysis terminable and interminable. SE vol 23, pp 209-253

Freud S (1937d) Constructions in analysis. SE vol 23, pp 255-269
Freud S (1940a) An outline of psycho-analysis. SE vol 23, pp 139-207
Freud S (1940b) Some elementary lessons in psycho-analysis. SE vol 23, pp 279-286
Freud S (1955a [1907-08]) Original record of the case ('rat man'). SE vol 10, pp 251-318
Frick EM (1985) Latent and manifest effects of audiorecording in psychoanalytic psychotherapy. Yearbook Psychoanal Psychother 1: 151-175
Fromm E (1973) The anatomy of human destructiveness. Holt, Rinehardt and Winston, New York
Gadamer HG (1965) Wahrheit und Methode. Anwendung einer philosophischen Hermeneutik. Mohr, Tübingen
Gardiner M (1971) The wolf-man. Basic, New York
Garfield SL, Bergin AE (eds) (1986) Handbook of psychotherapy and behavior change, 3rd edn. Wiley, New York
Gaus E, Köhle K (1986) Psychosomatische Aspekte intensivmedizinischer Behandlungsverfahren. In: Uexküll T von (ed) Psychosomatische Medizin, 3rd edn. Urban and Schwarzenberg, Munich, pp 1157-1172
Gay P (1987) A godless Jew. Yale University Press, New Haven
Gebsattel V von (1954) Prologemena einer medizinischen Anthropologie. Springer, Berlin
Gedo JE (1983) Saints of scoundrels and the objectivity of the analyst. Psychoanal Inquiry 3: 609-622
Geist WB, Kächele H (1979) Zwei Traumserien in einer psychoanalytischen Behandlung. Jahrb Psychoanal 11: 138-165
Geleerd E (1963) Evaluation of Melanie Kleins "Narrative of a Child analysis". Int J Psychoanal 44: 493-513
Gill MM (1982) Analysis of transference. Vol I: Theory and technique. International Universities Press, New York
Gill MM (1983) The point of view of psychoanalysis. Energy discharge or person. Psychoanal Contemp Thought 6: 523-551
Gill MM (1984) Transference: a change in conception or only in emphasis? Psychoanal Inquiry 4: 489-523
Gill MM (1985) Discussion. A critique of Robert Lang's conception of transference. Yearbook Psychoanal Psychother 1: 177-187
Gill MM, Hoffman IZ (1982) A method for studying the analysis of aspects of the patient's experience in psychoanalysis and psychotherapy. J Am Psychoanal Assoc 30: 137-167
Gill MM, Simon J, Fink G, Endicott NA, Paul IH (1968) Studies in audio-recorded psychoanalysis. I. General considerations. J Am Psychoanal Assoc 16: 230-244
Giovacchini PL (1972) Tactics and techniques in psychoanalytic therapy. Hogarth, London
Glover E (1952) Research methods in psycho-analysis. Int J Psychoanal 33: 403-409
Glover E (1955) The technique of psychoanalysis. Baillière Tindall and Cox, London
Goffman E (1974) Stigma. Notes on the management of spoiled identity. Aronson, New York
Goudsmit W (1986) Delinquenz und Gesellschaft. Vandenhoeck and Ruprecht, Göttingen
Goudsmit W (1987) Bemerkungen zu ambulanten Behandlung von Persönlichkeitsstörungen. Z Psychoanal Theorie Praxis 2: 148-164
Gould RL (1970) Preventive psychiatry and the field theory of reality. J Am Psychoanal Assoc 18: 440-461
Göbel P (1980) Das Erleben in der Sprache und die Funktion der Metaphorik. Z Psychosom Psychoanal 26: 178-188
Göbel P (1986) Symbol und Metapher. Z Psychosom Med 32: 76-88
Görres A, Kasper W (1988) Tiefenpsychologische Deutung des Glaubens? Herder, Freiburg
Grassi E (1979) Die Macht der Phantasie. Zur Geschichte abendländischen Denkens. Athenäum, Königstein im Taunus
Grawe K (1988) Zurück zur psychotherapeutischen Einzelfallforschung. Z Klin Psychol 17: 4-5
Grey A, Fiscalini J (1987) Parallel processes as transference-countertransference interaction. Psychoanal Psychol 4: 131-144
Greenacre P (1953) Certain relationships between fetishism and the faulty development of the body image. Psychoanal Study Child 8: 79-98
Greenson RR (1959) Phobia, anxiety and depression. J Am Psychoanal Assoc 7: 663-674

Greenson RR (1967) The technique and practice of psychoanalysis, vol I. International Universities Press, New York

Grinberg L (1962) On a specific aspect of countertransference due to the patients projective identification. Int J Psychoanal 43: 436-440

Grinberg L (1979) Projective counteridentification and countertransference. In: Epstein L, Feiner AH (eds) Countertransference. Aronson, New York, pp 169-191

Groddeck G (1977 [1925]) The meaning of illness. In: Groddeck G (ed) The meaning of illness. Hogarth, London, pp 197-202

Grosskurth P (1986) Melanie Klein. Her world and her work. Maresfield Library, London

Grunberger B, Chasseguet-Smirgel (1979) Freud oder Reich? Psychoanalyse und Illusion. Ullstein, Frankfurt am Main

Grünbaum A (1984) The foundations of psychoanalysis. A philosophical critique. University of California Press, Berkeley

Grünbaum A (1985) Explications and implications of the placebo concept. In: White L, Tursky B, Schwartz GE (eds) Placebo: theory, research and mechanisms. Guilford, New York, pp 9-36

Grünbaum A (1987a) Psychoanalyse in wissenschaftstheoretischer Sicht. Zum Werk Sigmund Freuds und seiner Rezeption. Universitätsverlag, Konstanz

Grünbaum A (1987b) Psychoanalysis and theism. The Monist 70: 150-192

Guntrip H (1975) My experience of analysis with Fairbairn and Winnicott. Int Rev Psychoanal 2: 145-156

Gurman AS, Kniskern DP, Pinsof WM (1986) Research on process and outcome of material and family therapy. In: Garfield S, Bergin AE (eds) Handbook of psychotherapy and behavior change, 3rd edn. Wiley, New York, pp 565-624

Habermas J (1968) Knowledge and human interests. Beacon, Boston

Habermas J (1981) Theorie des kommunikativen Handelns. Suhrkamp, Frankfurt am Main

Haegglund TB (1978) Dying. A psychoanalytical study with special reference to individual creativity and defensive organization. International Universities Press, New York

Haesler L (1985) Zur Psychodynamik der Anniversery Reactions. Jahrb Psychoanal 17: 211-266

Häfner H (1987) Angst als Chance und als Krankheit. Fundamenta Psychiatrica 1: 196-204

Häfner H, Veiel H (1986) Epidemiologische Untersuchungen zu Angst und Depression. In: Helmchen H, Linden M (eds) Die Differenzierung von Angst und Depression. Springer, Berlin Heidelberg New York, pp 65-74

Hahn P, Jacob W (eds) (1987) Viktor von Weizsäcker zum 100. Geburtstag. Springer, Berlin Heidelberg New York

Hamilton NG (1986) Positive projective identification. Int J Psychoanal 67: 489-496

Hand I, Wittchen HU (eds) (1986) Panic and phobias. Empirical evidence of theoretical models and longterm effects of behavioral treatments. Springer, Berlin Heidelberg New York

Hartmann H (1939) Ich-Psychologie und Anpassungsproblem. Int Z Psychoanal 24: 62-135, reprinted in: Psyche 14: 81-164

Hartmann H (1960) Psychoanalysis and moral values. International Universities Press, New York

Hastedt H (1988) Das Leib-Seele-Problem. Suhrkamp, Frankfurt am Main

Head H (1920) Studies in neurology, vol 2. Oxford University Press, London

Heigl F, Heigl-Evers A (1984) Die Wertprüfung in der Psychoanalyse. Z Psychosom Med 30: 27-82

Heigl-Evers A (1966) Einige psychogenetische und psychodynamische Zusammenhänge beim Krankheitsbild des endogenen Ekzems. Z Psychosom Med 12: 163-178

Heimann P (1950) On countertransference. Int J Psychoanal 31: 81-84

Heimann P (1969) Gedanken zum Erkenntnisprozeß des Psychoanalytikers. Psyche 23: 2-24

Heimann P (1989 [1966]) Comments on the psychoanalytic concept of work. In: Tonnesmann M (ed) About children and children-no-longer. Collected papers 1942-1980 of Paula Heimann. Tavistock/Routledge, London, pp 191-205

Heimann P (1989 [1978]) On the necessity for an analyst to be natural with his patient. In: Tonnesmann M (ed) About children and children-no-longer. Collected papers 1942-1980 of Paula Heimann. Tavistock/Routledge, London, pp 311-323

Heinrich K (1986) „Anthropomorphe“. Stern, Frankfurt am Main

Heising G, Brieskorn M, Rost WD (1982) Sozialschicht und Gruppenpsychotherapie. Vandenhoeck and Ruprecht, Göttingen

Henseler H (1981) Behandlungsprobleme bei chronisch-suizidalen Patienten. In: Reimer C (ed) Suizid-Ergebnisse und Therapie. Springer, Berlin Heidelberg New York
Hilgard JR, Fisk F (1960) Disruption for adult ego identity as related to childhood loss of a mother through hospitalisation for psychosis. J Nerv Ment Dis 131: 47-57
Hilgard JR, Newman M, Fisk F (1960) Strength of adult ego following childhood bereavement. Am J Orthopsychiatry 30: 788-798
Hirsch ED jr (1967) Validity in interpretation. Yale University Press, New Haven
Hirsch ED jr (1976) The aims of interpretation. University of Chicago Press, Chicago
Hoffer A (1985) Toward a definition of psychoanalytic neutrality. J Am Psychoanal Assoc 33: 771-795
Hoffer W (1950) Three psychological criteria for the termination of treatment. Int J Psychoanal 31: 194-195
Hoffmann SO (1983) Die niederfrequente psychoanalytische Langzeittherapie. Konzeption, Technik und Versuch einer Abgrenzung gegenüber dem klassischen Verfahren. In: Hoffmann SO (ed) Deutung und Beziehung. Kritische Beiträge zur Behandlungskonzeption und Technik in der Psychoanalyse. Fischer, Frankfurt am Main, pp 183-193
Hoffmann SO (1986) Die Ethologie, das Realtrauma und die Neurose. Z Psychosom Med 32: 8-26
Hoffmann SO (1987) Buchbesprechung von Panic and Phobias. Hand I, Wittchen HU (eds). Nervenarzt 58: 528
Hohage R (1986) Geschenke in der psychoanalytischen Therapie. Prax Psychother Psychosom 31: 138-144
Hohage R, Thomä H (1982) Über das Auftauchen von Erinnerungen als Ergebnis fokussierter Traumdeutung. Z Psychosom Med Psychoanal 28: 385-392
Hohage R, Kübler C (1987) Die Veränderung von emotionaler Einsicht im Verlauf einer Psychoanalyse. Z Psychosom Med Psychoanal 33: 145-154
Holland NN (1975) An identity for the Rat Man. Int Rev Psychoanal 2: 157-169
Hübner K (1985) Die Wahrheit des Mythos. Beck, Munich
Isaacs S (1939) Criteria for interpretation. Int J Psychoanal 20: 853-880
Jacob P jr (1981) Application: the San Francisco Project - the analyst at work. In: Wallerstein RS (ed) Becoming a psychoanalyst. A study of psychoanalytic supervision. International Universities Press, New York, pp 191-210
Jacobson E (1953) Contribution to the metapsychology of cyclothymic depression. In: Greenacre P (ed) Affective disorders. International Universities Press, New York, pp 49-83
Jacobson E (1971) Depression. International Universities Press, New York
Jiménez JP (1988) Die Wiederholung des Traumas in der Übertragung. Katharsis oder Durcharbeiten? Forum der Psychoanalyse 4: 190-204
Joas H (1985) Das Problem der Intersubjektivität. Suhrkamp, Frankfurt am Main
Jones E (1916) The theory of symbolism. Br J Psychol 9: 181-229
Jones E (1927) The early development of female sexuality. Int J Psychoanal 8: 459-472
Jones E (1954, 1955, 1957) The life and work of Sigmund Freud, vols 1-3. Hogarth, London
Joraschky P (1983) Das Körperschema und das Körper-Selbst als Regulationsprinzipien der Organismus-Umwelt-Interaktion. Minerva Publikation Saur, Munich
Joseph ED (1979) Comments on the therapeutic action of psychoanalysis. J Am Psychoanal Assoc 27: 71-80
Joseph ED (1984) Psychoanalysis: the vital issues. International Universities Press, New York
Junker H (1972) Ehepaargruppentherapien mit Patienten aus der oberen Unterschicht. Psyche 5: 370-388
Junker H (1987) General comments on the difficulties of retranslating Freud into English, based on the reading experiences of a German analyst with the Standard Edition (Strachey). Int Rev Psychoanal 14: 317-320
Kächele H (1981) Zur Bedeutung der Krankengeschichte in der klinisch-psychoanalytischen Forschung. Jahrb Psychoanal 12: 118-178
Kächele H (1982) Pflanzen als Metaphern für Selbst- und Objektrepräsentanzen. In: Schempp D, Krampen M (eds) Mensch und Pflanze. Müller, Karlsruhe, pp 26-28
Kächele H (1985) Mißerfolge in der Psychotherapie aus psychoanalytischer Sicht. Verhaltensmodifikation 5: 235-248

Kächele H (1988a) Spezifische und unspezifische Wirkfaktoren in der Psychotherapie. Prax Psychother Psychosom 33: 1-11
Kächele H (1988b) Clinical and scientific aspects of the Ulm process model of psychoanalysis. Int J Psychoanal 69: 65-73
Kächele H, Fiedler I (1985) Ist der Erfolg einer psychotherapeutischen Behandlung vorhersehbar? Psychother Med Psychol 35: 201-206
Kächele H, Schaumburg C, Thomä H (1973) Verbatimprotokolle als Mittel in der psychotherapeutischen Verlaufsforschung. Psyche 27: 902-927
Kächele H, Wolfsteller H, Hössle I (1985) Psychotherapie im Rückblick - Patienten kommentieren ihre Behandlung. Prax Psychother Psychosom 30: 309-317
Kächele H, Thomä H, Ruberg W, Grünzig HJ (1988e) Audio-recordings of he psychoanalytic dialogue: scientific, clinical and ethical problems. In: Dahl H, Kächele H, Thomä H (eds) Psychoanalytic process research strategies. Springer, Berlin Heidelberg New York, pp 179-194
Kafka JS (1977) On reality. An examination of object constancy, ambiguity, paradox and time. Psychiatry Human 2: 133-158
Kant I (1965 [1781]) The critique of pure reason. St. Martins, New York
Kanzer M, Glenn J (eds) (1980) Freud and his patients. Aronson, New York
Kaplan HF (1982) Ist die Psychoanalyse wertfrei? Huber, Bern
Keller-Bauer F (1984) Metaphorisches Verstehen. Eine linguistische Rekonstruktion metaphorischer Kommunikation. Linguistische Arbeiten, vol 142. Niemeyer, Tübingen
Kernberg OF (1965) Notes on countertransference. J Am Psychoanal Assoc 13: 38-56
Kernberg OF (1972) Critique of the Kleinian school. In: Giovacchini PL (ed) Tactics and techniques in psychoanalytic therapy. Hogarth, London, pp 62-93
Kernberg OF, Bursteine ED, Coyne L, Appelbaum A, Horwitz L, Voth H (1972) Psychotherapy and psychoanalysis. Final report of the Menninger Foundation. Bull Menn Clin 36: 3-275
Kernberg OF (1977) The structural diagnosis of borderline personality organization. In: Hartocollis P (ed) Borderline personality disorders. International Universities Press, New York, pp 87-121
Kernberg OF (1987) Projection and projective identification: developmental and clinical aspects. J Am Psychoanal Assoc 35: 795-819
Kerz JP (1987) Verkehrte Einsicht. Forum Psychoanal 3: 328-331
Kettner M (1987) Erwachen aus dem dogmatischen Schlummer. Psyche 41: 749-760
Khan MMR (1974 [1963]) The concept of cumulative trauma. In: Khan MMR (ed) The privacy of the self. International Universities Press, New York, pp 42-58
Kierkegaard S (1957) Die Krankheit zum Tode. Diederichs, Düsseldorf
Klann G (1979) Die Rolle affektiver Prozesse in der Dialogstruktur. In: Flader D, Wodak-Leodolter R (eds) Therapeutische Kommunikation. Scriptor, Königstein, pp 117-155
Klauber J (1966) Die Struktur der psychoanalytischen Sitzung als Leitlinie für die Deutungsarbeit. Psyche 20: 29-39
Klauber J (1987) Illusion and spontaneity in psychoanalysis. Free Association Books, London
Klein DF (1981) Anxiety reconceptualized. In: Klein DF, Rabkin J (eds) Anxiety: new research and changing concepts. Raven, New York, pp 235-265
Klein DF, Ross DC, Cohen P (1987) Panic and avoidance in agoraphobia. Arch Gen Psychiatry 44: 377-385
Klein DF (1988) Reply. Arch Gen Psychiatry 45: 389-392
Klein GS (1976) Psychoanalytic theory. An exploration of essentials. International University Press, New York
Klein M (1932) The psycho-analysis of children. The International Psycho-Analytical Library, No 22. Hogarth, London
Klein M (1935) A contribution to the psychogenesis of manic-depressive states. Int J Psychoanal 16: 145-274
Klein M (1946) Notes on some schizoid mechanisms. Int J Psychoanal 27: 99-110
Klein M (1957) Envy and gratitude. A study of unconscious sources. Basic, New York
Klein M (1961) Narrative of a child analysis. Hogarth, London
Klein M (1952) Some theoretical conclusions regarding the emotional life of the infant. In: Klein M, Heimann P, Isaacs S, Riviere J Developments in psycho-analysis. The International Psycho-Analytical Library, No 43. Hogarth, London

Klein M, Heimann P, Isaacs S, Riviere J (1952) Developments in psycho-analysis. The International Psycho-Analytical Library, No 43. Hogarth, London
Klerman GK, Weissman MM, Rounsaville BJ, Chevron ES (1984) Interpersonal psychotherapy of depression. Basic, New York
Köhle K, Simons C, Kubanek B (1986) Zum Umgang mit unheilbar Kranken. In: Uexküll T von (ed) Psychosomatische Medizin, 3rd edn. Urban and Schwarzenberg, Munich, pp 1203-1241
Köhler L (1982) Neuere Forschungsergebnisse psychoanalytischer Mutter/Kind-Beobachtungen und ihrer Bedeutung für das Verständnis von Übertragung und Gegenübertragung. Psychoanalyse 3: 238-265
Köhler L (1985) On selfobject countertransference. Annu Psychoanal 12/13: 39-56
Köhler L (1988) Probleme des Psychoanalytikers mit Selbstobjektübertragungen. In: Kutter P, Paramo-Ortega R, Zagermann P (eds) Die psychoanalytische Haltung. Internationale Psychoanalyse, Munich, pp 331-348
Kohut H (1959) Introspection, empathy, and psychoanalysis. An examination of the relationship between mode of observation and theory. J Am Psychoanal Assoc 7: 459-483
Kohut H (1971) The analysis of the self. A systematic approach to the psychoanalytic treatment of narcisstic personality disorders. International Universities Press, New York
Kolakowski L (1974) Die Gegenwärtigkeit des Mythos. Piper, Munich
Köller W (1986) Dimensionen des Metaphernproblems. Z Semiotik 8: 379-410
König K (1981) Angst und Persönlichkeit. Vandenhoek and Ruprecht, Göttingen
Kordy H, Senf W (1985) Überlegungen zur Evaluation psychotherapeutischer Behandlungen. Psychother Med Psychol 35: 207-212
Körner J (1985) Vom Erklären zum Verstehen in der Psychoanalyse. Vandenhoeck and Ruprecht, Göttingen
Krause R (1983) Zur Onto- und Phylogenese des Affektsystems und ihrer Beziehungen zu psychischen Störungen. Psyche 37: 1016-1043
Krause R, Lütolf P (1988) Facial indicators of transference processes within psychoanalytic treatment. In: Dahl H, Kächele H, Thomä H (eds) Psychoanalytic process research strategies. Springer, Berlin Heidelberg New York, pp 241-256
Kris E (1947) The nature of psychoanalytic propositions and their validation. In: Hook S, Konvitz MR (eds) Freedom and experience: essays presented to Horace M. Kallen. Cornell University Press, New York, pp 239-259
Kris E (1956) On some vicissitudes of insight in psychoanalysis. Int J Psychoanal 37: 445-455
Krueger DW (ed) (1986) The last taboo. Money as symbol and reality in psychotherapy and psychoanalysis. Brunner/Mazel, New York
Kubie LS (1952) Problems and techniques of psychoanalytic validation and progress. In: Pumpian-Mindlin E (ed) Psychoanalysis as science. The Hixon lectures on the scientific status of psychoanalysis. Basic, New York, pp 46-124
Kubie LS (1953) The central representation of the symbolic process in psychosomatic disorders. Psychosom Med 15: 1-15
Kubie LS (1958) Research into the process of supervision in psychoanalysis. Psychoanal Q 27: 226-236
Kubie L (1974) The drive to become both sexes. Psychoanal Q 43: 349-426
Küchenhoff J (1984) Dysmorphophobie. Nervenarzt 55: 122-126
Kuhns R (1983) Psychoanalytic theory of art. Columbia University Press, New York
Kuiper PC (1969) Liebe und Sexualität im Leben der Studenten. Huber, Bern
Küng H (1979) Freud and the problem of God. Yale University Press, New Haven
Küng H (1987) Freud und die Zukunft der Religion. Piper, Munich
Kurz G (1982) Metapher, Allegorie, Symbol. Vandenhoeck and Ruprecht, Göttingen
Kutter P (1981) Der Basiskonflikt der Psychosomatose und seine therapeutischen Implikationen. Jahrb Psychoanal 13: 93-114
Lacan J (1937) The looking-glass phase. Int J Psychoanal 18: 78
Lacan J (1949) Le stade du miroir comme formateur de la function de je. Revue francaise de Psychanalyse 13: 449-455
Lacan J (1975) Schriften 1. Suhrkamp, Frankfurt am Main
Lacan J (1980) A Lacanian psychosis. Interview by Jacques Lacan. In: Schneiderman S (ed) Returning to Freud. Yale University Press, New Haven, pp 19-41

Lampl-de Groot J (1953) Re-evaluation of the role of the oedipus complex. Int J Psychoanal 33: 333

Lampl-de Groot J (1976) Personal experience with psychoanalytic technique and theory during the last half century. Psychoanal Study Child 37: 283-296

Lang H (1986) Die Sprache und das Unbewußte. Jacques Lacans Grundlegung der Psychoanalyse, 2nd edn. Suhrkamp, Frankfurt am Main

Langer SK (1957) Philosophy in a new key. Harvard University Press, Cambridge

Laplanche J, Pontalis JB (1973) The language of psycho-analysis. Hogarth, London

Lasch C (1979) Haven in a heartless world. The family besieged. Basic, New York

Laufer M (1984) Adolescence and developmental breakdown. A psychoanalytic view. Yale University Press, New Haven

Leary DE (ed) (1990) Metaphors in the history of psychology. Harvard University Press, Cambridge

Leavy SA (1980) The psychoanalytic dialogue. Yale University Press, New Haven

Lelliott P, Marks I (1988) The cause and treatment of agoraphobia. Arch Gen Psychiatry 45: 388-392

Leodolter R (1975) Das Sprachverhalten von Angeklagten bei Gericht. Scriptor, Kronberg

Lerner RM (1984) Jugendliche als Produzenten ihrer eigenen Entwicklung. In: Olbrich E, Todt E (eds) Probleme des Jugendalters. Neuere Sichtweisen. Springer, Berlin Heidelberg New York, pp 69-88

Leuzinger-Bohleber M (1988) Veränderungen kognitiver Prozesse in Psychoanalysen. Fünf Einzelfallstudien. PSZ-Drucke. Springer, Berlin Heidelberg New York

Lewin BD (1933) The body as phallus. Psychoanal Q 2: 24-47

Lewin BD (1971) Metaphor, mind, and manikin. Psychoanal Q 40: 6-39

Lewin BD, Ross H (1960) Psychoanalytic education in the United States. Norton, New York

Lewy E, Rapaport D (1944) The psychoanalytic concept of memory and its relation to recent memory theories. Psychoanal Q 13: 16-42

Lichtenberg J (1983a) Psychoanalysis and infant research. Analytic Press, Hillsdale

Lichtenberg J (1983b) The influence of values and value judgement on the psychoanalytic encounter. Psychoanal Inquiry 3: 647-664

Lichtenstein H (1961) Identity and sexuality. J Am Psychoanal Assoc 9: 179-260

Lipowski ZJ (1976) Psychosomatic medicine: an overview. In: Hill OW (ed) Modern trends in psychosomatic medicine, III. Butterworths, London, pp 1-20

Lipowski ZJ (1977) Psychosomatic medicine in the seventies: an overview. Am J Psychiatry 134: 233-242

Lipton SD (1982) Essays on Paul Dewald's "The psychoanalytic progress". Contemp Psychoanal 18: 349-372

Little M (1951) Counter-transference and the patient's response to it. Int J Psychoanal 32: 32-40

Loewald HW (1960) On the therapeutic action of psychoanalysis. Int J Psychoanal 41: 16-33

Loewald HW (1980a) Papers on psychoanalysis. Yale University Press, New Haven

Loewald HW (1980b) Regression: some general considerations. In: Nedelmann C, Jappe G (eds) Zur Psychoanalyse der Objektbeziehungen. Fromann-Holzboog, Stuttgart, pp 189-206

London NJ, Rosenblatt AD (eds) (1987) Transference neurosis evolution or obsolescence. Psychoanal Inquiry 7: 587-598

Lorenz K, Leyhausen P (1968) Antriebe tierischen und menschlichen Verhaltens. Piper, Munich

Lorenzer A (1970) Sprachzerstörung und Rekonstruktion. Vorarbeiten zu einer Metatheorie der Psychoanalyse. Suhrkamp, Frankfurt am Main

Lorenzer A (1986) Tiefenhermeneutische Kulturanalyse. In: Lorenzer A (ed) Kultur-Analysen. Psychoanalytische Studien zur Kultur. Fischer, Frankfurt am Main, pp 11-98

Löw-Beer M (1988) Ist die Leugnung von Willensfreiheit eine Selbsttäuschung? In: König T (ed) Satre, ein Kongress. Rowohlt, Reinbek, pp 55-73

Löw-Beer M, Thomä H (1988) Zum Verhältnis von Einsicht und Veränderung. Forum Psychoanal 4: 1-18

Luborsky L (1967) Momentary forgetting during psychotherapy and psychoanalysis: a theory and a research method. In: Holt RR (ed) Motives and thought. Psychoanalytic essays in honor of David Rapaport. Psychological issues, vol V, no 2-3, monograph 18/19. International Universities Press, New York, pp 175-217

Luborsky L (1984) Principles of psychoanalytic psychotherapy. A manual for supportive-expressive treatment. Basic, New York

Luborsky L, Schimek J (1964) Psychoanalytic theories of therapeutic and developmental change implications for assessment. In: Worchel P, Byrne D (eds) Personality change. Wiley, New York

Luborsky L, Spence DP (1978) Quantitative research on psychoanalytic therapy. In: Garfield SL, Bergin AE (eds) Handbook of psychotherapy and behavior change: an empirical analysis, 2nd edn. Wiley, New York , pp 331-368

Luckmann TH (1979) Persönliche Identität, soziale Rolle und Rollendistanz. In: Marquardt O, Stierle K (eds) Identität. Fink, Munich, pp 293-313

M'Uzan M de (1977) Zur Psychologie des psychosomatisch Kranken. Psyche 31: 318-332

MacFarlane K, Waterman J, Conerly S, Durfee M, Long S (eds) (1986) Sexual abuse of young children: evaluation and treatment. Guilford, New York

Mahler MS, Pine F, Bergmann A (1975) The psychological birth of the human infant. Basic, New York

Mahony PJ (1977) The place of psychoanalytic treatment in the history of discourse. Psychoanal Contemp Thought 2: 77-111

Mahony PJ (1984) Cries of the Wolf Man. International Universities Press, New York

Mahony PJ (1986) Freud and the Rat Man. Yale University Press, New Haven

Mahony PJ (1987) Freud as a writer. Yale University Press, New Haven

Mahony PJ, Singh R (1975) The interpretation of dreams, semiology and chomskian linguistics: a radical critique. Psychoanal Stud Child 30: 221-241

Mahony PJ, Singh R (1979) Some issues in linguistics and psychoanalysis. Reflections on Marshall Edelson's Language and interpretation in psychoanalysis. Psychoanal Contemp Thought 2: 437-446

Margolin SG (1953) Genetic and dynamic psychophysiological determinants of pathophysiological processes. In: Deutsch F (ed) The psychosomatic concept in psychoanalysis. International Univrsities Press, New York, pp 3-34

Margraf J, Ehlers A, Roth W (1986) Panic attacks: theoretical models and empirical evidence. In: Hand I, Wittchen HU (eds) Panic and phobias. Springer, Berlin Heidelberg New York Tokyo, pp 31-43

Marquard O (1987) Transzendenter Idealismus. Romantische Naturphilosophie, Psychoanalyse. Verlag für Philosophie, Köln

Marten R (1983) Die psychoanalytische Situation und der Augen-Blick. In: Hoffmann SO (ed) Deutung und Beziehung. Kritische Beiträge zur Behandlungskonzeption und Technik in der Psychoanalyse. Fischer, Frankfurt am Main, pp 44-70

Marten R (1988) Der menschliche Mensch. Schöningh, Paderborn

Martini P (1953) Methodenlehre der therapeutisch-klinischen Forschung. Springer, Berlin Göttingen Heidelberg

Marty P (1968) A major process of somatization: the progressive disorganization. Int J Psychoanal 49: 243-249

Marty P (1969) Notes clinique et hypotheses à propos de l'économie de l'allergie. Rev Franc Psychoanal 33: 244-253

Marty P (1974) Die „allergische Objektbeziehung". In: Brede K (ed) Einführung in die Psychosomatische Medizin: klinische und therapeutische Beiträge. Fischer Athenäum, Frankfurt am Main, pp 420-445

Marty P, M'Uzan M de (1963) La „pensée opératoire". Rev Franc Psychoanal 27: 345-356

Marty P, M'Uzan M de, David C (1963) L'investigation psychosomatique. Presses Universitaires de France, Paris

Masling J (ed) (1983) Empirical studies of psychoanalytical theories. Vol I. Analytic Press, Hillsdale

Masling J (ed) (1986) Empirical studies of psychoanalytical theories. Vol II. Analytic Press, Hillsdale

Maurer Y (1987) Körperzentrierte Psychotherapie. Hippokrates, Stuttgart

Mayman M, Faris M (1960) Early memories as expressions of relationship paradigms. Am J Orthopsychiat 30: 507-520

McDougall J (1974) The psychosoma and the psychoanalytic process. Int Rev Psychoanal 1: 437-459

McDougall J (1985) Plädoyer für eine gewisse Abnormalität. Suhrkamp, Frankfurt am Main
McDougall J (1987) Ein Körper für zwei. Forum Psychoanal 3: 265-287
McDougall J, Lebovici S (1969) Dialogue with Sammy. Hogarth, London
McDougall W (1928) Grundlagen einer Sozialpsychologie. Fischer, Jena
McLaughlin JT (1982) Issues stimulated by the 32nd Congress. Int J Psychoanal 63: 229-240
McLaughlin JT (1987) The play of transference: some reflections on enactment in the psychoanalytic situation. J Am Psychoanal Assoc 35: 557-582
Mead GH (1934) Mind, self, and society. From the standpoint of a social behaviorist. University of Chicago Press, Chicago
Meehl PE (1983) Subjectivity in psychoanalytic inference: the nagging persistence of Wilhelm Fliess's Achensee question. In: Earman J (ed) Testing scientific theories. Minnesota Studies in the Philosophy of Science, vol 10. University of Minnesota Press, Minneapolis, pp 349-411
Meerwein F (1987) Bemerkungen zur Metapsychologie schwerer Krebserkrankungen. Bulletin der schweizerischen Gesellschaft für Psychoanalyse 23: 2-12
Meissner WW (1980) A note on projective identification. J Am Psychoanal Assoc 28: 43-67
Meissner WW (1983) Values in the psychoanalytic situation. Psychoanal Inquiry 3: 577-598
Meissner WW (1984) Psychoanalysis and religious experience. Yale University Press, New Haven
Meltzer D (1967) The psychoanalytic process. Heinemann, London
Meltzer D (1978) The Kleinian development: Part II, Richard week-by-week. Clunie, Perthshire
Mendelson M, Hirsch S, Weber CS (1956) A critical examination of some recent theoretical models in psychosomatic medicine. Z Psychosom Med 18: 363-373
Menne K, Schröter K (eds) (1980) Psychoanalyse und Unterschicht. Soziale Herkunft - ein Hindernis für die psychoanalytische Behandlung? Suhrkamp, Frankfurt am Main
Menninger KA, Holzman PS (1958) Theory of psychoanalytic technique. Basic, New York
Mentzos S (ed) (1985) Angstneurose. Fischer, Frankfurt am Main
Mergenthaler E (1985) Textbank systems. Springer, Berlin Heidelberg New York
Merlan P (1945) Brentano and Freud. J Hist Ideas 6: 375-377
Merleau-Ponty M (1965) Primacy of conception. Northwestern University Press, Chicago
Mester H (1982) Der Wunsch einer Frau nach Veränderung der Busengröße. - Ein Beitrag zur Frage der Dysmorphophobie. Z Psychosom Med Psychoanal 28: 69-91
Meyer AE (1981) Psychoanalytische Prozeßforschung zwischen der Skylla der „Verkürzung" und der Charybdis der „systematischen akustischen Lücke". Z Psychosom Med Psychoanal 27: 103-116
Meyer AE (1985) Vergleich psychosomatischer Modelle. Mitteilungen des DKPM 8: 46-57
Meyer AE (1987) Das Leib-Seele-Problem aus der Sicht eines Psychosomatikers. Modelle und ihre Widersprüche. Psychother Med Psychol 37: 367-375
Meyer AE (1988) What makes psychoanalysts tick? In: Dahl H, Kächele H, Thomä H (eds) Psychoanalytic process research strategies. Springer, Berlin Heidelberg New York, pp 273-290
Miall DS (ed) (1982) Metaphor: problems and perspectives. Harvester, Sussex/ Humanities Press, Atlantic Highlands
Michels R (1988) The future of psychoanalysis. Psychoanal Q 57: 167-185
Miller JA (ed) (1988) The seminar of Jacques Lacan, vol 1 and 2. Cambridge University Press, Cambridge
Mintz J (1971) The anniversary reaction: a response to the unconcious sense of time. J Am Psychoanal Assoc 19: 720-735
Minuchin S (1977) Familie und Familientherapie. Lambertus, Freiburg
Mitscherlich A (1966) Krankheit als Konflikt. Studien zur psychosomatischen Medizin, vol 1. Suhrkamp, Frankfurt am Main
Mitscherlich A (1967) Krankheit als Konflikt. Studien zur psychosomatischen Medizin, vol 2. Suhrkamp, Frankfurt am Main
Mitscherlich M (1983) Zur Theorie und Therapie des Torticollis. In: Studt HH (ed) Psychosomatik in Forschung und Praxis. Urban and Schwarzenberg, Munich, pp 401-410
Mittelstraß J (1984) Versuch über den sokratischen Dialog. In: Stierle K, Warning R (eds) Das Gespräch. Fink, Munich, pp 11-27
Momigliano LN (1987) A spell in Vienna - but was Freud a Freudian? Int Rev Psychoanal 14: 373-389

Morgenthaler F (1978) Technik. Zur Dialektik der psychoanalytischen Praxis. Syndikat, Frankfurt am Main
Moser T (1986) Das erste Jahr. Eine psychoanalytische Behandlung. Suhrkamp, Frankfurt am Main
Moser T (1987) Der Psychoanalytiker als sprechende Attrappe. Eine Streitschrift. Suhrkamp, Frankfurt am Main
Moser U (1962) Übertragungsprobleme in der Psychoanalyse eines chronisch schweigenden Charakterneurotikers. Psyche 15: 592-624
Moser U (1984) Beiträge zu einer psychoanalytischen Theorie der Affekte. Ein Interaktionsmodell, part 2. Berichte aus der Interdisziplinären Konfliktforschungsstelle, Universität Zürich, no 14
Moser U, Zeppelin I von, Schneider H (1981) Objektbeziehungen, Affekte und Abwehrprozesse. Aspekte einer Regulierungstheorie mentaler Prozesse. Berichte aus der interdisziplinären Konfliktforschungsstelle, Universität Zürich, no 9
Müller-Braunschweig H (1986) Psychoanalysis and body. In: Brähler E (ed) Body experience. Springer, Berlin Heidelberg New York, pp 19-33
Murphy C, Messer D (1979) Mothers, infants and pointing: a study of gesture. In: Schaffer H (ed) Studies in mother-infant interaction. Academic, New York, pp 325-354
Muschg W (1930) Freud als Schriftsteller. Die psychoanalytische Bewegung 2: 467-509
Nase E, Scharfenberg J (1977) Psychoanalyse und Religion. Wissenschaftliche Buchgesellschaft, Darmstadt
Nedelmann C (1980) Behandlungsziel und Gesundheitsbegriff der Psychoanalyse. In: Bach H (ed) Der Krankheitsbegriff in der Psychoanalyse. Bestimmungsversuche auf einem Psychoanalytiker-Kongreß der Deutschen Gesellschaft für Psychotherapie, Psychosomatik und Tiefenpsychologie 1980. Vandenhoeck and Ruprecht, Göttingen, pp 55-67
Needles W (1959) Gesticulation and speech. Int J Psychoanal 40: 291-294
Neisser U (1979) Kognition und Wirklichkeit. Prinzipien und Implikationen der kognitiven Psychologie. Klett-Cotta, Stuttgart
Nemiah JC, Sifneos PE (1970) Psychosomatic illness: a problem in communication. Recent research in psychosomatic. Psychother Psychosom 18: 154-160
Neudert L, Grünzig HJ, Thomä H (1987) Change in self-esteem during psychoanalysis: a single case study. In: Cheshire NM, Thomä H (eds) Self, symptoms and psychotherapy. Wiley, New York, pp 243-265
Neumann H (1987) Ein Ohr für den Partner. Forum Psychoanaly 3: 112-126
Niederland WG (1959) The "miracled up" world of Schreber's childhood. Psychoanal Study Child 14: 383-413
Nietzsche F (1973) Sämtliche Werke, vol 1, Morgenröte. Wissenschaftliche Buchgesellschaft, Darmstadt
Ogden TH (1979) On projective identification. Int J Psychoanal 60: 357-373
Olbrich E, Todt E (1984) Probleme des Jugendalters. Neuere Sichtweisen. Springer, Berlin Heidelberg New York
Olinick SL (1964) The negative therapeutic reaction. Int J Psychoanal 45: 540-548
Ornston D (1982) Strachey's influence. A preliminary report. Int J Psychoanal 63: 409-426
Ornston D (1985a) Freud's conception is different from Strachey's. J Am Psychoanal Assoc 33: 379-412
Ornston D (1985b) The invention of "cathexis" and Strachey's strategy. Int Rev Psychoanal 12: 391-412
Ortony A (ed) (1979) Metaphor and thought. Harvard University Press, Cambridge
Ostow M (1962) Drugs in psychoanalysis and psychotherapy. Basic, New York
Overbeck G (1977) Das psychosomatische Symptom. Psyche 31: 333-354
Paivio A (1971) Imagery and verbal processes. Holt, Rinehardt and Winston, New York
Palazzoli Selvini M (1986a) Towards a general model of psychotic family games. J Marital Family Therapy 12: 339-349
Palazzoli Selvini M (1986b) Rejoinder to Anderson. J Marital Family Therapy 12: 355-357
Parin P, Parin-Matthèy G (1983) Medicozentrismus in der Psychoanalyse. Eine notwendige Revision der Neurosenlehre und ihre Relevanz für die Theorie der Behandlungstechnik. In: Hoffmann SO (ed) Deutung und Beziehung. Kritische Beiträge zur Behandlungskonzeption und Technik in der Psychoanalyse. Fischer, Frankfurt am Main, pp 86-106

Perrez M (1972) Ist die Psychoanalyse eine Wissenschaft? Huber, Bern
Perrez M, Otto J (eds) (1978) Symptomverschiebung. Ein Mythos oder ein unklar gestelltes Problem? Müller, Salzburg
Peterfreund E (1983) The process of psychoanalytic therapy. Models and strategies. Analytic, Hillsdale
Peterfreund E (1986) Reply to Eagle and Wolitzky. Psychoanal Contemp Thought 9: 103-124
Petermann F (1982) Einzelfalldiagnose und klinische Praxis. Kohlhammer, Stuttgart
Petzold E (1979) Familienkonfrontationstherapie bei Anorexia nervosa. Verlag für Medizinische Psychologie, Göttingen
Pfandl L (1935) Der Narzißbegriff. Versuch einer neuen Deutung. Imago 21: 279-310
Pfeffer AZ (1959) A procedure for evaluating the results of psychoanalysis. A preliminary report. J Am Psychoanal Assoc 7: 418-444
Pfeffer AZ (1961) Follow-up study of a satisfactory analysis. J Am Psychoanal Assoc 9: 698-718
Pfeffer AZ (1963) The meaning of the analyst after analysis. A contribution to the theory of therapeutic results. J Am Psychoanal Assoc 11: 229-244
Pfeifer R, Leuzinger-Bohleber M (1986) Applications of cognitive science methods to psychoanalysis: a case study and some theory. Int Rev Psychoanal 13: 221-240
Pfister O (1944) Das Christentum und die Angst. Artemis, Zürich
Pfister O (1977 [1928]) Die Illusion einer Zukunft. In: Nase E, Scharfenberg J (eds) Psychoanalyse und Religion. Wissenschaftliche Buchgesellschaft, Darmstadt, pp 101-141
Philippopoulos GS (1979) The analysis of a case of dysmorphophobia (psychopathology and psychodynamics). Can J Psychiatry 24: 397-401
Philipps JH (1962) Psychoanalyse und Symbolik. Huber, Bern
Pines M (1985) On the question of revision of the Standard Edition of Freud's writing. Int J Psychoanal 66: 1-2
Plato (nd) Sämtliche Werke, vol 1. Das Gastmahl. Schneider, Berlin
Pollock GH (1971) Temporal anniversary manifestations: hour, day, holiday. Psychoanal Q 40: 123-131
Pollock GH (1977) The psychosomatic specificity concept: its evolution and re-evaluation. Annu Psychoanal 5: 141-168
Porder MS (1987) Projective identification: an alternative hypothesis. Psychoanal Q 56: 431-451
Pribilla O (1980) Arztrechtliche Fragen und Probleme in der Psychotherapie. Dt Ärztebl 38: 2250-2254
Pulver SE (1987a) Prologue to "How theory shapes technique: perspectives on a clinical study". Psychoanal Inquiry 7: 141-145
Pulver SE (1987b) Epilogue to "How theory shapes technique: perspectives on a clinical study". Psychoanal Inquiry 7: 289-299
Quervain PF de (1978) Psychoanalyse und dialektische Theologie. Huber, Bern
Racker H (1957) The meanings and uses of countertransference. Psychoanal Q 26: 303-357
Racker H (1968) Transference and countertransference. International Universities Press, New York
Rad M von (1987) Diskussionsbemerkung. In: Hahn P, Jacob W (ed) Viktor von Weizsäcker zum 100. Geburtstag. Springer, Berlin Heidelberg New York, pp 163-165
Rager G (1988) Das Menschenbild im materialistischen Emergentismus von Bunge. Z Klin Psychol, Psychopath, Psychother 36: 368-373
Rangell L (1959) The nature of conversion. J Am Psychoanal Assoc 7: 632-662
Rangell L (1968) A further attempt to resolve the "problem of anxiety". J Am Psychoanal Assoc 16: 371-404
Rangell L (1984) The analyst at work. The Madrid congress. Synthesis and critique. Int J Psychoanal 65: 125-140
Rank O (1914) Der Doppelgänger. Imago 3: 97-164
Rank O (1924) Eine Neurosenanalyse in Träumen. Internationaler Psychoanalytischer Verlag, Leipzig
Rapaport D (1942) Emotions and memory. Williams and Wilkins, Baltimore
Rapaport D (1953) Paul Schilder's contribution to the theory of thought-processes. Translator's foreword. In: Schilder P (ed) Medical psychology. International Universities Press, New York, pp 7-16

Rapaport D (1960) The structure of psychoanalytic theory: a systematizing attempt. Psychol Issues, no 6. International Universities Press, New York
Rapaport D (1967) A theoretical analysis of the superego concept. In: Gill MM (ed) The collected papers of David Rapaport. Basic Books, New York, pp 685-709
Redlich FC, Hollingshead AB (1958) Social classes and mental illness: a community study. Wiley, New York
Reed GS (1987) Scientific and polemical aspects of the term "transference neurosis" in psychoanalysis. Psychoanal Inquiry 7: 465-483
Rehberg KS (1985) Die Theorie der Intersubjektivität als eine Lehre vom Menschen. In: Joas H (ed) Das Problem der Intersubjektivität. Neuere Beiträge zum Werk GH Meads. Suhrkamp, Frankfurt am Main
Reich W (1958 [1933]) Character analysis. Vision, London
Reider N (1972) Metaphor as interpretation. Int J Psychoanal 53: 463-469
Reiter L (1973) Zur Bedeutung der Sprache und Sozialisation für die Psychotherapie von Patienten aus der sozialen Unterschicht. In: Strotzka H (ed) Neurose, Charakter, soziale Umwelt. Kindler, Munich, pp 157-179
Rentrop E, Straschill M (1986) Der Einfluß emotionaler Faktoren beim Auftreten des idiopathischen Torticollis spasmodicus. Z Psychosom Med Psychoanal 32: 44-59
Richards IA (1936) The philosophy of rhetoric. Oxford University Press, London
Richter HE (1976) Flüchten oder Standhalten. Rowohlt, Reinbek
Richter HE, Beckmann D (1969) Herzneurose. Thieme, Stuttgart
Rivers WHR (1920) Instinct and the unconscious. A contribution to a biological theory of the psycho-neuroses. Harvard University Press, Cambridge
Robbins M (1988) Use of audiotape recording in impasses with severely disturbed patients. J Am Psychoanal Assoc 36: 61-75
Rogers R (1942) The use of electrically recorded interviews in improving psychotherapeutic techniques. Am J Orthopsychiatry 12: 429-434
Rogers R (1978) Metaphor: a psychoanalytic view. University of California Press, Berkeley
Roheim G (1917) Spiegelzauber. Imago 5: 63-120
Roiphe H, Galenson E (1981) Infantile origins of sexual identity. International Universities Press, New York
Rosen VH (1969) Sign phenomena and their relationship to unconscious meaning. Int J Psychoanal 50: 197-207
Rosenfeld H (1971) Contribution to the psychopathology of psychotic states: the importance of projective identification in the ego structure and the object relation of the psychotic patient. In: Foucet P, Laurin C (eds) Problems of psychosis. Exerpta Medica, The Hague, pp 115-128
Rosenfeld H (1981) Zur Psychopathologie der Hypochondrie. In: Rosenfeld H (ed) Zur Psychoanalyse psychotischer Zustände. Suhrkamp, Frankfurt am Main, pp 209-233
Rosenfeld H (1987) Impasse and interpretation. Tavistock, London
Rothstein A (1983) The structural hypothesis. An evolutionary perspective. International Universities Press, New York
Rubinstein BB (1972) On metaphor and related phenomena. Psychoanal Contemp Sci 1: 70-108
Rubinstein BB (1973) On the logic of explanation in psychoanalysis. Psychoanal Contemp Sci 2: 338-358
Rubovits-Seitz P (1986) Clinical interpretation, hermeneutics and the problem of validation. Psychoanal Contemp Thought 9: 3-42
Rüger U (1976) Tiefenpsychologische Aspekte des Verlaufs phasischer Depressionen unter Lithium-Prophylaxe. Nervenarzt 47: 538-543
Rüger U (1986) Psychodynamische Prozesse während einer Lithium-Langzeitmedikation. In: Müller-Oerlinhausen B, Greil W (eds) Die Lithiumtherapie. Springer, Berlin Heidelberg New York
Sacks S (ed) (1979) On metaphor. University of Chicago Press, Chicago
Sandler J (1962) The Hampstead Index as an instrument of psychoanalytic research. Int J Psychoanal 43: 289-291
Sandler J (1976) Countertransference and role-responsiveness. Int Rev Psychoanal 3: 43-47
Sandler J (1983) Reflections on some relations between psychoanalytic concepts and psychoanalytic practice. Int J Psychoanal 64: 35-45

Sandler J, Sandler AM (1984) The past unconscious, the present unconscious and interpretation of the transference. Psychoanal Inquiry 4: 367-399
Sandler J, Dare C, Holder A (1973) The patient and the analyst: the basis of the psychoanalytic process. Allen and Unwin, London
Sander LW (1962) Issues in early mother-child interaction. J Am Acad Child Psychiat 1: 141-166
Sargent HD, Horwitz L, Wallerstein RS, Appelbaum A (1968) Prediction in psychotherapy research. Method for the transformation of clinical judgements into testable hypothesis. Psychological issues, vol 6, no 1, monograph 21. International Universities Press, New York
Sartre JP (1969) Der Narr mit dem Tonband. Neues Forum 16: 705-725
Schalmey P (1977) Die Bewährung psychoanalytischer Hypothesen. Scriptor, Kronberg
Scharfenberg J (1968) Sigmund Freud und seine Religionskritik als Herausforderung für den christlichen Glauben. Vandenhoeck and Ruprecht, Göttingen
Schaumburg C, Kächele H, Thomä H (1974) Methodische und statistische Probleme bei Einzelfallstudien in der psychoanalytischen Forschung. Psyche 28: 353-374
Scheidt CE (1986) Die Rezeption der Psychoanalyse in der deutschsprachigen Philosophie vor 1940. Suhrkamp, Frankfurt am Main
Schilder P (1923) Das Körperschema. Ein Beitrag zur Lehre vom Bewußtsein des eigenen Körpers. Springer, Berlin
Schilder P (1933) Das Körperbild und die Sozialpsychologie. Imago 19: 367-376
Schilder P (1935) The image and appearance of the human body. Studies in the constructive energies of the psyche. Kegan, London
Schleiermacher FDE (1977) Hermeneutik und Kritik. Suhrkamp, Frankfurt am Main
Schlesier R (1981) Konstruktionen der Weiblichkeit bei Sigmund Freud. Europäische Verlagsanstalt, Frankfurt am Main
Schlessinger N, Robbins FP (1983) A developmental view of the psychoanalytic process. Follow-up studies and their consequences. International Universities Press, New York
Schmidl S (1955) The problem of scientific validation in psychoanalytic interpretation. Int J Psychoanal 36: 105-113
Schneider E (1972) Die Theologie und Feuerbachs Religionskritik. Vandenhoeck and Ruprecht, Göttingen
Schneider H (1983) Auf dem Weg zu einem neuen Verständnis des psychotherapeutischen Prozesses. Huber, Bern
Schneider PB (1976) Zum Verhältnis von Psychoanalyse und psychosomatischer Medizin. Psyche 27: 21-49
Schneider PB (1977) The observer, the psychosomatic phenomenon and the setting of the observation. Psychother Psychosom 28: 36-46
Schneider W (1987) Deutsch für Kenner. Gruner and Jahr, Hamburg
Schönau W (1968) Sigmund Freud's Prosa. Literarische Elemente seines Stils. Metzlersche Verlagsbuchhandlung, Stuttgart
Schonecke O, Herrmann J (1986) Das funktionelle kardiovaskuläre Syndrom. In: Uexküll T von (ed) Psychosomatische Medizin, 3rd edn. Urban and Schwarzenberg, Munich, pp 503-522
Schopenhauer A (1974) Sämtliche Werke. Suhrkamp, Frankfurt am Main
Schröter K (1979) Einige formale Aspekte des psychoanalytischen Dialogs. In: Flader D, Wodak-Leodolter R (eds) Therapeutische Kommunikation. Ansätze zur Erforschung der Sprache im psychoanalytischen Prozeß. Scriptor, Königstein, pp 179-185
Schüffel W, Uexküll T von (1986) Ulcus duodeni. In: Uexküll T von (ed) Psychosomatische Medizin, 3rd edn. Urban and Schwarzenberg, Munich, pp 761-782
Schultz H (1973) Zur diagnostischen und prognostischen Bedeutung des Initialtraumes in der Psychotherapie. Psyche 27: 749-769
Schur M (1955) Comments on the metapsychology of somatization. Psychoanal Study Child 10: 119-164
Schwaber EA (1987) Models of the mind and data-gathering in clinical work. Psychoanal Inquiry 7: 261-275
Schwarz HJ (1987) Illness in the doctor: implications for the psychoanalytic process. J Am Psychoanal Assoc 35: 657-692
Searles HF (1965) Collected papers on schizophrenia and related subjects. International Universities Press, New York

Segal H (1964) Introduction to the work of Melanie Klein. Basic, New York
Segal H (1973) Introduction to the work of Melanie Klein, rev edn. Hogarth, London
Seiffke-Krenke I (1985) Problembewältigung im Jugendalter. Z Pädagogische Entwicklungspsychologie 18: 122-152
Sellschopp A (1988) Das Dilemma der Psycho-Onkologie. Mitteilungen der Deutschen Krebsgesellschaft 3: 10-19
Shakow D (1960) The recorded psychoanalytic interview as an objective approach to research in psychoanalysis. Psychoanal Q 29: 82-97
Shakow D, Rapaport D (1964) The influence of Freud on American psychology. Psychological Issues, vol 4. International Universities Press, New York
Shane E (1987) Varieties of psychoanalytic experience. Psychoanal Inquiry 7: 199-205; 241-248
Shapiro T (1984) On neutrality. J Am Psychoanal Assoc 32: 269-282
Sharpe EF (1940) Psycho-physical problems revealed in language: an examination of metaphor. Int J Psychoanal 21: 201-213
Sheehan DV, Sheehan KH (1983) The classification of phobic disorders. Int J Psychiat Med 12: 243-266
Shengold L (1971) More about rats and rat people. Int J Psychoanal 52: 277-288
Sherwood M (1969) The logic of explanation in psychoanalysis. Academic, New York
Sherwood M (1973) Another look at the logic of explanation in psychoanalysis. Psychoanal Contemp Sci 2: 359-366
Siegelmann EY (1990) Metaphor and meaning in psychotherapy. Guilford, New York
Sifneos PE (1973) The prevalence of "alexithymic" characteristics in psychosomatic patients. Psychother Psychosom 22: 255-262
Silberschatz G (1978) Effects of the therapist's neutrality on the patient's feelings and behavior in the psychoanalytic situation. Dissertation, New York University
Silverman MA (1987) Clinical material. Psychoanal Inquiry 7: 147-165
Simon J, Fink G, Gill MM, Endicott NA, Paul IH (1970) Studies in audio-recorded psychoanalysis. II. The effect of recording upon the analyst. J Am Psychoanal Assoc 18: 86-101
Smith HF (1990) Cues: the perceptual edge of the transformance. Int J Psychanal 71: 219-228
Spence DP (1976) Clinical interpretation: some comments on the nature of evidence. Psychoanal Contemp Sci 5: 367-388
Spence DP (1981) Psychoanalytic competence. Int J Psychoanal 62: 113-124
Spence DP (1982) Narrative truth and historical truth. Meaning and interpretation in psychoanalysis. Norton, New York
Spence DP (1983) Narrative persuasion. Psychoanal Contemp Thought 6: 457-481
Spence DP (1986) When interpretation masquerades as explanation. J Am Psychoanal Assoc 34: 3-22
Spence DP (1987) The Freudian metaphor. Toward paradigm change in psychoanalysis. Norton, New York
Spence DP, Lugo M (1972) The role of verbal clues in clinical listening. Psychoanal Contemp Sci 1: 109-131
Sperling E, Massing A (1970) Der familiäre Hintergrund der Anorexia nervosa und die sich daraus ergebenden therapeutischen Schwierigkeiten. Z Psychosom Med Psychoanal 16: 130-141
Spielberger CD (1980) Streß und Angst. Beltz, Weinheim
Spillius EB (1983) Some developments from the work of Melanie Klein. Int J Psychoanal 64: 321-332
Spitz RA (1973) Die Evolution des Dialogs. Psyche 27: 697-717
Spitz RA (1976) Vom Dialog. Studien über den Ursprung der menschlichen Kommunikation und ihre Rolle in der Persönlichkeitsbildung. Klett, Stuttgart
Stein MH (1985) Irony in psychoanalysis. J Am Psychoanal Assoc 33: 35-57
Steiner R (1985) Some thoughts about tradition and change arising from an examination of the British Psychoanalytical Society's Controversial Discussions (1943-1944). Int Rev Psychoanal 12: 27-72
Steiner R (1987) Some thoughts on "La vive voix" by I. Fonagy. Int Rev Psychoanal 14: 265-272
Stepansky PE (1977) A history of aggression in Freud. Psychol Issues, vol X, no 3. International Universities Press, New York
Sterba RF (1929) Zur Dynamik der Bewältigung des Übertragungswiderstandes. Int Z Psychoanal 15: 456-470

Sterba RF (1934) Das Schicksal des Ichs im therapeutischen Verfahren. Int Z Psychoanal 20: 66-73
Stern DN (1977) The first relationship. Mother and infant. Fontana, London
Stern DN (1985) The interpersonal world of the infant. Basic, New York
Stern MM (1970) Therapeutic playback, self objectification and the analytic process. J Am Psychoanal Assoc 18: 562-598
Stevenson RL (1967 [1886]) Dr. Jekyll and Mr. Hyde. Bantam, New York
Stiemerling D (1974) Die früheste Kindheitserinnerung des neurotischen Menschen. Z Psychosom Med Psychoanal 20: 337-362
Stierlin H (1975) Von der Psychoanalyse zur Familientherapie. Klett-Cotta, Stuttgart
Stierlin H, Weber G, Simon FB (1986) Zur Familiendynamik bei manisch-depressiven und schizoaffektiven Psychosen. Familiendynamik 11: 267-282
Stoller RJ (1968) Sex and gender. Vol I: On the development of masculinity and feminity. Vol II: The transsexual experiment. Hogarth, London
Stoller RJ (1985) Presentations of gender. Yale University Press, New Haven
Stoller RJ (1986a [1979]) Sexual excitement. Dynamics of erotic life. Maresfield Library, London
Stoller RJ (1986b [1975]) Perversion. The erotic form of hatred. Maresfield Library, London
Stolorow RD, Lachmann FM (1984/85) Transference: the future of an illusion. Annu Psychoanal 12/13: 19-37
Stone L (1961) The psychoanalytic situation. An examination of its development and essential nature. International Universities Press, New York
Strachey J (1934) The nature of the therapeutic action of psycho-anaylsis. Int J Psychoanal 15: 127-159
Straus E (1952) The upright posture. Psychiatr Q 26: 529-561
Strian F (1983) Angst. Grundlagen und Klinik. Ein Handbuch zur Psychiatrie und medizinischen Psychologie. Springer, Berlin Heidelberg New York
Strupp HH (1973) Psychotherapy. Clinical, research, and theoretical issues. Aronson, New York
Strupp HH (1978) Psychotherapy research and practice: an overview. In: Garfield SL, Bergin AE (eds) Handbook of psychotherapy and behavior change: an empirical analysis, 2nd edn. Wiley, New York, pp 3-22
Strupp HH, Binder J (1984) Psychotherapy in a new key. A guide to time-limited dynamic psychotherapy. Basic, New York
Strupp HH, Wallach MS, Wogan M (1964) Psychotherapy experience in retrospect: questionnaire survey of former patients and their therapists. In: Kimble GA (ed) Psychological monographs general and applied 78, Whole No 558
Stunkard AJ (1986) Adipositas. In: Uexküll T von (ed) Psychosomatische Medizin, 3rd edn. Urban and Schwarzenberg, Munich, pp 583-599
Szecsödy I (1981) The supervisory process. Theory and research in psychotherapy supervision (a research project). Report 3, University Stockholm
Szecsödy I (1986) Feedback in psychotherapy and in training. Nord Psych Tidsk 40: 193-200
Szecsödy I (1990) The learning process in psychotherapy supervision. Kongl. Carolinska Medico Chirurgiska Institute, Stockholm
Szondi F (1975) Einführung in die literarische Hermeneutik. Suhrkamp, Frankfurt am Main
Teller V (1981) Book Review: Rogers R: Metaphor: a psychoanalytic view. Psychoanal Rev 68: 458-460
Teller V, Dahl H (1986) The microstructure of free association. J Am Psychoanal Assoc 34: 763-798
Thomä H (1953) Traitment d'une hypertension considère comme exemple d'un "refoulement bèphas". L'Evolution psychiatrique III:443-456. Dt: (1953/54) Über einen Fall schwerer zentraler Regulationsstörung als Beispiel einer zweiphasigen Verdrängung. Psyche 7: 579-592
Thomä H (1954) Über die psychoanalytische Behandlung eines Ulcuskranken. Psyche 9: 92-125
Thomä H (1957) Männlicher Transvestitismus und das Verlangen nach Geschlechtsumwandlung. Psyche 11: 81-124
Thomä H (1962/63) Bemerkungen zu neueren Arbeiten über die Theorie der Konversion. Psyche 16: 801-813
Thomä H (1967a) Anorexia nervosa. International Universities Press, New York
Thomä H (1967b) Konversionshysterie und weiblicher Kastrationskomplex. Psyche 21: 827-847

Thomä H (1977) Psychoanalyse und Suggestion. Z Psychosom Med Psychoanal 23: 35-55
Thomä H (1978) Von der „biographischen Anamnese" zur „systematischen Krankengeschichte". In: Drews S et al (ed) Provokation und Toleranz. Festschrift für Alexander Mitscherlich zum 70. Geburtstag. Suhrkamp, Frankfurt am Main, pp 254-277
Thomä H (1981) Schriften zur Praxis der Psychoanalyse: Vom spiegelnden zum aktiven Psychoanalytiker. Suhrkamp, Frankfurt am Main
Thomä H (1983) Erleben und Einsicht im Stammbaum psychoanalytischer Techniken und der „Neubeginn" als Synthese im „Hier und Jetzt". In: Hoffmann SO (ed) Deutung und Beziehung. Kritische Beiträge zur Behandlungskonzeption und Technik in der Psychoanalyse. Fischer, Frankfurt am Main
Thomä H (1991) Idee und Wirklichkeit der Lehranalyse. Psyche 45: 385-433, 481-505
Thomä H, Cheshire N (1991) Freud's „Nachträglichkeit" und Strachey's "deferred action": trauma, constructions and the direction of causality. Int Rev Psychoanal 18: 407-427
Thomä H, Hohage R (1981) Zur Einführung einiger kasuistischer Mitteilungen. Psyche 35: 809-818
Thomä H, Houben A (1967) Über die Validierung psychoanalytischer Theorien durch die Untersuchung von Deutungsaktionen. Psyche 21: 664-692
Thomä H, Kächele H (1973) Problems of metascience and methodology in clinical psychoanalytic research. Annu Psychoanal 3: 49-119
Thomä H, Kächele H (1987) Psychoanalytic practice, vol 1. Principles. Springer, Berlin Heidelberg New York
Thomä H, Rosenkötter L (1970) Über die Verwendung audiovisueller Hilfsmittel in der psychotherapeutischen Ausbildung. Didacta Medica 4: 108-112
Thomä H, Thomä B (1968) Die Rolle der Angehörigen in der psychoanalytischen Technik. Psyche 22: 802-822
Thomä H, Grünzig HJ, Böckenförde H, Kächele H (1976) Das Konsensusproblem in der Psychoanalyse. Psyche 30: 978-1027
Ticho EA (1971) Termination of psychoanalysis; treament goals, life goals. Psychoanal Q 41: 315-333
Ticho EA (1974) DW Winnicott, Martin Buber and the theory of personal relationships. Psychiatry 37: 240-253
Tölle R (1983) Ärztliche Überlegungen zum Einsichtsrecht des Patienten. Dt Ärzteblatt 18: 47-53
Tugendhat E (1979) Selbstbewußtsein und Selbstbestimmung. Sprachanalytische Interpretationen. Suhrkamp, Frankfurt am Main
Tugendhat E (1984) Probleme der Ethik. Reclam, Stuttgart
Uexküll T von (1985) Der Körperbegriff als Problem der Psychoanalyse und der somatischen Medizin. Praxis Psychother Psychosom 30: 95-103
Uexküll T von (ed) (1986) Psychosomatische Medizin, 3rd edn. Urban and Schwarzenberg, Munich
Van Dam H (1987) Countertransference during an analyst's brief illness. J Am Psychoanal Assoc 35: 647-655
Vogt R (1986) Psychoanalyse zwischen Mythos und Aufklärung oder Das Rätsel der Sphinx. Campus, Frankfurt am Main
Wachtel PL (1982) Vicious circles. The self and the rhetoric of emerging and unfolding. Contemp Psychoanal 18: 259-273
Waelder R (1930) Das Prinzip der mehrfachen Funktion. Bemerkungen zur Überdeterminierung. Int Z Psychoanal 16: 285-300. Engl: (1936) The principle of multiple function. Observations on overdetermination. Psychoanal Q 5: 45-62
Waelder R (1960) Basic theory of psycho-analysis. International Universities Press, New York
Walker LEA (ed) (1988) Handbook on sexual abuse of children. Springer Publishing, New York
Wallerstein RS (1973) Psychoanalytic perspectives on the problem of reality. J Am Psychoanal Assoc 21: 5-33
Wallerstein RS (1981) Becoming a psychoanalyst. A study of psychoanalytic supervision. International Universities Press, New York
Wallerstein RS (1983) Reality and its attributes as psychoanalytic concepts: an historical overview. Int Rev Psychoanal 10: 125-144
Wallerstein RS (1986) Forty-two lifes in treatment. A study of psychoanalysis and psychotherapy. Guilford, New York

Wangh M (1987) The genetic sources of Freud's difference with Romain Rolland on the matter of religious feelings. In: Blum H, Kramer Y, Richards AK, Richards AD (eds) Fantasy, myth and reality. International Universities Press, New York
Weber JJ, Elinson J, Moss IM (1966) The application of ego strength scales to psychoanalytic clinic records. In: Goldman GS, Shapiro D (eds) Developments in psychoanalysis at Columbia University. Hafner, New York, pp 215-273
Weber M (1949 [1904]) The meaning of "ethical neutrality" in sociology and economics. In: Weber M (ed) The methodology of the social sciences. Free Press, New York
Weber M (1921) Soziologische Grundbegriffe. Mohr, Tübingen
Weiner H (1977) Psychobiology and human disease. Elsevier, New York
Weinrich H (1968) Die Metapher. Poetica 2: 100-130
Weinrich H (1976) Sprache in Texten. Klett, Stuttgart
Weiss E (1988) Symbolischer Interaktionismus und Psychoanalyse. Zur Geschichte und Bedeutung ihres theoretischen Verhältnisses. Psyche 42: 795-830
Weiss J, Sampson H (1986) Symbolischer Interaktionalismus und Psychoanalyse
Weizsäcker CF von (1987) Viktor von Weizsäcker zwischen Physik und Philosophie. In: Hahn P, Jacob W (eds) Viktor von Weizsäcker zum 100. Geburtstag. Springer, Berlin Heidelberg New York, pp 163-165
Weizsäcker V von (1950a) Diesseits und jenseits der Medizin. Köhler, Stuttgart
Weizsäcker V von (1950b) Zwei Arten des Widerstandes. Psyche 4: 1-16
Weizsäcker V von (1951) Fälle und Probleme, 2nd edn. Thieme, Stuttgart
White RW (1963) Ego and reality in psychoanalytic theory. A proposal regarding independend ego energies. Psychological issues, vol 3, no 3, monograph 11. International Universities Press, New York
Wilson E jr (1987) Did Strachey invent Freud? Int Rev Psychoanal 14: 299-315
Winnicott DW (1949) Hate in the countertransference. Int J Psychoanal 30: 69-74
Winnicott DW (1956) Zustände von Entrückung und Regression. Psyche 10: 205-215
Winnicott DW (1965) The maturational processes and the facilitating environment. Studies in the theory of emotional development. International Universities Press, New York
Winnicott DW (1972) Fragment of an analysis. In: Giovacchini PL (ed) Tactics and techniques in Psychoanalytic therapy. Hogarth, London, pp 455-693
Wirsching M, Stierlin H (1982) Krankheit und Familie. Klett-Cotta, Stuttgart
Wirsching M, Stierlin H, Haas B, Weber G, Wirsching B (1981) Familientherapie bei Krebsleiden. Familiendynamik 6: 2-23
Wittgenstein L (1984) Werkausgabe, vol 8. Suhrkamp, Frankfurt am Main
Wodak-Leodolter R (1979) Probleme der Unterschichttherapie. Aspekte einer empirischen Untersuchung therapeutischer Gruppen. In: Flader D, Wodak-Leodolter R (eds) Therapeutische Kommunikation. Ansätze zur Erforschung der Sprache im psychoanalytischen Prozeß. Scriptor, Königstein, pp 186-207
Wolf ES (1979) Transferences and countertransferences in the analysis of disorders of the self. Contemp Psychoanal 15: 577-594
Wolf ES (1983) Empathy and countertransference. In: Goldberg A (ed) The future of psychoanalysis. International Universities Press, New York, pp 309-326
Wolff HG (1977) The contribution of the interview situation to the restriction of phantasy, life and emotional experience in psychosomatic patients. Psychother Psychosom 28: 58-67
Wurmser L (1977) A defense of the use of metaphor in analytic theory formation. Psychoanal Q 46: 466-498
Wurmser L (1987) Flucht vor dem Gewissen. Springer, Berlin Heidelberg New York
Wyss D (1982) Der Kranke als Partner, vols 1,2. Vandenhoeck and Ruprecht, Göttingen
Wyss D, Bühler KE (1985) Von der Daseinsanalyse zur anthropologisch-integrativen Psychotherapie. Nervenheilkunde 4: 222-226
Yalom ID, Elkin G (1974) Every day gets a little closer. A twice-told therapy. Basic, New York
Zenz H, Brähler E, Braun P (1975) Persönlichkeitsaspekte des Kommunikationserlebens im Erstinterview. Z Psychosom Med Psychoanal 21: 376-389
Zeppelin I von (1987) Outline of a process model of psychoanalytic therapy. In: Cheshire N, Thomä H (eds) Self, symptoms and psychotherapy. Wiley, New York, pp 149-165
Zerssen D von, Möller HJ, Baumann U, Bühringer G (1986) Evaluative Psychotherapiefor-

schung in der Bundesrepublik Deutschland und West-Berlin. Psychother med Psychol 36: 8-17
Zetzel ER (1966) Additional notes upon a case of obsessional neurosis: Freud 1909. Int J Psychoanal 47: 123-129
Zulliger H (1957) Bausteine zur Kinderpsychotherapie und Kindertiefenpsychologie. Huber, Bern

Name Index

D

E

F

G

H

I

J

K

Z

Subject Index

B

C

D

Q

R

S

U

MIX
Papier aus verantwortungsvollen Quellen
Paper from responsible sources
FSC® C105338

If you have any concerns about our products,
you can contact us on
ProductSafety@springernature.com

In case Publisher is established outside the EU,
the EU authorized representative is:
Springer Nature Customer Service Center GmbH
Europaplatz 3, 69115 Heidelberg, Germany

Printed by Libri Plureos GmbH
in Hamburg, Germany